ANNUAL REVIEW OF
PUBLIC HEALTH

EDITORIAL COMMITTEE (1986)

ANNUAL REVIEW OF PUBLIC HEALTH

VOLUME 7, 1986

LESTER BRESLOW, *Editor*

University of California at Los Angeles

JONATHAN E. FIELDING, *Associate Editor*

University of California at Los Angeles

LESTER B. LAVE, *Associate Editor*

Carnegie Mellon University

ANNUAL REVIEWS INC.   4139 EL CAMINO WAY   PALO ALTO, CALIFORNIA 94306 USA

ANNUAL REVIEWS INC.
Palo Alto, California, USA

International Standard Serial Number: 0163–7525
International Standard Book Number: 0–8243–2707-1

Typesetting by Kachina Typesetting Inc., Tempe, Arizona; John Olson, President
Typesetting coordinator, Janis Hoffman

PRINTED AND BOUND IN THE UNITED STATES OF AMERICA

Annual Review of Public Health
Volume 7, 1986

RA
421
A66
v. 7

CONTENTS

(Note: Titles of chapters in Volumes 1–7 are arranged by category on pages 562–66.)

SYMPOSIUM ON NUTRITION

INDEXES

SOME RELATED ARTICLES IN OTHER *ANNUAL REVIEWS*

From the *Annual Review of Genetics*, Volume 19 (1985)

  Population Genetics, R. C. Lewontin

From the *Annual Review of Medicine*, Volume 37 (1986)

  Clinical Pharmacology of Nicotine, N. L. Benowitz
  Involuntary Treatment in Medicine, A. R. Jonsen
  Treatment of Hypercholesterolemia, J. P. Kane and R. J. Havel

From the *Annual Review of Nutrition*, Volume 6 (1986)

  Nutrition and Infection, G. T. Keusch and M. J. G. Farthing
  Mutagens and Carcinogens in Foods, C. Furihata and T. Matsushima
  Calcium and Hypertension, N. Karanja and D. A. McCarron
  The Impact of Culture on Food-Related Behavior, M. L. Axelson
  Diet and Human Behavior: How Much Do They Affect Each Other?, M. J. P. Kruesi
    and J. L. Rapoport

From the *Annual Review of Psychology*, Volume 37 (1986)

  The Regulation of Body Weight, R. E. Keesey and T. L. Powley
  Program Evaluation: The Worldly Science, T. D. Cook and W. R. Shadish, Jr.

From the *Annual Review of Sociology*, Volume 12 (1986)

  Alternatives to Bureaucracy: Democratic Participation in the Economy, J.
    Rothschild-Whitt and R. Russell
  The Shifting Social and Economic Tides of Black America, 1950–1980, W. R.
    Allen and R. Farley

ANNUAL REVIEWS INC. is a nonprofit scientific publisher established to promote the advancement of the sciences. Beginning in 1932 with the *Annual Review of Biochemistry*, the Company has pursued as its principal function the publication of high quality, reasonably priced *Annual Review* volumes. The volumes are organized by Editors and Editorial Committees who invite qualified authors to contribute critical articles reviewing significant developments within each major discipline. The Editor-in-Chief invites those interested in serving as future Editorial Committee members to communicate directly with him. Annual Reviews Inc. is administered by a Board of Directors, whose members serve without compensation.

ANNUAL REVIEWS OF		SPECIAL PUBLICATIONS
Anthropology	Medicine	Annual Reviews Reprints:
Astronomy and Astrophysics	Microbiology	Cell Membranes, 1975–1977
Biochemistry	Neuroscience	Cell Membranes, 1978–1980
Biophysics and Biophysical Chemistry	Nuclear and Particle Science	Immunology, 1977–1979
Cell Biology	Nutrition	
Earth and Planetary Sciences	Pharmacology and Toxicology	Excitement and Fascination
Ecology and Systematics	Physical Chemistry	of Science, Vols. 1 and 2
Energy	Physiology	
Entomology	Phytopathology	History of Entomology
Fluid Mechanics	Plant Physiology	
Genetics	Psychology	Intelligence and Affectivity,
Immunology	Public Health	by Jean Piaget
Materials Science	Sociology	
		Telescopes for the 1980s

A detachable order form/envelope is bound into the back of this volume.

Ann. Rev. Public Health. 1986. 7:1–12

IS THERE A PUBLIC HEALTH FUNCTION?

Abel Wolman

The Johns Hopkins University, Baltimore, Maryland 21218

The world is full of science and technology assessments, performed to prove that what we do has social significance. In recent decades the pressure to pursue this intellectual exercise has had a more important purpose. People must be convinced that what we do will not harm them. Perhaps of greater relevance, people must be made aware of what we are not, but should be, doing.

The subject has the tacit blessing of a distinguished public health practitioner. In February 1984, Susan S. Addiss, then President of the American Public Health Association, asked not too innocently (1):

> Has anyone noticed what has happened to the meaning of the word "health" lately? How well I remember my days at public health school, absorbing repeated strictures on the differences between "public health" and "medical care". . . . We were admonished never to forget that difference, lest we be co-opted by "sickness concerns". . . . Perhaps it is time for us to return to the strictures of our days in schools of public health, to be careful to say "hospital costs" when we mean "hospital costs," "medical care" when we mean "medical care," and reserve the word "health" to describe a positive state which does not generate "costs."

What do we do in the name of what we call "public health" and its corollary "public health research"—aptly designated "the gold-dust twins" because it is in these pursuits that the money is? Samples of our fields of actual battle, culled from some current literature on public health practice and research, are:

Is an educated wife hazardous to your health? Apparently she produces increased risk of coronary heart disease. Do your children, 5 or 6 years old, feel badly—why? Battered women; child abuse; health care finance; loneliness; alienation; lack of privacy in high rise apartments; stove design in the upper Volta; when the forests are gone, so is the firewood for cooking; the physiology of water loss in desert high temperatures.

1

0163-7525/86/0510-0001$02.00

These are fascinating issues to any inquiring mind. Some even say their choice, under the aegis of "public health," is validated by none other than William H. Welch, in his address years ago for the charter of the Johns Hopkins University School of Hygiene and Public Health. "It is a well-known fact that there are no social, no industrial, no economic problems which are not related to problems of health." But he added: "It is of vital importance that health activities should be based upon accurate knowledge of the cause and spread of disease."

Perception Versus Reality

Since the driving force today is public perception—a compound of fear and sometimes hysteria—we are drawn to sources of public and private money. The impact of a worried and sincere public, and some "paraders," cannot be gainsaid in creating public policy and hence public money. Like sunlight, this source is both good and bad. What is so often lacking is scientific validation of priority. An impatient public is not too friendly to those who suggest selectivity and sometimes slow motion in the absence of scientific evidence.

The antithesis to doing everything to revolutionize the universe is brusquely stated by a retired professor at Yale University (2). "Don't let the tastes of the American public set your standards for you. Spend time only on what is good. . . . Spot rubbish as rubbish and sweep it out." This is easy to say. Officials under attack suffer a traumatic experience just to stay alive.

The Thrust Toward Primary Health Care

As sure as the seasons alternate, an annual announcement appears of the long expected priority of preventive over curative medicine. The latest incentive to academic training and subsequent practice was given a major fillip in the famous 1977 Alma-Ata unanimous resolution, to provide "health for all by the year 2000." The vehicle was Primary Health Care, of which preventive medicine was an integral part of a wider approach. Accompanying the goal was the slogan, "quality of life," which was variously defined by the new proselytizers. Attainment of goals demanded a profound change in human behavior to reduce the familiar excessive use of smoking, alcohol, and food. Changes in life-long habits turn out to be less than easy. In spite of this, in the western world life expectancy has risen astonishingly to the middle 70s. A half a century ago it was about 50 at birth.

The desire to bestow this longevity upon the rest of the world has received the blessing of the world's ministries of health. What has been the fate of this desire in a world now caught unfortunately in one of the worst world-wide economic collapses in modern history?

An authoriative assessment of progress toward longer life via primary health care is by Halfdan Mahler, Director General of the World Health Organization. His views (5) were published in 1984 in a report on monitoring progress world-wide.

> A high level of political sensitization has taken place and the political will to achieve the goal of health for all exists in a large majority of the countries that have reported. Real implementation of objective is less than satisfying. While these themselves [the "will"—A. W.] are important achievements, made in a short time, a number of observations on the relative lack of progress may also be made. Few countries seem to have developed well-defined plans of action that include specific targets and objects, a time-frame, and data on the projection and allocation of resources. Even fewer countries can assess the resource flow from national and external sources to support their strategies.

Public health objectives, as Mahler points out, are not high on the national priority lists, in spite of the grand resolutions from Alma-Ata. A similar dilemma is demonstrated by the faltering International Water and Sanitation Decade of 1980–1990, discussed below. Both situations led Mahler to add to his review the following provocative questions:

> Was it too early to start this monitoring process, which was aimed not just at collecting information, but at identifying the progress made and the issues that need to be further addressed? . . . We need to identify the factors that are facilitating or impeding the development of national health systems and the areas to which supportive, developmental, and corrective action can be directed.

In spite of the differences between so-called developed and developing countries, the issues Mahler poses confront both. The money drought has made the questions universal, and the solutions are being battled throughout the world. In these debates, the voice of health departments is mute, while medical care and hospitalization hold the stage. Their costs have skyrocketed, not only because these services are of high importance, but because human expectations likewise apparently have no limit. In the United States we have been urged to "get the best," and it has become far more costly to do so in recent times.

Money shortage, real or impending, often drives decisions toward reality. Health-care costs in the US have now reached 10.5% of the gross national product, while Medicare is approaching 2%. All segments of society are in a rush to control costs—some of these efforts are good for, some are probably damaging to, the consumer.

One careful and highly experienced investigator in this field, Anne R. Somers (10), succinctly poses the dilemma and a possible solution by a marriage between prevention and health care:

> What is distressing is the continued lack of attention to what is potentially the most effective of all cost-control strategies: the prevention or minimization of disease and disability. . . . Perhaps even more discouraging is the lack of attention on the part of thoughtful students of health-care reform.

Some rays of sunshine appear in practicable suggestions for the linkage. Somers herself presents a series of thoughtful actions, which are supplemented by proposals by Lester Breslow. Simultaneously, officialdom, via the Department of Health and Human Services, is testing devices coupling the two routes. Even some schools of public health are buttressing their health care emphases by a resurgence of inquiry into the realities of disease prevention. Aside from lip-service, most health departments do not yet display a militant recapture of their responsibilities in prevention—lost so many decades ago.

The Question of Priorities—A New World

The examples noted prompt one to ask what has become of selectivity of purpose and program in the public health field. A few current issues illustrate the profession's hesitation to confront complex health issues of clear socio-political interest and concern. The less than favored world is now beginning to share these issues with the industrial west.

The physical, biological, and chemical threats of the past three quarters of a century were reasonably well met in the west. They remain to be conquered everywhere else. In the meantime, a new and perplexing challenge has come upon us. Each year about 1000 new chemicals are added to the 60,000 already marketed. Most are not yet tested for their potential or alleged health hazard. The search proceeds apace to test them all more rapidly, more cheaply, and more convincingly than at present. In these circumstances, where does the profession stand?

Mercier and Draper (7) recently posed the problem of chemical safety in nicely phrased lay terms:

> What is it? Animal, vegetable or mineral? The old guessing game for children thus catego-rised all the substances that people were likely to encounter in their daily lives. In other words, most items were derived with relatively little modification from the earth's substance and the growing things upon it. Today a fourth category can be added, a class of substances that had not existed until they were created by human scientific and industrial effort. These are the synthetic chemicals that play an increasingly dominant role in human affairs throughout the world. Their number, importance and pervasiveness are seldom appreciated.

The toxicologists are busily engaged in "establishing the precise way by which a toxic substance brings about its deleterious action." Mercier & Draper elaborate upon this simple statement:

> For a chemical what is important is: firstly, the knowledge that a particular substance has in certain circumstances harmful properties; secondly, whether it occurs in the environment; thirdly, the possibilities of human or animal exposures; and fourthly, how the latter can be prevented or reduced to harmless levels.

Great progress is already apparent on this whole front. Chemists have demonstrated their amazing capability not only to synthesize new products, but to convert old toxic ones into harmless and more rapidly biodegradable substances.

Negativism can be found in public health officialdom. It is easy to escape real responsibility by climbing on the present bandwagon of the hazardous waste "Superfund"—now at 1.9 billion dollars. Recent testimony at Congressional hearings proposes that this be amplified by $850 million annually for the next five years—totaling an additional $4,250 million. Some senators suggested raising the 1.9 to 9.0 billion dollars for the next ten years. What a marvelous bait for action, under the guise of a presumed public health threat! Does this "threat" in fact pose a reasonably demonstrable health impact?

Action-minded people are greatly annoyed when someone suggests that the terms need to be realistically defined before the gold rush to the Washington till. Our own associates, not to be forgotten, stand in line either by invitation or by chasing the holy grail—money. What impact do these waste dumps have upon morbidity and mortality? Does it make sense to dig them up and expose their contents somewhere else—so far nowhere else being acceptable to the public?

Some experienced toxicologists hesitantly suggest that it would be better to leave many of them where they are, treat them for esthetic improvement, prepare them for recreational areas, avoid them as places for housing. Reshuffling their contents may in fact create greater health hazards than if left in situ. Many are dangerous in their contamination of underground and surface waters used for drinking. The ground water situation is particularly stressful, because of increasing evidence of chemical, septic tank, and pesticide contamination. For the future, decent industry housekeeping is of course a policy must. Past practice is a poor guide.

Much public fear has its origin in the Love Canal "time bomb" created by a newspaper reporter, unfortunately aided and abetted by officials, including the President of the United States. The Love Canal dump is a symbol of ancient, sloppy industry housekeeping—certainly not to be condoned today.

The National Centers for Disease Control released its report in March 1984 on toxic wastes at Love Canal. Exposure to these wastes did not cause significant chromosome damage to residents in the area near Niagara Falls, New York. The findings replace a discredited 1980 report by the Environmental Protection Agency that terrified local residents. Chronic disease effects, however, seem to be appearing. The health "time bomb" has not yet been detonated. Its destructive impact upon public policy has been well on time.

Asbestos and Some Other Chemical Threats

Prevention of in-house industrial public health hazards is another example of public pressure often winning over scientific justification. The subject is a tender one, especially if you are running for office. If one dare not ask about black-lung, "white-lung" now dominates the scene. Impressive posters on the next asbestos symposium reach my desk every week. They disclose a country-wide problem. Asbestosis has taken too great a toll of human lives in the past. Residual, but important, unanswered questions remain. What is the public health warrant for indiscriminately tearing up schools, highways, houses, and office buildings to prevent the malignancies of asbestos?

Country-wide "corrective" activity goes forward by and large without technical guidance as to significance of effects, sources of money to recover costs, determination of long-term manifest effects of prior exposure, and ultimate legal responsibilities. In March, 1984, a US Court of Appeals in New Orleans found inadequate an emergency regulation proposed by the Occupational Safety and Health Administration and denied its issuance. In this ocean of ignorance, prospective symposia have a responsibility to maintain a difficult equilibrium between sheer propaganda and scientific verity.

If there is any evidence buried somewhere that health departments in this country have been examining buildings to determine significant differences in the health effects of different asbestos or asbestos-like minerals—and that somebody should have been distinguishing between them—it is not discernible.

Malcolm Ross (9), a US Geological Survey mineralogist, has recently stressed,

> Of the commercial asbestos used in the United States, about 95 per cent has been chrysotile, or "white" asbestos, about 2 per cent crocidolite, or "blue" asbestos. Chrysotile asbestos, some insist, poses minimal hazard to man compared with crocidolite. Despite the wide dissemination of white asbestos in our environment—in schools, homes, public buildings, brake lining emissions, etc—there is no evidence that the very frequent non-occupational exposures to this form of asbestos have caused any harm. On the other hand, non-occupational exposure to blue asbestos has been conclusively proven to have caused significant mortality. The different health effects of the various forms of asbestos require different regulatory responses and remedial actions.

Other practitioners, however, do not accept Ross's conviction regarding the minimal hazard of chrysotile. They contend that all forms should be banned. In many instances, they seem to ignore the conclusions of the Ontario, Canada, and Great Britain special commissions, which support Ross's position.

Regardless of which school of thought prevails, wholesale "stripping" is creating a threat that did not exist before. The dollar cost for this grand game has been estimated probably to exceed 3.0 billion dollars.

Still unresolved is the significance of chrysotile asbestos in ground and surface waters used for potable purposes. It occurs at levels above one million fibers per liter in more than 80 of 426 selected water supplies in the US. Where the watersheds include serpentine rock, the frequency of asbestos occurrence is high, as in many parts of California. California has completed perhaps the most elaborate survey (4) of any of the states of these contaminants. The public health significance in potables remains a complex research challenge (8).

Two more ubiquitous chemicals are dioxin and PCB. They engender ignorance, fear, and hysteria of the public. They wait upon sober evaluation.

The findings by the Harvard study of clusters of leukemia in Woburn, Massachusetts, suggest that potable well water is definitely incriminated as a probable cause of this unusual phenomenon. The Centers for Disease Control indicates that such clusters of disease are turning up with increasing frequency in other parts of the United States.

One need not extend the list of toxic chemicals to gain the impression that practitioners, confronted with unknowns, have taken refuge in benign silence. Part of this delinquency is undoubtedly caused by their forces having been stripped in the last decades by the shift to medical care and federal actions having virtually destroyed agencies responsible historically for the protection of the environment against disease. Some health departments are consciously struggling to recapture and exercise these responsibilities long in abeyance.

The Views of the American Public Health Association

The American Public Health Association, a voluntary association spokesman for public health, recently (July 26, 1984) invited tens of thousands of its members to prioritize concerns. The questionnaire listed some 42 options. Perhaps only three of them fall within the rubric of the toxic chemical world. The remaining 39 range from medical care, insurance, unemployment, and inflation to affirmative action for minorities and women. A more modest array might contribute some more revealing public health assessments in those challenges where society waits upon our disclosures. Are we drowning in a psychological morass of toxic chemical impacts or floundering in a true physiologic or genetic one? The public deserves help from the informed scientist-technologist as to what is fact or myth and what priority of action is warranted.

The issue has been squarely stated by Richard Wilson at Harvard, in the following terms:

> The public has to be able to distinguish between fact and myth. To that end, the scientific community has a duty to present data accurately. Academic journals rely on peer review, so scientists seldom publicly refute nonsense: The bad research simply goes unpublished. In matters of public policy, however, nonsense can gain a hearing, and scientists must be willing to speak out when it does.

The Dilemma of Science

One should not underestimate the scientific difficulties in determining the public health implications of toxic chemicals. Congress belatedly has been authoritatively informed of the intricacies of its legislative assignment to the executive agencies for protection of public health. Recognition of the task's complexity and the consequent adjustment of time scale for correctives is less than obvious. The warning of Congress is crystal clear (11):

Faced with an enormous universe of chemicals (63,000 chemicals in daily use, 43,000 have been listed by the Environmental Protection Agency . . . subject to regulation under the Toxic Substances Control Act of 1976) and a broad array of toxicological impacts, environmental and human health experts have been all but hamstrung in their efforts to establish standards that would safeguard human and aquatic environments. Limited data and financial resources, limitations in analytical technology, the multi-year periods necessary to conduct toxicological and epidemiological research, led members of the scientific community to advise the Subcommittee that far more is unknown than is known about the subject at hand.

In the new legislation, Congress requires definition of toxic wastes that are not to be deposited in the ground. If the legislation passes, many months will be required to accomplish any real compliance.

What part health departments should or must play in the arenas here noted is given new significance, because of calamitous accidents in 1984 in Mexico and India. Both accidents killed thousands of people. In India (December 3, 1984), several thousand people were killed by methyl isocyanate poisoning and tens of thousands perhaps permanently maimed. I am uncertain as to what the responsibility of the health department in such cases should be or might have been, but I know that it must be determined as soon as possible. We should not in the meantime accept wholeheartedly the dictum by one official of a US state health department, in commenting on the catastrophe in India, that "there is no reason for us to get involved in monitoring or reviewing such plants in the US." Do not the tragedies warrant a sanhedrin of health officials at least to consider appropriate policy?

Forgotten Environmental Issues

Since biblical times, some people have been aware that living with one's physiological wastes invites disease—the list of which is familiar and formidable. It has also been clear during the centuries, with periods of varying recognition, that these consequences are preventable. Many such consequences have been avoided in much of the western world but still are far too little avoided in the less favored world. In the latter, cholera continues, even now, though disguised in reports as diarrheas!

A major category of these offenses are water borne or water associated, or from water used for development. It would be captious to list them here. Nowhere on earth have any of these communicable diseases been eliminated, except that major killer and devastator, smallpox. The rest remain still to be recognized, prevented, and controlled.

The routes for these maneuvers are well known, tested, and efficient. They are in water, air, and land. Safe potable water, water to bathe in, excreta removal, and personal hygiene are simple means by which to reduce morbidity and mortality. Billions of people still lack these amenities. The entire 4.8 billion are plagued by deterioration of existing systems, collapse of maintenance and operation, and by recurring epidemics of diseases that were supposedly laid to rest in history books. Some no longer are even mentioned in current public health texts—as though the tens of thousands of cholera cases and hundreds of deaths did not occur in Africa in the mid 1970s and 1980s.

Water-borne giardiasis, infectious hepatitis, guinea worm, pathogenic coli, schistosomiasis, the diarrheas, even typhoid, periodically remind us, or should, that the water-borne disease utopia is not yet around the corner, or even visible by the year 2000.

The same accusation may be made against the failure to prevent an impressive list of causes of illness and death via air, food, and house pollution. Troubling examples are Legionnaires disease, salmonella, and Chagas' disease. Recrudescence of most of these continue to trouble us.

Progress is slow in alleviation, even though pride may well be taken in reduced infant mortality and increased life expectancy in a number of countries. So much yet remains to be done in a world now at low economic ebb.

Renewed Hopes and Expectations

The cliche that "every cloud has a silver lining" bears considerable truth. This is now being demonstrated by events in Washington. The Department of Health and Human Resources, a decade after the disappearance of environmental health activity within the agency, is taking on new vigor. Substantial increases in budget have been afforded by Congress to the National Institute of Environmental Health Sciences and Toxicology programs.

The creation of an Office of Disease Prevention and Health Promotion is still another marker of a belated recognition that law enforcement requires a bolstering of scientific understanding of disease causation. The CDC Center for Environmental Health is finally gearing up to stimulate state health departments to recapture an active role in environmental health. At one of its recent conferences on environmental public health, Dr. Vernon Houk, the Director of this division, repeated the forgotten formulation of public health in these terms:

> The public health role is one of prevention. Even in the absence of conclusive evidence that harm to humans has occurred, if the data and evidence from laboratory animal studies are sufficiently strong that harm may occur, then preventing exposure to future populations is a reasonable action. Here the policymaker must address what the potential harm is, what the potential remedial action is, the cost of the remedial action and is it warranted?

Congress has suddenly discovered the obvious—that we know far too little of the health implications of the thousands of chemical dumps dotting the US. The reluctance of EPA to share any superfund responsibilities with DHHS is familiar, but the General Accounting Office stresses that the necessity for disclosing health effects is long overdue. CDC is about ready to initiate the necessary research to provide these disclosures.

Mr. Ruckelshaus, recently retired (former) Administrator of the Environmental Protection Agency, finally adds important consolation to beleaguered health departments in a speech to the American Public Works Association in September 1984. He ventured the comment:

> What we have to remember. . . . The real mission of the hazardous waste control programs . . . is to protect human health. . . . We might look at the vast tonnage of waste more calmly if we reflect that only a portion of it is highly toxic.

International concerns have resulted in a variety of research undertakings, not only in the new world of chemical threats, but in the more familiar diseases still plaguing hundreds of millions of people. Simultaneously, new approaches to prevention and control of the communicable diseases go forward. Such diseases were presumably laid to rest in the western world, but still take an enormous toll of lives in the less fortunate world. Ten years ago, May 1974, the World Health Assembly requested the Director-General to do the following:

1. to intensify WHO activities in the field of research on the major tropical parasitic diseases (malaria, onchocerciasis, schistosomiasis, the trypanosomiases, etc), taking into consideration that such activities be carried out in endemic areas whenever possible and feasible;
2. to define the priorities in research on the problem of tropical parasitic diseases in the various regions of the world, bearing in mind the primary needs of the developing countries;
3. to extend cooperation with national institutions and other governmental and nongovernmental organizations in regard to the coordination of research in this field.

The list of familiar diseases under scrutiny is impressive. Investigators promise vaccines for many insults, wider use of oral rehydration, and simpler and less costly reconstruction of dilapidated houses harboring the carriers of Chagas' disease. The public, ever alert to the possibility of "instant enzymes" produced by research, as by a flood of money, rapidly turns away from other successful preventatives. Governments reduce these budgets, awaiting the miracles on the horizon. History teaches us that vaccines provide marvelous additional tools for the battle. They have not succeeded in mass prevention of any disease. Where these have been largely removed, it has been accomplished by reducing vectors, by physical, chemical, and biological means, accompanied by effective vaccines.

Prospect

The present state of affairs has been neatly stated by Professor Edward A. Emmett, M. D., of the Johns Hopkins University. He volunteers a diagnosis in these terms (personal communication):

The public health and medical communities may be silent because they have really little information and that leads to the second issue. Although a very large amount of money is being spent on dioxins, hazardous waste sites, asbestos removal and other such activities, there is virtually no sound information which allows us to quantitate the risk which is posed by these agents, and, indeed, much of the so-called risk assessment performed currently is fictional. The situation then calls for more understanding, rather than vast remedial measures, which may be better directed elsewhere. Unfortunately, virtually no money is being spent for meaningful work on the health consequences of these particular exposures. Thus, we are taking extraordinarily expensive remedial action without information as to the likely effectiveness and without any system of evaluation of the effectiveness that these measures may have had when we look back in the future. It would seem that meaningful research efforts must be increased and that these must primarily focus on the medical and health implications rather than merely on the technicologic ways to remove materials.

Some straws in the wind indicate that public health agencies may be on the way to recapture primary functions and responsibilities. This is apparent, not only in the vast environmental arena, but as a result of many disease manifestations. Less than ten years ago the presumed multiple cancer types appeared to pose interminable barriers to diagnosis, therapy, and prevention. Due to rapid, exciting disclosures by eager young investigators, some now believe that the probable causes are not multiple and may soon be sufficiently identified as to produce broad potential bases for cure and even prevention.

No closure of this manifesto could be more appropriate than to recognize that no real revival of public health impact control is likely to occur without a far better public understanding than now exists. Internecine warfare between people and their officials must not be continued. The striking advice of a wise lady (3) should top off the valedictory!

Lois Marie Gibbs, the President of the Love Canal Homeowners Association, Inc., registered important suggestions for officialdom—from the President of the US to the field representatives of federal, state, and local agencies. She recommended, in summary:

1. The creation of a team of experts in the effects of chemical exposures. It should consist of two separate units: one to evaluate health problems, the other to determine the extent of environmental damage. [It is not clear why two—A.W.]
2. One administrator should coordinate the activities of the two units.
3. An outside group of experts should review the findings.
4. It is crucial that the citizens or their representatives from the affected areas be included as full participants at each phase of the studies.
5. The affected community should have one specialist in environmental health who is responsible only to the community residents.

The public health official should have the last word. Here I turn to Great Britain (6). The observations are universally applicable.

Why is it that although as a nation we claim to be well educated and well informed, and proudly boast about the number of micro-computers to be seen in British homes, we are still a nation of illogical thinkers? And a large amount of our illogicity is centered around health? If we do not like the word illogical, the best we can use is conviction or faith, so putting our views on a par with politics or religion. One of the avowed objects of the Royal Institute of Public Health and Hygiene is to put health on a logical, scientific footing, but is it succeeding?

Literature Cited

1. Addiss, S. S. 1984. President's column. Am. Public Health Assoc. *The Nation's Health* 14:2
2. Am. Assoc. Univ. Professors. 1983. *Survey of the Views of Retired Professors.*
3. Gibbs, L. M. 1981. The need for effective governmental response to hazardous waste sites. *J. Public Health Policy*
4. Hayward, S. B. 1984. Field monitoring of chrysolite asbestos in California waters. *J. Am. Water Works Assoc.* 76:3
5. Mahler, H. 1984. Health 2000, the monitoring process has been set in motion. *World Health Forum* 5(2)
6. Lucas, B. 1984. Editorial. *J. R. Inst. Public Health Hyg.* 5(3)
7. Mercier, M., Morrell, D. 1984. Chemical safety: The international outlook. *World Health (WHO Mag.)* Aug./Sept., pp. 4–6
8. Polissar, L., Boatman, E. S. 1984. A case-control study of asbestos in drinking water and cancer risk. *Am. J. Epidemiol.* 119:3
9. Ross, M. 1984. *Environ. Health Lett.* 23(12):3
10. Somers, A. R. 1984. Why not try preventing illness as a way of controlling medical costs? *New Engl. J. Med.* 311(13):853–56
11. US Congress, House of Representatives, Comm. on Public Works and Transportation, Subcomm. on Oversight and Review. 1980. *Report, Implementation of the Federal Water Pollution Control Act,* p. 34. Washington DC: GPO

Ann. Rev. Public Health. 1986. 7:13–34

BEHAVIORAL AND ENVIRONMENTAL INTERVENTIONS FOR REDUCING MOTOR VEHICLE TRAUMA

Leon S. Robertson

Yale University School of Medicine, Department of Epidemiology and Public Health, New Haven, Connecticut 06510

INTRODUCTION

The interest of public health professionals in motor vehicle trauma has increased in recent years. This interest is almost entirely the result of seeds planted by William Haddon, Jr., whose memorial service I attended two days before beginning this chapter in March, 1985. In addition to originating much of the conceptual framework for the field and a considerable body of empirical research, Haddon also provided much of the funding for the more distinguished work of investigators in the 1970s and early 1980s through the good offices of the Insurance Institute for Highway Safety.

The federal safety standards for motor vehicles, most of which Haddon wrote with Robert Brenner in 1968–1969 when Haddon was head of what is now the National Highway Traffic Safety Administration, had by 1982 saved something on the order of 100,000 persons from premature death (68). Therefore, the story of the public health approach to motor vehicle trauma is, in large part, a memorial to William Haddon, Jr.

Haddon gave credit to his intellectual predecessors, such as Hugh DeHaven and John Stapp. It was DeHaven (13) who, in the 1940s, investigated the ability of human beings to survive mechanical energy insults. Stapp (77) demonstrated first with animals, and then with human volunteers, including himself, that human beings could tolerate up to 40 times gravity in deceleration forces without injury if those forces were distributed over a sufficient area of the body.

13

0163-7525/86/0510-0013$02.00

Haddon, Suchman & Klein (29) gathered the extant evidence in the 1960s into a book that came to the attention of the Congress. It was that evidence, along with a scandal created by General Motor's snooping into Ralph Nader's private life (41), that led to the federal safety agency and Haddon's leadership in the issuance of the first federal safety standards.

The fundamental public health principle that Haddon recognized in the work of DeHaven and Stapp was to think of trauma in two largely separable problems: (a) prevention of the incidence of events called accidents, and (b) reduction of their severity. While the incidence may be a result of a complex web of biological, psychological, social, and economic forces, the severity is a rather simple function of the mass and velocity of moving objects and the energy-absorbing properties of the materials impacted in crashes.

Indeed one can think of the problem of injury severity as an environmental issue. Virtually all of the world's population now lives in an environment of kinetic pollution created by the manufacture and use of motorized vehicles. In only a few places on the planet, such as Venice, Italy, can one leave one's residence without being exposed to the energy generated by the movement of such vehicles, and penetration of residences by crashing vehicles is not totally unheard of. The result in the industrialized countries is a loss of productive years of life on a par with either cancers or heart diseases (6). While these two diseases kill more people in the US, more than half of those who die of heart disease are more than 76 years old and more than half of cancer victims are 68 years old or older. In contrast, half of those who die in, or are struck by, motor vehicles are less than 27 years old (64). Motor vehicles are by far the leading cause of death from age 1 to 44 years (7).

COMPONENTS OF THE PROBLEM

Motor vehicle injury is viewed by public health researchers as analogous to infectious disease. The damaging agent—mechanical energy—is conveyed to a host by one or more carriers. The vehicles involved include cars, trucks, motorcycles, mopeds, minibikes, and road building and repair equipment. The precrash movement of nonmotorized bicycles in collisions with motorized vehicles adds somewhat to the energy exchange with the host bicyclist in a crash. The vehicles involved are usually operated by human vectors who may or may not be the host of the injury in a given crash.

Theoretically, the energy agent, the vehicles, or vectors or the hosts are subject to modification to lower the frequency or severity of trauma. The attributes of each are variable and the extent of our ability to change any one has not been totally explored scientifically. Nevertheless, we have the technical knowledge to prevent the vast majority of deaths and severe disabilities. Whether we have the ability to put the technical knowledge to use in the nihilistic socio-political environments that prevail remains to be seen.

TECHNICAL CHOICES

Fifteen years ago, Haddon published a systematic analysis of the technical choices available to reduce environmental hazards (24). He and others have given detailed examples of each in a variety of publications (6, 15, 25, 26, 64). Haddon emphasized that one should attempt to consider the full range of technical choices before choosing on the basis of other factors such as public acceptability, political feasibility, or costs. The following is an incomplete list of some available choices to reduce motor vehicle injuries suggested by Haddon and others.

1. Prevent the creation of the hazard in the first place. If motor vehicles had never been manufactured, and if the production and importation of fuel were now stopped, there would be no motor vehicle injuries. At the least, manufacture and present use of the most hazardous vehicles that are used mainly for recreation or for which there are much less hazardous substitutes, such as motorcycles and the Jeep CJ5, could be discontinued. These vehicles account for about 10% of the annual fatalities.

2. Reduce the amount of the hazard brought into being. The kinetic pollution of motor vehicles could be lowered by reductions in speed or mass. Reductions in mass have been confused both in professional and public circles with reductions in size. It has been argued that reductions in mass for fuel economy are incompatible with safety (37), but mass is related to weight, not size. The formula for kinetic energy is mass times velocity squared over two. It is well within the range of possibility to reduce energy-generating and fuel-consuming mass while retaining internal space to decelerate occupants of crashing vehicles. Unfortunately, we too often assume that what was done was all that it was possible to do. The maximum speed capability of most vehicles is twice the maximum legal speed limit. Such capability is contrary both to goals of safety and fuel economy. Vehicles capable of 120 miles per hour in the hands of 16-year-old males will, at least occasionally, be driven at that speed.

3. Prevent the release of the hazard that already exists. The rates and amounts of kinetic energy that reach people in motor vehicle crashes can be reduced by increased skid resistance of road surfaces, improved visibility of vehicles and road signs, more efficient handling and braking capabilities of vehicles, and improved driver knowledge and skills, or prohibited use of vehicles by high risk drivers. As noted below, the limits of human abilities to perceive and react to motion and the transient variation in human responses to stimuli place severe limits on approaches to behavioral change or the screening out of high risk drivers.

4. Modify the rate or spatial distribution of release of the hazard. Use of child restraints and seat belts by occupants of motor vehicles is an example of primary importance. We know from Newton's laws of motion, discovered some 300 years ago, that an occupant of a crashing motor vehicle will continue

to move at the precrash speed until slowed by contact with the interior of the vehicle, or the environment if ejected. The seat belt or child restraint keeps the occupant's deceleration more uniform with that of the vehicle and reduces contacts of vital organs with hostile surfaces. Failure of voluntary use and lack of compliance with laws regarding use of seat belts and child restraints, particularly by higher risk groups, diminishes their usefulness.

5. Separate, in time or space, the hazard and that which is to be protected. This approach is especially relevant to injuries to pedestrians and bicyclists. The obvious fact that pedestrians and bicyclists would not be struck by motor vehicles if their paths did not intersect is largely ignored except on certain limited access roads. Bicycle and pedestrian paths can be separated from roads. Vehicles of widely varying mass, such as 88,000-pound 18-wheel trucks and 3000 to 5000 pound cars, could be assigned to separate roads or to use of the same roads at different times. Rigid roadside objects such as trees and poles that concentrate energy in a crash are typically a few feet or inches from the roadside. About a third of the deaths occur from collisions with such objects. They could be removed, particularly from identifiable high risk sites.

6. Separate the hazard and that which is to be protected by interposition of a material barrier. This approach includes energy-absorbing material in the exterior areas of the vehicle; particularly important are the front end and doors. Inside the vehicle, cushions that inflate in a severe frontal crash automatically between the occupants and the dash and/or steering column have been feasible for 15 years, but have only been sold to the general public on expensive luxury cars. These so-called air bags spread the load over larger surfaces of the occupants' body than do seat belts. Use of crash helmets, particularly by motorcyclists and bicyclists who have no exterior vehicle structure to take up energy, is also an effective application of this approach. Structures in the medians of roads that prevent vehicles from crossing into the paths of oncoming vehicles are effective, especially when the design facilitates the guidance of a vehicle back into its lane without turning it over or sharply forcing it into a second lane or off the road. Energy-absorbing material can also be placed in front of rigid roadside objects such as bridge abutments that it is unfeasible to remove (35).

7. Modify the basic qualities of the hazard. The front ends of many vehicles have unnecessarily sharp edges and points that exacerbate injuries to pedestrians and bicyclists that are struck. The vehicle interiors also have protrusions from instrument panels and dashboards that taper to an edge in the direction of the vehicle occupants. Medical examiners are familiar with the impressions that these designs make on the heads, necks and chests of people in crashes. Along the sides of roads, utility, light, and sign posts can be made to break away when struck rather than standing rigid and concentrating all the energy exchange into the passenger compartment of vehicles that strike them.

8. Make that to be protected more resistant to damage from the hazard. This approach is limited to reducing the threshold to injury severity of persons made more vulnerable by debilitating physical conditions. Providing blood clotting factor to persons with hemophilia and reduction of osteoporosis by calcium consumption, hormones, or exercise are primary examples.

9. Begin to counter the damage already done by the environmental hazard. For those who survive the immediate forces of a crash, the quickness and quality of emergency response may mean the difference between eventual survival or degree of disability. This involves emergency communication systems such as frequently placed roadside telephones, and teams of persons well trained in life support at nearby, accessible locations. Reduction of shock, cleared breathing passages, control of hemorrhage, and prevention of post-crash exacerbation of spinal cord injury by inappropriate movement are important elements of emergency response.

10. Stabilize, repair, and rehabilitate the object of the damage. This includes skilled surgeons available at designated trauma centers who are sufficiently trained and experienced in the treatment of acute injury. Coordination of acute treatment and long-range rehabilitation is essential; for example, such treatment can preclude or make difficult the use of certain prosthetic devices. For the disabled, brain and spinal cord rehabilitation centers, burn centers, job training centers, and the like are important elements in the return of a greater proportion of the disabled to independent living.

STRATEGIES FOR IMPLEMENTATION

Control of motor-vehicle-induced trauma is obviously not for lack of choices that are technically sound and available. Some of those mentioned have been used to some degree, but there is not yet a comprehensive program that weighs the advantages and disadvantages of the choices available and implements those chosen. That statement is true for vehicle manufacturers that could implement many of the mentioned approaches, state governments that have authority over roads and traffic laws, and the National Highway Traffic Safety Administration (NHTSA). Such a program was begun at NHTSA under Haddon, but the agency subsequently has been headed by several people whose ideologies, lack of knowledge, or lack of political skill have resulted in dilution of the effort. In some instances, intervention from the White House or the Secretary of Transportation has altered the course of NHTSA efforts. For example, the 30-mile-per-hour automatic protection standard first scheduled for the early 1970s was delayed after a meeting of Lee Iaccoca and Henry Ford II with Richard Nixon and John Ehrlichman (4). It is now scheduled to be phased in during the late 1980s, contingent on state action on seat belt laws or additional political interference.

Three general strategies are available to implement public health policy:

1. Change the risky or self-protective behavior of the population at risk by some form of education or other persuasive tactic.
2. Change the risky or self-protective behavior of the population at risk by requiring the behavior change through the force of law or administrative rule.
3. Change the hazard, carrier vehicle, or environment in such a way as to decrease risk automatically (58).

Probably the most basic problem is that the most effective implementation strategies are frequently unacceptable ideologically (at least among those with the authority for implementation), while those that are ideologically acceptable are of less, or often no, effectiveness. Aside from the studies documenting the extent of incidence and severity, most of the research in recent years has attempted to measure the effects of the above strategies in implementing some of the mentioned technical choices.

Individual Voluntary Behavioral Change

The traditional attempts to change voluntary behavior for reduction of motor vehicle injury included driver education in public schools, special courses for adults either self-selected or required by employers or courts, and media advertising urging people to "think safety" or to take specific protective action such as using seat belts. The lack of adequate research designs, in those rare cases when these approaches were studied, sometimes misled their proponents into thinking they were effective when actually they were ineffective at best and, in the case of high school driver education, harmful in the aggregate.

Some automobile insurers give discounts for driver education based on the false inference that driver education causes the lower incidence crashes of drivers who have had the course. Research in the 1960s found that those students who took the course subsequently drove somewhat fewer miles per student than those who were licensed without the course. Self-selection into the course by drivers (or their parents) at lower risk was found to account for the supposed effect of the course (10, 42).

Experiments in which students were assigned to the course or to a control group found no difference in individual risk of crashes during subsequent years. The more recent of these experiments included two treatment groups, one similar to the usual high school course and one designed by psychologists and educators that approximately doubled the classroom and driving hours usually offered. Special off-road driving ranges were constructed and the best teachers were recruited from around the country. Despite the unusual effort put into this course, the risk of crashes in general and those involving injury in particular were the same in the two groups as in the control group after two and one half years of follow-up study of crash records (54).

The first controlled study of driver education found an adverse effect of the course, which the second attempted to avoid. While teenaged drivers assigned to take the course had no better or worse records per mile driven subsequently than the control group, substantially larger numbers obtained licenses earlier and thus drove more in the aggregate. Their total crashes as a group were more than in the control group (76). In the second study, only students who intended to be licensed were allowed in the study (54).

Among 27 states in the late 1960s and early 1970s (when driver education in public schools was being expanded rapidly, supplemented by increased federal funds), the death rates per population in the 16–17-year-old age group increased in those states that increased numbers trained in the public schools (69). In Connecticut, the state eliminated funding for driver education in 1975 and nine school districts dropped the course. Others retained it with increased fees or local tax funds. The communities that dropped the course experienced a substantial decline in 16–17 year olds licensed and a comensurate reduction in crashes of drivers in that age group. About 75% of the students who would have taken the course in those communities waited until they were 18 or older to be licensed, despite the fact that they could be licensed if parents certified that they had been trained by a licensed adult (62).

The role of federal funding in increasing the crash rate of teenagers is suggested by a recent study of the correlation of funding for high school driver education and fatality rates among the states. States that used larger amounts of federal funds for driver education during the late 1970s had increases in fatal crash rates, whereas those that used federal funds for such programs as spot improvements at high risk sites on roads had reductions in fatal crash rates (66).

These results illustrate the principle that any program directed at training people to engage in a hazardous activity must reduce the individual risk sufficiently to offset any increase in the activity promoted by the program. High school driver education has little or no effect on individual risk, but increases vehicle use in an age group that has the highest fatal crash rate per mile driven (64). Although not directed primarily at injury consequences of alcohol and other drug use, experimental study of self-reported use suggests that alcohol and drug education in the public schools increases use of both as well as dealing in illegal drugs (79). Simply informing people about risks or training in skills related to risk does not necessarily reduce risky behavior.

Among adults, little effect of education on subsequent crash records has been found when self-selection into programs is adequately controlled. One of the studies of the National Safety Council's "defensive driving" course cleverly avoided the selection bias. Crash records in the same two-year time period were compared between persons who had the course at the beginning of the two years and persons who had the course at the end of the two years. No difference in average crash rates between the groups was found (45). Nevertheless, many companies and government agencies require drivers of their vehicles to take "defensive driving."

Persons who have been convicted of particular offenses, such as driving while intoxicated, or accumulate a series of convictions for moving violations, are assigned to education courses in some courts as an alternative to license suspension or other sanctions. Follow-up study of the crash records of a group assigned to the "defensive driving" course and a second group given the usual court treatment found no difference in subsequent crashes (30). In Nassau County, New York, individuals convicted of driving while impaired by alcohol were assigned randomly to an education-rehabilitation program or to the usual court treatment, which usually included license suspension. The subsequent crash rate was greater in the education-rehabilitation group than in the comparison group (52). Apparently a program with less effect than license suspension was substituted for that sanction. The literature on education and rehabilitation programs for persons convicted of alcohol-related driving is voluminous, and some small successes have been claimed in some instances (40). The usefulness of this approach, to the extent that efficacy can be demonstrated in controlled experiments, is limited by the extent of identification of alcohol-impaired drivers before the fact of severe crashes. I recently examined the prior convictions of drivers in fatal crashes in the counties in the US where more than 90% of fatally injured drivers are tested chemically for blood alcohol concentration. Only 14% of those with illegal alcohol concentration had a prior conviction for alcohol-impaired driving. Thus, the remaining drivers would not have been identified for special education or rehabilitation before the fatal crash.

The effect of education and other persuasive techniques on the adoption of self-protective behaviors is related primarily to the amount of effort necessary for self-protection (58) and somewhat to the technique and who is using it. In injury control and other public health programs, education and counseling have been demonstrated effective in programs where a single action or a few actions will increase protection. It is possible to persuade the majority of the population to obtain immunizations or purchase smoke detectors (e.g. 43). However, many self-protective actions that must be performed very frequently, such as seat belt use, or with substantial effort, such as use of child restraints in motor vehicles, have proved enormously resistant to education and other forms of persuasion.

Because they reach large audiences repeatedly, the mass media have been used to convey messages urging people to use seat belts. Carefully controlled studies of media campaigns that included actual observation of belt use by persons exposed to the media found no effect of such campaigns. These studies have included comparisons among communities with a variety of media used with differential intensity (19) and comparisons of persons exposed to a multi-million dollar television campaign on one cable of a dual cable television system used for marketing studies (70). While these efforts cannot prove that no media campaign could have an effect, they did suggest that experimental-control study of effectiveness of such efforts is essential to avoid waste of vast amounts of money on their distribution. Nevertheless, such multimillion dollar campaigns by the National Highway Traffic Administration and state governments continue without prior proof of efficacy.

Counseling regarding self-protection has a small effect under certain conditions. An experiment in a hospital setting to promote use of infant restraints in cars had no effect, but an effort based in pediatricians' offices did result in increased use of restraints.

In the hospital study, neither literature given to new mothers nor literature in combination with counseling by a health educator resulted in increased use of child restraints greater than that of a control group during follow-up observations (57). Those given literature and a free restraint did have a few percent greater use than the control group. Apparently, removal of the cost barrier had some effect.

In a separate controlled experiment, pediatricians counseled new parents in their practices about the importance of child restraints, gave them a prescription for a restraint, and demonstrated how to properly restrain the child in the device and anchor the restraint to the vehicle with the seat belt. The counseling was reinforced at follow-up visits. Observed restraint use increased by 23% in the first month, even more in the second, but was up by only 9 to 12% at the fourth- and twelfth-month visits, respectively (56). Thus, intensive persuasion can have an effect on behavior, even a behavior that requires substantial effort. Sole reliance on such persuasion, however, leaves a large proportion of the population unprotected.

Industry-based health promotion activities have had some effect on seat belt use of employees. In a controlled study in one industry, employees were given reminder stickers for their cars, and were faced daily with reminder cards on cafeteria tables and signs at parking lot exits. Belt use increased 19% at one entrance and 10% at another during the morning, but less so during the afternoon (85).

Several studies of lottery-like efforts in industries and in communities have also had a positive effect on belt use. The general method is to announce that belt use will be observed and that license numbers of users will identify those eligible for a prize. A drawing is held periodically and prizes awarded. The increased belt use obtained by this method varies from a few percent to as much as 40–50% (17, 21, 22). Blue collar workers are much less persuaded than white collar workers, and use of seatbelts by both groups returns to near pre-lottery levels when the effort is discontinued.

Incentives in the form of adjustment of payment of benefits after the fact of injury if belts are used have not proved effective in increasing belt use. Nationwide Insurance Company for many years offered a 50% increment in benefits for anyone injured while seat belts were in use. In 1983, the company increased the benefit to double an injury award if belts were in use and offered a $10,000 death benefit to the estate of anyone killed while using seat belts. Policyholders were informed by mail and media advertisements of the increment in benefits for injured belt users insured by the company. Follow-up observations of belt use linked to motor vehicle records of declared insurer indicated no greater belt use among Nationwide's policyholders compared to drivers insured by other companies (67). General Motors gained a lot of free advertising in the media for a more limited offer, $10,000 to the estate of anyone killed while wearing a seat belt during the first year of ownership of a GM car. Given the limits of the plan and the results of the Nationwide offer, it is doubtful that the GM plan had any effect on belt use. For a post-injury incentive to have an effect on pre-injury behavior, vehicle users would have to acknowledge vulnerability, which many if not most are loath to do.

Another Approach to Driver Behavior

Studies of errors by drivers and other road users (18, 23, 32, 74) in the perception of and reactions to motion, as well as some attempts to enhance such perceptions and reactions, suggest that more research effort should be devoted to this approach. A change in the rear lighting of cars will be required on 1986 model cars as a result of one such set of experiments. An extra brake light mounted in the center of the vehicle above the trunk resulted in a 50% reduction in rear-end collisions when the front vehicle was braking, compared to randomly assigned control cars in the same fleets (e.g. 55). Recent research has demonstrated substantial reductions in crash incidence of cars equipped with a relay that automatically turns on the front running lights with increased candlepower, when the car's engine is running (78).

Comparison of crashes at signalized intersections indicate that the length of the delay between a green light in one direction and that on the cross street greatly affects the crash rate. Intersections with delays 10% below those recommended by traffic engineering standards had average crash rates six times those at intersections with delays 10% longer than the recommended standards for the speeds and numbers of lanes on the intersecting roads (92).

Stripes across a road at an exponentially decreasing distance creates the illusion of acceleration when crossed at constant speed (14). Installation of such stripes at high speed approaches to traffic circles in England resulted in an average 66% reduction in crashes at such sites.

Research comparing the point at which a vehicle left a road and hit a fixed object with a point a mile in the direction from which the vehicle traveled identified road curvature and grade as factors in such crashes: 50% of crash sites had curvature greater than 6 degrees compared to 25% of comparison sites; 25% of crash sites involved greater than 6 degree curvature combined with down hill gradation of greater than 2%. Only 8% of comparison sites had the combined characteristics (90). Using these criteria for site selection, the state highway department in Georgia placed reflectorized markers on the center line to enhance the perception of curvature at night. Nighttime crashes were subsequently reduced by 20% compared to those in the daytime during the same period (91).

One can ask in almost any community and find where the local "dead man's" curve is located. What is not so easily found are public officials who understand that there are remedies, such as enhanced perception of curvature, energy absorbing guardrails, and removal of rigid objects. In a recent discussion of these issues with public health officials in one community, the writer, expecting some enthusiasm for approaches that reduced injury, was told that the drivers should take more responsibility for their actions. Ignored is the evidence of severe limitations in human ability to perceive motion and maintain constant vigilance (64). The attitude too often seems to be that human beings who are not perfect deserve the death penalty when they make a mistake.

Laws Directed Toward Individual Behavior Change

In addition to education, the traditional approach to control of motor vehicle injury has included major emphasis on laws directed at behavior of drivers and other road users. The older laws have the mixed purpose of control of traffic flow and injury prevention. More recently, some laws have included required use of self-protective equipment such as motorcycle helmets, child restraints, and seat belts.

The effect of law on individual behavior and accompanying injury rates cannot be studied as definitively as other behavioral change programs because legislators will not enact laws to comply with the requirements of a randomized experiment. Quasi-experimental and correlational studies have been done in sufficient numbers, however, to suggest some principles for the effectiveness of laws directed at individual behavior.

Traditional legal approaches to behavior were largely oriented toward deterrence of behaviors that were thought or known to increase the risk of injury, such as prohibitions against drunk driving, speeding, failing to stop at stop signs or red lights, and the like. More recently, this approach has been augmented in numerous jurisdictions with laws requiring the use of protective equipment, such as helmets by motorcyclists and seat belts or child restraints by vehicle occupants. The latter laws have been more controversial. Lowering of speed limits in the 1970s was also hotly debated.

Based on a review of the research on laws, I have proposed ten factors that contribute to increased or decreased effectiveness of laws directed toward individual behavior:

1. The law is irrelevant because people are behaving in the prescribed manner.
2. High individual propensity to conform to laws or rules on moral or other grounds.
3. High probability of detection and conviction.
4. Compliance does not interfere with personal comfort, convenience, and pleasure.
5. Few, if any, exceptions are allowed in the law.
6. Enforcement can be augmented by persons other than the police.
7. Observation of the regulated behavior by authorities is obviously easy.
8. A perception of increased concentration of enforcement to detect nonconformity affects behavior.
9. Conviction occurs soon after detection.
10. Conviction results in relatively severe punishment (64).

This is not intended as a ranking of the effect of these factors on compliance with law; the ranking could not be precise because the research is not complete enough to compile a perfect ranking. One interesting aspect of such a list is that sociological theory and legislative energy tends to be concentrated on debate over the effects of arrest, conviction, and punishment to the neglect of the other factors.

The first factor is obvious and negates the need for law or other formal rule. The second factor probably contributes the most to conformity with laws and rules where the behavior would not otherwise occur. To the extent that there is compliance with essentially unenforceable laws such as those limiting blood alcohol concentration when driving, the propensity of some people to conform with any law, simply because it is the law and the moral overtones of failure to comply is a potent force for compliance.

The success of enforcement and punishment in reducing injury associated with driving while intoxicated by alcohol is very limited, contrary to popular belief. Roadside surveys of drivers stopped at random and asked to give a breath sample, when compared with arrest rates for driving while impaired in the same area, find a low probability of arrest. The highest ever found in such studies is 1 in 200 (8). The more common finding is about 1 in 2000. Data on the correlation of crime rates to arrest rates suggest that the arrest rate would have to be increased to greater than 1 in 3 for the law to begin to reduce the alcohol-related crash rate (83).

Such an arrest rate is unlikely because of another factor on the list; the behavior is not easily observable. Persons with relatively high blood alcohol concentrations often can operate a vehicle so as to appear that nothing is awry. They mainly have difficulty when they have to respond to multiple cues from different senses (44).

Crackdowns in law enforcement that create the illusion of greatly increased probability of arrest have temporary effects on death rates. The initial reaction to the British Road Safety Act of 1967 was empty pubs in the countryside and a 25% reduction in motor vehicle fatality rates. Within three years, when the publicity declined drastically and the drinkers learned that arrest was unlikely and conviction less so, the mortality rate returned to the pre-crackdown level (72). This experience has been repeated in numerous jurisdictions around the world (71).

The effect of the movement against drunk driving in the US in the 1980s is yet to be adequately evaluated, but previous experience portends a temporary effect, if indeed any effect can be demonstrated. My analysis of the data from counties where more than 90% of fatally injured drivers are tested for alcohol indicates no decrease in alcohol-involved fatal crashes through 1982 that is not paralleled or exceeded by a decrease in mortality without alcohol involvement. About half of fatally injured drivers in 1982 had blood alcohol above the legal limit, about the same as in the studies during the 1950s and 1960s (48). Police reports of alcohol involvement are highly inaccurate when compared to laboratory tests of alcohol in blood (5, 28) and should not be believed when used in court or research.

Severe punishment for alcohol-impaired driving has been advocated based on claimed effects of jail sentences in the Scandinavian countries. One analyst, who did extensive studies of the Scandinavian laws and their correlation to motor vehicle fatalities, labeled the claimed effectiveness "the Scandinavian Myth" (73). Visitors to the Scandinavian countries have claimed the laws are effective because, in drinking situations, one of their hosts will abstain and drive afterward. Perhaps moderate social drinkers with foreign visitors are deterred by the threat of an embarrassing arrest and jail sentence. But the best evidence suggests that the hard-drinking population is not so deterred (73). One of the extraordinary aspects of doing research in this field is that one's colleagues will argue a point on the basis of anecdotal evidence that the same persons would find totally unacceptable as evidence in their own areas of research.

One alcohol policy that has been found consistently effective in reducing fatal crashes is a high minimum age for purchase of alcoholic beverages.

Fatalities involving drivers less than 21 years old increased in states that reduced their minimum purchasing ages in the 1960s, compared to those that did not (87), and the reverse effect occurred recently as states increased the minimum age for purchase of alcohol (88). The likely reason for the effect of these laws is that their enforcement is augmented by the community, in this case, retail outlets, and there are means of identifying those under age who attempt to violate the law.

Another important law that is probably enforced by the community more than the police is the minimum driving age law. In New Jersey, where the licensing age is 17, 16-year-olds have about 66 to 80% fewer fatal crashes than in Connecticut, where teenagers can be licensed on their sixteenth birthdays (86). Parents are unlikely to allow use of the family car by an unlicensed teenager, and the youngster cannot rent a car without showing a license. A few steal cars or drive their friends' cars on occasion, but the licensing age remains a major deterrent to vehicle use by under-aged drivers. Similarly, prohibition in several states of driving during certain hours of the night by persons less than a specified age is associated with substantially lower fatal crash rates by drivers in the specified age groups during the specified hours, with no offsetting increase during legal driving hours (53). Again, it is likely that parents are the main enforcers of those laws.

Laws regarding speeding are more enforceable than drinking driver laws apparently because the law prohibits a directly observable behavior. In the 1970s, the effects of speeding laws were dramatically illustrated when energy shortages motivated the US Congress to require states to enact a maximum speed limit of 55 miles per hour in order to qualify for federal highway funds. The motor vehicle deaths declined 20% in a single year, partly because of reduced availability of fuel and partly because of reduced speeds and more uniform speeds. Since the total reduction cannot be apportioned to the speed limits, a small research industry developed around dissecting the relative contribution of each factor. A National Research Council/National Academy of Sciences report summarized the evidence and estimated about a 10% reduction—4500 fewer fatalities per year—as a result of the 55 mile per hour limit (46). The decline in deaths was primarily on roads where the maximum speed limit was lowered (36).

A second change in law, related to the energy shortages, probably resulted in increased pedestrian injuries. Increases in intersections where right turn on red is allowed were associated with an increment in pedestrian injuries (93).

Several laws requiring use of protective equipment have been associated with reductions in fatal injury. States that enacted laws requiring helmet use by motorcyclists experienced a 30% reduction in motorcyclist fatalities compared to adjacent states without the laws at the time. Observed use of helmets by motorcyclists on the road was virtually 100% in states where they were required, compared to 25 to 50% use in states without the requirement (59). The behavior is easily observable by police and the behavior cannot be changed easily while in transit when the police are out of sight, thus probably accounting for the high degree of compliance with the law.

Motorcycle helmet laws have been repealed in many states after a vocal minority of motorcyclists lobbied the state legislatures. Increases in deaths in the states that repealed their helmet laws were predictable from the effects when the original laws were enacted (84).

By 1985 all of the states in the US had some form of law requiring use of child restraints for infants and young children in moving motor vehicles. The laws vary regarding the upper age limit and exemptions dependent on seating position and other factors. Studies of child restraint use among children to whom the law applied in Tennessee, the first state to enact such a law, found about 28% compliance (89). More recent evidence of use in crashes suggests a use rate of about 40% following increased enforcement efforts. The injury rate to child occupants is associated with the laws (12), although the studies thus far have not included adequate comparison with areas not having such laws to assess the precise magnitude of the effect. Since motor vehicle fatalities fluctuate in relation to economic and other secular trends (7), before-after comparisons are inadequate for precise estimates.

Laws requiring seat belt use have been in effect in several countries for more than a decade and have begun to be enacted in the US. In New York, the first US state with such a law, belt use ranged from 10 to 20% in 1984 prior to the law and varied from 45 to 70% among various communities after the law went in force in early 1985 (31). This is similar to the experience of the first large jurisdiction to require belt use, Victoria, Australia in the early 1970s (3). Reductions accompanying belt use laws in deaths to vehicle occupants vary from 10% in rural areas of Australia (20) to 25% in England (50).

The effect of allowing exemptions to a law was illustrated in Ontario, Canada when a belt use law was enacted there in the mid-1970s. The public complained that belts in pre-1974 cars without inertial reels were uncomfortable, so the government exempted shoulder belt use in pre-1974 cars within two months after the original law was in force. Belt use, which had initially risen to 70% declined to 50%, including declines in vehicles not exempted (61). Belt use has fluctuated with enforcement campaigns in Ontario, but a consistently high belt use such as that achieved in Australia and New Zealand has not yet been attained.

The reduction in deaths associated with belt use laws is less than the estimated effects of belts would predict. If belts reduce deaths to wearers by 60%, Australia should have experienced a 35% reduction in occupant deaths

(65). Several observations have explained the less-than-expected effectiveness. Belt use does not increase as much among the young, alcohol-impaired, or nighttime drivers as among drivers at less risk (11, 50, 61).

Automatic Protection

Despite these findings, the US Department of Transportation (DOT) has falsely depicted seat belt laws as the equivalent of increased automatic crash protection in cars and has promised to exempt the automobile manufacturers from any requirements for such protection if two thirds of the population is covered by seat belt use laws meeting certain criteria by 1989. Two thirds of the population covered by belt laws with the maximum effectiveness observed in England, 25%, would result in approximately 3700 fewer deaths per year ($0.66 \times 0.25 \times 22000$ car occupant deaths per year, approximately). Air bags that inflate in the more severe frontal crashes would reduce deaths some 9000 per year with no increase in belt use. Furthermore, since half those 3700 deaths reduced by seat belt laws would be in nonfrontal crashes, less than 2000 of the 9000 lives prevented by air bags, during the average ten year life of any model year of car, would be prevented by the seat belt laws.

By the mid-1970s, motor vehicle safety regulations were subjected to cost-benefit analyses in which lives to be saved by one method were equated to lives to be saved by another method, irrespective of whether or not they were the same lives. By the mid-1980s, decisions were being made primarily to circumvent the Supreme Court's decision that the earlier recision of the automatic protection standard was illegal (80). The dream of William Haddon, Jr., and the framers of the 1966 Motor Vehicle Safety Act, for an orderly increment in motor vehicle safety standards commensurate with sound research into the effectiveness of developed technology has been transformed by a federal agency into an attempt to substitute controls on individual behavior in lieu of forcing the use of technically proven technology that manufacturers, in the vast majority, have refused to use voluntarily.

This change is largely the result of the antifederal government ideology that developed as a result of the Viet Nam War and the Watergate scandals. It is aided by the claim of neoclassic economic theory that people decide what level of safety they desire by their market decisions and any government imposition of standards will be inefficient and offset by human behavior. Empirical test of this theory has proved it false.

Aside from a few consensus standards for headlamps and the like imposed by the states, motor vehicle manufacture was unregulated until 1964. A few states passed laws requiring lap seat belt installation in the early 1960s and enough had done so by 1964 that manufacturers installed them routinely in most cars. The purchasing arm of the government required energy-absorbing steering assemblies and other safety features in vehicles sold to the government in 1966.

Manufacturers with a large volume of sales of certain models to government began to include these features on those and a few other models sold to the public as well as the government. The 1968 standards required all new vehicles offered for sale in the US to have shoulder belts in front outboard seats, energy-absorbing steering assemblies, padded dashboards, high-penetration-resistant windshields, improved doorlocks to reduce ejection, redundant braking systems, reduced glare in driver's eyes, side marker lights, minimum tire performance, and several other requirements (64). Revisions of the standards, new standards for head restraints, fuel tanks, etc were issued in subsequent years.

Initial comparisons of vehicles that met specific standards compared to those that did not indicated substantial reductions in severity of injury associated with the changes in equipment (27, 38). In a highly publicized article, however, an economist argued that drivers would offset the increased protection by driving more riskily to keep constant their "demand for risk." He claimed that his time-series analysis showed an increase in fatalities to "pedestrians" that offset the 20% reduction in occupant deaths that occurred by 1972 (51).

A reanalysis of the data used to support those claims found that the study was faulty. The model did not accurately project trends in fatalities prior to regulation. Motorcyclists' deaths were counted as "pedestrians" during a period when motorcycle registrations were doubling every five years with a commensurate increase in deaths. Regulated cars were not separated from unregulated cars or trucks. Correction of the model resulted in less than projected deaths to nonoccupants as well as occupants (60). Subsequent analysis of disaggregated data indicated that regulated vehicles killed fewer pedestrians, bicyclists, and motorcyclists than unregulated vehicles. This result is consistent with the fact that crash avoidance standards (windshield glare, running lights, brakes) were included in the standards (63). By 1982, the US had about 14,000 to 15,000 fewer deaths per year than would have been expected without the motor vehicle safety standards (68).

The theory that increased occupant crash protection results in driving behavior that increases risk has also been discredited by actual observation of several relevant behaviors before and after the increased belt use that accompanies belt use laws. There is no observed change in speed on curves, following distance by a driver moving in tandem with a forward vehicle, or moving through intersections when lights are red (39, 50).

Despite the lack of evidence of some sort of risk thermostat in people's brains, or any credible evidence of offsetting behavior when risk is reduced, it is not uncommon for those of us who labor in this vineyard to be greeted with that theory, particularly in presentations to academic audiences. Apparently many academics prefer cute theories to empirical evidence. Actually, the theory did not originate with its modern academic proponents, but was used by nineteenth century railroad owners to forestall the use of automatic braking, signaling, and coupling systems on their trains (1). That and other arguments delayed widespread adoption of the technology for 40 years. When it was finally required by the Congress, railroad deaths declined 80% (81).

A second myth that pervades the debate regarding regulation is that manufacturers will provide safer vehicles if there is sufficient demand. In 1979, a previously withheld 1970 marketing study by General Motors regarding air bags was discovered. Several more done during the 1970s were forthcoming from GM at the request of Congress. These studies showed that General Motors had known from 1970 that at least half their customers wanted air bags and were willing to pay the quoted costs for them (2). Yet GM would offer air bags only on its most expensive cars in 1974–1976 with little advertising, long delays in delivery, and dealer discouragement of customers who requested them (34). A study of GM's air bag marketing noted that GM sold more air bags in the first year of their availability than they had sold comparably priced air conditioning when it first appeared (9). The company continued to market air conditioners to the point that they are now on more than half of cars sold, but it dropped the air bag.

Should the standard requiring criteria for automatic protection in frontal crashes up to 30 miles per hour into a barrier be adopted in the late 1980s, it will be long out of date technologically. In the 1970s, several contractors to the National Highway Traffic Safety Administration developed research safety vehicles that demonstrated the feasibility of survivable frontal crashes into test barriers up to 45 miles an hour. One of these vehicles could be manufactured in mass production of one million copies or more and sold profitably for about the price of current compact cars (16). Contrary to popular myth, it is not cost that determines the safety of vehicles.

Even when manufacturers are required to meet federal safety standards, they do not necessarily respond with the most efficacious or the least expensive approach to crash protection. In the 1960s, tests of head restraints to reduce injury to the head and neck resulted in recommendations that seat backs high enough to reach the back of the head of the tallest males were more effective in injury reduction than adjustable head restraints (75). This was reinforced by a 1971 study that found the majority of adjustable restraints observed in traffic were not adjusted behind the head (49). Despite the evidence, the manufacturers have continued to market the majority of cars with adjustable restraints. Furthermore, the adjustable restraints cost $28 more per car, on average, than high seat backs. A recent study found that high seat backs are 70% more effective in preventing neck injury than adjustable restraints, as the previous studies predicted, but that 72% of vehicles manufactured from 1969 through 1981 had adjustable restraints (33).

Frustrated by the lack of response of appeals to reason directed to the manufacturers and DOT, a few activists in the legal and public health communities have advocated product liability lawsuits against the manufacturers who have failed to provide technologically and economically feasible crash protection (82). The American Public Health Association and the Association for Public Health Policy have joined in cases regarding air bags as *amicus curiae*. Should large numbers of these cases be successful, the motor vehicle manufacturers will be in a position similar to that of the asbestos producers, in economic difficulty because of recalcitrance and neglect.

CONCLUSION

For decades, tens of thousands of lives were lost and millions were injured by motor vehicles annually with little notice in public health circles. The problem was left mainly to educators, law enforcement, liability lawyers, and insurance adjusters. The number of researchers and teachers in schools of public health who devote more than half their time to epidemiology and prevention of trauma of any origin, including that involving motor vehicles, can be counted on one's fingers. Only at The Johns Hopkins University is there a graduate program with sufficient breadth for students to obtain the necessary credentials in the area. Most of the professionals who have done research in this area were trained in research on other subjects. Most are self-educated with respect to trauma research. Despite the much greater productive years of life lost from trauma compared to cancers, a report from the National Research Council/National Academy of Sciences recently noted that 11¢ is devoted to trauma research for every dollar devoted to cancer research (47). With little training of researchers and shortage of research funds, the productivity in recent trauma research, as outlined in this chapter, is all the more remarkable.

Literature Cited

1. Adams, C. F. 1879. *Notes on Railroad Accidents*. New York: Putnam
2. Advertising and Marketing Section. 1971. *Consumer Opinions Relative to Automotive Restraint Systems*. Detroit: General Motors Corp.
3. Andressand, D. C. 1976. Victoria and the seat belt law. *Hum. Fact.* 18:593–600
4. Archives of the United States. 1982. Part of a conversation among President Nixon, Lide Anthony Iacocca, Henry Ford II, and John D. Ehrlichman in the oval office on April 27, 1971, between 11:08 and 11:43 A.M. *Aut. Lit. Rep.* Nov. 18, pp. 1784–98
5. Baker, S. P., Fisher, R. S. 1977. Alcohol and motorcycle fatalities *Am. J. Public Health* 14:187–96
6. Baker, S. P., Dietz, P. E. 1979. Injury prevention. In *Healthy People, The Surgeon General's Report on Health Promotion And Disease Prevention, Background Papers*. Washington DC: US DHEW
7. Baker, S. P., O'Neill, B., Karpf, R. 1984. *The Injury Fact Book*. Lexington, Mass.: Heath
8. Beitel, G. A., Sharp, M. C., Glauz, W. D. 1975. Probability of arrest while driving under the influence of alcohol. *J. Studies Alcohol* 36:109–16
9. Booz-Allen & Hamilton 1983. *A Retrospective Analysis of the General Motors Air Cushion Restraint System Marketing Effort 1974–1976*. Washington, DC: Natl. Highway Traffic Safety Admin.

10. Conger, J. J., Miller, W. C., Rainey, R. V. 1966. Effects of driver education: The role of motivation, intelligence, social class, and exposure. *Traf. Safe. Res. Rev.* 10:67–71
11. Dalgaard, J. B. 1977. Experiences with the new seat belt law on fatal lesions of car occupants in Denmark. In *Proc. 6th Int. Assoc. Accident and Traffic Med.* Melbourne: Royal Australasian Coll. of Surgeons
12. Decker, M. D., Dewey, M. J., Hutcheson, R. H. Jr., Schaffer, W. 1984. The use and efficacy of child restraint devices: The Tennessee experience. *J. Am. Med. Assoc.* 252:2571–75
13. DeHaven, H. 1942. Mechanical analysis of survival in falls from heights of fifty to one hundred and fifty feet. *War Med.* 2:586–96
14. Denton, G. G. 1980. The influence of visual pattern on perceived speed. *Perception* 9:393–402
15. Dietz, P. E., Baker, S. P. 1974. Drowning: Epidemiology and prevention. *Am. J. Public Health* 64:303–12
16. DiNapoli, N. 1977. *Research Safety Vehicle Phase II, Volume II; Comprehensive Technical Results.* Springfield, Va.: Natl. Tech. Inform. Serv.
17. Ellman D., Killebrew, T. J. 1978. Incentives and seat belts: Changing a resistant behavior through extrinsic motivation. *J. Appl. Soc. Psychol.* 8:72–83
18. Evans, L. 1970. Speed estimation from a moving automobile. *Ergonomics* 13:219–30
19. Fleischer, G. A. 1972. *An experiment in the use of broadcast media in highway safety.* Los Angeles: Univ. So. Calif. Dept. Indust. Systems Engineering
20. Foldvary, L. S., Lane, J. C. 1974. The effectiveness of compulsory wearing of seat-belts in casualty reduction. *Accident Anal. Prevent.* 6:59–81
21. Geller, E. S., Johnson, R. P., Pelton, S. L. 1982. Community-based interventions for encouraging safety belt use. *Am. J. Commun. Psychol.* 10:183
22. Geller, E. S., Davis, L., Spicer, K. 1983. Industry-based incentives for promoting seat belt use: Differential impact on white-collar versus blue-collar employees. *J. Organiz. Behav. Manag.* 5:17–29
23. Gordon, D. A., Mast, T. M. 1970. Driver's judgment in overtaking and passing. *Hum. Fact.* 12:341–46
24. Haddon, W. Jr. 1970. On the escape of tigers: An ecologic note. *Tech. Rev.* 72:44
25. Haddon, W. Jr. 1975. Reducing the damage of motor vehicle use. *Tech. Rev.* 77:53–59
26. Haddon, W. Jr. 1980. Advances in epidemiology of injuries as a basis for public policy. *Public Health Rep.* 95:411–21
27. Haddon, W. Jr. 1970. What we're talking about. In *Key Issues In Highway Loss Reduction,* ed. C. W. Wixom. Washington DC: Insurance Inst. Highway Safety
28. Haddon, W. Jr., Bradess, V. A. 1959. Alcohol in the single vehicle fatal accident, experience of Westchester County, New York. *J. Am. Med. Assoc.* 169:1587–93
29. Haddon, W. Jr., Suchman, E. A., Klein, D., Eds. 1964. *Accident Research: Methods and Approaches.* New York: Harper & Row
30. Hill, P. S., Jamieson, B. D. 1978. Driving offenders and the defensive driving course—an archival study. *J. Psychol.* 98:117–27
31. Insurance Inst. for Highway Safety. 1985. Early New York results show belt use varies from 43 to 80 percent. *Stat. Rep.* 20:3
32. Johansson, G., Rumar, K. 1971. Driver's brake reaction times. *Hum. Fact.* 13:23–27
33. Kahane, C. J. 1982. *An Evaluation of Head Restraints: Federal Motor Vehicle Standard 202.* Washington DC: Natl. Highway Traffic Safety Admin.
34. Karr, A. R. 1976. Saga of the air bag, or the slow deflation of a car-safety idea. *Wall Street J.* Nov. 11, p. 1
35. Kelley, A. B. 1972. *Boobytrap* (film). Washington DC: Insurance Inst. for Highway Safety
36. Kemper, W. J., Byington, S. R. 1977. Safety aspects of the 55 MPH speed limit. *Public Roads* 41:58–67
37. Lave, L. 1981. Conflicting objectives in regulating the automobile. *Science* 202:893
38. Levine, D. N., Campbell, B. J. 1971. *Effectiveness of Lap Seat Belts and the Energy Absorbing Steering System in the Reduction of Injuries.* Chapel Hill: Univ. North Carolina Safety Res. Cent.
39. Lund, A. K., Zador, P. L. 1984. Mandatory belt use and driver risk taking. *Risk Anal.* 4:41–53
40. Mann, R. E., Leigh, G., Vingilis, E. R., De Genova, K. 1983. A critical review of the effectiveness of drinking-driving rehabilitation programmes. *Accident Anal. Prevent.* 15:441–61
41. McCarry, C. 1972. *Citizen Nader.* New York: Saturday Review Press
42. McGuire, F. L., Kersh, R. C. 1969. *An*

Evaluation Of Driver Education. Berkley, CA: Univ. Calif. Press

43. Miller, R. E., Reisinger, K. S., Blatter, M. M., Wucher, W. 1982. Pediatric counseling and subsequent use of smoke detectors. *Am. J. Public Health* 72:392–93

44. Moskowitz, H. 1971. A behavioral mechanism of alcohol related accidents. *Proc. 1st Ann. Conf. Natl. Inst. Alcohol Alcohol Abuse.* Washington DC: US DHEW

45. Mulhern, T. 1977. *The National Safety Council's defensive driving course as an accident and violation countermeasure.* Phd dissertation. College Station, TX: Texas A and M Univ.

46. Natl. Res. Counc. 1984. *55: A Decade of Experience.* Washington DC: Natl. Acad. Sci.

47. Natl. Res. Council. 1985. *Injury in America: A Continuing Public Health Problem.* Washington DC: Natl. Acad. Sci.

48. *1968 Alcohol and Highway Safety Report.* 1968. Washington DC: US House of Representatives Committee on Public Works (Committee Print)

49. O'Neill, B., et al. 1972. Automobile head restraints: Frequency of neck injury claims in relation to the presence of head restraints. *Am. J. Public Health* 62:399

50. O'Neill, B., Lund, A. K., Zador, P. L., Ashton, S. 1984. Mandatory belt use and driver risk taking: An empirical evaluation of the risk-compensation hypothesis. (mimeo) Washington DC: Insurance Inst. Highway Safety

51. Peltzman, S. 1975. The effects of automobile safety regulation. *J. Polit. Econ.* 83:677

52. Preusser, D. F., Ulmer, R. G., Adams, J. R. 1976. Driver record evaluation of a drinking driver rehabilitation program. *J. Safe. Res.* 8:98–105

53. Preusser, D. F., Williams, A. F., Zador, P. L., Blomberg, R. D. 1984. The effects of curfew laws on motor vehicle crashes. *Law and Policy* 6:115–28

54. Ray, H. W., Weaver, J. K., Brink, J. R., Stock, J. R. 1982. Safe Performance Secondary School Education Curriculum. Washington, D.C.: Natl. Highway Traffic Safety Admin.

55. Reilly, R. E., Kurke, D. S., Bukenmaier, C. C. Jr. 1980. Validation of the Reduction of Rear-End Collisions by a High Mounted Auxiliary Stoplamp, Washington, DC: Natl. Highway Traffic Safety Admin.

56. Reisinger, K. S., Williams, A. F., Wells, J. A. K., John, C. E., Roberts, T.

R., Podgainy, H. J. 1981. The effect of pediatricians counseling on infant restraint use. *Pediatrics* 67:201–6

57. Reisinger, K. S., Williams, A. F. 1978. Evaluation of programs designed to increase protection of infants in cars. *Pediatrics* 62:280–87

58. Robertson, L. S. 1975. Behavioral research and strategies in public health: A demur. *Soc. Sci. Med.* 9:165

59. Robertson, L. S. 1976. An instance of effective legal regulation: Motorcyclist helmet and daytime headlamp laws. *Law Soc. Rev.* 10:456–77

60. Robertson, L. S. 1977. A critical analysis of Peltzman's "The effects of automobile safety regulation." *J. Econ. Issues* 11:587

61. Robertson, L. S. 1978. The seat belt use law in Ontario: Effects on actual use. *Can. J. Public Health* 69:154–57

62. Robertson, L. S. 1980. Crash involvement of teenaged drivers when driver education is eliminated from high school. *Am. J. Public Health* 70:599–603

63. Robertson, L. S. 1981. Automobile safety regulations and death reductions in the United States. *Am. J. Public Health* 71:818–22

64. Robertson, L. S. 1983. *Injuries: Causes, Control Strategies and Public Policy.* Lexington, Mass.: Heath

65. Robertson, L. S. 1983. Public perception and behavior in relation to vehicle passenger restraints. In *The Analysis of Actual Versus Perceived Risk,* ed. V. T. Covello. New York: Plenum

66. Robertson, L. S. 1984. Federal funds and state motor vehicle deaths. *J. Public Health Policy* 5:376–86

67. Robertson, L. S. 1984. Insurance incentives and seat belt use. *Am. J. Public Health* 74:1157–58

68. Robertson, L. S. 1984. Automobile safety regulation: Rebuttal and new data. *Am. J. Public Health* 74:1390–94

69. Robertson, L. S., Zador, P. L. 1978. Driver education and fatal crash involvement of teenaged drivers. *Am. J. Public Health* 68:959–65

70. Robertson, L. S., Kelley, A. B., O'Neill, B. Wixom, C. W., Eiswirth, R. S., Haddon, W. Jr. 1974. A controlled study of the effect of television messages on safety belt use. *Am. J. Public Health* 64:1071–80

71. Ross, H. L. 1982. *Deterring the Drinking Driver: Legal Policy and Social Control.* Lexington, Mass.: Heath

72. Ross, H. L. 1973. Law, science and accidents: The British Road Safety Act of 1967. *J. Legal Studies* 2:1–78

73. Ross, H. L. 1975. The Skandinavian myth: The effectiveness of drinking-and-driving legislation in Sweden and Norway. *J. Leg. Stud.* 1:285–310

74. Schmidt, F., Tiffin, J. 1969. Distortion of drivers' estimates of automobile speed as a function of speed adaptation. *J. Appl. Psychol.* 53:536–39

75. Severy, D. M., Brink, H. M., Baird, J. D. 1968. Backrest and head restraint design for rear-end collision protection. Detroit: Soc. of Automotive Engineers

76. Shaoul, J. 1975. The Use of Accidents and Traffic Offenses as Criteria for Evaluating Courses in Driver Education, Salford, England: Univ. Salford

77. Stapp, J. P. 1957. Human tolerance to deceleration. *Am. J. Surg.* 93:734–40

78. Stein, H. 1984. Fleet experience with daytime running lights in the United States—preliminary results. (mimeo.) Washington DC: Insurance Inst. Highway Safety

79. Stuart, R. B. 1974. Teaching facts about drugs: Pushing or preventing. *J. Educ. Psychol.* 66:189–201

80. Supreme Court of the United States. 1983. *Motor Vehicle Manufacturers Association, Inc., et al. v. State Farm Mutual Automobile Insurance Co., et al.* No. 82–354

81. Swain, P. L. 1980. Labor market contracting and the provision for workplace hazards: a historical study. Unpublished doctoral dissertation, Cambridge, MA: Mass. Inst. Technol.

82. Teret, S. 1981. Injury control and product liability. *J. Public Health Policy* 2:49–57

83. Tittle, C. R., Rowe, A. R. 1974. Certainty of arrest and crime rates: A further test of the deterrence hypothesis. *Soc. Forces* 2:455–62

84. Watson, G. F., Zador, P. L., Wilks, A.

1980. The repeal of helmet use laws and increased motorcyclist mortality in the United States, 1975–1978. *Am. J. Public Health* 70:579–92

85. Weinstein, N. D., Grubb, P. D., Vautier, J. S. 1984. Increasing automobile seat belt use: An intervention emphasizing risk susceptability. (mimeo.) New Brunswick, NJ: Rutgers Univ.

86. Williams, A. F., Karpf, R. S., Zador, P. F. 1983. Variations in minimum licensing age and fatal motor vehicle crashes. *Am. J. Public Health* 73:1401–3

87. Williams, A. F., Rich, R. F., Zador, P. L., Robertson, L. S. 1975. The legal minimum drinking age and fatal motor vehicle crashes. *J. Legal Studies* 4:219–39

88. Williams, A. F., Zador, P. L., Harris, S. S., Karpf, R. S. 1983. The effect of raising the legal minimum drinking age on fatal crash involvement. *J. Legal Studies* 12:169–79

89. Williams, A. F., Wells, J. A. K. 1981. The Tennessee child restraint law in its third year. *Am. J. Public Health* 71:163

90. Wright, P. H., Robertson, L. S. 1976. Studies of roadside hazards for projecting fatal crash sites. *Trans. Res. Rec.* 609. Washington DC: Natl. Acad. Sci.

91. Wright, P. H., Zador, P. L., Park, C. Y., Karpf, R. S. 1982. Effect of pavement markers on nighttime crashes in Georgia. (mimeo.) Washington DC: Insurance Inst. Highway Safety

92. Zador, P. L., Stein, H., Shapiro, S., Tarnoff, P. 1984. The effect of signal timing on traffic flow and crashes at signalized intersections. (mimeo.) Washington DC: Insurance Inst. Highway Safety

93. Zador, P. L. 1984. Right turn on red law and motor vehicle crashes: A review of the literature. *Accident Anal. Prevent.* 16:241–45

Ann. Rev. Public Health. 1986. 7:35–58

RELATIVE RISK AND ODDS RATIO REGRESSION

R. L. Prentice and V. T. Farewell

Division of Public Health Sciences, Fred Hutchinson Cancer Research Center, Seattle, Washington 98104

INTRODUCTION

Consider a cohort of nearly 20,000 residents of Hiroshima and Nagasaki who have undergone biennial clinical examinations for the past 20 years under the auspices of the Radiation Effects Research Foundation. Suppose that one would like to use a series of blood pressure measurements on an individual to assess the risk of a subsequent cardiovascular disease event. This type of assessment is complicated by a number of features: the "risk factors" of interest are evolving over time, risk factor data may be missing, there may be many other "confounding" factors, and endpoint events may be censored due to competing risks or dropout.

During the past 15 years a vast biostatistical literature has developed on the regression analysis of "failure" time data. This literature is relevant to a range of problems in medicine and public health as well as in other areas. For example "failure time" may refer to time-to-relapse in a clinical trial, or to the age of disease diagnosis in an epidemiologic cohort study or in a disease prevention trial. Often interest will center on the dependence of failure rate on individual characteristics, exposures, or treatment assignments, which are collectively referred to here as "covariates." In the above example the covariates may include the sequence of preceding blood pressure readings, along with such control factors as age at cohort selection and sex. Relative risk regression models express the ratio of instantaneous failure rates (i.e. hazard rates) as a function of covariates. A chief accomplishment of the literature alluded to above is the demonstration that such relative risks, or more generally relative

35

risk processes, can be efficiently estimated under a variety of sampling schemes without making any assumptions about the "baseline" disease rates; that is, about the rates corresponding to a standard covariate history. For example, in the analyses described below of the Hiroshima and Nagasaki data the standard covariate history was defined by systolic and diastolic blood pressure readings of 110/70 with stratification on age and sex. The results described are, in fact, unaffected by the choice of blood pressure standard.

Sometimes it will be convenient to model and estimate the probability of failure during a specified time period, rather than modeling instantaneous failure rates. For example, in the Japanese cohort illustration one may wish to examine the relationship between baseline blood pressure readings and cardiovascular disease incidence during the first 15 years of cohort follow-up. Odds ratio regression methods are natural for such modeling and estimation, since the odds ratio is itself fairly readily interpreted and typically closely approximates the relative risk if the failure accession period is short.

The current state of development of relative risk and odds ratio regression methods are reviewed in subsequent sections. The next section introduces the regression models mentioned above. Subsequent sections describe the methodology of their application under cohort sampling, case-control sampling, and some hybrid sampling schemes, respectively. In general, model-fitting procedures and asymptotic distribution theory are quite well established for these methods. Further work on small sample estimation procedures and on model checking is needed.

This review concentrates wholly on regression models for *ratios* of either failure rates or failure odds. Regression models for absolute risk, for example, may provide additional useful insights and more parsimonious models in some circumstances. Such models have, however, received comparatively little attention in the literature and, for example, are not well suited to case-control sampling.

RELATIVE RISK AND ODDS RATIO REGRESSION MODELS

Relative Risk Models

Consider a large, conceptually infinite population about which inferences are to be drawn (e.g. inference on the predictive value of blood pressure in respect to cardiovascular disease incidence in the previously mentioned Japanese population). Let $Z(u)$ denote the covariate value for a subject in this population at u units of time after a certain point in chronological time (e.g. the subjects blood pressure measurements during the uth biennial examination period). As time progresses the subject will generate a covariate history $[Z(u), 0 \leqslant u < t]$ that consists of all covariate measurements on the subject prior to time t (e.g. the sequence of blood pressure measurements from the first to $(t-1)$st biennial examination). Suppose now that one is interested in the relationship between aspects of covariate history prior to time t and the subsequent frequency of "failure" in the population (e.g. the relationship between cardiovascular disease incidence in examination cycle t and blood pressure in the immediately preceding examination period). Let T denote the time of failure for a subject. The population frequency of failure in a time period t to $t + \Delta$, given preceding covariate history $[Z(u), 0 \leqslant u < t]$ and lack of failure prior to time t, will be written

$$pr[t \leqslant T < t + \Delta \mid Z(u), 0 \leqslant u < t; T \geqslant t].$$ 1.

With conceptually infinite populations it will be reasonable to suppose that failure times arise continuously in time, and to consider the instantaneous failure rate in the population

$$\lambda[t; Z(u), 0 \leqslant u < t] = \lim_{\Delta \downarrow 0} pr[t \leqslant T < t + \Delta \mid Z(u), 0 \leqslant u < t; T \geqslant t] \Delta^{-1}.$$ 2.

Expression 2 is often referred to as the *hazard rate* or *force of mortality* for the population. The population relative risk process is defined here to be the ratio of the hazard rate 2 at a general covariate history $[Z(u); 0 \leqslant u < t]$ to that at some standard covariate history $[Z_0(u), 0 \leqslant u < t]$. The standard covariate may, for example, be chosen to correspond to lack of exposure in a population occupationally exposed to a toxic substance, or to the control group in a therapeutic or a prevention trial. The hazard rate process 2 can be written

$$\lambda[t; Z(u), 0 \leqslant u < t] = \lambda_0(t) \, RR[t; Z(u), 0 \leqslant u < t]$$ 3.

where $\lambda_0(t) = \lambda[t; Z_0(u), 0 \leqslant u < t]$ and $RR(\cdot)$ denotes the relative risk process mentioned above.

Relative risk regression models attempt to describe the population rates 3 by the modeling of $\lambda_0(\cdot)$ and $RR(\cdot)$. The class of models to be discussed here presumes a parametric form

$$RR[t; Z(u), 0 \leqslant u < t] = r[X(t)\beta]$$ 4.

for the relative risk process. In 4 the "relative risk form" $r(\cdot)$ is a fixed function, usually $r(\cdot) = \exp(\cdot)$ or $r(\cdot) = 1 + (\cdot)$ standardized so that $r(0) = 1$; $X(t) = [X_1(t), \cdots, X_p(t)]$ is a "modelled regression vector" consisting of functions of $[Z(u), 0 \leqslant u < t]$ and product terms between such functions and t, defined so that $X(t) \equiv 0$ for the standard covariate history $[Z_0(u), 0 \leqslant u < t]$; and β is a column p-vector of relative risk parameters to be estimated. For example, in the Japanese cohort one may define $X(t)$ to consist of systolic and diastolic blood pressure readings in examination cycle $t-1$, in which case β will consist of two parameters that quantitatively express the dependence of cardiovascular disease incidence on these blood pressure measurements.

Expression 4 requires the parametric modeling of the entire relative risk process. A useful relaxation arises from a stratification of the population frequencies, followed by the modeling of stratum-specific relative risks. Specifically, suppose that the population at time t is divided into q strata denoted by $s = s(t) \in \{1,\cdots,q\}$. Such strata may involve functions of $[Z(u), 0 \leq u < t]$ or product terms between such functions and t. Typically stratification factors would be chosen from covariates that are thought to relate importantly to failure rate, but whose relationship to failure rate is not currently the object of study. A standard covariate history $[Z_{0s}(u), 0 \leq u < t]$ is then defined for each stratum $s \in \{1,\cdots,q\}$, along with a stratum-specific baseline failure rate $\lambda_{0s}(t) = \lambda[t; Z_{0s}(u), 0 \leq u < t]$ and a stratum-specific relative risk model

$$RR_s[t; Z(u), 0 \leq u < t] = \lambda[t; Z(u), 0 \leq u < t]/\lambda_{0s}(t)$$

$$= r[X(t)\beta_s]. \qquad\qquad 5.$$

In the Japanese cohort analyses described below, strata are defined on the basis of sex and age in 1960 in 5-year intervals. The subscript s on the regression parameter β then permits the relative risk associated with specific blood pressure levels $X(t)$ to vary with sex and age. In subsequent sections we take the relative risk process 4, or more generally 5, as the target of estimation.

Note that a range of failure rate models, of the type 4 or 5, could be also defined for

$$\lambda[t; Z(u), 0 \leq u < x] = \lim_{\Delta t \downarrow 0} pr[t \leq T < t + \Delta \mid Z(u), 0 \leq u < x; T \geq t]\Delta^{-1}$$

for $x \leq t$.

Chronological time holds a special position in the above model specification. While it is natural for some time variable to play such a role, other choices, such as subject age or time from a certain lifetime event, may be more natural in some circumstances. Relative risk regression models, of the type described above, can be defined for other such time specifications. Some additional issues may arise however, as we describe below.

The relative risk, as defined above, is an attractive target of estimation. Ratios of failure rates often provide a natural means of communicating a dependence of failure rate on covariate histories. Furthermore, relative risks can be conveniently estimated under a variety of important sampling schemes, as reviewed below. The relative risk regression models introduced above have the desirable feature that such estimation can take place without imposing any assumptions on the baseline failure rates $\lambda_0(\cdot)$ or $\lambda_{0s}(\cdot)$.

Odds Ratio Models

Some procedures for sampling from the population do not allow identification of hazard ratios. Sampling procedures that note only whether failure occurs during a specified time period Δ, rather than noting the precise time of failure T for a subject, allow only for the identification of certain other functions of the population frequencies 1. For example, for a given Δ one could specify a model for the population frequency ratio

$$pr[t \leq T < t + \Delta | Z(u), 0 \leq u < t; T \geq t]/pr[t \leq T < t + \Delta | Z_0(u), 0 \leq u < t; T \geq t],$$

which is sometimes referred to as the *population rate ratio,* or even as the *relative risk,* in common epidemiologic parlance. This ratio process is not amenable to estimation under certain prominent sampling schemes. The population odds ratio, however, is identifiable under a range of sampling plans. It is defined by

$$OR[t;Z(u),0 \leq u<t,\Delta] = \frac{pr\{t \leq T<t+\Delta|Z(u),0 \leq u<t;T \geq t\}/pr\{T \geq t+\Delta|Z(u),0 \leq u<t;T \geq t\}}{pr\{t \leq T<t+\Delta|Z_0(u),0 \leq u<t;T \geq t\}/pr\{T \geq t+\Delta|Z_0(u),0 \leq u<t;T \geq t\}} \quad 6.$$

Expression 6 can be recognized as the ratio of odds of failure in the time period $(t, t + \Delta)$ at a general covariate history to that at the standard covariate history. Odds ratio regression models

$$OR[t;Z(u);0 \leq u < t,\Delta] = r[X(t)\beta] \quad 7.$$

may be specified with definitions exactly as in 4. Using 6, such an odds ratio model can be written as

$$pr[t \leq T < t + \Delta | Z(u); 0 \leq u < t; T \geq t] = \lambda_0(t)r[X(t)\beta]/\{1 + \lambda_0(t)r[X(t)\beta]\}, \quad 8.$$

where $\lambda_0(t)$ is the denominator of 6. Expression 8 can be recognized as a rather general form of a binary logistic regression model. The model is most frequently used with $\lambda_0(t) = \exp(\alpha)$ and $r[X(t)\beta] = \exp[X(t)\beta]$.

It is a disadvantage that the interpretation of the odds ratio model 7 depends on the time period Δ. Hence, for example, odds ratio estimates from distinct studies will be strictly comparable only if the corresponding Δ values are equal. For this reason special attention focuses on odds ratios in circumstances in which 6 is a good approximation to $RR\{t;Z(u),0 \leq u < t\}$.

Odds ratio models are readily extended to allow stratification, as in 5 above.

RELATIVE RISK AND ODDS RATIO ESTIMATION IN COHORT STUDIES

Sampling Requirements

A cohort study consists of random sampling, or stratified random sampling, from the above conceptually infinite population, and a follow-up of sampled individuals for occurrence of failure. Suppose first that subjects $i = 1, \cdots, n$ are selected independently and randomly at time $t = 0$, without stratification. Let $P(\cdot)$ denote the probability distribution induced by such independent random sampling. Also let the "counting process" N_i be defined so that $N_i(t)$ has value zero prior to an observed failure on subject i and value one thereafter, $i = 1, \cdots, n$. It is convenient to require the sample paths of each N_i to be right continuous. In the absence of censorship, independent random sampling will imply, for any (i, Δ), that

$$P\{t \leq T_i < t + \Delta \mid Z_i(u),0 \leq u < t;T_i \geq t;[N_j(u),Z_j(u);0 \leq u < t, j \neq i]\}$$
$$= P[t \leq T_i < t + \Delta \mid Z_i(u),0 \leq u < t;T_i \geq t],$$

so that the "intensity" process (instantaneous failure rate given preceding counting and covariate histories on the cohort) for the ith subject is precisely

$$\lambda_i(t) = \lambda[t;Z_i(u);0 \leq u < t],$$

$i = 1, \cdots, n$, where λ is the population hazard rate defined in 2.

Censorship arises because some subjects in the cohort may not be under observation for failure at certain times. For example, a subject may enter the cohort late at a time $t > 0$ (in which case the cohort may be referred to as *dynamic*), or subjects may be lost to follow-up or may die without experiencing the failure event of interest. It may even be necessary to censor some subjects intermittently if the necessary covariate data are unavailable. Such varied censorship patterns are conveniently denoted by introducing for the ith cohort member $(1 = 1, \cdots, n)$, a censoring process Y_i such that $Y_i(t) = 1$ at times at which the ith subject is "at risk" for failure—that is, is without failure and under active monitoring for failure—and $Y_i(t) = 0$ otherwise. It is convenient to require the sample paths of each Y_i to be left continuous. Independent censorship requires that cohort members at risk at any time t are representative of the population without failure prior to t, given their corresponding $Z(t)$ values.

Such an assumption therefore precludes the selective censoring of subjects thought to be at unusual risk of failure given their corresponding covariate histories, but allows the censoring rate to depend on such preceding covariate histories. An independent censorship assumption may be defined precisely by the requirement that the "intensity process" (instantaneous failure rate given preceding counting, covariate and censoring processes on the cohort) is given $(i = 1, \cdots, n)$ by

$$\lambda_i(t) = Y_i(t)\lambda[t; Z_i(u); 0 \leq u < t]. \qquad 9.$$

An independent sampling (sometimes referred to as *independent failure time*) and an independent censoring condition then jointly imply that the population hazard rates 2 are identifiable in a cohort study. The collective data on the ith subject can be denoted $[F_i(t), t \geq 0]$, where $F_i(t) = [N_i(t), Y_i(u), Z_i(u); 0 \leq u < t]$ and the collective data on the entire cohort by $[F(t), t \geq 0]$, where $F(t) = [F_1(t), \cdots, F_n(t)]$. Independent failure and censorship conditions imply

$$
\begin{aligned}
\lambda_i(t) &= \lim_{\Delta \downarrow 0} P[t \leq T_i < t + \Delta \mid F(t)]\Delta^{-1} \\
&= \lim_{\Delta \downarrow 0} P[t \leq T_i < t + \Delta \mid F_i(t)]\Delta^{-1} \\
&= Y_i(t) \lim_{\Delta \downarrow 0} P\{t \leq T_i < t + \Delta \mid [Z_i(u); 0 \leq u < t], T_i \geq t\}\Delta^{-1} \\
&= Y_i(t)\lambda[t; Z_i(u); 0 \leq u < t].
\end{aligned}
$$

The above presentation is very general in respect to the covariate processes. A cautionary note seems appropriate in dealing with evolutionary covariates (i.e. covariates that evolve over time) along with time definitions other than chronological time. In such circumstances, in order that 9 apply, one must be careful that the covariates histories up to time t on some subjects do not convey future failure information (i.e. at times $t' > t$) on other cohort members.

Since the above rates are defined conditionally on baseline covariate histories $Z(0)$, it is evident that the above requirements can be relaxed to allow sampling rates to depend on $Z(0)$.

Relative Risk Estimation

Suppose now that a relative risk regression model 5 applies to $\lambda[t; Z(u), 0 \leq u < t]$. Because of technicalities that may arise if counting and covariate processes jump at the same time instant, the sample paths for the modeled covariate $X(\cdot)$ are required to be left continuous with right-hand limits. A valuable method for estimating the relative risk regression parameter β can be based on the following observation: At a time t of failure, denoted $N(t) \neq N(t^-)$ where $N(t) =$

$[N_1(t), \cdots, N_n(t)]$, the probability that failure occurs on subject i, given all counting, censoring, and covariate information prior to t, is easily shown to be

$$P[N_i(t) \neq N_i(t^-) \mid F(t), N(t) \neq N(t^-)] = Y_i(t)\lambda_0(t)r[X_i(t)\beta] / \sum_{l=1}^{n} Y_l(t)\lambda_0(t)r[X_l(t)\beta]$$

$$= Y_i(t)r[X_i(t)\beta] / \sum_{l=1}^{n} Y_l(t)r[X_l(t)\beta]. \qquad 10.$$

Estimation of β can then be based on a "partial likelihood" function, which is the product of terms 10 over all distinct failure times in the cohort. Note that because the baseline rate $\lambda_0(\cdot)$ drops out of the ratio 10 this partial likelihood function will not involve $\lambda_0(\cdot)$. Let $t_i = \min[t \mid Y_i(u) = 0, \text{ all } u > t]$ denote the time of failure or terminal right censorship (during the prescribed follow-up period) for the ith subject, while the corresponding censoring indicator δ_i takes value one if $N_i(t_i) \neq N_i(t_i^-)$ and value zero otherwise. The partial likelihood function can now be written

$$L(\beta) = \prod_{i=1}^{n} \{r_{ii} / \sum_{l=1}^{n} r_{li}\}^{\delta_i} \qquad 11.$$

where $r_{li} = Y_l(t_i)r[X_l(t_i)\beta]$. $L(\beta)$ can be manipulated as if it were an ordinary likelihood function in respect to asymptotic likelihood inference on β.

In order to facilitate the exposition, literature citations were omitted from the above presentation. This will be partly remedied by noting some references while simultaneously listing some of the properties of estimation based on 11. The relative risk regression model 4 represents a generalization to evolutionary covariates and nonexponential relative risk forms of a life table regression model proposed by Cox (13). The discussion following Cox's paper pointed out that expression 11 is not an ordinary conditional likelihood function [see also Kalbfleisch & Prentice (26)]. Hence Cox (14) introduced the notion of partial likelihood. His argument shows that the score statistic

$$U(\beta) = \partial \log L(\beta)/\partial\beta = \sum_{i=1}^{n} U_i(\beta) = \sum_{i=1}^{n} \delta_i\{c_{ii} - \sum_{l=1}^{n} b_{li} / \sum_{l=1}^{n} r_{li}\}, \qquad 12.$$

where

$$b_{li} = Y_l(t_i)X_l(t_i)r'[X_l(t_i)\beta], \quad c_{li} = b_{li}r^{-1}[X_l(t_i)\beta] \quad \text{and} \quad r'(u) = dr(u)/du,$$

has mean zero and that the score statistic contributions from distinct failure times are uncorrelated. These facts follow easily from the conditional expectations

$$E[U_i(\beta) \mid F(t_i), N(t) \neq N(t_i^-)] = \delta_i \sum_{l=1}^{n} (c_{li} - B_i R_i^{-1}) r_{li} = 0,$$

and, for $t_i < t_j$,

$$E[U_i(\beta) U_j(\beta) \mid F(t_j), N(t_j) \neq N(t_j^-)] = U_i(\beta) E[U_j(\beta) \mid F(t_j), N(t_j) \neq N(t_j^-)] = 0,$$

where

$$B_i = \sum_{l=1}^{n} b_{li}, R_i = \sum_{l=1}^{n} r_{li}.$$

Hence, Cox (14) argued that a central limit result could be expected to show $n^{-1/2}U(\beta)$ to converge in distribution to a normal variate with mean zero and variance estimated by $n^{-1}I(\beta) = n^{-1}[-\partial^2 \log L(\beta)/\partial\beta^2]$. A standard Taylor series expansion of $U(\beta)$ about the true parameter value, evaluated at the maximum partial likelihood estimate $\hat{\beta}$, defined by $U(\hat{\beta}) = 0$, then causes one to expect convergence in distribution of $n^{1/2}(\hat{\beta}-\beta)$ to a normal distribution with mean zero and variance estimated by $nI^{-1}(\hat{\beta})$. Precise conditions for these asymptotic results are given in Tsiatis (59) for non-time-dependent-covariates and exponential relative risk form, by Andersen & Gill (3) for general covariates with exponential relative risk form, and by Prentice & Self (49) for general covariates with a general relative risk form. The approach of Andersen & Gill is particularly noteworthy. They decompose the counting processes N_i into the sum of the cumulative intensity process and a local square integrable martingale. Powerful martingale convergence results then yield the asymptotic results indicated above under quite general conditions. Specifically it is not even necessary that the data (N_i, Y_i, Z_i), $i = 1, \cdots, n$ be identically distributed.

Since 11 is not an ordinary likelihood function, the efficiency properties of $\hat{\beta}$ require special study. Efficiency properties with evolutionary covariates have not received much attention. The special case in which $X(t)$ involves only functions of baseline covariates $Z(0)$ or product terms between such functions and t and $r(\cdot) = \exp(\cdot)$, has been studied by a number of authors. For example, Efron (17) and Oakes (40) show, in such circumstances, that it is not possible to improve on the efficiency of $\hat{\beta}$ without placing restrictions on the baseline rates $\lambda_0(\cdot)$. Furthermore they show $\hat{\beta}$ to have generally acceptable efficiency properties relative to maximum likelihood estimates arising from parametric submodels of the above relative risk regression models. This comment applies even relative to parametric models that specify $\lambda_0(\cdot)$ up to a single scale parameter.

To date study has been rather limited of the sample sizes and data configurations necessary to ensure a good approximation by the asymptotic theory mentioned above. Johnson et al (25) describe simulation studies that imply good approximations with 40 or more failures in situations with well-behaved time-independent covariates and exponential-form relative risk. The score statistic $U(\beta)$ may adhere to its asymptotic distribution in the special case $r(\cdot) = \exp(\cdot)$ even with smaller numbers of failures. Such appeared to be the case, for example, in simulation studies by Latta (30) that included the log-rank statistic (35, 41). [The statistic, $U(0)$, given above includes both the log-rank and time-dependent log-rank statistic as special cases.] Case reports in the literature make it clear that certain asymptotic distributional approximations may be much poorer with relative risk forms other than the exponential [e.g. Thomas (57)]. In such circumstances it is, however, reasonable to expect likelihood ratio statistics based on 11 to have distributions that are well approximated by their asymptotic distributions, even with moderate numbers of failures. Further study of these issues is merited.

With cohort data the cumulative baseline hazard function $\Lambda_0(t) = \int_0^t \lambda_0(u)du$ is also readily estimated by

$$\hat{\Lambda}_0(t) = \int_0^t \{\sum_{i=1}^n Y_i(u)r[X_i(u)\hat{\beta}]\}^{-1}d\overline{N}(u) \qquad 13.$$

where $\overline{N}(u) = N_1(u) + \cdots + N_n(u)$, which generally converges to a Gaussian process (3, 49). Accordingly, one can also use relative risk regression models to estimate cumulative excess risks

$$\int_0^t \lambda_0(u)r\{X(u)\beta\}du - \Lambda_0(t)$$

associated with a covariate history $Z(t)$ as compared to the standard $Z_0(t)$, and related quantities. Procedures that directly model excess risk may, however, be more convenient for such purposes.

Expressions 11 and 13 as they stand can accommodate tied failure times, as may arise from a grouping of the underlying continuous times. Such grouping, however, will generally introduce bias in the regression parameter estimation, since the desired processes $\{N_i, Y_i, Z_i\}$ are not precisely known. As a rule of thumb the bias is not likely to be severe if not more than 5% of the subjects "at risk" fail at any specific failure time.

Introduction of stratification into the relative risk model does not introduce conceptual change in the above estimation procedure, even if stratum assignments are time-dependent. (If stratum assignments for an individual vary over time, stratum sample paths should be left continuous.) The partial likelihood function for $\beta = (\beta_1, \cdots, \beta_q)$ in 5 can be written

$$L(\beta) = \prod_{i=1}^n \prod_{s=1}^q [r_{sii}/\sum_{l=1}^n r_{sli}]^{\delta_{si}} \qquad 14.$$

where, now, $r_{sli} = Y_{sl}(t_i)r[X_l(t_i)\beta_s];Y_{sl}(t)$ takes value one if subject l is at risk in stratum s at time t and value zero otherwise, and $\delta_{si} = 1$ if the ith subject is uncensored and in stratum s at time t_i and $\delta_{si} = 0$ otherwise. Stratum-specific cumulative baseline hazard functions can be estimated in a manner similar to 13.

The choice of the time scale for $\lambda_0(\cdot)$ will primarily depend on the application. Breslow et al (9) consider the choice in the context of cohort studies of occupational risks. Formal statistical consideration of the choice is examined in (19).

Illustrations

The biomedical literature contains many examples of the use of models 4 and 5. Many applications, particularly in clinical trials, have involved time-independent covariates $X(t) = X$, in which case these models have a proportional hazards interpretation. See (47) for an example in which the time-dependent feature of the modeled regression vector was used to explore relative risk form in a large animal carcinogenesis dataset. For applications to occupational mortality cohorts see, for example, (6, 9). Most applications to date assume an exponential relative risk form. See (50, 57) for cohort applications using the linear relative risk form $r(\cdot) = 1 + (\cdot)$.

Consider now in more detail the above mentioned cohort of nearly 20,000 residents of Hiroshima and Nagasaki followed by the Radiation Effects Research Foundation. As indicated above, systolic and diastolic blood pressure, along with a number of other cardiovascular disease risk factors and potential confounding factors, were measured during the course of biennial examinations beginning in 1958. The analyses described in Prentice et al (53) make use of data on 16,711 subjects examined at least once during the period 1958–1974, from whom 108 incident cases of cerebral hemorrhage, 469 incident cases of cerebral infarction, and 218 incident cases of coronary heart disease developed. Specific objectives of these analysis concerned the relative importance of systolic and diastolic blood pressure as risk indicators for these three major cardiovascular disease categories, and the relative importance of blood pressure levels two or more biennial exam periods before a risk period, given the blood pressure measurements from the immediately preceding examination period. The application of relative risk regression methods described in (53) used model 5 with t defined as the examination cycle (i.e. $t = 1$ in 1958–1960, $t = 2$ in 1960–1962, . . .) with 32 strata defined on the basis of sex and 16 five-year, age-at-baseline categories and with relative risk form $r(\cdot) = \exp(\cdot)$. Note that with this exponential relative risk form inferences on the regression parameters are independent of the choice of standard covariate history $X_0(t)$. The modeled regression vector $X(t)$ was taken to consist of systolic and diastolic blood pressure levels in examination cycles $1,2,\cdots,t-1$ or functions thereof. Naturally, in order that $X(t)$ be defined it is necessary that certain preceding examinations have been attended and that the desired blood pressure measurements have been taken. In order to accommodate missing covariate data it is necessary to assume that the set of subjects at risk in examination cycle t with available covariate $X(t)$ are representative of all subjects at risk in examination cycle t that would give rise to this same covariate value. Provided the censoring processes $Y(\cdot)$ are defined to take the value zero at times t at which $X(t)$ is missing, this assumption is subsumed in the independent censorship assumption described above.

Table 1 shows the results of relative risk regression analyses with $X(t) = \{SBP(t-1), DBP(t-1)\}$ the systolic and diastolic blood pressure measurements in examination cycle $t-1$, and with common regression parameters across strata ($\beta_s \equiv \beta$). Note that previous cycle diastolic blood pressure is the important disease risk predictor for cerebral hemorrhage, whereas the corresponding systolic blood pressure is the more important predictor for cerebral infarction and for coronary heart disease. This observation has clinical implications and provides insight into the three disease processes.

Table 2 gives results of analyses in which a sequence of blood pressure measurements is related to subsequent disease incidence. The regression vector is now defined as $X(t) = \{(DBP(t-1), DBP(t-2), DBP(t-3)\}$ for cerebral hemorrhage and $X(t)$ equal to the corresponding SBP values from the three preceding cycles for cerebral infarction and coronary heart disease. Note that for a subject to contribute to the risk set in examination cycle t, all three previous biennial examinations need to have been attended. From Table 2 one can note that the most recent systolic blood pressure measurement is highly predictive of cerebral infarction risk, while the next most recent makes some additional contribution to risk prediction. With coronary heart disease, however, a recent elevated systolic blood pressure measurement is not predictive, or is possibly even negatively predictive, of risk, given the levels of SBP in the two

Table 1 Relative risk regression of cardiovascular disease incidence in relation to previous examination cycle systolic and diastolic blood pressure measurements; the analyses stratify on age and sex

Regression variable	Cerebral hemorrhage $\hat{\beta}^a (\times 10^2)$	Cerebral infarction $\hat{\beta}(\times 10^2)$	Coronary heart disease $\hat{\beta}(\times 10^2)$
SBP($t-1$)	0.58	1.77	1.15
	$(0.30)^b$	(<0.0001)	(0.003)
DBP($t-1$)	5.48	0.46	-0.46
	(<0.0001)	(0.36)	(0.56)
Cases	92	406	187

[a] $\hat{\beta}$ values are maximum partial likelihod estimates.
[b] Asymptotic significance levels for testing $\beta = 0$ are given in parentheses.

Table 2   Relative risk regression of cardiovascular disease incidence in relation to blood pressure measurements from the three preceding examination cycles; the analyses stratify on age and sex

Regression variable	Cerebral hemorrhage $\hat{\beta}^a(\times 10^2)$	Cerebral infarction $\hat{\beta}(\times 10^2)$	Coronary heart disease $\hat{\beta}(\times 10^2)$
SBP($t-1$)		1.13	−1.06
		(0.001)	(0.06)
DBP($t-1$)	3.23		
	(0.01)[b]		
SBP($t-2$)		0.80	1.46
		(0.03)	(0.007)
DBP($t-2$)	−1.07		
	(0.45)		
SBP($t-3$)		0.35	0.64
		(0.30)	(0.22)
DBP($t-3$)	4.77		
	(<0.0001)		
Cases	48	207	97

[a] β values are maximum partial likelihood estimates.
[b] Asymptotic significance levels for testing $\beta = 0$ are given in parentheses.

preceding cycles. One explanation for this result might be that hypertensive medication brings about blood pressure control without a corresponding reduction in coronary heart disease risk. The analysis for cerebral hemorrhage indicates that both elevated diastolic blood pressure and the duration of elevation are strong risk predictors.

These analyses involve an approximation in that the continuous disease incidence date were, for numerical convenience, grouped into biennial exam periods. Such grouping can be expected to have little effect on relative risk parameter estimation, since the fraction of the cohort failing in any grouping interval is small (i.e. < 0.05).

An interesting technical point in the use of evolutionary covariates relates to the fact that the disease rate process being modeled, namely $\lambda[t;Z(u),0 \leqslant u < t]$, conditions on the subject's entire preceding covariate history. Risk factor associations of interest may, however, involve the relationship between disease rate and a subset of the preceding covariate history. For example, Table 1 is concerned with cardiovascular disease rates in relation to previous blood pressure measurements, but only blood pressure measurements recorded in the immediately preceding examination cycle. An application of the asymptotic results mentioned above to Table 1 would then implicitly require one to assume disease rates to be independent of earlier blood pressure measurements, given the most recent measurements—an assumption not substantiated by Table 2. To address this issue, S. G. Self and R. L. Prentice, in a submitted paper, have generalized the above results to allow aspects of preceding covariate history to be excluded from the conditioning at the division points of a time axis partition. The relative risk parameter is then chosen to maximize a pseudo-likelihood function that is the product of partial likelihoods over the elements of the time axis partition. The maximum pseudo-likelihood function is identical to that which would be obtained by specifying an oversimplified intensity process model that involves only selected aspects of the preceding covariate history. An adjustment is required, however, to give a consistent variance estimator for this maximum pseudo-likelihood estimator. Fortunately, however, this variance adjustment appears to be unimportant in situations of practical interest.

Odds Ratio Estimation

Suppose the cohort of the previous section is followed from time zero to time Δ without censorship. The odds ratio model 8 with parameters $\lambda = \lambda_0(0)$ and β may be applied using standard parametric procedures [e.g. Cox (12), Anderson (5)] in order to relate the odds of failure in $(0,\Delta)$ to baseline covariates. If, for example, age rather than chronological time is taken as the time variable in 8, then $\lambda_0(\cdot)$ would need to be specified parametrically prior to the use of standard likelihood methods. The use of such logistic regression methods has played a fundamental role in the analysis of data on large epidemiologic cohorts, for example, in the analysis of the well-known Framingham study.

Some disadvantages of such an approach compared to the relative risk regression methods previously described are obvious. Specifically, the method is not well suited to varying follow-up durations among cohort members. Such variations may arise because subjects die or are lost to follow-up without experiencing the type of failure under study. The method also does not permit study of evolutionary covariates. Furthermore, the regression parameter interpretation depends on Δ. These limitations can be partially circumvented by dividing the follow-up period into intervals—for example, intervals of fixed length—and applying an odds ratio regression model of the form 8 in each such interval. If such intervals are required to be short, such an approach is virtually identical to the relative risk regression approach previously described. In fact, even with a moderately long follow-up period, the logistic regression model 8 will often give parameter estimates (corresponding to functions of baseline covariates) quite similar to those from a corresponding model 4, provided the fraction of the cohort experiencing failure is small (e.g. less than 0.10). Matthews (36) formally examines this issue.

Generalizations and Topics Meriting Further Attention

Suppose that multiple failure events may occur on individual subjects. The hazard rate 2 can be generalized by including in the conditioning event the counting process history $[N(u); 0 \leq u < t]$ for the subject, where now $N(u)$

denotes the number of failures at or before time u. Relative risk regression models 4 or 5 can again be specified, where both the modeled regression vector $X(t)$ and the stratum specifications $s = s(t)$ may involve functions of $[Z(u), N(u); 0 \leq u < t]$ and product terms between such functions and t. Partial likelihood expressions are readily developed for the application of such models to cohort data [Prentice et al (52), Gail et al (22)]. The asymptotic distributional results previously cited (3, 49) are general enough to include such multivariate failure time problems.

A second class of models (52), in which the hazard rate is given by

$$\lambda\{t; [Z(u), N(u); 0 \leq u < t]\} = \lambda_{0s}(t - t^*) r\{X(t)\beta_s\},$$

where t^* is the most recent failure time on the subject prior to time t, also gives rise to partial likelihood estimation, provided that the stratification is fine enough to require the subject to move to a new stratum following each of its failure occurrences; for example, one could define $s(t) = N(t) + 1$. See also Voelkel & Crowley (60) for inference in a related class of models.

Multivariate failure times data that arise as correlated univariate failure times within experimental units or blocks are not so conveniently handled by relative risk regression methods, largely because of the need to accommodate censorship on some block members while others continue at risk. Regression generalizations of the model of Clayton (10) that reduce to 4 in the special case of block of size one would be well worth studying. See, in particular, the interesting models considered by Clayton & Cuzick (11). Generalization of the odds ratio regression model 8 to multivariate failure times is somewhat problematic, since for any $\Delta > 0$ one can expect with positive frequency two or more failures in $(t, t + \Delta)$.

Competing risk generalizations of relative risk regression models have also been described (46). Specifically, if m distinct disease categories arise in a cohort study, a relative risk regression model

$$\lambda_{0j}(t) r\{X(t)\beta_j\}$$

may be specified for the rate of type j failure, for selected values of $j \in \{1, 2, \cdots, m\}$. Straightforward partial likelihood estimation of the disease-j relative risk regression parameters β_j proceeds by regarding failure occurrences of types other than j as censored. Some work (43) has also taken place to allow relative risk regression parameter estimation and testing in the presence of random measurement errors in the covariate processes, a topic of obvious practical importance in many cohort settings, and one that merits further work. A full regression approach, of course, requires not only suitable model fitting and estimation procedures, but also a range of procedures for model criticism. In general the area of model criticism is at a rather early stage of development for relative risk regression methods. Some relevant works include proposals in respect to test of fit [Schoenfeld (54)], residuals [Kalbfleisch & Prentice (27), Lagakos (29), Schoenfeld (55), Andersen (2)], regression diagnostics [Storer & Crowley (56)], and choice of relative risk form [Thomas (57), Tibshirani & Ciampi (58), Breslow & Storer (9a)]. Further information on relative risk regression methods can be found in recent books on survival data (e.g. 27, 15).

RELATIVE RISK AND ODDS RATIO ESTIMATION IN CASE-CONTROL STUDIES

Sampling Procedures

Suppose now that all failures, or a random sample thereof, can be ascertained in the large, conceptually infinite population described above. Such ascertainment may take place by means of a disease register or a mortality index, for example. Identification of a suitable cohort and assembly of covariate histories on cohort members would often be prohibitively expensive, particularly if the failure rates are small. If the cohort is to be followed prospectively, a long period of time may be required before sufficient failure experience accumulates. Furthermore, if failure rates are low, the covariate data on many of the subjects who do not fail are largely redundant for purposes of relative risk and odds ratio estimation.

The case-control design provides a valuable and much used alternative in such circumstances. In general terms, this design involves the selection of a random sample of failures *(the cases)* occurring in the population during some specified case accession period. A corresponding comparison group *(the controls)* are selected who are without failure during some or all of the case accession period. Covariate histories pertaining to times up to case or control ascertainment are then obtained retrospectively. The comparison of such histories between cases and controls can lead to relative risk and odds ratio estimation. Major methodologic concerns relate to (*a*) the ability to construct accurate covariate histories retrospectively, and to do so equally for cases and controls *(recall bias)* and (*b*) the ability to sample randomly from case and control populations *(ascertainment bias)*.

There are many variations on the case-control design involving, for example, the degree of matching of cases to controls and, particularly, the matching or lack thereof on the primary time variable. Very often in epidemiologic applications time will be defined as study subject age. In particular, relative risk estimation under population models 4 or 5 can take place by time-matching controls to cases. Specifically, controls corresponding to a failure at time (e.g.

age) t should be selected to be representative of the subset of the population that is at risk at t. Matching on other potential confounding characteristics may also be included. More conventionally, odds ratio estimation under a population model 8 can take place by selecting controls that are without failure at the end of a case accession period of duration Δ. Such case accession periods should be short in respect to the range of possible failure times. The odds ratios will then closely approximate the corresponding relative risks. See, however, Greenland et al (24) for a cautionary note.

Relative Risk Estimation

Suppose now that a randomly sampled case is time-matched to a set of $n-1$ controls who are randomly sampled from the population at risk and without failure at the time, t, of case occurrence. Suppose also that cases and controls are independently sampled. In the same notation as above one can readily calculate [Prentice & Breslow (45)] under relative risk model 4

$$P[N_i(t) \neq N_i(t^-) \mid F(t), N(t) \neq N(t^-)] = Y_i(t)r[X_i(t)\beta] / \sum_{l=1}^{n} Y_l(t)r[X_l(t)\beta], \quad 15.$$

precisely as above. Expression 15 gives the probability that subject i is the case where $F(t)$ represents the counting, censoring, and covariate processes on the n subjects in the matched set, and where $N(t) \neq N(t^-)$ denotes that a failure within the matched set occurs at time t. Note that $Y_l(t) = 1$, $i = 1, \cdots, n$ under the above sampling requirements. The assumption of a conceptually infinite population implies that the matched sets at distinct failure times can be assumed disjoint, whence a conditional likelihood for β can be obtained by multiplying probabilities of the form 15 over distinct failure times. This product can be written

$$L(\beta) = \prod_{s=1}^{q} \{ r[X_{s1}(t_{s1})\beta] / \sum_{l=1}^{n_s} r[X_{sl}(t_{s1})\beta] \}, \quad 16.$$

where subscript s denotes the sth matched set of size n_s, and a value of 1 for the second subscript denotes the case in matched set s that occurs at failure time t_{s1}. The same expression, with β replaced by β_s, applies under the stratified relative risk model 5, provided controls are both time- and stratum-matched to cases.

Since 16 has a conditional likelihood interpretation, standard asymptotic likelihood results can be expected to apply under mild conditions (1). Because 16 can be viewed formally as a special case of 14, few new concepts arise in model fitting or in model criticism. In fact, some simplifications occur, since a given subject contributes to at most one term in the product 16, thus giving rise to convenient regression diagnostics [Moolgavkar et al (39)].

Odds Ratio Estimation

As is more usual, suppose now that one draws an independent random sample of cases occurring in our large population during a case accession period of duration Δ. Suppose further that an independent random control sample is selected from population members at risk and without failure at the end of the case accession period. An odds ratio regression model 7 or 8 may be considered to relate failure probability to baseline covariates, that is to covariates pertinent to the beginning of the case accession period or earlier. The prospective model 8 cannot be directly applied to such case-control data, but it turns out [Anderson (4), Prentice & Pyke (48), Farewell (18)] that, upon specifying a parametric form for $\lambda_0(\cdot)$ and assuming no censorship, the model 8 can be directly applied to such case-control data for the purpose of maximum likelihood estimation of the odds ratio parameter β and its asymptotic distribution. The exponential odds ratio form was used exclusively in the results just cited, but generalization to other odds ratio forms appears to be straightforward. Generalization to include stratification of cases and corresponding controls in either the design or the analysis is also straightforward. With fine stratification (e.g. less than 20 cases and controls in certain strata) it would be desirable to condition out, rather than maximize over the stratum specific parameters in $\lambda_0(\cdot)$. This reduces bias in the estimation of β with little loss of efficiency (18, 20, 21, 32, 42). See Gail et al (23) for details of this approach, which does have some computational limitations. The book by Breslow & Day (8) gives considerable further detail on the above estimation procedures.

Illustration

Consider the study of Weiss et al (61), which aims to relate exposure to exogenous estrogens, primarily used for the treatment of menopausal symptoms, to subsequent risk of endometrial cancer. This study identified and interviewed 322 cases of endometrial cancer occurring among white women in western Washington during the period January 1975 to April 1976. A random sample of 288 white women in the same age range were selected using area sampling methods and were interviewed. Personal interviews ascertained information on prior hormone use and on endometrial cancer risk factors. Women who had undergone hysterectomy, and thus were not at risk for endometrial cancer, were excluded from the analysis.

Table 3 gives results of applying a logistic model 8 to these data, with stratification on baseline age in one year intervals. As noted above, with such fine stratification it is important to condition out the stratum parameters, rather than jointly maximizing $\{\lambda_{0s}, \beta\}$. Table 3 makes use of the exponential form $r(\cdot) = \exp(\cdot)$ for the odds ratio. The regression vector, X, defined for each subject, includes a variable indicating whether ($X_1 = 1$) or not ($X_1 = 0$) the subject had a

Table 3   Odds ratio regression of endometrial cancer incidence in relation to exposure to exogenous estrogens and other factors; the analyses stratify on baseline age

Regression variable			$\hat{\beta}$	SE[a]	Sig. level[b]
Estrogen use:	1 if duration of use between 1–8 yr; 0 otherwise	(x_1)	1.37	0.24	<0.0001
	1 if duration of use 8 yr or greater; 0 otherwise	(x_2)	2.60	0.25	<0.0001
Obesity:	1 if weight greater than 160 lbs; 0 otherwise	(x_3)	0.50	0.25	0.04
Hypertension:	1 if history of high blood pressure; 0 otherwise	(x_4)	0.42	0.21	0.05
Parity:	1 if number of children 2 or greater; 0 otherwise	(x_5)	0.81	0.21	0.0001

[a]Estimated standard error of $\hat{\beta}$.
[b]Estimated significance level for testing $\beta = 0$.

duration of use of exogenous estrogen of between 1 and 8 years at baseline, a variable indicating whether ($X_2 = 1$) or not ($X_2 = 0$) the subject had a duration of estrogen use in excess of 8 years at baseline, and indicator variables for obesity, hypertension, and parity. Note that estrogen use of between 1 and 8 years is associated with an estimated odds ratio for endometrial cancer of $\exp(1.37) = 3.94$, with an associated asymptotic 95% confidence interval of (2.46, 6.30). The corresponding estimate and asymptotic 95% confidence interval associated with 8 years or more of estrogen use are $\exp(2.60) = 13.46$ and (8.25, 21.98), respectively. These analyses make an accommodation for the observed dependence of endometrial cancer risk on obesity, hypertension, and parity.

Logistic models are not restricted to the use of indicator covariates. For example, a model that uses log (estrogen duration use in years + 1) as an exposure variable fits the data of Weiss et al (61) as well as the model in Table 3, without any arbitrary grouping of the exposure variable. The grouping of a continuous exposure variable is useful for presentation purposes, however, and is a convenient way of checking assumptions made in modeling continuous variables.

More refined regression analyses that include product terms among estrogen use variates and obesity, hypertension, parity, and age group indicators could examine whether the odds ratios associated with the use of exogenous estrogen depend on such characteristics. Because of the short case-accession period and the fine stratification on age, the odds ratios estimated in this analysis are likely to be virtually indistinguishable from relative risk estimates based on an age-matched case control study.

Discussion

Case-control designs are very frequently used in observational studies, in which appropriate control of confounding factors is often crucially important. Miettinen (37) and Breslow & Day (8, Chapter 3) provide general discussions of confounding. Epidemiologic tradition dating from the seminal paper by Mantel & Haenszel (35) very much concentrates on the use of stratification to control confounding.

Models 4–8 allow the data analyst the choice of stratification or regression modeling for the control of confounding factors. Such models therefore allow one to avoid the excessive stratification that sometimes poses a problem in direct application of the Mantel-Haenszel technique, but also avoids the unnecessary restrictions or unwieldy regression models that may arise in the absence of stratification. In short, 4–8 allow one to extract the best from traditional epidemiologic methods and modern failure time data methods. Note also that Day & Byar (16) establish a formal equivalence between Mantel-Haenszel type statistics and score statistics based on logistic models.

Subjects experiencing failure of types other than that under study are sometimes selected as "controls" in view of the difficulty of selecting population-based disease-free controls in some settings. Independent random samples from both case and control failure types along with relative risk models 4–5 for each such failure type can lead to convenient estimation of the ratio of relative risk processes for case to control failure types (45, 51). Whittemore and colleagues (62, 63) have noted that efficiency properties for the relative risk estimator under the time-matched case-control estimation procedure described above are somewhat poorer than are corresponding efficiencies for odds ratio parameters under unmatched case-control sampling. This presumably arises because "time" is not an ordinary stratification factor in the sense that a given subject may properly serve as a member of the control group for cases occurring at a range of times during a case accession period. The time-matched case-control analysis, however, aligns each control with only a single case.

RELATIVE RISK AND ODDS RATIO ESTIMATION IN CASE-COHORT STUDIES

Sampling Requirements

Suppose now that a cohort is independently and randomly selected from the large population, and covariate data are assembled for cohort members and for an independent random sample of failures in the population, during a defined case accession period. Such a design is subject to the same concerns over recall bias as the case-control design. It does, however, allow individual cohort members to serve in the comparison group at a range of failure times in the case accession period, with potentially valuable efficiency gains, particularly if the follow-up period is relatively lengthy. Kupper et al (28) and Miettinen (38) consider similar designs under the labels "hybrid retrospective design" and "case-base design," respectively. Prentice (44) gives a more detailed account of this design and its relative risk estimation, under the label "case-cohort design."

Relative Risk and Odds Ratio Estimation

Briefly, under a relative risk model 4 for the population one can conveniently estimate the relative risk parameter β by maximizing a likelihood function that is formally identical to 11 with the product being over all failures, whether occurring within or outside of the selected cohort, and with the ith denominator summation over the subject failing at t_i along with all cohort members at risk. This function is no longer a partial likelihood, since "score statistic" contributions at distinct failure times are generally correlated. Such correlations can be conveniently estimated, however, thus giving rise to a suitable means of estimating the distribution of the relative risk parameter estimate. Extensions to allow baseline stratification at either the design or analysis stage are straightforward. Some limited simulation results (44) suggest that case-cohort estimation efficiency properties will agree closely with corresponding unmatched case-control estimation efficiencies, though further study is indicated.

Odds ratio estimation under a case-cohort design is similar indeed to that indicated above for a case-control design. In fact, one can estimate the odds ratio parameters merely by applying 8 with parametric specification of $\lambda_0(\cdot)$ as though a prospective study had been conducted (44), at least as far as asymptotic likelihood inference on the odds ratio parameter β is concerned.

CASE-CONTROL AND CASE-COHORT DESIGNS WITHIN A DEFINED COHORT

Sampling Requirements

It is sometimes desirable to sample within the context of a cohort study in order to simplify the computational aspects of model fitting and regression parameter estimation or, perhaps more importantly, in order to reduce the number of subjects for whom covariate histories need be assembled. Often covariate assembly will involve expensive analysis of stored specimens (e.g. blood serum) or the coding of detailed questionnaire data. Recall bias will typically not be an issue if covariate histories are assembled from prospectively collected raw materials.

A number of authors [Mantel (34), Liddell et al (31), Breslow & Patton (7), Oakes (40a), Whittemore & McMillan (63), Breslow et al (9)] have suggested the imposition of case-control sampling procedures on the cohort, sometimes under the name "synthetic case-control design." These authors suggest that controls be time-matched to cases by selecting controls for a given case randomly and without replacement from cohort members at risk and without failure at the time the case occurs. Control selections at distinct failure times are required to be statistically independent. Lubin & Gail (33) discuss biases that arise if subjects are excluded from the control selection process on the basis of their subsequent failure experience.

The case-cohort design mentioned above is particularly well suited to relative risk and odds ratio regression within a cohort since cohort follow-up periods tend to be relatively longer than case ascertainment periods in the designs of previous sections. The case-cohort approach merely requires the selection of a random subcohort, or stratified random subcohort, which then serves as the comparison group for all cases arising in the cohort, whether or not such cases are subcohort members.

Relative Risk and Odds Ratio Estimation

The "case-control within cohort design" described above yields a likelihood function of the form 11, with the denominator summation, for i such that $\delta_i = 1$, over the case occurring at t_i and its matched controls. In fact, this expression can be seen to be a partial likelihood function [Oakes (40a)] by extending the definition of $F(t)$ to include the identity of the matched sets at all $u \leq t$, and by noting that control selections are statistically independent at distinct failure times.

Procedures to estimate relative risk based on a case-cohort design within the context of a defined cohort are unchanged from those outlined above. Procedures for estimating odds ratios with cases and controls, or cases and subcohort, randomly selected from the entire cohort are unchanged from the case-control or case-cohort results, respectively, given previously. It is worth commenting that the case-cohort design in this context also admits an estimator of the form 13 for the cumulative baseline incidence.

ACKNOWLEDGMENTS

This work was supported by grants GM 24472, GM 28314, and CA 34847 from the National Institutes of Health.

Literature Cited

1. Andersen, E. B. 1970. Asymptotic properties of conditional maximum likelihood estimators. *J. R. Statist. Soc. B* 32:283–301
2. Andersen, P. K. 1982. Testing goodnenss of fit of Cox's regression and life model. *Biometrics* 38:67–78
3. Andersen, P. K., Gill, R. D. 1982. Cox's regression model for counting processes: A large sample study. *Ann. Statist.* 10:1100–20
4. Anderson, J. A. 1971. Separate sample logistic discrimination. *Biometrika* 59:19–35
5. Anderson, J. A. 1983. Robust inference using logistic models. *Bull. Int. Statist. Inst.* 48(2):35–53
6. Breslow, N. E. 1978. Some statistical models useful in the study of occupational mortality. In *Environmental Health: Quantitative Methods*, ed. A. Whittemore, pp. 88–103. Philadelphia: SIAM
7. Breslow, N. E., Patton, J. 1979. Case-control analysis of cohort studies. In *Energy and Health*, ed. N. E. Breslow, A. S. Whittemore, pp. 226–42. Philadelphia: SIAM
8. Breslow, N. E., Day, N. E. 1980. *Statistical Methods in Cancer Research I. The Analysis of Case-Control Studies.* Lyon: IARC
9. Breslow, N. E., Lubin, J. H., Marek, P., Langholz, B. 1983. Multiplicative mod-

els and cohort analysis. *J. Am. Statist. Assoc.* 78:1–12

9a. Breslow, N. E., Storer, B. S. 1985. General relative risk functions for case-control studies. *Am. J. Epidemiol.* 122:149–62

10. Clayton, D. G. 1978. A model for association in bivariate life tables and its application in epidemiologic studies of familiar tendency in chronic disease incidence. *Biometrika* 65:141–51

11. Clayton, D. G., Cuzick, J. 1985. Multivariate generalizations of the proportional hazards model (with discussion). *J. R. Statist. Soc. A.* In press

12. Cox, D. R. 1970. *The Analysis of Binary Data.* London: Methuen

13. Cox, D. R. 1972. Regression models and life tables (with discussion). *J. R. Statist. Soc. B* 34:187–220

14. Cox, D. R. 1975. Partial likelihood. *Biometrika* 62:269–76

15. Cox, D. R., Oakes, D. 1984. *Analysis of Survival Data.* New York: Chapman & Hall

16. Day, N. E., Byar, D. P. 1979. Testing hypotheses in case-control studies—equivalence of Mantel-Haenszel statistics and logit score tests. *Biometrics* 35:623–30

17. Efron, B. 1977. Efficiency of Cox's likelihood function for censored data. *J. Am. Statist. Assoc.* 72:557–65

18. Farewell, V. T. 1979. Some results on the estimation of logistic models based on retrospective data. *Biometrika* 66:27–32

19. Farewell, V. T., Cox, D. R. 1979. A note on multiple time scales in life testing. *Appl. Statist.* 28:73–75

20. Farewell, V. T., Prentice, R. L. 1980. The approximation of partial likelihood with emphasis on case-control studies. *Biometrika* 67:273–78

21. Farewell, V. T., Dahlberg, S. 1983. On the comparison of procedures for testing the equality of survival curves. *Biometrika* 70:707–9

22. Gail, M. H., Santner, T. J., Brown, C. C. 1980. An analysis of comparative carcinogenesis experiments based on multiple times to tumor. *Biometrics* 36:255–66

23. Gail, M. A., Lubin, J. H., Rubinstein, L. V. 1981. Likelihood calculations for matched case-control studies and survival studies with tied death times. *Biometrika* 68:703–7

24. Greenland, S., Thomas, D. C., Morgenstein, H. 1985. The rare disease assumption revisited: A critique of 'Estimates of relative risk for case-control studies' and a review of case-cohort design. *Am. J. Epidemiol.* In press

25. Johnson, M. E., Tolley, H. D., Bryson,

M. D., Goldman, A. S. 1982. Covariate analysis of survival data: A small-sample study of Cox's model. *Biometrics* 38:685–98

26. Kalbfleisch, J. D., Prentice, R. L. 1973. Marginal likelihoods based on Cox's regression and life model. *Biometrika* 60:267–78

27. Kalbfleisch, J. D., Prentice, R. L. 1980. *The Statistical Analysis of Failure Time Data.* New York: Wiley

28. Kupper, L. L., McMichael, A. J., Spirtas, R. 1975. A hybrid epidemiologic study design useful in estimating relative risks. *J. Am. Statist. Assoc.* 70:524–28

29. Lagakos, S. W. 1981. The graphical evaluation of explanatory variables in proportional hazards regression models. *Biometrika* 68:93–98

30. Latta, R. 1981. A Monte Carlo study of some two-sample rank tests with censored data. *J. Am. Statist. Assoc.* 76:713–19

31. Liddell, F. D. K., McDonald, J. C., Thomas, D. C. 1977. Methods of cohort analysis: Appraisal by application to asbestos mining. *J. R. Statist. Soc. A* 140:469–91

32. Lubin, J. H. 1981. An empirical evaluation of the use of conditional and unconditional likelihoods for case-control data. *Biometrika* 68:567–71

33. Lubin, H. J., Gail, M. H. 1984. Biased selection of controls for case-control analyses of cohort studies. *Biometrics* 40:63–75

34. Mantel, N. 1973. Synthetic retrospective studies and related topics. *Biometrics* 29:479–86

35. Mantel, N., Haenszel, W. 1959. Statistical aspects of the analysis of data from retrospective studies of disease. *J. Natl. Cancer Inst.* 22:719–48

36. Matthews, D. E. 1984. Efficiency considerations in the analysis of a competing-risk problem. *Can. J. Stat.* 12:207–10

37. Miettinen, O. S. 1974. Confounding and effect modification. *Am. J. Epidemiol.* 100:350–53

38. Miettinen, O. S. 1982. Design options in epidemiologic research. An update. *Scand. J. Work Environ. Health 8, Suppl.* 1:7–14

39. Moolgavkar, S. H., Lustbader, E. D., Venzon, D. J. 1984. A geometric approach to nonlinear regression diagnostics with application to matched case-control studies. *Ann. Statist.* 12:816–26

40. Oakes, D. 1977. The asymptotic information in censored data. *Biometrika* 64:441–48

58   PRENTICE & FAREWELL

40a. Oakes, D. 1981. Survival times: Aspects of partial likelihood. *Int. Statist. Rev.* 49:235–64
41. Peto, R., Peto, J. 1972. Asymptotically efficient rank invariant test procedures (with discussion). *J. R. Statist. Soc. A* 135:185–206
42. Pike, M. C., Hill, A. P., Smith, P. G. 1980. Bias and efficiency in logistic analysis of stratified case-control studies. *Int. J. Epidemiol.* 9:89–95
43. Prentice, R. L. 1982. Covariate measurement errors and parameter estimation in Cox's failure time regression model. *Biometrika* 69:331–42
44. Prentice, R. L. 1986. A case-cohort design for epidemiologic cohort studies and disease prevention trials. *Biometrika.* In press (Part 1)
45. Prentice, R. L., Breslow, N. E. 1978. Retrospective studies and failure time models. *Biometrika* 65:153–58
46. Prentice, R. L., Kalbfleisch, J. D., Peterson, A. V., Flournoy, N., Farewell, V. T., et al. 1978. The analysis of failure times in the presence of competing risks. *Biometrics* 34:541–54
47. Prentice, R. L., Peterson, A. V., Marek, P. 1982. Dose mortality relationship in RFM mice following 136Cs gamma irradiation. *Radiat. Res.* 90:57–76
48. Prentice, R. L., Pyke, R. L. 1979. Logistic disease incidence models and case-control studies. *Biometrika* 66:403–12
49. Prentice, R. L., Self, S. G. 1983. Asymptotic distribution theory for Cox-type regression models with general relative risk form. *Ann. Statist.* 11:804–13
50. Prentice, R. L., Shimizu, Y., Lin, C. H., Peterson, A. V., Kato, H., et al. 1982. Serial blood pressure measurements and cardiovascular disease in a Japanese cohort. *Am. J. Epidemiol.* 116:1–28
51. Prentice, R. L., Vollmer, W. M., Kalbfleisch, J. D. 1984. On the use of case series to identify disease risk factors. *Biometrics* 40:445–58
52. Prentice, R. L., Williams, B. J., Peter-

son, A. V. 1981. On the regression analysis of multivariate failure time data. *Biometrika* 68:373–79
53. Prentice, R. L., Yoshimoto, Y., Mason, M. W. 1983. Relationship of cigarette smoking and radiation exposure to cancer mortality in Hiroshima and Nagasaki. *J. Natl. Cancer Inst.* 70:611–22
54. Schoenfeld, D. 1980. Chi-squared goodness of fit tests for the proportional hazards regression model. *Biometrika* 67:145–53
55. Schoenfeld, D. 1982. Partial residuals for the proportional hazards regression model. *Biometrika* 69:239–42
56. Storer, B., Crowley, J. 1985. A diagnostic for Cox regression and conditional likelihoods. *J. Am. Statist. Assoc.* 80:139–47
57. Thomas, D. C. 1981. General relative risk models for survival time and matched case-control analysis. *Biometrics* 37:673–86
58. Tibshirani, R. J., Ciampi, A. 1983. A family of proportional and additive hazard models for survival data. *Biometrics* 39:141–47
59. Tsiatis, A. A. 1981. A large sample study of Cox's regression model. *Ann. Statist.* 9:93–108
60. Voelkel, J. G., Crowley, J. 1984. Nonparametric inference for a class of semi-Markov processes with censored observations. *Ann. Statist.* 12:142–60
61. Weiss, N. S., Szekeley, D. R., English, D. R., Schweid, A. J. 1979. Endometrial cancer in relation to patterns of menopausal estrogen use. *J. Am. Med. Assoc.* 242:261–64
62. Whittemore, A. S. 1981. The efficiency of synthetic retrospective studies. *Biometrics. J.* 23:73–78
63. Whittemore, A. S., McMillan, A. 1982. Analyzing occupational cohort data: Application to U.S. uranium miners. In *Environmental Epidemiology: Risk Assessment,* ed. R. L. Prentice, A. S. Whittemore, pp. 65–81. Philadelphia: SIAM

Ann. Rev. Public Health. 1986. 7:59–75

MEDICAL CARE AT THE END OF LIFE: The Interaction of Economics and Ethics

A. A. Scitovsky

Health Economics Department, Research Institute, Palo Alto Medical Foundation, Palo Alto, California 94301

A. M. Capron

University of Southern California Law Center, Los Angeles, California 90089-0071

INTRODUCTION

The rising cost of medical care in the United States over the past quarter century has become a matter of growing concern for both private citizens and government at all levels. National health expenditures increased almost 12-fold between 1960 and 1982, from $26.9 billion to $322.4 billion, or from 5.3% of the gross national product (GNP) to 10.5%. Only a small part of this increase is attributable to the increase in the population, which grew by only about 30% during this period. The major factors accounting for the increase in spending for medical care are the steady rise in medical care prices, which increased at a faster pace than did the prices of all other goods and services; greater use of health services because of higher real incomes and more comprehensive health insurance coverage; changes in medical technologies, such as the introduction of new and more expensive forms of treatment; and last but not least, the increase in the number and proportion of persons aged 65 years and older, who have higher medical care expenses per capita than younger persons.

   It is this last problem, the high medical expenses of the elderly, which has been receiving special attention in recent years. One reason for this concern is the drain these expenses are putting on the Medicare Hospital Insurance Trust Fund, which is in danger of a deficit by the end of the century unless changes are

59

0163-7525/86/0510-0059$02.00

made in its benefit structure or financing or both. Various studies have shown another equally if not more important reason: A very large share of the elderly's medical care expenditures are incurred in the last year or even months of their lives; this has led to the question of whether scarce resources are being "wasted" on the dying, resources that could be spent more productively on other patients. Finally, doubts about the appropriateness of treatment are also voiced by people, like Eli Ginzberg, who are concerned "less with financial risk and more with the dangers threatening the aged from overtreatment in acute care hospitals" (17).

In this article we review the economic, ethical, and legal problems of the use and costs of medical care at the end of life. We begin with an overview of the general problem of health care and the elderly, their increasing numbers, their health status, their health care needs, and their health care expenditures. In the second section we examine what we know and do not know about medical expenditures of the elderly in their last years of life. We discuss in a final section the ethical and legal aspects of medical care of terminal patients as well as the more complex ethical problems posed by the growing number of elderly patients who are frail and sick but—despite the apparent assumptions of some studies—are not necessarily terminally ill.

HEALTH CARE AND THE ELDERLY

The Aging of the Population

More Americans are living to age 65 and over than ever before. In 1950, there were 12.4 million elderly people in the United States, or 8.2% of the total population. By 1981 their number had grown to 26.1 million, or 11.4% of the population. By the year 2000 their number is expected to reach 35.1 million, or 13.1% of the population. Moreover, the proportion of the very old—those aged 75 years and over—has grown even more rapidly than that of the "young" elderly, those aged 65 to 74 years. In 1950, the "old old" accounted for only 2.6% of the total population and 31.7% of the total number of elderly, but by 1981 had increased to 4.5% of the total population and 40.2% of the elderly population (12).

During the first half of this century the major cause of the aging of the population was the decline in fertility, which reduced the proportion of young persons to older persons. In the second half of the century, the leading factor has been the decline in mortality across all age groups, resulting from improved living standards and medical advances in the prevention and treatment of infectious diseases that formerly were often fatal (13). The age-adjusted mortality rate for all ages declined from 8.4 deaths per 1000 population in 1950 to 5.4 deaths in 1982. During the same period, the rate for persons aged 65 years and over dropped from 62.7 per 1000 to 50.5. Similar declines occurred for each of the over-65 year age groups.

As a result of the decline in mortality rates, life expectancy—both at birth and at age 65—has increased substantially in the course of the past three decades (12). A child born in 1982 could expect to live almost six years longer than one born in 1950 and reach age 74.5 years compared to 68.2 years for a child born in 1950. Similarly, a person aged 65 years in 1982 could expect to live another 16.8 years—almost three years longer than the 13.9 years expected for a person aged 65 years in 1950. Female life expectancy has especially increased—a woman aged 65 years in 1982 can expect to live an additional 18.8 years on average compared to 14.4 years for a 65-year-old male. Thus, an increasing proportion of the elderly, and especially of the very old, is female.

Health Status and Health Needs of the Elderly

Although life expectancy at age 65 is now almost 17 years, what has been termed "active life expectancy" is considerably less. "Active life expectancy" is the projected number of years of functional well-being; the end point of "active life expectancy" is not death but "the loss of independence in the activities of daily living (ADL)" (20). According to a study by the originators of the concept, a group of 65 to 69 year-old persons living in the community whose total life expectancy was 16.5 years had an "active life expectancy" of only 10.0 years. Moreover, they found that the proportion of dependent years increased with age, so that persons living independently at age 85 would need assistance for 60% of their remaining 7.3 years of life.

The reason for the increasing dependence of elderly people is the deterioration of their health due to the onset of chronic conditions that tend to become more disabling as they grow older. By every measure of health status, elderly people are worse off than younger people (33). National data show that almost half of all elderly people have some activity limitation, almost 40% are limited in their major activity, and almost 18% are unable to carry out their major activity. Elderly people average about 40 days of restricted activity per year, 14 of them bed disability days. Almost one third rate their health as fair or poor compared to that of others their age. The data also show the elderly's increasing dependence on others as they grow older (11). For example, while 53 of every 1000 persons aged 65 to 74 need some help in one or more basic activities of daily living, this number nearly triples (to 157) for those aged 75 and over.

Because the elderly suffer primarily from chronic conditions, they use more health care services than younger persons (33). In contrast to acute conditions, there is generally no cure for chronic conditions, but medical care can at least make symptoms more tolerable. As a result, the elderly's use of medical care tends to be high and to continue over many years. For example, persons aged 65 years and over average 6.3 physician visits per person per year compared to between four and five visits for those under 65 years. The differences in their use of hospital services are even more striking. The elderly average 396.5 hospital admissions and 4155.3 hospital days per 1000 population per year, more than twice the rate of hospital use of those under 65 years. Moreover, the use of hospital services by the elderly increases as they age. For example, the rate of hospital admissions of persons aged 75 and over is 51% higher than that of persons aged 65 to 74, and their rate of hospital days is 70% higher (National Center for Health Statistics, personal communication).

The elderly also are the principal users of nursing home services. The National Center for Health Statistics' most recent survey of nursing homes, conducted in 1977, found that almost 5% of persons aged 65 and over were in nursing homes, accounting for almost 90% of all nursing home residents (9). Again, use rises sharply with age: 21.6% of those aged 85 and over were in nursing homes, accounting for one third of all nursing home residents though constituting less than 1% of the total United States population.

Health Care Expenditures of the Elderly

In light of these health needs, it is hardly surprising that the elderly's share of total personal health care expenditures has risen faster than their proportion in the population, from 23.8% of total personal health care expenditures in 1965 to 29.4% in 1978 (14) and 34.4% in 1984, based on a preliminary estimate (42). In 1965, average expenditures of persons aged 65 years and over were 5.7 times those of persons less than 19 years old and 2.2 times those of persons aged 19 to 64 years. By 1978, these figures had risen to 7.1 and 2.7 times the expenditures of persons in the two younger age groups, respectively.

A major reason for the steeper rise in average health care expenditures of the elderly compared to that of younger persons is the aging of the elderly population itself, that is, the increase to nearly 9% in the proportion of the old who are over 85 years old. Although there are no data on *total* health care expenditures by age for the 65-year and over population, Medicare data show that reimbursements increase with age. In 1982 average reimbursements *per person served* amounted to $2960 for Medicare beneficiaries aged 85 years and older, compared to $2172 for beneficiaries aged 65 to 74 years, or 36% more (10). The difference in average reimbursements *per enrollee* is even greater, with average reimbursements of the 85-year and older group being 66% higher than those of the younger group ($2170 versus $1303). This difference reflects both the higher medical care expenditures of the older beneficiaries who have some medical expenses and the greater proportion of older beneficiaries who use Medicare services. The difference between *total* health care expenditures of the "old old" and those of the "young old" is likely to be even greater than these figures indicate, because Medicare covers only a small fraction of nursing home expenditures and, as shown above, nursing home utilization rises sharply with age.

A dramatic change has also occurred in the source of payment for the care of the elderly. In 1965, the year the Medicare and Medicaid programs went into effect, public sources—federal, state and local government programs—accounted for just under 30% of the health care expenditures of the elderly (14). By 1978, the share of public funds had risen to 63.2% (and is estimated to have risen to 67.2% in 1984). There has also been a major shift from state and local government sources to federal sources. In 1965, public funding for health care of the elderly was about evenly divided between federal sources, on the one hand, and state and local sources, on the other. By 1978, 86% of total public funding of care for the elderly came from federal sources, representing 54% of the total expended on health care for the elderly. Estimates for 1984 suggest that the federal share today may even be slightly higher (42).

To sum up, the aging of the population, and especially the increase in the number and proportion of the very old, has been an important cause of the increase in national health care expenditures in the United States and is largely responsible for the financial difficulties of the Medicare program. Because Medicare reimbursements increase with age, average annual reimbursements per enrollee have increased; and because elderly people live longer, Medicare payments per enrollee continue over a longer period of years than when the program was introduced in 1965.

THE ECONOMICS OF CARING FOR PATIENTS WHO DIE

Just as concern over the growing proportion of national expenditures devoted to health care often focuses on the major contribution made by the aging of the population, concern about the high cost of care for the elderly is heightened by the evidence from several studies that shows that a large part of these expenses is incurred in the last year or months of life. The most frequently cited statistic on this subject comes from a Health Care Financing Administration (HCFA) study by Lubitz & Prihoda (25), which found that the 5.9% of Medicare beneficiaries who died in 1978 accounted for 27.9% of Medicare expenditures. In fact, as Fuchs has pointed out, the high medical expenses of persons who die are the principal reason that medical care expenditures of the elderly rise with age (15). Using data on Medicare expenditures per enrollee by age and sex, he showed that adjusting for age-sex differences in survival status eliminates much of the age-related increase in expenditures, especially the very high expenditures of the 80-year and older group, for whom his figures actually show a decline rather than an increase in expenses. (It must be remembered, however, that the data on which these estimates are based are for Medicare reimbursements and thus do not include expenses for nursing home care, which are the heaviest for the oldest age group.)

To determine whether medical resources are being misused for the dying, a review and evaluation of the data on medical care use and expenditures at the end of life are essential. Studies of medical care at the end of life have been classified into two broad categories: (*a*) studies dealing specifically with use and costs of care at the end of life, and (*b*) studies of high-cost illness in general, which also provide some information about high-cost patients who died during the period under study (36).

Studies of the Use and Cost of Care

HOSPITAL DEATHS   One group of studies in the first category deals with the use of hospital services by patients who died. A study conducted in 1961 showed that 48% of all deaths (and 45% of the deaths of persons aged 65 years and over) occurred in short-stay hospitals (39); it also showed that 63% of all decedents (and 61% of decedents aged 65 and over) used some hospital care in the last year of life. A somewhat later study of hospital and institutional care in the last year of life of adults aged 25 and over who died in 1964 and 1965 found that although 73% of these decedents used some hospital and institutional care in their last year of life, only 13% of the living population used such services during a 12-month period (40). The study also found that the median hospital bill of decedents was almost three times higher than that of hospital patients who did not die. Yet another study estimated that in 1974 over 20% of all nonpsychiatric hospital and nursing home expenditures in nongovernment facilities were for the care of patients who died (28).

CANCER CARE   Another group of studies in this category examines the cost of care for terminal cancer patients. A study based on the Third National Cancer Survey found that in 1969 and 1970, hospital expenses of cancer patients who died within 24 months were almost twice as high as those of cancer patients who did not die (37). A study by Cancer Care found that in 1971 and 1972, total expenditures of patients who died of advanced cancer ranged from less than $5000 to more than $50,000 per patient, with an average cost of $21,718 (6). A more recent study of cancer patients under age 65 showed that expenditures averaged $21,219 for the terminal year and grew exponentially as death approached; $15,836 was spent in the last six months and $6161 in the last month (24).

MEDICARE BENEFICIARIES   There have been several studies of Medicare expenditures of beneficiaries who died. The most comprehensive of these is the study by Lubitz & Prihoda referred to above (25), which compares Medicare expenditures in the last 12 months of life of enrollees who died in 1978 with expenditures during a 12-month period of enrollees who survived. In addition to finding that the 5.9% of enrollees who died accounted for 27.9% of total Medicare expenditures, the study also showed that 92% of decedents compared to 58% of survivors had some Medicare reimbursements during the 12-month period; 74% of decedents compared to 20% of survivors had one or more hospitalizations in the course of the year; 32% of decedents compared to only 4% of survivors had expenses of $5000 or more; and total Medicare reimbursements were over six times higher for decedents than for survivors, and reimbursements for hospital services were seven times higher for decedents. A study by McCall of Colorado Medicare enrollees who died in 1978 showed much the same differences between reimbursements for decedents and survivors (27).

Lubitz & Prihoda also found that 77% of all expenses of decedents occurred in the last six months of life, 46% in the last 60 days, and 30% in the last 30 days; McCall likewise found that a large part of medical expenses in the decedents' last year of life were incurred in the final month and 67% of inpatient charges arose in the last three months of life.

Several other Medicare studies, although less detailed, have come up with similar findings. For example, a study of Medicare beneficiaries who died in 1967 showed that the 5% of beneficiaries who died accounted for 22% of Medicare expenditures in that year (30); and another study found that the 5% of Medicare beneficiaries who died in 1979 accounted for 21% of total Medicare expenditures in that year (18). (Unlike the Lubitz-Prihoda and the McCall studies, these two studies cover only Medicare payments in the calendar year of death, i.e. on the average for six months before a beneficiary's death.)

COMMUNITY RESIDENTS   Finally, a study of medical care expenditures of elderly people living in the community throughout 1980, based on actual expenditures rather than Medicare reimbursement data, found that although only 5% of these elderly people either died or were institutionalized during the year, their expenditures while they lived in the community accounted for 22% of total expenditures (even though on the average they were there for only six months) (21).

Studies of High-Cost Illness

In addition to the studies dealing specifically with medical care costs of patients who died, there have been numerous studies of high-cost illness, all of which show that a considerable portion of these costs was incurred by patients who died. For example, one study of high-cost patients in a number of San Francisco Bay Area hospitals found that 15% of these patients died while in the hospital (34), and a follow-up study found that two years after discharge 34% had died (35).

Several studies of patients in intensive care units also showed a high percentage of deaths. For example, one study found that only 62% of patients admitted to the critical care unit of a cancer center were discharged alive (41). Another study found that nonsurvivors treated in an intensive care unit incurred significantly higher costs than patients who survived hospitalization (8).

Evaluating the Studies

None of the studies tell the whole story of medical care use and costs at the end of life. Some of the studies cover only hospital care, others only one specific cause of death, cancer. The data on high-cost hospital patients—and especially those on patients treated in special care units—come mainly from tertiary care centers with the latest high-technology equipment, where treatment practices differ from those in community hospitals, which provide most of the hospital care in the United States. The Medicare studies are limited to expenses for services for which Medicare pays, mainly hospital care and to a lesser extent physician services, and exclude all expenses for nursing home care and out-patient drugs and prescriptions. The study of medical expenses of elderly people living in the community also does not include nursing home expenses for those who died or were institutionalized.

Nevertheless, taken together the studies leave little doubt that medical care expenditures at the end of life are indeed high. From some of the earlier studies one can see that this is not a recent development: For at least 20 years, medical care costs of persons who died have been high compared to those of survivors. The greater concern about these costs today than 15 or 20 years ago is tied to the general concern over constantly rising medical care expenses which threaten to consume an ever larger share of the GNP and to sink the Medicare fund in red ink, as well as to the great public awareness of the details of high-technology medicine. As one public official opined, "We've got a duty to die and get out of the way with all our machines and artificial hearts and everything else like that and let the other society, our kids, build a reasonable life" (22). However, although the studies establish that medical care costs at the end of life are high, this by no means proves that a "disproportionate" amount is being spent on terminally ill patients.

The assertion that the "dying elderly" are receiving "too much" health care could mean several different things. First, those concerned with controlling health care expenditures may mean that elderly patients who die absorb an "excessive" amount of the total public (and/or private) resources available for health care. Yet looking in the Lubitz-Prihoda study for decedents who probably received high-technology interventions in their last year of life—namely those with Medicare reimbursements of $20,000 or more—reveals that only 3% of all elderly decedents (24,000 patients) fell into this category (25). Even going to a lower threshold figure of $15,000 yields only 56,000 decedents, or 6% of the total. Thus, the number of elderly patients who died who appear to have received aggressive, intensive medical care is very small. Had all medical care been withheld from them (a highly improbable step), the savings to the Medicare program would have been small: $644 million (3.5% of total Medicare reimbursements for the decedents and survivors included in Lubitz &

Prihoda) if care had been withheld from those with reimbursements of $20,000 or more, or $1196 million (6.5% of total Medicare reimbursements) if the threshold had been $15,000. Thus, the bulk of Medicare reimbursements for all elderly patients who died is accounted for by patients other than those who received intensive medical care in their last year of life.

Alternatively, the claim of "too much" care may be that these patients are receiving care that is neither desired by, nor appropriate for, them. Rather than being an economic argument, this conclusion is explicitly framed in ethical terms. An analysis of the philosophical principles by which this assertion can be evaluated demonstrates, however, that the first version of the "disproportionality" claim also rests—and should be judged—on ethical as well as economic presuppositions.

ETHICAL IMPLICATIONS AND PROBLEMS

Among the teleological and deontological theories that might bear on the subject, three merit special attention. The funding of care at the end of life can be evaluated based upon principles of (a) justice, (b) utility, or (c) beneficence and autonomy.

Just Allocation

Justice is a complex concept, with meanings that range in different contexts from procedural fairness to the distribution of benefits and burdens by desert (3). Health care financing raises issues of comparative justice, that is, the fairness of one person or group receiving a resource at the expense of another person or group.

In a society in which most goods are distributed through marketplace mechanisms, the claim that a particular good (such as health care) is distributed unfairly could be collapsed into a complaint about the basic distribution of wealth and income. However, given the large role that public funding plays in health care, especially for the elderly, the claim that it is unfairly distributed need not be seen as an invitation to a wide-ranging debate about the entire organization of American society. What, then, are the criteria by which the fairness of health care's distribution might be judged? Three—equality, need, and equity—require examination.

EQUAL ALLOCATION   In many settings, justice is served by treating people equally (i.e. "one person, one . . ."). If this standard were applied to health care, it might mean that each person would be entitled to an equal amount of care over the course of a year or perhaps over the person's lifetime. Given the wide variations in health status among individuals, such a standard would almost certainly have unacceptable results: If the amount of care guaranteed were set high (so as to encompass those whose health is chronically poor), an enormous drain would be imposed on resources that could be used to meet other, non–health care needs; if, to avoid this problem, the level were set low (merely enough to meet the needs of persons in average health or better), services that could preserve life or restore health would be unavailable for some sick people. Indeed, if the equality standard were strictly applied, such services would have to be withheld from patients who wished to use their own resources to purchase health care rather than other goods and services. Thus, the fact that health care expenditures are not even among individuals or among groups in the population—such as the elderly versus the nonelderly—is not grounds for concluding that the distribution of care is unjust.

DISTRIBUTION BY NEED   To remedy the perverse effects of an equality standard, distribution according to need has been suggested as a preferable criterion for justice. Under this standard, the high incidence of chronic illness among the elderly would justify the greater proportion of health care provided to this group, just as a large percentage of education dollars is appropriately spent on the young. The problem with using need as the basis of an ethical theory of health care distribution is that it opens the door to unlimited spending on this one good, to the potential exclusion of many other individual and social goods.

EQUITABLE ACCESS   In light of the weaknesses in need and equality as standards, the President's Commission for the Study of Ethical Problems in Medicine and Biomedical and Behavioral Research concluded that the principle of justice required that everyone have *equitable* access to health care, which was interpreted to mean that society has an ethical obligation to ensure access to an adequate level of care for all without imposing undue burdens on anyone in obtaining that care (32). Thus, to decide whether an unfair amount of care was being provided to patients who die, one would have to determine (*a*) whether the provision of that care went beyond the adequate level, and (*b*) whether this allocation deprived others of obtaining an adequate level.

Application of the first of these points to expenditures on elderly patients should rest on a general assessment of the justice of the distribution of care, rather than singling out this one group. Distribution is not yet just: Millions of Americans are not ensured access to an adequate level of care, while public funds help secure far more than merely adequate care for others (32).

In the long run, a societal concensus about access to health care, including life-sustaining care, is needed. Rather than beginning with restrictions on life-sustaining care, however, it would be better to develop principles for equitable and acceptable limits on the use of health care generally, and then to apply those principles to issues at the end of life (31, p. 100).

The second aspect of equity—whether the allocation of resources to one deprives others of an adequate level of care—reveals that adequacy is a comparative concept, dependent on the cost of a particular type of treatment under particular circumstances in relation to alternative forms of care in achieving the goals that make health care of special moral significance (e.g. enhancing patients' welfare and opportunities, providing valuable information, and symbolizing mutual respect and empathy). If one concentrates solely on the physical aspects of health care (i.e. preserving life and restoring functioning), then resources would be most sensibly applied to younger rather than older patients, since the former will enjoy the prospect of benefitting from the results of successful treatment much longer than the latter. Indeed, Aaron & Schwartz discern this as a prime "principle" explaining the allocation process in Great Britain:

> The low incidence of chronic dialysis among the elderly with renal failure dramatizes such discrimination. The limitation of resources allocated to the treatment of terminal illness is another expression of this bias (1, p. 97).

As noted above, however, the study by Lubitz & Prihoda shows that health care expenditures on elderly patients who died after expensive ($20,000+) care amounted to only $644 million in 1978. If there are problems of distributional justice in the system, they are likely to be exacerbated rather than solved by the Draconian step of cutting off high cost care for older "dying patients."

Utilitarian Analysis

An alternative analysis of the concern over excessive expenditures at the end of life would turn to the principle of utility, under which the distribution of health care is examined in terms of its relative efficacy in producing the greatest net benefit for all persons affected. An initial difficulty in applying utilitarian analysis to the question at hand lies in deciding what counts as a benefit of a particular medical intervention (2). Especially when dealing with groups of people (e.g. those under 65 years old versus those over this age), it is extremely difficult to make valid comparisons: Is restoration of function in a 12 year-old valued the same as in a 72 year-old?

PROGNOSTIC LIMITATIONS   Even if (for the purposes of argument) continued life is taken to be an absolute value, a basic problem with a utilitarian evaluation remains: To be applicable, such a method would have to be able accurately to predict which patients will live (i.e. should be treated) and which will die (i.e. where treatment—beyond palliation of pain—would be "wasted"). The uncertainty and difficulty of medical prognosis are well-known. With the possible exception of cancer patients, for whom a prognosis of death can be made with reasonable accuracy beyond a certain point in the course of their disease, predicting imminent death is difficult in most cases, and predicting death 12, six, or even three months in advance is well-nigh impossible.

Practically all the studies dealing with medical care costs at the end of life fail to face the problem of how to determine in advance who will die. By necessity retrospective, they tend to equate patients who die with dying patients. Unfortunately but not surprisingly, none of the studies provide the kind of information about the patients who died (for example, about their medical and functional status prior to death) that would make it possible to estimate how many of them were terminally ill or how long before death they became terminal cases. Of the 49,000 patients with Medicare reimbursements of $20,000 or more in the Lubitz-Prihoda study, 24,000 died and 25,000 survived (25). How many of those who died, one wonders, were recognized as being terminal patients, and how long before death was their status clear? Conversely, how many of the survivors were regarded as hopelessly ill according to the best judgment of their physicians but surprised them by recovering? One has to be cautious, therefore, not to equate the high medical costs at the end of life with the high costs of terminal care.

Beneficence and Autonomy

As this analysis suggests, ethical analysis is needed to evaluate the concerns voiced about a disproportionate percentage of health care (and especially public) funds being expended for patients who die. Plainly, the topic's deeper resonance—and its involvement with other and at least equally perplexing ethical issues—derives from the widespread sense that, putting aside any effects on health care financing, many elderly patients receive more care than they want—or more than they would want if they knew what was good for them. Dr. Alexander Leaf, the chief of medicine at the Massachusetts General Hospital, spoke for many concerned physicians when he observed that in acute-care hospitals, the elderly "are too often subjected to the same management that might offer hope of benefitting a younger person with less extensive disease" (23, p. 888).

Although overtreatment of this sort, with its high incidence of morbidity as well as mortality, is taken to be a common problem, the Lubitz-Prihoda data previously cited suggest that only a small percentage of the decedents (about 3%) had Medicare reimbursements at a level one would expect to find in cases of aggressive treatment. Moreover, more elderly patients treated at this level survived than died, so it is not possible to know how realistic the prospect of continued life was for at least some of those who died despite treatment.

TWO GROUPS   Further data are thus needed to ascertain whether a substantial number of cases occur in which the medical profession's moral duty of beneficence (to help others further their important and legitimate interests) is violated through overtreatment. Some preliminary data on 216 elderly decedents from a study we are currently conducting on medical care costs in the last year of life (which includes information on functional status during the 12 months preceding death) suggest that over one half fall into one of two distinct groups.

First are the elderly who were in good functional shape as indicated by measures such as the Activities of Daily Living (ADL) and the Instrumental Activities of Daily Living (IADL) during most of this period until they were struck by a serious illness: a heart attack, a stroke, or a fractured hip, for example. Because of their favorable previous history, they are not the kind of patients, even if they are quite old, for whom "No Code" (i.e. no cardiopulmonary resuscitation) orders are likely to be written or whom physicians are likely to "allow to die" in the absence of such explicit orders. Most of these patients therefore received relatively intensive care, often involving hospitalization, with the result that their medical costs were high in the last weeks or months of life.

The second group of elderly patients who die are frail, debilitated, and mostly very old—yet patients who despite their poor health are not clearly dying. According to our preliminary findings, such patients are given mainly supportive care—but such care, given over many months, is expensive, a fact not revealed by studies of Medicare expenditures alone. We found that their expenditures in the last 12 months of life averaged about $21,000, compared to about $23,000 for the group who were relatively unimpaired until just before death. But whereas 96% of the expenses of this latter group were for hospital and physician services, only 25% of the expenses of the former were for these services, and the rest were mainly for supportive care such as home and nursing home care. That such patients can have high expenses is also shown by Ginzberg's account of the expenses incurred by his 93-year-old mother in the last six months of life, which amounted to $31,000 (16). Although she received some hospital care, it was purely palliative, not "heroic," and like the patients in our study, she had high costs for home care.

It is this second group of patients who, we believe, pose the most difficult ethical problems for their physicians, families, and society as a whole. Indeed, the ethical problems in decision making about patients in the second group are likely to grow more pronounced, as their numbers increase and as means are implemented to allow decisions to be made better and more easily by and for terminally ill patients (and even by and for patients in the first group).

IMPROVING DECISIONS   The means developed in recent years to further the interests of all patients have particular importance for very sick or dying patients whose condition prevents them from participating in decisions about their own care. The objective of most of these mechanisms is to promote goals associated with the ethical principle of autonomy—namely, that all treatments be based upon the patient's individual value preferences and definition of what serves his or her goals.

The first of these mechanisms, under the title of the "Living Will," provides a means for a person, while still competent, to instruct his or her physician, family, and other advisors about the limits of treatment if the person becomes incompetent and there is no reasonable prospect of recovery from extreme physical or mental disability. Although nearly 40 states have recently adopted so-called Natural Death Acts (meant to give instructions of this sort binding legal effect when executed under certain, narrow conditions), the statutes are more useful in stimulating discussion among patient, physician, and others than in providing precise guidance. Indeed, people are seldom able to know enough in advance about their final illness to describe with the necessary precision which treatments they would want or not want; moreover, the passage of time, and particularly the process of an illness itself, may cause a change in previously expressed wishes.

Recently, another alternative—a patient's appointment of someone to make choices on his or her behalf—has been recommended as a more realistic and flexible tool to ensure that the patient receives treatment of a type and scope desired, even when the patient has lost the capacity to participate in decision making (31). Most states have so-called Durable Power of Attorney statutes that permit the appointment of someone (such as spouse, child, or friend) to act regarding the person or property of another after that person becomes incompetent. When used in conjunction with instructions about care, the Durable Power of Attorney removes the decision-making paralysis that many physicians feel when faced with the question of withholding or withdrawing life-sustaining treatment from an incompetent patient for whom such treatment does not promise to restore functioning. Thus, it provides a means (much simpler and more expeditious than judicial appointment of a guardian) to serve the goals both of autonomy and beneficence. Further, some hospitals have recently appointed Institutional Ethics Committees to improve the quality of decisions made in certain difficult cases and to ensure that the best interests of very sick (and usually incapacitated) patients are served.

REMAINING PROBLEMS   Such mechanisms are not widely employed by patients and physicians, nor yet incorporated into the ethos of the medical profession; therefore, practical questions about the extent and vigor appropriate in treating acute illness in elderly patients remain. These questions are especially perplexing regarding the frail and debilitated elderly who require only modest medical and nursing interventions.

While there has been no systematic study of the type of care given to such elderly and debilitated patients, there is some evidence that the very old and sick are treated less aggressively than the "young old" (4). The experiences of one physician are supported by the preliminary evidence from our current study:

> In my own practice and in the practices I see around me, the old, chronically ill, debilitated, or mentally impaired do not receive the same level of aggressive medical evaluation and treatment as do the young, acutely ill, and mentally normal (19, p. 717).

Furthermore, data from the study by Lubitz & Prihoda point to the same conclusion that the very old are treated less aggressively. They found that Medicare reimbursements for decedents decreased with age while they increased for survivors. This decrease appears to be due mainly to a decrease in the use of hospital services, with admissions, discharges, and days of hospital care per 1000 enrollees steadily decreasing with age. (It must be remembered that nursing home expenses are not covered by Medicare, and that therefore total expenses may have risen with age.) Finally, a study not of the frail and debilitated elderly but of terminal cancer patients also found an inverse relationship between expenses in the last six months of life and age, expenses decreasing on the average by $151 for each year of age (38).

CONCLUSION

In sum, although the available data are not conclusive, it appears unlikely that more than a relatively small part of the high medical expenses at the end of life, and of the elderly in general, are due to excessively aggressive care of terminally ill patients. Most of these expenses seem to be for the care of very ill but not necessarily dying patients, care that, especially in the case of the very old and chronically ill, is relatively conservative yet expensive.

This last group thus creates a double dilemma. On the one hand, the care of these patients is costly and probably accounts for far more than the costs of care of "terminally ill" patients, as that term is commonly used. On the other hand, the decision-making mechanisms (such as Durable Powers of Attorney) that are available to avoid unwanted or futile treatment in the case of the patients who maintain their vigor and powers of thought until near the time of their fatal illness, are less likely to be effective with chronically ill, debilitated patients, whose incapacity to participate in decisions is often of long standing, thus making it unlikely that they will have expressed their current wishes about the extent of care they desire.

Moreover, the fact that this second group of patients is not "dying" raises grave questions in the minds of many about the application to them of the substantive standards for withdrawal of "life-sustaining" treatment that have recently come to be widely accepted regarding more gravely ill patients. Many people may share the sentiments of the respected journalist, Alan Otten, who publicly expressed concern over the fate of his 90-year-old mother and others like her in nursing homes, "enduring barren year after barren year, with chronic diseases that unfortunately do not kill but merely irrevocably waste the body and destroy the mind" (29).

> Doctors, nursing homes and hospitals work to keep these old people alive with tube feeding, nutritional supplements, antibiotics at the first sign of infection. For what? Are we really doing these people any favor by fighting so hard to prolong their lives?

Yet, despite the prevalence of such views (26), society has only just begun to address this problem. Thus far, only one state's highest court has sanctioned the withdrawal of supportive care (including artificially provided nutrition and fluids) from debilitated elderly patients, based upon their previously expressed wishes or on an "objective" assessment of their "best interests" (7), and respected ethicists remain troubled by the analogy drawn between artificial respirators and artificial feeding (5). Until firmer guidance emerges from professional bodies, the courts, and the legislatures for the treatment of these patients, including true alternatives to the "all-or-nothing" stance of most acute-care facilities (23), physicians may be left with a felt ethical compulsion to "do something"—even halfhearted and ineffective measures that make "no medical or ethical sense at all" (19, p. 717). Thus, until medical prognostic powers improve substantially and ethical and legal standards emerge to allay fears that any failure to "do everything possible" for these patients would send the country sliding into the abyss of active euthanasia, medical treatment will continue to be provided that possibly wastes resources and that may harm rather than help some patients.

Literature Cited

1. Aaron, H. J., Schwartz, W. B. 1984. *The Painful Prescription.* Washington DC: Brookings Inst. 161 pp.
2. Avorn, J. 1984. Benefit and cost analysis in geriatric care: Turning age discrimination into health policy. *New Engl. J. Med.* 310:1294–1301
3. Beauchamp, T. L., Childress, J. F. 1983. *Principles of Biomedical Studies,* pp. 183–220. New York/Oxford: Oxford Univ. Press. 364 pp.
4. Brown, N. K., Thompson, D. J. 1979. Nontreatment of fever in extended-care facilities. *New Engl. J. Med.* 300:1246–50
5. Callahan, D. 1983. On feeding the dying. *Hastings Cent. Rep.* 13(5):22
6. Cancer Care. 1973. *The Impact, Costs and Consequences of Catastrophic Illness on Patients and Families.* New York: Nat. Cancer Found.
7. Conroy, *in re.* 1985. 98 N.J. 321, 486 A.2d 1209
8. Detsky, A. S., Stricker, S. C., Mulley, A. G., Thibault, G. E. 1981. Prognosis, survival, and the expenditure of hospital resources for patients in an intensive care unit. *New Engl. J. Med.* 305:667–72
9. DHEW, Natl. Cent. Health Stat. 1979. The National Nursing Home Survey: 1977 Summary for the United States. *Vital and Health Statistics,* Ser. 13, No. 43. Hyattsville, MD: DHEW, Natl. Cent. Health Stat. DHEW Publ. No. (PHS) 79-1794
10. DHHS, Health Care Financing Admin. 1984. *Annual Medicare Program Statistics 1982.* Baltimore, MD: Health Care Financ. Admin. HCFA Publ. No. 03189
11. DHHS, Natl. Cent. Health Stat. 1983. Americans needing help to function at home. *Advance Data,* No. 92. Hyattsville, MD: Natl. Cent. Health Stat. DHHS Publ. No. (PHS) 83-1250
12. DHHS, Natl. Cent. Health Stat. 1984. *Health—United States 1984.* Hyattsville,

MD: Natl. Cent. Health Stat. DHHS Publ. No. (PHS) 85-1232

13. Fingerhut, L. A. 1982. Changes in mortality among the elderly: United States, 1940–79. *Vital and Health Statistics,* Ser. 3, No. 22. Hyattsville, MD: Natl. Cent. Health Stat. DHHS Publ. No. (PHS) 82-1406

14. Fisher, C. R. 1980. Differences by age groups in health care spending. *Health Care Fin. Rev.* 1(4):65–90

15. Fuchs, V. R. 1984. Though much is taken: Reflections on aging, health, and medical care. *Milbank Mem. Fund Q.* 62:151–54

16. Ginzberg, E. 1980. The high cost of dying. *Inquiry* 17:293–95

17. Ginzberg, E. 1984. The elderly are at risk. *Inquiry* 21:301

18. Helbing, C. 1983. Medicare: Use and reimbursement for aged persons by survival status, 1979. *Health Care Financing Notes,* November. Washington, DC: Off. of Res. and Demonstrat., Health Care Financing Admin.

19. Hilfiker, D. 1983. Allowing the debilitated to die: Facing our ethical choices. *New Engl. J. Med.* 308:716–19

20. Katz, S., Branch, L. G., Branson, M. H., Papsidero, J. A., Beck, J. C., et al. 1983. Active life expectancy. *New Engl. J. Med.* 309:1218–24

21. Kovar, M. G. 1983. Expenditures for the medical care of elderly people living in the community throughout 1980. *National Medical Care Utilization and Expenditure Survey, Data Report No. 4.* Hyattsville, MD: Natl. Cent. Health Stat. DHHS Publ. No. (PHS) 84-20000

22. Lamm, R. D., Governor of Colorado. 1984. Speech before Colorado Health Lawyers Association, Denver, CO, March 27, 1984 (corrected transcript, *Denver Post*)

23. Leaf, A. 1977. Medicine and the aged. *New Engl. J. Med.* 297:887–90

24. Long, S. H., Gibbs, J. O., Crozier, J. P., Cooper, D. I. Jr., Newman, J. F. Jr., et al. 1984. Medical expenditures of terminal cancer patients during the last year of life. *Inquiry* 21:315–27

25. Lubitz, J., Prihoda, R. 1984. The use and costs of Medicare services in the last two years of life. *Health Care Fin. Rev.* 5(3):117–31

26. Malcolm, A. H. 1984. Many see mercy in ending empty lives. *NY Times,* Sept. 23, p. 1, col. 3

27. McCall, N. 1984. Utilization and costs of Medicare services by beneficiaries in their last year of life. *Med. Care* 22:329–42

28. Mushkin, S. J. 1974. Terminal illness and incentives for health care. In *Consumer Incentives for Health Care,* ed. S.

J. Mushkin, pp. 183–216. New York: N. Watson

29. Otten, A. L. 1985. Can't we put my mother to sleep? *Wall St. J.,* June 5, p. 34, col. 3

30. Piro, P. A., Lutins, T. 1973. Utilization and reimbursement under Medicare for persons who died in 1967 and 1968. *Health Insurance Stat.,* Oct. 17. DHEW Publ. No. (SSA) 74-11702

31. President's Commission for the Study of Ethical Problems in Medicine and Biomedical and Behavioral Research. 1983. *Deciding to Forego Life-Sustaining Treatment.* Washington DC: US GPO. 554 pp.

32. President's Commission for the Study of Ethical Problems in Medicine and Biomedical and Behavioral Research. 1983. *Securing Access to Health Care.* Washington DC: US GPO. 223 pp.

33. Rice, D. P., Estes, C. L. 1984. Health of the elderly: Policy issues and challenges. *Health Affairs* 3(3):25–49

34. Schroeder, S. A., Showstack, J. A., Roberts, H. E. 1979. Frequency and clinical description of high-cost patients in 17 acute-care hospitals. *New Engl. J. Med.* 300:1306–9

35. Schroeder, S. A., Showstack, J. A., Schwartz, J. 1981. Survival of adult high-cost patients. *J. Am. Med. Assoc.* 245:1446–49

36. Scitovsky, A. A. 1984. "The high cost of dying": What do the data show? *Milbank Mem. Fund Q.* 62:591–608

37. Scotto, J., Chiazze, L. 1976. *Third National Cancer Survey: Hospitalization and Payments to Hospitals. Part A: Summary.* DHEW Publ. No. (NIH) 76-1094

38. Spector, W. D., Mor, V. 1984. Utilization and charges for terminal cancer patients in Rhode Island. *Inquiry* 21:328–37

39. Sutton, G. F. 1965. Hospitalization in the last year of life, United States—1961. *Vital and Health Statistics,* Ser. 22, No. 1. Washington DC: DHEW, Natl. Cent. Health Stat.

40. Timmer, E. J., Kovar, M. G. 1971. Expenses for hospital and institutional care during the last year of life for adults who died in 1964 or 1965. *Vital and Health Statistics,* Ser. 22, No. 11. Hyattsville, MD: DHEW, Natl. Cent. Health Stat.

41. Turnbull, A. D., Carlon, G., Baron, R., Sichel, W., Young, C., Howland, W. 1979. The inverse relationship between cost and survival in the critically ill cancer patient. *Critical Care Med.* 7:20–23

42. Waldo, D., Lazenby, H. C. 1984. Demographic characteristics and health care use and expenditures by the aged in the United States: 1977–1984. *Health Care Financ. Rev.* 6(1):1–29

Ann. Rev. Public Health. 1986. 7:77–104

OCCUPATIONAL ERGONOMICS—Methods to Evaluate Physical Stress on the Job

W. Monroe Keyserling and Don B. Chaffin

Center for Ergonomics, The University of Michigan, Ann Arbor, Michigan 48109-2117

INTRODUCTION

Ergonomics—An Emerging Discipline in Occupational Health

The word "ergonomics" is of Greek origin, and literally means "work laws." The term is not new—it was used by the prominent Polish labor science educator, Professor Jastrzebowski (1799–1882), to describe studies of work (41). Though the term was not used, the detailed studies of manual activities in United States industry by Frederick Taylor and Frank and Lillian Gilbreth during the period 1880 to 1930 are often referred to as providing the early methodological foundations for ergonomic evaluations of jobs today. They emphasized how one must carefully observe, measure, and analyze human behavior during work if one wishes to improve the productive capability of an organization. Further, the experimental studies performed by these early pioneers in the field showed that the level of human performance can be positively or negatively affected by relatively small changes in the work environment and work methods. These studies also showed a large variance in the performance capability of worker populations.

During World War II the need to select and train men quickly and effectively emphasized the importance of understanding human behavior under a variety of extreme working conditions. Human errors were documented as the cause of a majority of system failures. The military began studies of how such errors could be minimized, and thus the concept of "predictable human error" emerged. In other words, it was proposed that if a defined set of unreasonable physical and

77

0163-7525/86/0510-0077$02.00

mental demands on a human operator are given, there will arise a reasonable probability that the operator will err.

Studies of the cause and prevention of human errors involved experimental psychologists working with engineers during World War II, and resulted in teams of "human engineers." These studies have resulted in many military standards regarding the design of displays and controls. Since the 1950s, similar inquiries in the United States have resulted in a variety of human-engineered consumer products, such as push-button telephones, automobile interiors, kitchen appliances, and cameras. The psychologists and engineers who were mainly responsible for these developments organized themselves in 1957 for the purpose of sharing their experiences and officially formed the Human Factors Society. The HFS currently has over 4000 members in all 50 states.

In a parallel development in Europe, industrial managers and engineers also recognized that the improvement of future manufacturing systems would rely on how well the industrial system designer considered the worker's capabilities and limitations. By considering known human attributes in the design of a manufacturing system, not only would the probability of human error be reduced, but an improvement in the performance of the system could be realized (i.e. productivity and quality of finished goods could be improved). In Europe, and particularly in Great Britain, this larger goal involved people of varied disciplines, including engineers, physiologists, anatomists, and psychologists. These individuals formed the Ergonomics Research Society of Great Britain in 1950. The term "ergonomics" was thereby resurrected in an eclectic effort to draw upon a variety of disciplines in an effort to understand the effects of work on people and vice versa. Thus, the European orientation has differed from that of the United States, in that a broad disciplinary base was established for ergonomic studies and a majority of the activity in Europe has direct application to industrial operations.

In 1961, the International Ergonomics Association was formed to bring together various factions from around the world. The Association now has over 9000 members in 23 different affiliated organizations (including the Human Factors Society).

Today, ergonomists pursue the science of designing work environments that will be compatible and wholesome for a variety of people. They do this by studying the interaction of people with machines, tools, and work methods to determine how the interaction can be designed to improve performance and minimize human suffering as the result of error or chronic overstress. Such study requires a broadly educated individual with a background in human physiology, anatomy, and psychology as well as modern manufacturing technology and organization. Fortunately, the past research in the field has yielded sufficient literature and academic expertise to form a growing educational effort at many universities throughout the world.

The ergonomist is a specialist who works with engineers, industrial hygienists, safety professionals, and occupational health nurses and physicians to develop a better match between worker and job attributes. The ergonomist is concerned with optimizing both the physical and mental interaction required to perform a task in industry. This is depicted in Figure 1. The information flow between worker and hardware must be structured so the worker can quickly and correctly perceive, recognize, and respond appropriately without becoming mentally overstressed. Similarly, the physical interaction must be designed to accommodate the large variation in the strength, size, mobility, dexterity, and endurance of normal working populations. Many other conditions affect workers' health and safety as well. The ergonomist must be aware of these environmental hazards, as they often are synergistic in their effects on the worker-hardware system.

Ergonomics—Why Is It of Concern to So Many?

Many occupational injuries and illnesses are not being controlled by traditional safety and health strategies. This is particularly true regarding occupationally caused or aggravated musculoskeletal disorders (MSDs), which are ranked by the National Institute for Occupational Safety and Health (NIOSH) as one of the most serious health problems affecting US workers. In a recent report prepared by NIOSH (37), the following statements were made regarding musculoskeletal disorders:

1. MSDs rank first among health problems in the frequency with which they affect the quality of life, as indicated by the extent of activity limitation.

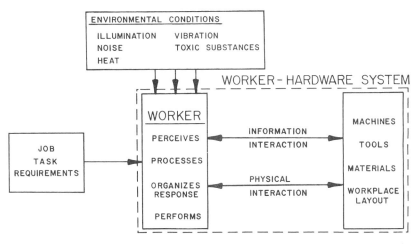

Figure 1   Diagram of two types of Worker-Hardware Interaction of concern to ergonomics. The study of these primary interactions is confounded by a variety of other environmental conditions that alter the effects on the worker-hardware system.

2. MSDs are the leading cause of disability of people in their working years, afflicting 19 million, especially in high risk industries including manufacturing, construction, and food processing. Nearly one half of the nation's work force are affected at some time during their working life.

3. MSDs also represent a significant accessory or causal factor in a large number of acute traumatic injuries.

4. Cost of MSDs, based on lost earnings and worker compensation payments, exceed that of any single health disorder. Back problems alone cost American industry an estimated 14 billion dollars per year.

5. MSDs, such as inflamed joints, or sprains/strains, account for one third of annual worker compensation claims. Sprains and strains are the most prevalent, with the back accounting for almost 50% of such disorders.

6. The frequency and impact of musculoskeletal conditions on the work force is expected to increase over the next several decades as the average age of the work force increases.

The projected increase in musculoskeletal disorders is already evident, despite the move toward more sophisticated automation and the shift away from physical to mental work, i.e. the processing of information. It is remarkable that the introduction of modern office technology (e.g. video display terminals) has generated new, pervasive, and even more insidious sources of biomechanical stress to the musculoskeletal system. The new technology has already increased the incidence of cumulative trauma disorders (CTDs) due to localized chronic repetitive motion of the upper extemity, and localized musculoskeletal fatigue syndromes due to prolonged static and constrained postures of the neck and torso. The magnitude of these problems is only now beginning to emerge.

Also ranked very high by NIOSH is the need to prevent acute trauma (e.g. cuts, abrasions, contusions, fractures, and amputations) caused by human error. Ergonomists believe that many of these errors are predictable by using established human factors job evaluation methods and databases.

A second important reason for ergonomics in industry stems from the recent legislation in many countries requiring improved accommodation to workers with diverse physical and mental capabilities and impairments. Simple rules denying people of certain age, gender, race, or apparent disability a fair opportunity to perform a job are no longer valid (35). Recent studies have shown that people who were not able to demonstrate an isometric strength sufficient to perform adequately the tasks in the various jobs assigned to them had a three-fold increase in both the incidence and severity of musculoskeletal injuries compared to their stronger peers (8, 11, 28). The development and validation of appropriate functional capacity tests of both job applicants and people seeking to return to work after suffering a musculoskeletal injury is a major occupational biomechanics effort within ergonomics.

A third reason for ergonomics' importance to industry is its comprehensive, rational approach to improving the work environment.

Ergonomics in the Prevention of Musculoskeletal Disorders in Industry

Two types of situations cause harm to workers. One occurs when a worker makes an error due to confusion, slow or imprecise response, or failure to perceive or recognize an appropriate signal. A second occurs when a worker is incapable of performing a particular manual task without great risk or injury to the musculoskeletal system. Because of the growing concern over musculo-skeletal disorders and their consequences in public health planning, in the rest of this paper we discuss ergonomic factors associated with the development of occupational musculoskeletal disorders. A broader perspective on the whole of ergonomics can be gained from reviewing recent books by McCormick & Sanders (31), Grandjean & Vigliani (18), and the Eastman Kodak Human Factors Section (15).

TRADITIONAL APPROACHES TO JOB EVALUATION

Work Measurement and Methods Analysis

Many different contemporary job evaluation systems have evolved from the work measurement systems developed in the United States during the late nineteenth century. As a result of managements' desire to reduce the cost of direct labor in manufacturing operations, the early job analysis schemes were designed to measure the time required to perform a job and to assist in the development of more efficient work methods [see Niebel (39), Barnes (6), and Polk (42) for additional information].

TIME STUDY   Time study was the first work measurement technique to be widely used in the United States. Developed by Taylor (47) in 1881, the method is still widely used by industrial engineers to improve work methods and to establish the standard time allowed to perform a job.

The process of time study has several applications to occupational ergonom-ics. The preliminary analysis of the workstation and the resulting sketch can reveal possible ergonomic deficiencies such as bench heights that require awkward working posture or machine locations that require excessive reaches. The observation of work methods and the resulting task descriptions can reveal potential biomechanical stresses associated with activities such as lifting or carrying heavy loads. In short, time study is a structured observational tech-nique that can be used to describe work activities and identify *potential* ergonomic stresses. Time study cannot be used, however, to quantify the level of ergonomic stress, or to evaluate a work activity to determine whether it is excessively strenuous.

MOTION STUDY   Motion study was developed during the early twentieth century by Frank and Lillian Gilbreth as a system for finding the best way to perform a manual operation (6, 17, 39, 42). Many of the methods and principles developed by the Gilbreths are still used today by industrial or production engineers. Like time study, the first step in motion study is to observe the job and to develop a description of the workstation and operator actions. However, whereas time study results in a task-based description of the standard method, motion study results in a highly detailed description of the body actions required to perform an operation. [For example, the task of manually moving a part from one location to another would be described as the following sequence: (*a*) reach, (*b*) grasp, (*c*) move, (*d*) position, and (*e*) release.]

A major contribution of the Gilbreths was the introduction of high-speed cinematography as a method for analyzing work motions. Following their extensive frame-by-frame analysis of films representing a wide variety of manufacturing jobs, they developed a system for classifying manual work into 17 fundamental motions, called *therbligs* (17). The Gilbreths also developed "rules of motion economy" to be used when designing work stations and work methods. When these rules were applied to the bricklaying trade, operator efficiency was increased from 120 bricks laid per hour to 350 bricks laid per hour. Video documentation of work motions and subsequent therblig analysis has been used by Armstrong et al (5) to study work motions associated with carpal tunnel syndrome and other repetitive motion disorders of the upper extremities.

PREDETERMINED TIME SYSTEMS   Predetermined time systems such as Work-Factor (43) and Methods Time Measurement (MTM) (34) were developed during the 1930s as an alternative to time study for predicting the time required to perform a job. These systems resulted from experimental studies that measured the time required for people to perform generic, fundamental work motions (such as reach, grasp, position, walk, etc) under a variety of conditions typically found in industry. By describing a job as a sequence of fundamental motions (each with a known time requirement), the normal time required to complete the job can be predicted by summing the time values for each of the fundamental motions.

Predetermined time systems have gained wide acceptance in recent years because they offer several advantages over time study (6, 39, 42). First, they do not require that the job actually exists, nor do they require physical simulation of a job in order to perform a comparative evaluation of two or more alternate methods. Hence, work methods can be evaluated and perfected "on paper" prior to starting up a new operation. Second, they can be used to estimate labor requirements to assure that adequate human resources are available when a new facility becomes operational. Finally, because they predict the normal time required to perform a job, the subjective and sometimes controversial exercise of performance rating is not required.

LIMITATIONS OF TRADITIONAL WORK MEASUREMENT   The systems described above were designed to predict the time required to perform a job or to improve the efficiency of work methods. Although these systems provide very useful methods for observing and describing work activities, their ability to measure and evaluate ergonomic stress is limited in several ways:

1. The traditional work measurement systems do not record the exact loads that workers must handle during strenuous tasks such as lifting or carrying. Accurate assessment of biomechanical stresses cannot be made without precise measurement of weights lifted, hand forces exerted, etc, during strenuous work activities (discussed further below).

2. Traditional work measurement systems do not require an accurate description of posture. While a sketch of a workstation may provide preliminary insight to the postural demands of a job, it does not describe the extreme or awkward postures that can result from the interaction of workstation layout, tool design, work methods, and operator size. Because extreme posture can result in musculoskeletal injury or contribute to fatigue, this layout sketch should be augmented with photographs or sketches of selected work activities that cause the stressful postures.

3. Because the primary objective of the traditional schemes is to predict the time required to perform a job, irregular activities that account for only a small fraction of the workday may be completely ignored. Examples of such activities include lifting a heavy totepan to replenish a bin of small parts, changing a 55 gallon drum, and leaning into a machine to remove scrap. Although tasks of this nature may account for less than 5 or 10% of the operator's workday (and are therefore relatively unimportant from the standpoint of improving methods to increase time efficiency), they may be the most stressful activities performed by the worker.

4. Perhaps most importantly, the traditional systems were designed to improve time efficiency with relatively little concern for ergonomics. In some cases, work methods designed to be the most efficient may not be the best in terms of ergonomics and worker safety.

An example of this situation frequently occurs in materials handling when a worker must reach to his left or right to transfer the load from one location to another. Traditional work measurement suggests that the most efficient method for performing this task is to rotate the body and twist the spine because this requires less time than a sidestep. Ergonomics favors the sidestep due to the high biomechanical stresses associated with twisting.

Physical Stress Surveys

Due to labor shortages in the United States during World War II, a large number of women were hired into industrial jobs previously held by males. An early advocate of achieving a better match between workers and jobs was Dr. Bert Hanman (22), who in 1945 defined selective placement as:

> the process whereby the worker is chosen and assigned to that job which (a) will afford the greatest utilization of his skills and aptitudes, and (b) which at the same time will be compatible with his physical capacities and protect his health and safety.

Dr. Hanman advocated the use of physical stress checklists to describe job demands. The results of a job analysis would be summarized on this checklist so that an industrial physician could make an informed decision when assigning a worker to a new job.

Various types of checklists have been developed since the early work of Dr. Hanman, each attempting to describe the physical demands of a job. Virtually all were designed to describe the weights that a worker would be expected to lift, and other stressful activities such as carrying or pushing loads, climbing ladders or stairs, or working in awkward postures. One of the most sophisticated checklists was developed in 1973 by Koyl & Marsters-Hanson (30). This checklist recorded the number of hours per day that each activity was performed as well as whether the left or right hand performed the activity. By comparing the results of the job analysis with a clinical evaluation of mobility and strength, a better job–worker match could be achieved.

Weight Lifting Limits

In 1962, the International Labor Organization (ILO) proposed that a proportion of work-related musculoskeletal injuries could be prevented by limiting occupational weight lifting to maximal "safe" weights. The ILO weight limits recognized variations of strength in the population by assigning different limits based on age group and gender. The ILO concept was not new; at the time of its adoption, virtually all states in the US had adopted occupational weight lifting limits, particularly for female workers. As a result of civil rights legislation passed during the 1960s and 1970s that prohibited arbitrary discrimination based on age or gender, all of the state laws were either rescinded or declared unconstitutional (7).

From the standpoint of ergonomics, the concept of a maximum "safe" weight is overly simplistic. Factors such as body posture during lifting, workstation layout, and lifting frequency contribute to lifting stress and may increase the risk of musculoskeletal injury. Nonlifting tasks that require awkward or sustained posture can also increase the risk of musculoskeletal injury. Fortunately, more sophisticated methods have been recently developed for evaluating occupational lifting and postural stresses.

CONTEMPORARY ERGONOMIC APPROACHES TO JOB EVALUATION

Recent Developments in Evaluation and Design of Jobs Requiring Manual Handling of Materials

It is estimated by NIOSH (38) that approximately one third of workers in the United States must exert significant strength in lifting, pushing, or pulling on objects as part of their jobs. This same report by NIOSH also presented the following statistics based on worker's compensation records:

1. Overexertion was claimed as the cause of lower back pain by over 60% of people suffering from it.
2. Overexertion injuries of all types in the US occurred to about 500,000 workers per year (about 1 in 200 workers each year).
3. If the overexertion injuries involved low-back pain resulting in significant lost time, less than one third of the patients eventually returned to their previous work.
4. Overexertion injuries accounted for about one fourth of all reported occupational injuries in the United States; some industries reported that over half of the total reported injuries were due to overexertion.
5. Approximately two thirds of overexertion injury claims involved lifting loads, and about 20% involved pushing or pulling loads.

Collectively, these observations indicate that manual handling of materials is now, and will continue to be, prevalent in many industries, and that such activity is associated with either causing or aggravating preexisting musculoskeletal disorders in a large number of workers.

Herrin et al (23) concluded that of all the different types of manual materials handling acts performed in industry, research findings were most conclusive regarding the act of manually lifting of loads that are symmetrically balanced in front of the body. Based on this, a multidisciplinary team of specialists in epidemiology, biomechanics, work physiology, and ergonomics were assembled by NIOSH to develop a *Work Practices Guide for Manual Lifting* (38). This *Guide* represents the first comprehensive approach to the control of the adverse effects of manual materials handling in industry.

NIOSH GUIDE FOR MANUAL LIFTING   The *Guide* focuses on those task and material/container characteristics that best define a hazardous lifting act. These factors are defined and given a variable designation, as follows:

1. Weight of object lifted (L).
2. Location of object center of mass (or hand grip center) measured horizontally from a point on the floor midway between the ankles at the origin and destination of a lifting motion (H).

3. Vertical location of object center of mass (or hand grip center) measured at beginning (origin) of lift from the floor (V).
4. Vertical travel distance of hands from origin to destination (release) of object (D).
5. Frequency of lifting (in lifts per minute) averaged over period of lifting (F).
6. Duration of the period during which lifting takes place (less than one hour, or on an eight-hour basis).

As an example, consider the lifting of a 44 lb stock reel from the floor to a spindle on top of a small press (see Figure 2). The data from the analysis of this lifting task is:

Object weight (L) = 44 lb
Horizontal hand location (H) at origin = 20 inches
Vertical hand location (V) at origin = 15 inches
Horizontal hand location at destination = 20 inches
Vertical hand location at destination = 63 inches
Task frequency (f) = 0.

The "zero" entry for task frequency denotes that the stock reel is loaded less than once every five minutes.

From population studies of strength, anthropometry, and aerobic work capacity, it is obvious that a large variation in lifting capability exists in any normal group of workers. Because of this, the NIOSH recommendations are based on two levels of hazard. The first level establishes an *Action Limit* (AL), wherein an increased risk of injury and fatigue for *some* individuals exists if they are not carefully selected and trained for the lifting task found to exceed the limit. Specifically, the *Action Limit* is based on:

1. Epidemiological data indicating that *some* workers would be at increased risk of injury on jobs exceeding the AL.
2. Biomechanical studies indicating the L5/S1 disc compression forces can be tolerated by most (but not all) people at about the 770 lb level, which would be created by conditions at the AL.
3. Physiological studies disclosing that the average metabolic energy requirement would be 3.5 kcal/min for jobs performed at the AL.
4. Psychophysical studies showing that over 75% of women and 99% of men could lift loads at the AL.

The second level of hazard in the *Guide* establishes a *Maximal Permissible Limit* (MPL). This limit is based on:
1. Epidemiological data indicating that musculoskeletal injury rates and severity rates are significantly higher for *most* workers placed on jobs exceeding the MPL.

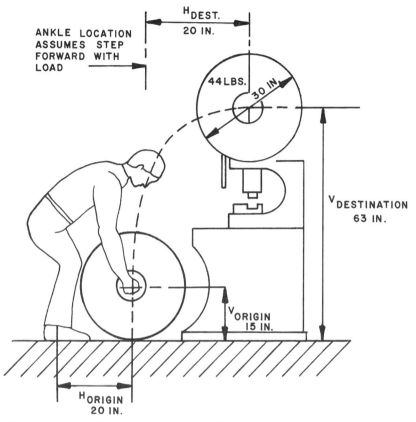

Figure 2 Example of lifting stock reel into punch press. It is assumed that the worker steps forward with the load to place it atop the press.

2. Biomechanical studies indicating that L5/S1 disc compression forces cannot be tolerated over the 1430 lb level in most workers, which would be created at the MPL.
3. Physiological studies disclosing that the metabolic energy expenditure rate would exceed 5.0 kcal/min for most workers lifting loads at the MPL.
4. Psychophysical studies showing that only about 25% of men and less than 1% of women workers have the muscle strength to be able to perform lifting above the MPL.

Thus, the AL and MPL permit lifting tasks to be classified into three hazard categories for control planning:

1. Those above the MPL should be considered as unacceptable, and engineering controls should be sought to redesign the lifting conditions.

2. Those between the AL and MPL are unacceptable without administrative or engineering controls, thus requiring careful employee selection, placement, and training, or job redesign.
3. Those conditions below the AL are believed to represent nominal risk to most workers.

The magnitude of the AL and MPL values for a job are estimated by an algebraic equation, or graphically, using the concept that the AL for occasional lifts, close to the body, and standing erect is 90 lbs (40 kg). If any lifting is performed in other conditions, then the 90 pound limit is reduced by a factor. This results in a multiplicative discounting procedure, in which the AL (in pounds of force that can be lifted) is estimated by:

$$AL = 90(HF)(VF)(DF)(FF) \text{ lbs}$$

where HF is the discounting factor due to the *horizontal* location at the beginning of the lift, VF is the discounting factor due to the *vertical* location of the load at the beginning of the lift, DF is the discounting factor due to the *distance* the load is lifted, FF is the discounting factor due to the *frequency* of the lifts.

All of the discounting variables have maximum values of 1.0, which are achieved at the optimum conditions described above. The values of the discounting factors are given in Figure 3. Inspection of the graphs reveals that the horizontal location H and frequency of lift F factors can exhibit the greatest discounting effect. Thus, job evaluations must give these two factors careful consideration. The next most important factor is the vertical location of the load V at the initiation of the vertical lift, followed by the distance D that the load is moved.

The Maximum Permissible Level MPL for a load is simply:

$$MPL = 3AL.$$

Using this procedure on the stock lifting example described above in Figure 3 results in:

$HF = 0.28$ (where $H = 20$ inches)
$DF = 0.76$ (where $D = 63 - 15 = 48$ inches)
$VF = 0.85$ (where $V = 15$ inches)
$FF = 1.00$ (where F once every five minutes).

The Action Limit is:

$$AL = 90(.28)(.76)(.85)(1.00) = 15 \text{ lbs}$$

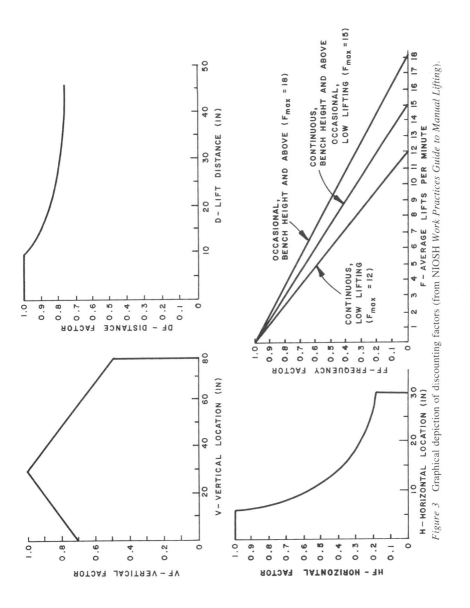

Figure 3 Graphical depiction of discounting factors (from NIOSH *Work Practices Guide to Manual Lifting*).

and the Maximum Permissible Level is:

$$MPL = 3(15) = 45 \text{ lbs.}$$

Because the stock reel lifted in this example weighed 44 lbs, its weight exceeds the 15 lb AL value, and thus lifting it is considered hazardous to some individuals. This would mean administrative controls should be used, i.e. careful selection and placement of persons with enough strength to handle the loads and training of such workers to minimize the lifting stresses. Because the load is almost equal to the 45 lb MPL value in this case, an engineering change would certainly be suggested to (a) reduce the load, (b) use a mechanical handling aid (hoist), or (c) arrange the workplace to allow the person to lift the reel from the side (reducing the H distance). If the stock reel weighed more than the 45 lb MPL value, then these engineering controls would be strongly recommended, not simply suggested.

The NIOSH *Guide* is a recent effort to control one aspect of manual materials handling problems—namely, that associated with the simple act of lifting loads in the sagittal plane. It attempts to be more comprehensive than previous efforts relative to (a) job evaluation methods, (b) criteria used for the limits, and (c) control strategies. It differs from past attempts in that it synthesizes data from many different studies, and advocates both engineering and administrative controls.

Though it is too early to tell whether it has had a positive effect on reducing occupational musculoskeletal disorders, it is being widely promoted and used by various safety and health professional groups, insurance companies, and NIOSH. In fact, the *Guide* is being considered as the basis for a new Federal Safety Standard by the Occupational Safety and Health Administration.

BIOMECHANICAL STRENGTH MODELS OF MANUAL EXERTIONS   The NIOSH *Guide* and other such tabular recommendations pertaining to how much workers can lift are quite empirical and are thus limited in scope, however. More fundamental models of the musculoskeletal system have been developed that allow a job analyst to input (a) specific postural data (angles of the body during an exertion), (b) anthropometry of the population (body weight and structure), and (c) load magnitude and direction operating on one or two hands. These models assume that the human body is a kinematic chain. Moments caused by the load in the hands and body segment weights are computed at each major articulation of the body for a given task. These load moments are compared to the strength moments produced by worker populations who have been isometrically tested. In addition, a gross estimate of the compression force acting on the L5/S1 disc is predicted and compared to the NIOSH limits of spinal compression force of 770 lbs for the AL value and 1430 lbs for the MPL value. The logic, assumptions, computational procedures, and validation of this modeling approach is described in detail by Chaffin & Andersson (10).

The practical implementation of this strength prediction method has been facilitated by the wide-scale use and computational power of the personal computer. As an example, consider the act of lifting the stock reel from the floor as shown in Figure 2. The input data to a Biomechanical Strength Model are:

Load:	44 lb in magnitude acting vertically down ($-90°$ from horizontal) and lifted with both hands.
Posture:	Angles (relative to horizontal) measured from a video or photograph of a person performing the lift are as follows:
Lower arm:	$-$ 68° (below horizontal)
Upper arm:	$-$ 87° (below horizontal)
Torso:	$+$ 32° (above horizontal)
Upper leg:	$+116°$ (above horizontal)
Lower leg:	$+$ 78° (above horizontal).
Anthropometry:	Depends on worker population, but average size male and female will be assumed for this example.

The Biomechanical Strength Model used for this analysis was developed by the Center for Ergonomics at The University of Michigan. It runs on any IBM-PC or compatible computer. In this model the above data are entered from the keyboard and displayed on the upper left quadrant of the screen shown in Figure 4. The upper right quadrant depicts the postural data in a graphical "stick figure" form. The evaluation of muscle strengths at each joint is given in the lower left quadrant of the screen for the posture and hand load conditions entered. In this particular lifting situation, the 44 lb reel would be difficult for almost half of the female workforce because of the large amount of muscle strength required at the hip joints, i.e. the model predicts that only 58% of women could perform the lift in this position. The results of the analysis indicate that the L5/S1 compression forces are also high, as shown in the lower right quadrant of Figure 4. Recall that if these values exceed 770 lbs (which is the NIOSH Action Limit), then special action would be needed either to reduce the load (e.g. use a hoist) or to select and train people to handle the load in a manner that would minimize such forces.

When the stock reel in this example is lifted to the top of the press, the limited female muscle strength in the shoulder muscles becomes even more of a problem. Only about 3% of women would be expected to have the shoulder strength to perform such a lift, and almost one out of four men would have difficulty with such a lift. Given these results, a job modification would certainly be recommended.

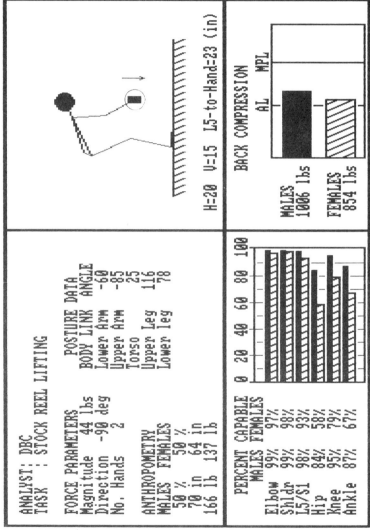

Figure 4 Output screen from The University of Michigan Static Strength Model depicting an evaluation of lifting a stock reel as shown in Figure 2.

Previous epidemiological studies by Chaffin & Park (12), Andersson (2), and Snook (45) have indicated that the handling of loads of this magnitude greatly increases the risk of developing low-back pain. With the advent of these newer, personal computer–based biomechanical strength analysis models, specific hazardous job conditions can be determined with much greater precision and sensitivity than was possible only a few years ago.

Recent Developments in Posture Analysis

The relationship between awkward postures of the trunk and shoulder and the development of fatigue and musculoskeletal disorders has been demonstrated in several recent investigations. Laboratory studies have demonstrated that trunk flexion, lateral bending, or twisting increases mechanical stresses on the spinal muscles and intervertebral discs (1, 44) and that prolonged trunk flexion causes extreme levels of muscle fatigue (9). Epidemiological studies have shown that sustained static postures of the trunk such as prolonged sitting or forward bending result in increased risk of low-back pain (27, 33). Bending and twisting of the trunk have also been cited as factors in the development of back pain (32).

Laboratory studies of shoulder posture have shown that prolonged elevation of the arms (shoulder flexion or abduction) causes extreme levels of muscle fatigue and, in some cases, acute tendinitis (9, 20). The relationship between shoulder elevation and increased risk of tendinitis has been demonstrated in a cross-sectional field study (21). Shoulder abduction and extension have been cited as postural stresses related to the development of thoracic outlet syndrome (16).

Several systems for measuring work posture have been developed during the past decade (26, 29). In order to identify specific causes of postural stress (e.g. poor workstation layout, improper tool selection, inappropriate work methods, etc), it is necessary to measure work activities and working posture on a common, continuous time scale. A computer-aided system with this capability has been recently developed by the authors to analyze the working posture of the trunk and shoulders on repetitive, assembly line jobs (publication under review). Because the computer simplifies data-recording activities and reduces analysis time, this system can be used to analyze postural stresses in the workplace quickly.

Posture Analysis Case Study

JOB DESCRIPTION   The case study job is a manual spotwelding operation performed in an automobile assembly plant. The purpose of this operation is to secure the roof panel to the car body with a series of spotwelds located along the windshield opening, the side drip rails, and the back window opening. The operation is performed by two workers, one on each side of the car body as it moves down the assembly line. The worker on the right side of the car obtains a roof panel from a shipping rack and places it on the car with the assistance of the worker on the left side. After the panel is properly positioned, spotwelds are made around its perimeter so that it becomes an integral part of the body structure. Because the activities of the left and right side workers are very similar, the remainder of the case study is limited to the left-side worker.

EQUIPMENT AND TOOLS   The principal tool used on this job is the manual spotwelding gun illustrated in Figure 5a. This gun is used to spotweld the roof along the left-side drip rail and along the opening for the back windshield. The gun is suspended from an overhead trolley system so that it can be moved in directions parallel or perpendicular to assembly line. This gun is called a C-type gun because of the shape of its electrodes.

A second spotwelding gun, illustrated in Figure 5b, is used to spotweld the roof panel above the windshield opening. This gun is suspended from overhead on a trolley system and balanced with a retractor. This design is called a P-type gun because its electrodes move together in a pinching action.

MAJOR TASKS   The following tasks are performed by the left-side operator during a typical work cycle:

1. Both operators work together to position the roof on the car body.

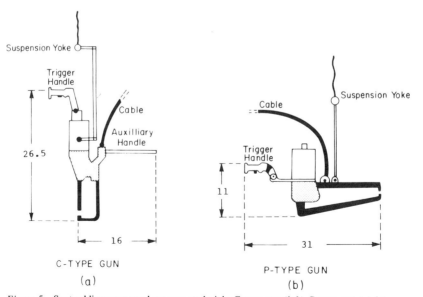

Figure 5 Spotwelding guns used on case study job: C-type gun *(left)*, P-type gun *(right)*.

2. The C-type spotwelding gun is used to bond the roof panel along the left-side drip rail. The gun is moved along the drip rail from the windshield opening to the rear window opening while making approximately 20 welds. While performing this task, the operator uses his right hand to position the electrodes and the left hand to activate the trigger. (See Figure 6.)
3. The gun is released and the operator walks to the front of the car body to remove a fixture that retracts to a position above the conveyor. The operator walks back to the rear of the body.
4. The operator grasps the C-type gun and uses it to weld the roof panel at the opening for the rear window. Approximately 10 welds are made between the left drip rail and the center of the rear window to secure the panel. During this task, the operator uses his right hand to position the electrodes and his left hand to activate the trigger.
5. The operator walks to the front of the car body to obtain the P-type gun for the final set of welds.
6. The P-type gun is used to secure the roof panel above the windshield opening with approximately 10 welds. To make these welds, the right hand is used to position the electrodes and the left hand is used to activate the trigger.
7. The operator grasps the fixture (suspended from a retractor above the assembly line) and walks back to the next unit. He then waits for the right-side operator to deliver the roof so that it can be positioned and secured.

RESULTS OF THE TASK ANALYSIS   The seven tasks performed by the left-side operator are summarized in Table 1. This table also presents the duration of each task (in seconds), and the elapsed time from the beginning of the work cycle. The time data in this table can be used with the results of the posture analysis to identify tasks associated with postural stress.

Table 1   Results of task analysis

Task description	Duration	Elapsed time (sec)
1. Position roof and secure with fixtures	5.6	5.6
2. Spotweld left drip rail	9.8	13.4
3. Release windshield fixture	7.3	22.6
4. Spotweld rear window opening	16.1	38.7
5. Walk to front of unit	4.2	42.9
6. Spotweld windshield opening	8.2	51.2
7. Walk to next unit and move fixtures	17.1	68.3

RESULTS OF POSTURE ANALYSIS   The results of the posture analysis for the
case study job are summarized in Table 2 and Figure 7. Table 3 presents the
posture profiles for the trunk, left shoulder, and right shoulder. Figure 7
presents the results of the task and posture analysis on the same time scale. This
figure can be used to track posture changes over the work cycle and to associate
work posture with specific tasks.

ERGONOMIC CONCERNS   The principal ergonomic concern on this job is the
overhead reach required to operate the trigger of the C-type gun while performing Tasks 2 and 4. The results presented in Figure 7 show that the left shoulder

Table 2   Posture profiles for the trunk and shoulders

	Freq (sec)	Min (sec)	Max (sec)	Mean (sec)	SD (sec)	Total time	% of cycle
Trunk							
Posture							
Neutral	4	2.3	31.4	14.9	13.6	59.5	87
Mild flex	3	1.6	3.7	2.7	1.1	8.0	12
Bent/twist	1	0.5	0.5	0.5	—	0.5	1

Number of posture changes = 8
Avg. time per posture = 8.5 sec
Work cycle duration = 68.1 sec

	Freq (sec)	Min (sec)	Max (sec)	Mean (sec)	SD (sec)	Total time	% of cycle
Left shoulder							
Posture							
Neutral	7	0.9	7.3	4.2	2.5	29.4	43
Mild flex	4	1.1	3.2	2.1	0.9	8.4	12
Bent/twist	3	3.0	16.9	10.8	6.9	30.2	45

Number of posture changes = 14
Avg. time per posture = 4.7 sec
Work cycle duration = 68.1 sec

	Freq (sec)	Min (sec)	Max (sec)	Mean (sec)	SD (sec)	Total time	% of cycle
Right shoulder							
Posture							
Neutral	8	0.5	5.9	3.4	2.2	27.5	40
Mild flex	8	0.7	11.2	4.2	3.8	33.5	49
Bent/twist	2	3.4	3.8	3.6	0.3	7.2	11

Number of posture changes = 18
Avg. time per posture = 3.8 sec
Work cycle duration = 68.1 sec

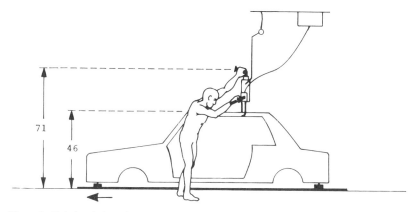

Figure 6   Existing design of workstation (i.e. conveyor height) and welding tool requires shoulder flexion during Task 2. (Dimensions in inches.)

remains in severe flexion for the duration of these two tasks. This extreme overhead reach is caused by a combination of the workstation layout and the design of the spotwelding gun. The height of the car body added to the height of the conveyor places the drip rail and the top of the rear window opening at a height of 46 inches above the floor. (See Figure 6.) The length of the gun, 26.5 inches, from electrode to trigger handle (see Figure 5a), and the fact that it must be held in a nearly vertical orientation, place the trigger handle at the height of about 71 inches above the floor when performing Tasks 2 and 4.

Anthropometric studies of the US civilian population show an average height of 69 inches for males and 63.5 inches for females (36). The corresponding shoulder height is 57 inches for the average male and 52 inches for the average female (14). Because of the difference in handle height and shoulder height, it is necessary during Task 2 to flex the left shoulder to an extreme angle in order to reach and grasp the trigger handle as illustrated in Figure 6. The amount of shoulder flexion is inversely related to the operator's height, i.e. a short person would have to flex the shoulder more than a tall person.

The posture profile presented in Table 2 provides additional insight to the potential shoulder problems on this job. The operator must hold his left shoulder in severe flexion for a total of 30 seconds (approximately 44% of the work cycle). Furthermore, the severe flexion posture is sustained for almost 17 seconds while performing Task 4 (see Figure 7). Due to the highly repetitive nature of this job, the extreme posture of the left shoulder while operating the trigger could result in the development of local muscle fatigue over the course of the workday, and could be a factor in the development of tendinitis and other cumulative trauma disorders (9, 20, 21).

Regarding the shoulder posture required to hold and activate the

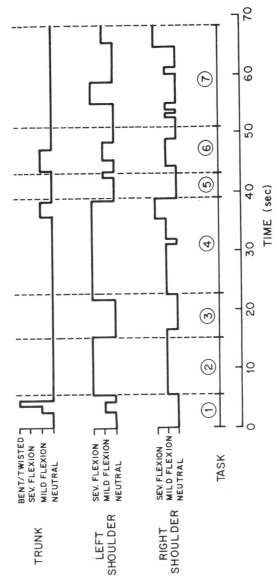

Figure 7 Posture changes at the trunk and shoulders during the work cycle.

trigger, Task 6 presents an interesting contrast to Tasks 2 and 4. Recall from the task description that Task 6 is performed with the P-type gun with the right hand positioning the electrodes and the left hand activating the trigger. Because of the design of the electrodes on the P-type gun (see Figure 5b), it can be held in a nearly horizontal orientation while welding the roof panel to the front wind-shield opening. This places the trigger handle at the height of the roofline, 46 inches, and substantially reduces the stresses on the shoulder.

The remaining instances of severe shoulder flexion occur when the worker handles the welding fixtures for the rear window and windshield openings during Tasks 4 and 7 (see Figure 7). These fixtures must remain clear of the car bodies when not in use, and are therefore suspended above the assembly line between work cycles. An overhead reach with the right hand is required to grasp these fixtures during movement.

In general, the trunk postures required for this job are relatively non-stressful. The posture profile results in Table 2 show that the trunk remains in a neutral position for 87% of the work cycle.

RECOMMENDATION FOR JOB DESIGN   The principal postural stress on this job occurs with use of the C-type gun to weld the roof panel along the drip rail and rear window opening. In order to position the electrodes in the proper orientation for welding, the gun handle is located at a height of 71 inches above the floor. This results in an extreme reach requirement for all but the tallest operators.

The objective of any design change should be to lower the height of the trigger handle relative to the position of the operator. This could be accomplished in several ways. One method would be to lower the height of the assembly line. Another method would be to utilize a P-type gun for Tasks 2 and 4. A third method would be to redesign the trigger handle so that it could be easily grasped without using an extreme posture. The third method is discussed below because it can include design features to accommodate operators of varying body size easily.

An alternative design for the C-type spotwelding gun and trigger mechanism is presented in Figure 8. The major design change is that the standard pistol-grip trigger handle has been replaced by a long cylindrical handle. The trigger button has been replaced by two trigger rings incorporated into the cylindrical handle. Either ring can be pressed from any location around its circumference to activate the gun.

Because the long handle is oriented vertically during use, it can accommodate workers of different heights. Small workers can grasp the handle at a low position whereas tall workers can grasp the handle at a high position. The location of the trigger rings is intended to accommodate workers of different heights. These locations correspond to the elbow heights of the fifth percentile

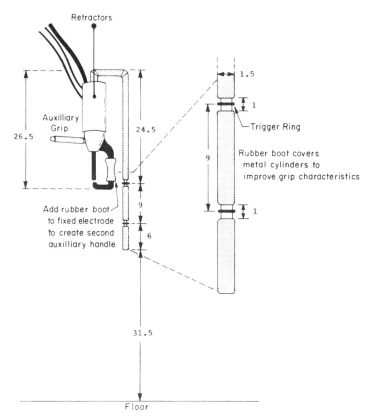

Figure 8 Proposed design for spotwelding gun features long vertical handle and recessed trigger rings. (Dimensions in inches.)

female and ninety-fifth percentile male so that both anthropometric extremes could activate the trigger ring with their trunk and shoulders in a neutral posture with an elbow angle of about 90°. An operator whose body size falls between the two extremes would select the ring that is more comfortable.

In summary, the new design eliminates the awkward posture associated with welding the roof panel along the drip rails and rear window. In addition, it accommodates operators within a wider range of body sizes than does the standard pistol-shaped handle.

Recent Developments in Evaluation of Upper Extremity Stresses

Upper extremity cumulative trauma disorders (CTDs) such as tendinitis, tenosynovitis, ganglionic cysts, and carpal tunnel syndrome are a major cause of lost time on jobs that require hand-intensive work (3). While the etiology of these disorders is quite complex, occupational factors such as highly repetitive hand exertions, forceful hand exertions, and awkward posture of the upper extremities are frequently reported as contributing factors (5a). Frequently, all three factors are present on jobs associated with elevated rates of CTD. Although a critical level for the repetitiveness of hand exertions has not been established, it is generally believed that the risk of CTD can be reduced by controlling the repetitiveness of work (4, 19, 48).

Forces on the tendons and nerves of the upper extremities are related to the magnitude of forces exerted by the hand and to hand posture. In the absence of a critical force level, there is general agreement that force is an important factor in the development of CTD (4, 19, 48). The force of hand exertions can some-times be effectively controlled by reducing the weight of the handled object or changing its size or shape so that it can be gripped at its center of gravity. Weight can also be reduced in some work situations by picking up fewer objects at a time or by lifting with two hands instead of one (5a). Internal muscle forces are lowest when an object can be held in a power grip (e.g. the posture used to grasp a tennis racket or suitcase handle). Four to five times as much force must be exerted to hold objects with a pinch grip than with a power grip (4, 46). Awkward posture such as flexion or extreme extension of the wrist is associated with tenosynovitis of the flexor and extensor tendons in the wrist and with carpal tunnel syndrome (4, 40, 48). Ulnar and radial deviation of the wrist are associated with tenosynovitis at the base of the thumb or "DeQuervain's Disease" (19, 48).

Work posture can usually be controlled through the location and orientation of the work surface or through the design of the object or tool held in the hand (4, 5, 5a). Figure 9 illustrates these relationships for two common handle designs for a powered screwdriver (5). To drive a horizontal screw located at elbow height into a vertical surface, a pistol-shaped tool is preferred because it can be used with a nondeviated wrist *(top left)*. The use of an in-line tool in this situation causes an ulnar deviation *(bottom left)*. To drive a vertical screw located at elbow height into a horizontal surface, the in-line tool is preferred *(bottom center)*. A pistol-shaped tool for this task results in substantial wrist flexion *(top center)*. The pistol-shaped tool is preferred again, however, when driving a vertical screw into a horizontal surface below waist height *(top right)*. The use of an in-line tool in this situation causes flexion or ulnar deviation *(bottom right)*. As these examples illustrate, tool selection is an important method for controlling upper extremity ergonomic stress.

OTHER RISK FACTORS IN OCCUPATIONAL CTD   Other risk factors associated with the development of upper extemity CTDs include mechanical pressure on musculoskeletal tissue or nerves, vibration, low temperature, and the use of

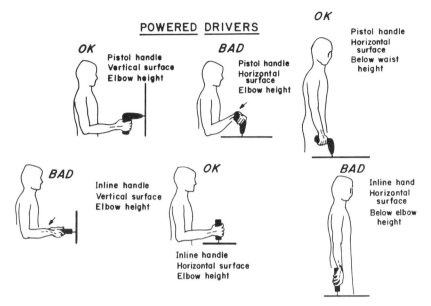

Figure 9   In order to avoid awkward wrist postures, one must consider the nature of the task and the workstation layout in selecting tools (4). The in-line driver is preferred in some situations (*top center, bottom left, bottom right*), whereas the pistol-shaped driver is preferred in other situations (*top left, top right, bottom center*).

gloves. A detailed description of these stresses and the appropriate analysis methods is beyond the scope of this paper. For additional information on this topic, refer to Armstrong (3).

SUMMARY

Ergonomics is the study of people at work to understand the complex relationships among people, machines, job demands, and work methods. All work, regardless of its nature, results in stress. As long as stress is kept within reasonable limits, work performance will be satisfactory and the worker's health and well-being will be maintained. However, if stress is excessive, undesirable outcomes may result in the form of accidents and injuries.

A variety of musculoskeletal injuries and disorders can be caused by physical stress in the work environment. Because of the high medical and compensation costs associated with these problems, it becomes essential in many manufacturing situations to implement programs for controlling physical stress.

An important part of any control program is job evaluation. We have presented several analytical methods for measuring and evaluating physical stress in the workplace. In almost all instances in which it is found to be excessive, stress can be reduced to acceptable levels by applying ergonomic principles to the design of facilities, processes, equipment, tools, and work methods. This design effort should be multidisciplinary, with inputs from medical personnel, engineers, ergonomists, and workers.

Literature Cited

1. Andersson, G., Ortengren, R., Herberts, P. 1977. Quantitative electromyographic studies of back muscle activity related to posture and loading. *Orthop. Clinic. North Am.* 8:85–96
2. Andersson, G. B. J. 1981. Epidemiologic aspects of low-back pain in industry. *Spine* 6(1):53–60
3. Armstrong, T. J. 1985. *Biomechanical Aspects of Upper Extremity Performance and Disorders.* Ann Arbor: Univ. Mich., Dept. Environ. Indust. Health
4. Armstrong, T. J. 1983. *An Ergonomics Guide to Carpal Tunnel Syndrome.* Akron, OH: Am. Indust. Hyg. Assoc.
5. Armstrong, T. J., Foulke, J., Joseph, B., Goldstein, S. 1982. An investigation of cumulative trauma disorders in a poultry processing plant. *Am. Indust. Hyg. Assoc. J.* 43:103–16
5a. Armstrong, T. J., Langolf, G. D. 1983. Ergonomics and occupational safety and health. In *Environmental and Occupational Medicine,* ed. W. N. Rom. Boston: Little, Brown
6. Barnes, R. M. 1968. *Motion and Time Study—Design and Measurement of Work,* pp. 10–20. New York: Wiley. 6th ed.
7. Bureau of National Affairs. 1973. *The Equal Employment Opportunity Act of 1972.* Washington DC: Bur. Natl. Affairs
8. Chaffin, D. B. 1974. Human strength capability and low-back pain. *J. Occup. Med.* 16(4):248–54
9. Chaffin, D. B. 1973. Localized muscle fatigue—definition and measurement. *J. Occup. Med.* 15:346–54
10. Chaffin, D. B., Andersson, G. B. J. 1984. *Occupational Biomechanics.* New York: Wiley
11. Chaffin, D. B., Herrin, G. D., Keyserling, W. M. 1978. Preemployment strength testing. *J. Occup. Med.* 206:403–8
12. Chaffin, D. B., Park, K. S. 1973. A longitudinal study of low-back pain as associated with occupational weight lifting factors. *Am. Indust. Hyg. J.* 34:513–25
13. Corlett, E. N., Madley, S., Manenica I. 1979. Posture targeting: A technique for recording working postures. *Ergonomics* 22:357–66
14. Drillis, R., Contini, R. 1966. *Body Segment Parameters.* Washington DC: USDEW Off. Vocational Rehab.
15. Eastman Kodak Company. 1983. *Ergonomic Design for People at Work,* Vol. 1. Belmont, Calif.: Lifetime Learning Publ.
16. Feldman, R., Goldman, R., Keyserling, W. 1983. Peripheral nerve entrapment syndromes and ergonomic factors. *Am. J. Indust. Med.* 4:661–81
17. Gilbreth, F. B. 1911. *Motion Study.* Princeton, NJ: Van Nostrand
18. Grandjean, E., Vigliani, E. 1983. *Ergonomic Aspects of Visual Display Terminals.* London: Taylor & Francis
19. Greenberg, L., Chaffin, D. B. 1976. *Workers and Their Tools.* Midland, Mich.: Pendell Publishers Press
20. Hagberg, M. 1982. Local shoulder muscular strain—symptoms and disorders. *J. Human Ergology* 11:99–108
21. Hagberg, M. 1984. Occupational musculoskeletal stress and disorders of the neck and shoulder: A review of possible pathophysiology. *Int. Arch. Occup. Environ. Health* 53:269–78
22. Hanman, B. D. 1945. Matching the physical characteristics of workers and jobs. *Indust. Med.* 14(5):405–23
23. Herrin, G. D., Chaffin, D. B., Mach, R. S. 1974. *Criteria for research on the hazards of manual materials handling.* Contract CDC-99-74-118. Cincinnati: US Dept. Health Human Serv. (NIOSH).
24. International Labor Organization. 1962. *Maximum Permissible Weight to be Carried by One Worker.* Geneva: I.L.O. Information Sheet No. 3
25. Deleted in proof
26. Karhu, O., Kansi, P., Kuorinka, I. 1977. Correcting working postures in industry: A practical method for analysis. *Appl. Ergonom.* 8:199–201
27. Kelsey, J., Hardy, R. 1975. Driving of motor vehicles as a risk factor for acute herniated lumbar intervertebral disk. *Am. J. Epidemiol.* 102:63–73

28. Keyserling, W. M., Herrin, G. D., Chaffin, D. B. 1980. Isometric strength testing as a means of controlling medical incidents on strenuous jobs. *J. Occup. Med.* 22(5):332–36

29. Kilbom, A., Persson, J., Jonsson, B. 1985. Risk factors for work-related disorders of the neck and shoulder—with special emphasis on working postures and movements. *Int. Symp. Ergonom. Working Posture, Zadar, Yugoslavia*

30. Koyl, F. F., Marsters-Hanson, P. 1973. *Age, Physical Ability, and Work Potential*. Washington DC: USDOL—Off. Manpower Admin.

31. McCormick, E. J., Sanders, M. S. 1982. *Human Factors in Engineering and Design*. New York: McGraw-Hill. 615 pp.

32. Magora, A. 1970. Investigation of the relation between low back pain and occupation, Part I. *Indust. Med. Surg.* 39:21–37

33. Magora, A. 1970. Investigation of the relation between low back pain and occupation, Part II. *Indust. Med. Surg.* 39:28–34

34. Maynard, H. B., Stegemorten, G. J., Schwab, J. L. 1948. *Methods Time Measurement*. New York: McGraw-Hill

35. Miner, M. G., Miner, J. G. 1978. *Employee Selection within the Law*. Washington DC: Bur. Natl. Affairs

36. Natl. Aeronautics and Space Admin. 1978. *Anthropometric Source Book—Volume 1: Anthropometry for Designers*. Washington DC: NASA Publ. No. 1024

37. Natl. Inst. for Occupational Safety and Health. 1985. *Prevention of Musculoskeletal Injuries: A Proposed Synoptic National Strategy*. Cincinnati: NIOSH

38. Natl. Inst. for Occupational Safety and Health. 1981. *A Work Practices Guide for Manual Lifting*. Cincinnati: Tech. Rep. 81-122, US Dept. Health and Human Serv. (NIOSH)

39. Niebel, B. W. 1982. *Motion and Time Study*, pp. 10–21. Homewood, IL: Irwin. 7th ed.

40. Phalen, G. 1966. The carpal tunnel syndrome. *J. Bone Joint Surg.* 48A:211–18

41. Polish Ergonomics Society. 1979. *Ergonomia* 2(1). 7th Int. Ergonomics Assoc. Congr.

42. Polk, E. J. 1984. *Methods Analysis and Work Measurement*, pp. 1–26. New York: McGraw-Hill

43. Quick, J. H., Duncan, J. H., Malcolm, J. A. 1962. *Work-Factor Time Standards*. New York: McGraw-Hill

44. Schultz, A., Andersson, G., Ortengren, R., Nachemson, A., Haderspeck, K. 1982. Loads on the lumbar spine: Validation of a biomechanical analysis: Measurements of interadiscal pressures and myoelectric signals. *J. Bone Joint Surg.* 64A:713–20

45. Snook, S. H. 1982. Low-back pain in industry. In *Symposium on Idiopathic Low Back Pain*, ed. A. A. White, S. L. Gordon, pp. 23–8. St. Louis: Mosby

46. Swansen, A., Mater, I., Groot, G. 1970. The strength of the hand. *Bull. Prosthet. Res.*, pp. 145–53

47. Taylor, F. W. 1911. *The Principles of Scientific Management*. New York: Harper

48. Tichauer, E. G. 1966. Some aspects of stress on forearm and hand in industry. *J. Occup. Med.* 8:63–70

Ann. Rev. Public Health. 1986. 7:105–25

CURRENT STATUS AND PROSPECTS FOR SOME IMPROVED AND NEW BACTERIAL VACCINES*

Frederick C. Robbins

Case Western Reserve University School of Medicine, Cleveland, Ohio 44106

John B. Robbins

Laboratory of Developmental and Molecular Immunity, National Institute of Child Health and Human Development, Washington DC 20418

INTRODUCTION

In this essay, we review some new bacterial vaccines, prospects for modification and improvement of existing products, and the implication of recent insights into the pathogenic mechanisms of bacterial infection that may have an impact on the development of products for immunoprophylaxis. This subject has been recently reviewed (1–4).

Innovation in the prevention of bacterial diseases by immunologic methods was in the doldrums for many years. Only two classes of bacterial vaccines were available until about a decade ago: toxoids for the prevention of toxin-mediated diseases, namely diphtheria and tetanus toxoids, and whole-cell vaccines for the prevention of pertussis, typhoid, anthrax, and plague. The efficacy of whole-cell bacterial vaccines has been questioned, and their standardization and reproducibility of production have been difficult to achieve.

An important advance in the prevention of bacterial diseases by immunologic methods evolved from the studies in the late 1930s by Felton and Macleod and their associates, using vaccines composed of the purified capsular polysacchar-

---

ides of pneumococci (5, 6). The advent of antibotics in the 1940s seemed to diminish interest in the subject because of the widespread notion that control of bacterial diseases had been achieved. Yet, a reexamination of the problems of pneumococcal and hospital-acquired infections, by Austrian and Finland and their associates, showed that the availability of antibiotics had not solved all the problems of bacterial diseases (7, 8). The elderly were found to be at particular risk, as were the increasing numbers of patients admitted to the hospital for extensive surgical and/or chemotherapeutic treatment. Many of the bacterial infections in these populations were caused by organisms that do not usually cause disease. Microorganisms resistant to a wide range of antibiotics have emerged. Thus, interest has rekindled in immunoprophylaxis of bacterial diseases.

Another important factor in this resurgence of interest in immunologic methods for the prevention of bacterial diseases has been the advances in our knowledge about virulence and immuno-protective factors of bacteria and the acquired immune mechanisms in the host that confer resistance.

PROSPECTS FOR IMPROVED DIPHTHERIA AND TENTANUS TOXOIDS

The success of toxoids, prepared by formalin inactivation of the exotoxins of *Corynebacterium diphtheriae* and *Clostridium tetani,* for the prevention of diphtheria and tetanus has been extraordinary. Diphtheria and tetanus have been recorded rarely in persons who have been properly immunized with these toxoids. Yet, there is a problem, albeit minor, whose solution could result in even more effective diphtheria and tetanus toxoid vaccines: Adverse reactions, primarily local but occasionally systemic, follow the use of these toxoids when administered to previously immunized older children and adults. The reactions, which are of the immediate-type hypersensitivity, are largely due to the small amount of nontoxoid antigens in the vaccine. These impurities are not removed by current methods of preparation of either toxoid because formalin is added to the intermediate products during the purification process to detoxify these lethal toxins. Formalin is an active compound and this treatment of the partially purified toxins results in the production of heterogeneous polymers that cannot be easily purified by commercial processes. Because of the adverse reactions produced by these minor impurities, the amount of toxoid that can be administered in one injection is limited. Since the antitoxin response (protective toxin-neutralizing antibodies) is directly related to the dose of toxoid administered, satisfactory immunization requires two or three injections in order to induce a protective response in most infants and children. It would be an important step, particularly for use in the developing countries, where tetanus and diptheria still account for many deaths, to have vaccines free of impurities that could be given at higher doses so that one or possibly two injections might be sufficient for a primary immunization. Two promising approaches toward this objective are being pursued.

One approach is the result of the discovery by Pappenheimer and his associates of a mutant strain of *C. diphtheriae* that is nontoxic but produces a protein CRM (cross-reacting mutant) 197, that is identical to diphtheria toxin except for a missense mutation in its A fragment (9). The CRM 197 protein is antigenically indistinguishable from the native toxin. Despite the fact the CRM 197 protein is nontoxic, formalinization is required in order to make it of comparable immunogenicity to the toxoid, presumably because the native protein is degraded by tissue enzymes more rapidly than the denatured product (10). Another mechanism to explain the enhancement of immunogenicity that follows treatment by formalin is that the native CRM 197 binds and preferentially reacts with nonlymphoid cells. Formalinization may reduce the binding specificity, thus making it more available to stimulate lymphocytes. *C. diphtheriae* strains have been constructed that produce high yields of the CRM 197 (11, 12). CRM 197 can be purified easily and economically by column chromatography to provide a highly purified diphtheria antigen that is less reactive and can be given safely in larger amounts and thus immunize with fewer doses than those required for the presently available toxoid. Its commercial possibilities are being actively explored.

Genetic manipulation of *C. tetani* is still under study, and CRMs of this strain are not yet available. However, affinity chromography is providing an approach to an improved tetanus toxoid vaccine. Tetanus toxin has been shown to interact with gangliosides of neural and other cells and most efficiently with the ganglioside GMD (13). Svennerholm and associates have been able to obtain this ganglioside in significant amounts and to affix it to an insoluble matrix. This method of preparing an affinity resin can now be used selectively to adsorb tetanus toxin from the culture filtrate of *c. tetani* (following fermentation) (14). The toxin can be dissociated from the affinity column free of other proteins of *C. tetani*. The resultant product has been shown to be a homogeneous protein. Toxoid prepared from this material has been found to be a superior immunogen to the one prepared by conventional means. Its clinical effectiveness is under study.

These advances have been made possible by the new techniques of genetic manipulation and affinity chromotography. Vaccines prepared by these methods will probably be more effective than those presently in use, require fewer injections, and be less costly.

PERTUSSIS VACCINES

Pertussis (whooping cough), a respiratory disease caused by *Bordetella pertussis,* remains a common and serious affliction throughout the world wherever pertussis vaccine is not in wide use. A vaccine composed of whole-inactivated

B. pertussis cells has been available since the 1940s and has proven effective in controlling pertussis. For instance, in the United States, only about 1000 to 2000 cases of pertussis, with about 30 deaths, are recorded each year, as compared to approximately 150,000 cases recorded in the early 1940s (15, 16). The vaccine is estimated to be 90% effective (15). In spite of its effectiveness, pertussis vaccine has posed special problems for control agencies and public health services. The whole-cell vaccine contains a large assortment of antigens. Until recently, little was known about which of these were significant in pathogenesis and immunity. Likewise, assessing protective immunity in the host has not been possible. This lack of understanding about the pathogenesis of and immunity to pertussis was the basis for the difficulty of assessing the composition of whole-cell vaccines for controlling and regulating the manufacture of pertussis vaccine. The standard test for vaccine potency is conducted in mice. Animals are immunized by intraperitoneal administration of varying dilutions of the vaccine to be tested. After an interval of two weeks the mice are inoculated intracerebrally with a lethal dose of live, virulent organisms. The amount of vaccine required to protect 50% of animals is calculated and expressed in a standardized fashion. The mouse potency test has been shown to have a relationship to the efficacy of the vaccine in humans and has served as the standard test for potency (17). Recent evidence suggests that it is a more relevant test than many had thought. *B. pertussis* organisms do not invade the substance of the mouse brain following the intracerebral challenge but localize on the ciliated ependymal cells; death occurs presumably as a result of the toxin elaborated by these bacteria. Support for this hypothesis is provided by the demonstration that passive immunization with monoclonal or polyclonal antipertussis toxin antibodies can protect mice inoculated intracerebrally with virulent organisms (18–20).

The most troublesome aspect of the pertussis vaccine has been the reactions experienced by children postinoculation. Fortunately, most of the reactions have not been serious, although some can be alarming, such as screaming fits that sometimes occur within a few hours after inoculation. Less frequently convulsions are seen. These reactions, alarming as they may be, have not been associated with sequelae (21). However, very rarely, in the order of 1 in 300,000–500,000 doses administered, recipients do experience an encephalopathy severe enough to produce long-term neurologic impairment (22). Although public health authorities and most physicians regard the risk-benefit ratio to be such that routine immunization should be continued, they also consider the rate of reactions to be undesirably high and the development of a less reactive product an urgent matter. The public is aware of the situation. In some countries where the dangers have been widely publicized, rates of vaccination have fallen to such low levels that epidemics of pertussis have occurred for the first time in many years (22–24).

Recently, prompted by public concern about the safety of the pertussis vaccine and the availability of the new techniques of molecular biology, there has been renewed interest in studying the pathogenesis of the disease and the development of safer and more effective vaccines. The direction of recent research has been much influenced by the ideas of Pittman, who, in 1979, on the basis of the information available then, proposed that pertussis was an infection localized to the respiratory tract and that the symptoms characteristic of whooping cough (systemic manifestations and the whooping characteristic of pertussis) were due to a toxin[1] elaborated by the bacterium (25, 26). The evidence cited by Pittman supplemented by newer data provide impressive support for her hypothesis that pertussis is a toxin-mediated disease. This evidence is summarized below.

B. pertussis attaches only to the cilia of the respiratory epithelial cells. The organism does not invade the tissues of the host. Although in the natural infection only the respiratory tract is involved, experimentally, *B. pertussis* also attaches to other ciliated cells, in the central nervous system and in the Fallopian tubes (27). Following its affixation to the respiratory mucosa, *B. pertussis* elicits symptoms of an upper respiratory infection. At this stage, the organism is readily recovered from the patient. The nonspecific respiratory symptoms progress in severity and gradually over several weeks develop into the typical clinical syndrome of whooping cough. By this time, the characteristic elevation of the peripheral blood lymphocytes is evident, but the organism can rarely be recovered from the patient. Early treatment of the noncharacteristic upper respiratory infection stage, by antibiotics shown to be effective in vitro against *B. pertussis,* can reduce the severity of pertussis. Treatment with these antibiotics is ineffective, however, when the classic symptoms of pertussis are evident (28–30).

Pertussis can be prolonged, lasting several months, and in many instances, the symptoms reappear with the acquisition of another unrelated respiratory pathogen.

These features of pertussis are all characteristic of a toxin-mediated disease. Symptoms caused by toxins usually occur distant from the site of infection and are unaffected by treatment with antibiotics once the toxin has affixed to the cells and exerted its metabolic effect. Toxin-mediated diseases are prolonged, and their duration depends presumably upon the duration of the life of intoxicated cells. Pertussis toxin is lethal for laboratory animals at doses comparable to those of diphtheria and tetanus toxins. It is not cytotoxic, so cells whose metabolism have been altered by this protein can persist for prolonged periods of time. The purified pertussis toxin induces a lymphocytosis in laboratory

---

[1]Pertussis toxin was formerly denoted as lymphocytosis-promoting factor, islet-cell activating factor, histamine-sensitizing factor, pertussingen.

animals that is indistinguishable from that observed in patients with pertussis. The lymphocytosis results from the release of pre-formed cells from the bone marrow and lymph nodes (31). These cells remain in the circulation probably because they have acquired a defective "homing" activity. The lymphocytosis of pertussis is the best evidence for the systemic release of pertussis toxin during clinical pertussis.

Pertussis toxin has been isolated in homogeneous form, and its mode of action has been characterized to a considerable degree (32). Many of the systemic effects of clinical pertussis as well as the numerous biologic activities exerted by the *B. pertussis* in laboratory animals can be elicited by the purified toxin. Pertussis toxin is a mitogen and a hemagglutinin, and it has enzymatic activity with specificity for its cell substrate similar to that of cholera toxin. It is composed of subunits with different structures and functions. The subunit denoted S-1 has ADP ribosylation activity. This enzymatic activity is directed toward a cell membrane regulatory protein called N1 that normally responds to external inhibitory compounds such as prostaglandins and adrenalin; following ADP ribosylation it is no longer reactive and thus the intoxicated cell is not subject to regulation by inhibitory hormones.

The other peptides of pertussis toxin are involved in the attachment to cell surfaces such as erythrocytes (hemagglutination). The specificity of this cell-binding activity has not been fully elucidated, but preliminary evidence indicates that the toxin has specificity for the complex mannose-containing oligosaccharide that is linked to asparagine residues. The *N*-acetyl glucosamine component of this mannose-containing peptide seems to be the critical binding moiety (32, 33).

For years it has been known that *B. pertussis* cells or partially purified supernates of cultures of *B. pertussis* exerted remarkable and different biologic activities, all of which can be initiated by the purified pertussis toxin. The most convincing evidence that pertussis toxin is released into the systemic circulation is provided by these effects upon organ systems other than the respiratory tract. The most characteristic systemic effect is the unusual and almost unique lymphocytosis that regularly accompanies clinical pertussis and can be repro-duced experimentally (31). Pertussis also affects glucose regulation, a phenom-enon extensively studied in experimental animals in which there appears to be an altered glucose-insulin relationship in the islet cells following their interac-tion with pertussis toxin (34–37). It is of interest that this toxicity of pertussis toxin can be potentiated by exposure of experimental animals to conditions that increase their adrenalin secretion or by actual administration of adrenalin or its analogues. The encephalopathy that may occur in infants after clinical pertussis and rarely after administration of whole-cell pertussis vaccines has been pro-posed to be due to hypoglycemia and/or to altered glucose regulation caused by the toxin (38).

Thus it is evident that any effective vaccine against pertussis must contain the toxin (as its toxoid). However, the extent to which pertussis toxin is responsible for the various reactions to the current whole-cell vaccine is still uncertain. Furthermore, debate remains about whether or not the toxoid molecule is all that is needed to confer immunity or whether other components of the *B. pertussis* cell are required in order to achieve full protection.

One of the other candidates for inclusion in the vaccine is the filamentous hemagglutinin (FHA). This protein, which has high specific hemagglutinating activity for mammalian cells, is composed of a number of identical 22,000 molecular weight subunits. When injected as a purified substance, it does not induce protection in mice against the intracerebral challenge, nor does passive immunization with monoclonal or polyclonal antibodies to this protein confer protection (18–20, 37). Yet, there has been interest in using this protein for at least two reasons:

1. An aerosol challenge model in laboratory mice has been devised by several laboratories. This model has many features of the respiratory disease as it occurs in humans, despite the fact that *B. pertussis* is truly pathogenic only for the latter. Active immunization with FHA or passive immunization with monoclonal antibodies to FHA induces an incomplete but definite protective response against pulmonary infection in the aerosol challenge model (18–20).
2. Sato & Sato have reported that the addition of FHA increases the effectiveness of pertussis toxin to induce immunity to the aerosol challenge model (20).

Much remains to be known about the FHA protein in the pathogenesis of disease. Although it is a hemagglutinin, its role in facilitating attachment of the organism to the cilia is yet undefined. The FHA can be purified and is highly immunogenic in laboratory animals.

Another candidate for inclusion in the vaccine is the pilus (fimbriae) of *B. pertussis,* which is another protein that is located at the surface of the bacterial cell. Several indirect experiments have suggested that attachment of *B. pertussis* to cilia is mediated by this surface protein (30). Although the evidence is incomplete at the time of writing, it has been proposed that antibodies to these fimbriae are the "agglutinogens" that have been indirectly correlated with effectiveness of the vaccine and convalesence from disease (17). The degree of antigenic heterogeneity of fimbriae is not yet determined. The protective effect of fimbriae in the mouse potency assay or aerosol challenge model is under study. The antigenic diversity and in vitro protective effects of this *B. pertussis* component requires further study, but its role in attachment suggests that fimbrae may be another antigen involved in inducing protection against pertussis (39).

In the hopes of producing a safer vaccine, Sato and his collaborators in Japan have led an industrial venture to produce an acellular preparation. Their vaccine is formalin-treated culture supernatant and is composed predominately of pertussis toxin and FHA. It induces comparable levels of antitoxin and anti-FHA antibody as the whole-cell vaccine and passes a modified mouse potency test (40). This vaccine has been administered to three to four million children, with only a few minor side reactions. At the time of writing, however, there have been no substantial reports of its effectiveness against disease. So far the vaccine has been administered only to two- to three-year-olds and not in infancy, the routine age for immunization against pertussis in most of the world.

The most difficult problem involved in introducing a new pertussis vaccine will be testing for clinical effectiveness. Curiously, our currently-used whole-cell vaccines have never been studied for their effectiveness by a case-controlled placebo method such as has been used to evaluate new viral and other bacterial vaccines. Effectiveness was assessed by comparison of attack rates of clinical pertussis among vaccinated and unvaccinated children exposed to cases within the home or to other conditions of intimate contact where the incidence among the controls can be expected to be high (17). A placebo control trial of a new pertussis vaccine is complicated by the ethical problem of having an effective pertussis vaccine already available as well as by the practical problem that there is very low incidence of clinical disease in this country. Some difficult decisions will have to be made soon by those responsible for licensure of vaccines as to what can be regarded as acceptable evidence for efficacy and effectiveness of new pertussis vaccines, since a high priority is placed by society upon the development of a less reactive preparation.

VACCINES COMPOSED OF BACTERIAL CAPSULAR POLYSACCHARIDES FOR THE PREVENTION OF INVASIVE DISEASES DUE TO ENCAPSULATED BACTERIA

Pneumococci, meningococci, and *Haemophilus influenzae* type b account for the majority of invasive diseases due to bacteria occurring in otherwise healthly individuals. The capsular polysaccharides of these encapsulated bacteria are essential for their virulence, which is due to the inhibition of the action of complement upon the surface of the bacteria. Immunity to invasive diseases caused by these organisms, therefore, requires the action of specific antibodies to initiate protective complement reactions. Only low levels of serum antibodies are required to confer immunity. Most polysaccharide antigens are good immunogens in healthy adults and regularly elicit protective levels of antibodies (1–4). These polysaccharides, however, fail to induce protective levels of antibodies in infants and young children, who suffer the highest attack rate of invasive disease due to encapsulated bacteria (41, 42). The immunologic properties of capsular polysaccharides differ from those of proteins such as toxoids and viral vaccines and have been conveniently termed "T-independent." Thus, reinjection of most polysaccharides does not result in booster or recall responses. The complex immunologic properties of polysaccharide vaccines is illustrated in Table 1.

Meningoccal Vaccines

There are now 11 serologically and chemically distinct capsular polysaccharides of the meningococci, called group-specific antigens (2, 41). Most meningoccocal disease is caused by meningococci-bearing serogroups A, B, and C; the remaining 10% of isolates from patients are of serogroup Y or W-135. Epidemics of meningoccal meningitis, such as occurred in Brazil and Finland in 1973 or which occur almost annually in the "meningitis" belt of Central and West Africa, have been caused by group A organisms. Group B organisms usually cause endemic meningitis but also may be the cause of unusually high attack rates of meningitis such as have occurred in Spain, Norway, and in South Africa in the past decade. Group C organisms cause endemic meningitis and were mainly responsible for the outbreaks of meningitis that occurred in Armed Forces recruits in the US during the late 1950s and the 1960s. The severity of meningitis caused by these serogroups is similar (2, 42–44).

A vaccine composed of serogroups A, C, W-135, and Y capular polysaccharides is currently in use. It induces bactericidal serum antibodies to the four capsular polysaccharides and has been shown to be safe and effective in preventing meningitis due to these serogroups under certain conditions:

1. Group C polysaccharide fails to elicit protective levels of antibodies in individuals less than two years of age (44).
2. Two doses of the Group A polysaccharide are required in infants and children less than two years of age in order to achieve protective levels of immunity (42–44).
3. Immunity in adults elicited by Group A and C polysaccharides is of long duration. However, in children ages two to approximately six years, antibody levels decline in several years so that a reinjection is required to maintain protective levels (44).
4. The duration of protective immunity in children and adults to Group A is not as long as is that to Group C. The Group A vaccine has been demonstrated to be highly effective in aborting epidemics in Brazil, Finland, and more recently in Nepal. The usefulness of Group A vaccine in Africa and certain other parts of the world may be limited because of the observed decrease in antibody responsiveness to the vaccine of persons who have concurrent

Table 1 Serum antibody responses elicited in humans by five representative bacterial capsular polysaccharide vaccines

Polysaccharide	Age-related response	Effect of reinjection
Pneumococcus type 3	Adult levels in infancy	No booster
H. influenzae type b	Slight response up to 18 mo, adult levels at 6 yr	No booster
Group A meningococcus	No response after first injection up to 2 yr. Adult levels at 6 yr	Booster after second injection up to 2 yr; thereafter no booster
Group C meningococcus	Response in infancy, protective levels at 2 yr. Adult levels at 6 yr	Suppression after second injection up to 18 mo; thereafter, no effect
Group B meningococcus & *E. coli* K1	Not studied in infants or children. Only 1/50 adults responded	Not studied

malaria or other chronic diseases that result in decreased immunologic responsiveness (43).

An important problem under active investigation concerning the polysaccharide vaccines generally is to find ways to increase their immunogenicity and confer the property of T-dependence, particularly in infant age groups and in adults with acquired immunodeficiency. The principal approach to this problem is to bond the polysaccharide chemically to an immunogenic and T-cell dependent protein. Various proteins and chemical means of binding have been explored and some promising results achieved with meningococcal, *H influenza type b* and pneumococcal polysaccharides *(vide infra)* (1–3, 45).

A special problem is the poor immunogenicity of the Group B meningococcal polysaccharide. The reasons for this are not well understood, but at least three factors may be involved, singly or together.

1. The Group B polysaccharide has been found to have similarities chemically to many of the sialic acid residues of ganglioside and glycoproteins, including recently discovered glycoproteins of fetal brain. This close relationship to "self" antigens may influence its antigenicity (46, 47).
2. Group B polysaccharide, a linear homopolymer of alpha 2→8 nacetylneuraminic acid, is more readily degraded by mammalian enzymes than the other capsular polysaccharides.
3. Finally, Group B polysaccharide seems to have a less stable tertiary structure than the other polysaccharides (48).

The problem with the Group B polysaccharides has stimulated a search for alternative surface components for this meningoccccal capsular antigen and for other encapsulated bacteria. Two groups of investigators have studied the immunogenicity of the major outer-membrane protein of Group B meningoccoci (49, 50). This protein is polymorphic within Group B organisms. At least 15 antigenic variants have been described, but only a few, including types 2 and 15, are responsible for most invasive disease due to Group B organisms; the other antigenic variants are most often isolated from asymptomatic carriers. Recently both laboratories have devised methods for increasing the immunogenicity of these membrane proteins so that they will regularly induce bactericidal antibodies in vaccinees. Clinical studies with these more immunogenic antigens are eagerly awaited.

Pneumococcal Vaccine

Since its licensure in the United States in 1977, the 14-valent pneumococcal vaccine has been the subject of increasing study. Based on a collaborative study that included the World Health Organization (WHO), a new, more comprehensive 23-valent formulation was recommended and licensed in the United

States and several other countries (1–3, 51). The choice of the 23 types was based upon an extensive surveillance involving over 13,000 isolates from patients and upon physicochemical and immunologic studies of the pneumococcal polysaccharides, with special reference to the cross-reactive types within groups. A series of studies, published by the Centers for Disease Control and investigators at Yale University, have confirmed the effectiveness of pneumococcal vaccine in the adult population (52, 53). Yet, the pneumococcal vaccine, similar to other polysaccharide vaccines, has limitations that have discouraged its routine use in populations at risk. The first limitation is its lack of immunogenicity in two groups at risk. The pneumococcal types that most frequently cause invasive diseases in children, especially those at unusually high risk, such as sickle-cell anemia and other patients with splenic deficiencies, fail to induce protective levels of antibodies in these subjects up to six years of age (54). Second, the pneumococcal vaccine fails to elicit protective levels of antibodies in patients with primary or acquired immune deficiencies, especially those involving malignancies of the lymphoid system treated with cytotoxic drugs such as Hodgkin's Disease (53, 55). These latter patients probably constitute much of the at-risk population for pneumococcal disease and its complications in the United States (56).

Two approaches have been used to improve the pneumococcal vaccine. The first is similar to that reported for *H. influenzae* type b, pneumoccocal type 6A, and meningoccocal polysaccharides Group C and Group A. Several pneumococcal polysaccharides, including pneumococci type 3 and type 6, have been covalently attached to T-dependent carrier proteins (1, 3, 45, 57). Pneumococcous type 6 is particularly important because it is the least immunogenic of the pneumococcal types in the vaccine and because it is such a frequent cause of pneumococcal disease in infants and adults (51, 53, 57). A pneumococcal type 6 tetanus toxoid protein conjugate was shown to have considerably increased immunogenicity over the polysaccharide alone when injected into adult volunteers (58). It is likely that clinical studies involving protein-polysaccharide conjugates of the critical pneumoccocal types will be conducted in infants and children and in patients with immunodeficiencies in the near future. Other carrier proteins of medical interest, such as *Escherichia coli* enterotoxins (heat-labile cholera-like toxin), *Campylobacter jejuni,* and other pertinent toxins, could serve as carrier proteins for the numerous pneumococcal polysaccharides that will be required to have an effective vaccine against pneumococcal disease in adults.

A second approach to preventing pneumoccocal disease by immunologic methods has been advocated by Briles and his associates (59). Briles recalled the observations of Tillett et al, who reported that an increase in immunity in rabbits and other laboratory animals to encapsulated pneumococci could be achieved by immunization with unencapsulated pneumococci. Briles showed that antibodies to phosphocholine could protect mice against lethal infection with several pneumococcal types. It is likely that the phosphocholine monoclonal antibodies will react with the cell wall polysaccharide of pneumococcus 4 (C-polysaccharide) that is present in all pneumococci. The C-polysaccharide contains phosphocholine, and protective phosphocholine antibodies have been shown to react with purified preparations of C-polysaccharide (60). Work is now underway in several laboratories to prepare the C-polysaccharide in a manner suitable for clinical investigation. It is possible that this vaccine could confer a species specific immunity to all pneumococci or, possibly, could act synergistically with capsular polysaccharide antibodies.

Haemophilus Influenza Type B (Hib)

Hib is the cause of several diseases, of which meningitis poses the most serious public health problem. Hib meningitis has been estimated to occur in about 1:250 to every 300 live births in the United States (61, 62). In some populations, such as patients with sickle-cell anemia, Alaskan Eskimos, and Navajo Indians, the attack rate of H. influenzae is higher (63, 64). The age distribution is similar to that reported by Fothergill & Wright in 1933; most of the cases occur in children between three months and two years of age, with the peak incidence ranging from about 6 to 15 months (1–4, 65). This age distribution is directly related to the prevalence of bactericidal antibodies in the general population. Newborns and adults have preexisting antibodies and therefore are immune. When the level of maternally acquired antibodies in the newborn falls to nonprotective levels due to catabolism, then the infants become susceptible. Bactericidal antibodies appear in the circulation of healthly children at about two to three years of age with increasing frequency and titer so that virtually all children have bactericidal antibodies at age five or six years. Most of the antibodies are directed toward the capsule and are stimulated by asymptomatic carriage with the homologous organism or by a continued interaction with cross-reacting nonpathogenic bacteria (66, 67). Capsular polysaccharide antibodies are protective in vitro and in laboratory animals (68, 69). The Hib polysaccharide (Hib Ps) has been purified and clinical trials have verified its effectiveness in preventing meningitis in children over the age of two years of age (1–3, 70, 71). It is precisely at this age that the polysaccharide begins to stimulate protective levels of antibodies in most recipients. By the time this article is published, the Hib Ps will probably be licensed and recommended for universal immunization of children at two years of age in the US (62). The use of the Hib Ps is based upon its excellent safety and effectiveness record and the morbidity and mortality of Hib diseases. The duration of this vaccine-induced immunity is at least one year, but it is still under study. Studies have shown that immunization with Hib Ps does not interfere with the natural age-related acquisition of Hib Ps antibodies (72, 73).

As with the pneumococcal and meningococcal polysaccharides, Hib Ps fails both to induce protective levels of antibodies in infants and young children and to induce a booster response. A considerable increase in immunogenicity and the property of T-cell dependence (booster effect) have been conferred on this antigen by preparing covalent conjugates with carrier proteins (57, 58, 74, 75). Several approaches have been used and have shown promise for conferring protective immunity in infants to Hib diseases. Studies with conjugates prepared with tetanus toxoid have shown that simultaneous injection of the carrier protein with the conjugate accelerates the polysaccharide antibody response (57). This indicates that polysaccharide protein conjugates composed of carrier proteins such as tetanus and diphtheria toxoid are compatible with our existing DPT formulation. Therefore, our future DTP will probably contain Hib and possibly other polysaccharide protein conjugates designed to prevent invasive diseases due to this organism in infancy.

PREVENTION OF HOSPITAL-ACQUIRED DISEASES CAUSED BY GRAM-NEGATIVE BACTERIA

Gram-negative organisms constitute a majority of the agents of the severe bacteremic infections associated with hospitalization and with certain chronic disease (7). The diversity of gram-negative species responsible for serious hospital-acquired infections and their serologic heterogeneity pose problems for immunoprophylaxis using capsular antigens or outer-membrane proteins. Another approach to active or passive immunization against gram negative bacteremia has been taken by Braude and McCabe and their associates (76, 77). These investigators noted that lipopolysaccharides (LPS or endotoxins) of most gram-negative bacteria have an antigenically-related core region. LPS are complex structures located in the outer membrane of gram-negative bacteria and are composed of three domains. The first domain, extending out from the bacterial surface, is the O-specific polysaccharide side chain. Antibodies to the O-specific side chain exert complement-dependent opsonic and bactericidal reactions. The wide antigenic diversity of these side chains and the presence of many gram-negative bacterial pathogens whose LPS do not contain these O-specific side chains make this region unsuitable as vaccine. The second domain of the LPS is the "core" region, which is structurally and antigenically similar in Enterobacteriaceae. The core region contains ketodeoctonate (KDO) and ethanolamine. Antibodies to this core region cross-react serologically with most-gram negative pathogens (78). The third domain is designated as lipid A composed of glucosamine dimers with fatty acids attached by ester and amide linkages. The lipid A is the portion of the LPS responsible for insertion of this macromolecule into the outer membrane. Lipid A is also responsible for many of the pharmacological properties of LPS (endotoxins) such as fever, vasomotor collapse, leukopenia, and leukocytosis. The serologic properties of this region of LPS are difficult to evaluate because of the insolubility of the lipid A region, but it is too toxic to be used as primary vaccine. Antibodies to the "core" region exert an "anti-endotoxin" effect, i.e. inhibition of fever and prevention of vasomotor collapse. Several clinical studies have provided evidence that antibodies to this region protect against serious gram-negative infections (76, 79). The alleged protective effects of antibodies directed toward the lipid A region are still controversial, however.

The preparation of LPS-protein conjugates is being investigated. Some LPS have comparatively low molecular weight and are not very immunogenic. The "endotoxic" properties of LPS must be reduced or removed before these molecules can be considered for clinical study. Removal of one or more of their fatty acid constituents reduces the "endotoxicity" of the LPS, thus making them suitable for clinical use (80, 81). The delipidated molecules, however, can no longer form micelles and thus their immunogenicity is considerably reduced. LPS-protein conjugates have been synthesized from so-called "deep" mutants of *Escherichia coli,* including the J5 strain used by Braude and his colleagues. Antibodies induced by this latter strain have been shown to confer protection in patients suffering from gram-negative bacteremia. LPS-protein conjugates have been synthesized and have been found to induce immunity against gram-negative infections of a wide variety of Enterobacteriaceae in laboratory animals.

Another potential use of LPS conjugates is to provide immunity against systemic infections caused by *Neisseria* species. The LPS of Group B meningococci are also being explored as potential vaccines (81). In addition, there is good evidence that LPS antibodies confer protection against invasive diseases caused by *Neisseria gonorrhea.* Preliminary evidence indicates that gonococcal LPS conjugates exert protection in laboratory animals (2).

It is unlikely that *active* immunization with LPS protein conjugates will be useful for hospital-acquired infections. Many patients who are at risk for hospital-acquired infections have therapy-induced immunodeficiencies and cannot be expected to react with a protective immune response. Furthermore, vaccination would have to be given in anticipation of hospitalization to patients expected to be at risk—not a practical procedure. Therefore, these experimental LPS conjugate vaccines probably will be first studied for their ability to elicit protective antibodies that can be used for passive immunization of patients at risk, such as older men undergoing prostatectomy, burned patients, and patients with lymphoid malignancies.

Attenuated Bacteria as Vaccines

A great deal of effort has been directed toward developing attenuated bacterial strains for inducing immunity to bacterial diseases of the intestinal tract (1–3). This development has been stimulated by at least three factors:

1. the failure of parenteral vaccines to induce immunity to enteric disease, such as cholera and shigellosis;
2. new information about the multiplicity of pathogenic mechanisms involved in enteric diseases such as severe diarrheal diseases caused by so-called enteropathogenic *E. coli;*
3. new methods of inducing and characterizing mutants by DNA recombinant technology.

Further, the study of attenuated strains of enteric bacterial pathogens has provided new insights into both the pathogenesis and immunity to these diseases.

Epidemiologic and controlled clinical studies provided evidence that convalescence from cholera confers immunity to further disease caused by this organism. The pathogenesis of the diarrhea of cholera is largely mediated by the cholera exotoxin. The structure of this protein and the mechanism of its toxicity have been elegantly elucidated. The failure of both parenteral immunization with "cholera toxoid" and peroral immunization with this vaccine alone or combined with the LPS of the organism to prevent cholera stimulated Finkelstein and his collaborators to isolate a mutant *Vibrio cholera* strain (from Tor Ogawa strain 3083 designated "Texas Star") that could only synthesize the binding subunits of cholera toxin (82). This mutant induced sustantial immunity against challenge with vibrios of both LPS serotypes in adult volunteers. The "Texas Star" strain, however, induced a mild and unexplained diarrhea in some of the recipients. Kaper and his associates, using this information, generated a *V. cholera* strain with its "tox" gene deleted (83). Unexpectedly, this tox(-) strain also elicited mild diarrhea but did confer an immunity comparable to the "Texas Star" strain in the recipients. The molecular basis for this slight diarrhea is as yet unknown. One possibility might be that the *V. cholera* strains induce a mild diarrhea in association with attachment to the small intestinal mucosa. Another is that *V. cholera* strains may possess more than one toxin; this "other toxin" may be similar or identical to "Shigella toxin." The genome for this toxin has been found in *E. coli* and in other gram-negative enterics, including *V. cholera.* The expression of this toxin and its role in producing diarrheal symptoms in *V. cholera* infection are under study (84).

Knowledge of the principles underlying the development of attentuated bacterial strains for preventing enteric diseases, including enteric fevers and diarrheal diseases, requires basic knowledge of the protective antigens of the microbes and immune mechanisms of the host. The regulation of intestinal antibody synthesis and cell-mediated reactions are not nearly as well characterized as the effects of parenteral immunization. The success of the oral attentuated strains for the prevention of typhoid fever, *S. typhi Ty21A,* should encourage further research on immunization with attentuated strains (1–3). Formal and his colleagues introduced DNA segments from *Shigella dysenteriae* that coded for virulence determinants into the *S typhi Ty21A*. The resultant strain remained virulent and conferred some immunity in volunteers against challenge (85–87).

CONCLUSION

We have limited this review to discussion of only some of the prospects for new and improved bacterial vaccines. Other opportunities will be provided by the use of recombinant DNA methods and greater exploitation of monoclonal antibodies and by our rapidly expanding knowledge of immunology. These techniques are only now being applied to the problems of bacterial vaccines, and they have much to offer.

In particular, the questions raised about the safety of the pertussis component of DTP have created a level of concern in the population that could seriously jeopardize the program of childhood immunization as a whole. For this reason, the development and testing of an improved pertussis vaccine assumes unusual importance and should be given first priority and expedited as rapidly as possible within reasonable bounds of safety.

Additionally, based on present technology it should be possible in the foreseeable future to have a multivalent vaccine for primary immunization of infants that contains several polysaccharide protein conjugates, including mennigococcus and *H. influenzae* antigens along with improved, less toxic diptheria and tetanus toxoids and selective pertussis antigens. To this could be added a formalin-killed polio preparation of high potency such as that developed recently in the Netherlands. Such a poly-valent vaccine should provide protection with two doses in infancy, with a booster some years later.

While these developments seem thoroughly possible scientifically, conducting appropriate field trials will present a major problem. Maintaining a manufacturing capacity in this country is also a problem, as most of the major US firms who develop and manufacture vaccines have discontinued this activity. This decline in manufacturing is caused by several factors, including the relatively poor return on investment derived from human vaccines and, perhaps most important, the manufacturer's concern about liability for injury suffered by vaccinees that may or may not have been caused by the vaccine. The frequency of suits and the size of some of the awards are clearly major factors in discouraging industrial research on vaccines and their production.

Finally, safe and effective vaccines are of little value unless they are used. Largely because of the legal requirement for vaccination in order to enter school, the school age population has a high rate of immunization. However, the rates are not so high in preschool children, particularly in certain segments of the population. The scientific and industrial community must develop vaccines of satisfactory effectiveness and safety, and the public health and medical care community must develop delivery systems that are publicly acceptable and reach all elements of the population.

Literature Cited

1. Robbins, J. B., Hill, J. C., Sadoff, J. C., Eds. 1982. *Seminars in Infectious Diseases.* New York: Thieme-Stratton
2. Germanier, R., Ed. 1984. *Bacterial Vaccines.* New York: Academic
3. Robbins, J. B., Schneerson, R., Klein, D., Sadoff, J. C., Eds. 1985. *Ontogeny of Immune Function and Pathogenic Mechanisms Involved in Bacterial Vaccine Development.* Philadelphia: Praeger
4. Sekura, R., Moss, J., Eds. 1985. *Pertussis Toxin.* New York: Academic
5. Ekwurzel, G. M., Simmons, J. S., Dublin, L. I., Felton, L. D. 1938. Studies on immunizing substances in pneumococci. VII. Report on field tests to determine the prophylactic value of a pneumococcus antigen. *Publ. Health Rep.* 53:1877–1900
6. MacLeod, C. M., Hodges, R. G., Heidelberger, M., Bernhard, W. G. 1945. Prevention of pneumococcal pneumonia by immunization with specific capsular polysaccharides. *J. Exp. Med.* 82:445–65
7. McGowan, J. E., Barnes, M. W., Finland, M. 1975. Bacteremia at Boston City Hospital; occurrence and mortality during 12 selected years (1935–1972), with special reference to hospital-acquired cases. *J. Infec. Dis.* 132:316–35
8. Austrian, R., Gold, J. 1964. Pneumococcal bacteremia with especial reference to bacteremia pneumococcal pneumonia. *Ann. Int. Med.* 60:757–76
9. Pappenheimer, A. M., Uchida, T., Harper, A. A. 1972. An immunological study of the diphtheria molecule. *Immunochemistry* 9:881–906
10. Porro, M., Saletti, M., Nencioni, L., Tagliaferri, L., Marsili, I. 1980. Immunogenic correlation between cross-reacting material (CRM 197) produced by a mutant of *Corynebacterium diphtheriae* and diphtheria toxoid. *J. Infect. Dis.* 142:716–24
11. Rappuoli, R., Michel, J. L., Murphy, J. R. 1983. Integration of Corynebacteriophages btox+, wtox+, and ytox+ into two attachment sites on the *Corynebacterium diphtheriae* chromosome. *J. Bacteriol.* 153:1202–10
12. Rappuoli, R., Michel, J. L., Murphy, J. R. 1983. Restriction endonuclease map

of Corynebacteriophage wctox+ isolated from the Park-Williams No. 8 strain of *Corynebacterium diphtheriae. J. Virol.* 45:524–30
13. van Heyningen, W. E. 1974. Gangliosides as membrane receptors for tetanus toxin, cholera toxin and serotonin. *Nature* 249:415–17
14. Tayot, J.-L., Holmgren, J., Svennerholm, L., Lindbad, M., Tardy, M. 1981. Receptor-specific, large-scale purification of cholera toxin on silica beads derivatized with LysoGM1 ganglioside. *Eur. J. Biochem.* 113:241–58
15. Broome, C. V., Fraser, D. W. 1981. Pertussis in the United States, 1979. A look at vaccine efficacy. 144:187–90
16. Mortimer, E. A., Jones, P. K. 1979. Pertussis vaccine in the United States: The benefit-risk ratio. In *Int. Symp. on Pertussis,* ed. C. R. Manclark, J. C. Hill, p. 270. DHEW (NIH) 79–1830. Washington DC: US GPO
17. Armitage, P., Cockburn, W. C., Evans, D. G., Irwin, J. O., Knowelden, A., Standfast, A. F. 1956. Vaccination against whooping cough: Relation between protection in children and results of laboratory tests. *Br. Med. J.* 2:454–62
18. Sato, Y., Izumiya, K., Sato, H., Cowell, J. L., Manclark, C. R. 1981. Role of antibody to leukocytosis-promoting factor hemagglutinin and filamentous hemagglutinin in immunity to pertussis. *Infect. Immun.* 31:1223–31
19. Munoz, J. J., Arai, H., Cole, R. L. 1981. Mouse-protecting and histamine-sensitizing activities of pertussigen and fimbrial hemagglutinin from *Bordetella pertussis. Infect. Immun.* 32:243–50
20. Sato, H., Ikto, A., Chiba, J., Sato, Y. 1984. Monoclonal antibody against pertussis toxin: Effect on toxin activity and pertussis infections. *Infect. Immun.* 46: 422–28
21. Cody, C. L., Baraff, L. J., Cherry, J. D., Marcy, S. M., Manclark, C. R. 1981. The nature and rates of adverse reactions associated with DTP and DT immunizations in children. *Pediatrics* 68:650–60
22. Committee on Safety of Medicines, Joint Committee on Vaccination and Immu-

nization. 1981. *Whooping Cough*, Chap. 3, pp. 25–75. London: HMSO
23. Kanai, K. 1980. Japan's experience in pertussis epidemiology and vaccination in the past thirty years. *Jpn. J. Med. Sci. Biol.* 33:107–43
24. Trollfors, B. 1984. *Bordetella pertussis* whole cell vaccines—Efficacy and toxicity. *Acta Pediatr. Scand.* 73:417–25
25. Pittman, M. 1979. Pertussis toxin: The cause of the harmful effects and prolonged immunity of whooping cough. A hypothesis. *Rev. Infect. Dis.* 1:401–12
26. Pittman, M. 1984. The concept of pertussis as a toxin-mediated disease. *Pediatr. Infect. Dis.* 3:467–86
27. Robbins, J. B. 1984. Towards a new vaccine for pertussis. In *Microbiology* pp. 176–83. Washington DC: Am. Soc. Microbiol.
28. Whooping Cough Subcommittee of the Antibiotics Clinical Trials. 1963. Treatment of whooping cough with antibiotics. *Br. Med. J.* 1:1110–12
29. Bass, J. W., Klenk, E. L., Kotheimer, J. B., Linneman, C. C., Smith, M. D. 1969. Antimicrobial treatment of pertussis. *J. Pediatr.* 75:768–81
30. Trollfors, B. 1981. Whooping cough in adults. *Br. Med. J.* 283:696–97
31. Morse, S. L., Morse, J. H. 1976. Isolation and properties of the leukocytosis- and lymphocytosis-promoting factor of *Bordetella pertussis. J. Exp. Med.* 143:1483–1502
32. Tamura, M. K., Nogimori, S., Murai, M., Yajima, K., Ito, T., Katada, M., Ui, M., Ishii, S. 1982. Subunit structure of islet-activating protein, pertussis toxin, in conformity with the A-B model. *Biochemistry* 21:5516–22
33. Sekura, R. D., Zhang, Y.-L., Quentin-Millet, M.-J. 1985. Pertussis toxin: Structural elements involved in the interaction with cells. In *Pertussis Toxin, A Symposium,* ed. R. D. Sekura, J. Moss. New York: Academic
34. Pittman, M., Furman, B. L., Wardlaw, A. C. 1980. *Bordetella pertussis* respiratory tract infection in the mouse: Pathophysiological response. *J. Infect. Dis.* 142:56–66
35. Furman, B. L., Wardlaw, A. C., Stevenson, L. Q. 1981. *Bordetella pertussis*-induced hyperinsulinemia without marked hypoglycemia: A paradox explained. *Br. J. Exp. Pathol.* 62:504–11
36. Katada, T., Ui, M. 1976. Accelerated turnover of blood glucose in pertussis-sensitized rats due to combined actions of endogenous insulin and adrenergic beta-stimulation. *Biochem. Biophys. Acta* 421:57–69

37. Bokoch, G. M., Katada, T., Northrup, J. K., Hewlitt, E. L., Gilman, A. G. 1983. Identification of the predominant substrate for ADP-ribosylation by islet cell activating protein. *J. Biochem.* 258:2072–75
38. Hannik, C. A., Cohen, H. 1979. Changes in plasma insulin concentration and temperature in infants after pertussis vaccination. See Ref. 16, pp. 297–99
39. Ashworth, L. A. E., Irons, L. I., Dorsett, A. B. 1982. Antigenic relationship between serotype-specific agglutinogen and fimbriae of *Bordetella pertussis. Infect. Immun.* 37:1278–81
40. Sato, Y., Kimura, M., Fukumi, H. 1984. Development of a pertussis component vaccine in Japan. *Lancet* 1:122–26
41. Bishop, C. T., Jennings, H. J. 1982. Immunology of polysaccharides. In *The Polysaccharides,* ed. G. O. Aspinall, 1:291–330. New York: Academic
42. Peltola, H. 1983. Meningococcal disease: Still with us. *Rev. Infect. Dis.* 5:71–91
43. Greenwood, B. M. 1984. Selective primary health care: Strategies for control of disease in the developing world. XII. Acute bacterial meningitis. *Rev. Infect. Dis.* 6:S374–S89
44. Gold, R., Lepow, M. L. 1976. Present status of polysaccharide vaccines in the prevention of meningococcal disease. *Adv. Pediatr.* 23:71–93
45. Beuvery, E. C., Rossum, F. V., Nagel, J. 1982. Comparison of the induction of immunoglobulin M and G antibodies in mice with purified pneumococcal type 3 and meningococcal group C polysaccharides and their protein conjugates. *Infect. Immun.* 37:15–22
46. Finne, J., Leinonen, M., Makela, P. H. 1983. Antigenic similarities between brain components and bacteria causing meningitis. Implications for vaccine development. *Lancet* 2:235–37
47. Soderstrom, T., Hansson, G., Larson, G. 1984. The *Escherichia coli* K1 capsule shares antigenic determinants with the human gangliosides GM3 and GD3. *New Eng. J. Med.* 310:726–27
48. Lifely, M. R., Gilbert, A., Moreno, C. 1984. Rate, mechanism, and immunochemical studies of lactonisation in serogroup B and C polysaccharides of *Neisseria meningitidis. Carb. Res.* 134:229–43
49. Wang, L. Y., Frasch, C. E. 1984. Development of a *Neisseria meningitidis* Group B serotype 2b protein vaccine and evaluation in a mouse model. *Infect. Immun.* 46:408–14
50. Zollinger, W. D., Mandrell, R. E., Grif-

fiss, J. M. 1982. Enhancement of immunologic activity by noncovalent complexing of meningococcal Group B polysaccharide and outer membrane proteins. See Ref. 1, pp. 254–62

51. Robbins, J. B., Austrian, R., Lee, C.-J., Rastogi, S. C., Schiffman, G., et al. 1983. Considerations for formulating the second-generation pneumococcal capsular polysaccharide vaccine with emphasis on the cross-reactive types within groups. *J. Infect. Dis.* 148:1136–59

52. Shapiro, E. D., Clemens, J. D. 1985. A controlled evaluation of the protective efficacy of pneumococcal vaccine for patients at risk for serious penumococcal infections. *Ann. Int. Med.* 101:325–40

53. Bolan, G., Broome, C. V., Facklam, R. R., Flikaytis, B. D., Fraser, D. W., Schlech, W. F. 1985. Pneumococcal vaccine efficacy in selected populations in the United States. *Ann. Int. Med.* In press

54. Austrian, R. 1981. Some observations on the pneumococcal vaccine and on the current status of pneumococcus disease and its prevention. *Rev. Infect. Dis.* 3:S1–S7

55. Siber, G. R., Weitzman, S. A., Aisenberg, A. C., Weinstein, H. J., Schiffman, G. 1978. Impaired antibody response to pneumococcal vaccine after treatment for Hodgkin's disease. *New Engl. J. Med.* 299:442–48

56. Recommendation of the Public Health Service Advisory Committee on Immunization Practices. 1981. *Pneumococcal polysaccharide vaccine. Morbid. Mortal Week. Rep.* 30:410–12, 417–19

57. Schneerson, R., Robbins, J. B., Chu, C.-Y., Sutton, A., Vann, W., et al. 1984. Serum antibody responses of juvenile and infant rhesus monkeys injected with *Haemophilus influenzae* type b and pneumococcus type 6A polysaccharide-protein conjugates. *Infect. Immun.* 45:582–91

58. Schneerson, R., Robbins, J. B., Wang, Z., Schlesselman, J. C., Feliciano, O., et al. 1985. Characterization of serum *Haemophilus influenzae* type b and pneumococcus type 6A antibodies elicited by polysaccharide-protein conjugates in adult volunteers. See Ref. 3, In press

59. Briles, D. E., Forman, C., Hudak, S., Clafin, J. L. 1982. Anti-phosphorylcholine antibodies of the T15 idiotype are optimally protective against *Streptococcus pneumoniae. J. Exp. Med.* 156:1177–85

60. Jennings, H. J., Lugowski, C., Young, N. M. 1980. Structure of the complex polysaccharide C-substance from *Strep-tococcus pneumoniae* type 1. *Biochemistry* 19:4712–19

61. Parke, J. C., Schneerson, R., Robbins, J. B. 1972. The attack rate, age incidence, racial distribution and case fatality rate of *Haemophilus influenzae* type b meningitis in Mecklenburg County, North Carolina. *J. Pediatr.* 81:765–69

62. Cochi, S. L., Broome, C. V., Hightower, A. W. 1985. Immunization of US children with *Hemophilus influenzae* type b polysaccharide vaccine. *J. Am. Med. Assoc.* 253:521–29

63. Ward, J. J., Lum, M. K. W., Margolis, H. S. 1981. *Haemophilus influenzae* in Alaskan Eskimos: Characteristics of a population with an unusual incidence of invasive disease. *Lancet* 1:121–25

64. Coulehan, J. L., Michaels, R. H., Hallowell, C., Schults, R., Welty, T. K., Kuo, J. S. C. 1984. Epidemiology of *Haemophilus influenzae* type b disease among Navajo Indians. *Publ. Health Rep.* 99:406–9

65. Fothergill, L. D., Wright, J. 1933. Influenzal meningitis: Relation of age incidence to the bactericidal power of blood against the causal organism. *J. Immunol.* 24:273–84

66. Schneerson, R., Robbins, J. B. 1975. Induction of serum *Haemophilus influenzae* type b antibodies in adult volunteers fed cross-reacting *Escherichia coli* O75:K100:H5. *New Engl. J. Med.* 292:1093–96

67. Insel, R. A., Anderson, P. W. 1982. Cross-reactivity with *Escherichia coli* K100 in human serum anticapsular antibody response of *Haemophilus influenzae* type b. *J. Immunol.* 128:1267–70

68. Schneerson, R., Rodrigues, L. P., Parke, J. C. Jr., Robbins, J. B. 1971. Immunity to *Haemophilus influenzae.* II. Specificity and some biological characteristics of "natural," infection-acquired and immunization-induced antibodies to the capsular polysaccharide of *H. influenzae* type b. *J. Immunol.* 107:1081–89

69. Smith, D. H., Peter, G., Ingram, D. L., Anderson, P. 1975. Responses of children immunized with the capsular polysaccharide of *Haemophilus influenzae* type b. *Pediatrics* 52:637–41

70. Peltola, H., Kayhty, H., Virtanen, M., Makela, P. H. 1984. Prevention of *Haemophilus influenzae* type b bacteremic infections with the capsular polysaccharide vaccine. *New. Engl. J. Med.* 310:1561–66

71. Robbins, J. B., Schneerson, R., Parke, J. C. Jr. 1982. A review of the efficacy trials with *Haemophilus influenzae* type b

polysaccharide vaccines. In *Haemophilus Influenzae: Epidemiology, Immunology, and Prevention of Disease*, ed. S. H. Sell, P. F. Wright, pp. 255–63. Nashville: Vanderbilt Univ. Press

72. Robbins, J. B. 1975. Acquisition of natural and immunization-induced immunity to *Haemophilus influenzae* type b Diseases. *Microbiology*, pp. 400–5. Washington DC: Am. Soc. Microbiol.

73. Kayhty, H., Karanko, V., Peltola, H., Makela, P. H. 1984. Serum antibodies after vaccination with *Haemophilus influenzae* type b capsular polysaccharide and responses to reimmunization: No evidence of immunologic tolerance or memory. *Pediatrics* 74:857–65

74. Schneerson, R., Barrera, O., Sutton, A., Robbins, J. B. 1980. Preparation, characterization and immunogenicity of *Haemophilus influenzae* type b polysaccharide-protein conjugates. *J. Exp. Med.* 152:361–76

75. Anderson, P. 1983. Antibody responses to *Haemophilus influenzae* type b and diphtheria toxin induced by conjugates of oligosaccharides of the type b capsule with the nontoxic protein CRM 197. *Infect. Immun.* 39:233–38

76. Ziegler, E. J., McCutchan, A., Fierer, J., Glauser, M. P., Sadoff, J. C., et al. 1982. Treatment of gram-negative bacteremia and shock with human antiserum to a mutant *Escherichia coli*. *New Engl. J. Med.* 307:1225–1330

77. McCabe, W. R., Kieger, B. E., Johns, M. 1972. Immunization with R mutants of *Salmonella minnesota*. I. Protection against challenge with heterologous gram-negative bacteria. *J. Immunol.* 108:601–10

78. Nelles, M. J., Niswander, C. A. 1984. Mouse monoclonal antibodies reactive with J5 lipopolysaccharide exhibit extensive serological cross-reactivity with a variety of gram-negative bacteria. *Infect. Immun.* 46:677–81

79. Pollack, M., Young, L. S. 1979. Protective activity of antibodies to exotoxin

A and lipopolysaccharide at the onset of *Pseudmonas aeruginosa* septicemia in man. *J. Clin. Invest.* 63:276–86

80. Seid, R. C., Sadoff, J. C. 1981. Preparation and characterization of detoxified lipolysaccharide-protein conjugates. *J. Biol. Chem.* 256:7305–10

81. Jennings, H. J., Lugowski, C., Ashton, F. E. 1984. Conjugation of meningococcal lipopolysaccharide R-type oligosaccharides to tetanus toxoid as route to a potential vaccine against Group B *Neisseria meningitidis*. *Infect. Immun.* 43: 407–12

82. Levine, M. M., Black, R. E., Clements, M. L., Lanata, C., Sears, S., et al. 1984. Evaluation in humans of attenuated *Vibrio cholerae* E. Tor Ogawa strain Texas Star-SR as a live oral vaccine. *Infect. Immun.* 43:515–22

83. Kaper, J. B., Lockman, H., Baldini, M. M., Levine, M. M. 1984. Recombinant nontoxingenic *Vibrio cholerae* strains as attenuated cholera vaccine candidates. *Nature* 308:655–58

84. O'Brien, A., LaVeck, G. D. 1983. Purification and characterization of a *Shigella dysenteriae* 1-like toxin produced by *Escherichia coli*. *Infect. Immun.* 40:675–83

85. Formal, S. B., Baron, L. S., Kopecko, D. J., Washington, O., Life, C. A. 1981. Construction of a potential bivalent vaccine strain: Introduction of *Shigella sonnei* form I antigen into the galE. *Salmonella typhi* Ty21a typhoid vaccine strain. *Infect. Immun.* 34:746–50

86. Tramont, E. C., Chung, R., Berman, S., Keren, D., Kapfer, C., Formal, S. B. 1984. Safety and antigenicity of typhoid-*Shigella sonnei* vaccine (strain 5076–1C). *J. Infect. Dis.* 149:133–36

87. Formal, S. B., Hale, T. L., Kapfer, C., Cogan, J. P., Snay, P. J., et al. 1984. Oral vaccination of monkeys with an invasive *Escherichia coli* K-12 hybrid expressing *Shigella flexneri* 2a somatic antigen. *Infect. Immun.* 46:465–69

Ann. Rev. Public Health. 1986. 7:127–49

LEGAL APPROACHES TO SMOKING DETERRENCE

Diana Chapman Walsh

Health Policy Institute, and School of Public Health, Boston University, Boston, Massachusetts 02215

Nancy P. Gordon

Division of Health Policy, Research, and Education, Harvard University, Cambridge, Massachusetts 02138

As a target of opportunity for public health action, smoking stands alone. The scientific indictment has been so compellingly constructed that it exemplifies how painstaking research can weave around an initially observed correlation, strand-by-strand, a web of causation so ineluctable that all it lacks is "a signed confession from the cigarette" (5). The health and human costs are so clear that most of the 55 million cigarette smokers in the United States freely voice the wish that they could stop. The economic trade-offs are so stark that the present lifetime value of quitting for heavily smoking men under age 45 is about $34,000 in reduced risks of lung cancer, coronary heart disease, and emphysema alone, according to one estimate (47a). And the political situation has evolved to the remarkable point where the Secretary of Health and Human Services in a most ardent free market and antitax administration could float the proposition that the government exact a kind of users' tax on cigarettes, to aid in the funding of the Medicare program (18).

Yet the disturbing observation, from a public health perspective, is how modest and ambivalent the political response has been to a product that annually kills over 300,000 Americans. To claim an equivalent share of lives, the airline industry would have to experience three jumbo jet crashes a day, every day of the year (79). Annual mortality attributable to cigarettes is seven times that of motor vehicle crashes and 100 times the rate for AIDS (49). For public health,

127

0163-7525/86/0510-0127$02.00

then, the target is unmistakable. Less clear, however, is along which of many available avenues the campaign should proceed.

A CLASSIFICATION SCHEME

At a low level of abstraction, smoking policies seem bewilderingly fluid and numerous. But raised to a higher level, they can be sorted into three enduring categories: government instruments, market mechanisms, and persuasive efforts. Our focus is the first: legal actions aimed at reducing the incidence, prevalence, intensity—and the harmful effects—of cigarette smoking. Employing the machinery of government, these actions are imposed by a politically organized society and are (or can be) enforced by threat of punishment, even if only vaguely implied. We confine our attention to the United States, and commend for an international perspective Ruth Roemer's monograph, available through the World Health Organization (51).

Some legal interventions aim directly at reducing smoking, while others work more indirectly by creating or enhancing market mechanisms or mobilizing persuasive efforts. These distinctions are summarized in Table 1. The growing number of restrictions on smoking in public places represent the direct approach; they foreclose opportunities to smoke. This both reduces the number of hours in a day available for smoking and (the primary emphasis) limits the "involuntary smoker's" exposure to "second-hand smoke." Less overtly it may also change the social norms, gradually transforming smoking into a deviant act (46).

Approaches working indirectly through the market increase the costs of cigarettes at any point from production, manufacture, and distribution to sale and ultimate use. These include straightforward devices like taxation, as well as more tortuous mechanisms seeking to reallocate the social and medical costs of tobacco-induced illness to influence decision makers, whether producers, consumers, or intermediaries: distributors of tobacco products, underwriters of insurance, and officials responsible for policies governing behavior in public places, as well as semiprivate places like the workplace. Also relevant are government policies that affect the economics of the tobacco and cigarette industries, the most important being the long-standing program of price supports for tobacco farming.

Persuasive efforts, finally, can be lent legal support, as by statutes that mandate school-based antismoking programs or earmark funds for them, by regulation of advertising, packaging and labeling, or marketing of cigarettes, or by public policies encouraging a wide range of programs aimed at producing or disseminating information that may convince people to remain or become nonsmokers.

Table 1 Types and targets of legal smoking deterrents, with illustrations

Category (mobilizing)	Direct-legal (behavior)	Indirect via market (incentives)	Indirect via persuasion (beliefs)
Demand side (Consumer)	Ban use Restrict use Require employers and others to restrict use Empower nonsmokers to demand restrictions	Increase excise (and other) taxes Mandate insurance incentives Establish employer's right to refuse to hire smokers	Mandate educational programs Earmark funds for educational programs Conduct legislative hearings Issue government reports Fund smoking-health research
Supply side (Grower, manufacturer, advertiser, distributor)	Ban manufacture and/or distribution Restrict manufacture and/or distribution 　—Age (minors) 　—Outlets (vending machines) Regulate composition of cigarettes	Increase taxes on growers, manufacturers, marketers Reduce/eliminate government price supports Provide other incentives to hasten diversification Establish legal liability of producers and/or advertisers Require employers to compensate disability of non-smokers exposed on the job to smoke	Ban advertising Restrict advertising (channels, content) Require package warnings Conduct tar and nicotine testing Require disclosure of additives, reporting of sales

Along a second dimension, legal approaches to the smoking problem can be divided into a dichotomy that reflects their primary target: buyer or supplier (broadly defined). Again, the pathways are more and less direct and sometimes overlap: normal business and sales taxes levied on the supplier's side are virtually indistinguishable in the consumer's eyes from excise taxes at the point of sale. But the distinction has policy relevance and helps organize the material for this review.

A massive literature on the smoking problem is accessible through the Office on Smoking and Health of the US Department of Health and Human Services (DHHS) and in materials available through organizations like the American Cancer Society, the American Lung Association, the World Health Organization, Action for Smoking and Health (ASH), the Group Against Smoking Pollution (GASP), the Coalition on Smoking and Health, and other such groups. The literature is of such scope and magnitude that all we can reasonably attempt here is to erect some guideposts through it, emphasizing the more recent developments that are less fully documented, and identifying major findings and trends as well as issues for the future.

DIRECT LEGAL DETERRENTS TO SMOKING OR TOBACCO SALES

An impressive array of federal administrative agencies has something to say about where and when consumers should be permitted to buy and use tobacco products, and how purveyors may market and distribute them. Conspicuous by their absence are the two agencies—the Food and Drug Administration (FDA) and the Consumer Products Safety Commission (CPSC)—whose strictures would doubtless be the toughest. Congress has proscribed them from acting on the smoking and health evidence; indeed one of the deals struck in 1906 to win acceptance of the Pure Food and Drug Act was to remove tobacco from the US *Pharmacopoeia,* where it had been listed at the turn of the century and has not reappeared since (12). ASH has petitioned the FDA to accept jurisdiction and has gone to court over this issue, so far without success; similar efforts directed at the CPSC by the American Public Health Association have likewise been rebuffed (12).

Demand-side Interventions to Restrict Smoking

To be all-inclusive, the total ban of cigarettes can be mentioned as a logical possibility, if not a political one. In conjunction with the moral crusade against alcohol at the turn of the century, several states did ban the purchase and use of cigarettes, but these laws went the way of the Volstead Act: none survived beyond 1927. After the first surgeon general's report in 1964 (69), bills were filed in Congress to amend the federal Food, Drug, and Cosmetic Act to bring cigarettes into its ambit, but they failed to pass. Then when the CPSC was created in 1973, its first chairman claimed the authority, under the Hazardous Substances Act, to set standards for cigarettes or ban them entirely (24). Congress responded with a 1976 law tying the Commission's hands.

Timing provides one explanation for the anomolies in governmental responses to addictive substances: tobacco as compared with illicit drugs like heroin. Tobacco products arrived on the market and established their social acceptability (and their economic and political power base) before their adverse properties were known. Breslow argues that currently available tests of mutagenicity and carcinogenicity would exclude them from the market today were they not, in effect, protected by an unspoken "grandfather" clause that places the very suggestion of a total ban in the realm of unthinkable governmental intrusion into the affairs of a strong, established industry (8).

FEDERAL ACTIONS TO RESTRICT SMOKING   With Congress tugging continuously at their reins, some 20 federal offices, agencies, and departments have tried in various ways to monitor and mitigate the harm that arises from smoking. Most of their efforts are informational or educational, but a direct legal intervention is occasionally tried. Smoking has been limited to some degree in all federal buildings by order of the General Services Administration, with special restrictions in some, such as facilities of DHHS. Regulations of the Interstate Commerce Commission require that smoking sections of buses constitute no more than 30% of seats (22) and that trains restrict smoking to designated areas (23). The airlines have attracted particular attention.

In 1972 the Civil Aeronautics Board (CAB) began requiring the designation on every commercial air flight of a nonsmoking section large enough to accommodate any passenger requesting a seat in it (25). This was in response to a decade of pressure by ASH, together with a government survey in which 60% of nonsmokers and 38% of smokers indicated that on airplanes they found smoke bothersome. Then, in 1983, the US Court of Appeals for the District of Columbia ruled that nonsmoking airline passengers were inadequately protected; and the CAB subsequently promulgated a smoking ban on any flight or flight segment of up to two hours. In eliminating smoking on over 80% of all scheduled flights, this regulation represented a major victory for the nonsmokers' movement; but within hours of its announcement, it was reversed at the insistence of lobbyists and powerful members of Congress (9). Experiences such as this have led analysts to conclude that although the federal government could in a single stroke enact comprehensive legislation for smoke-free indoor air, the more feasible route through which to achieve the same objective is a state-by-state approach, using model or uniform statutes (62).

STATE AND LOCAL SMOKING RESTRICTIONS   Nearly 50 years after the first generation of state laws restricting smoking, a second began to emerge around 1972. In that year, the surgeon general's second report on smoking and health mentioned, among other new findings, the possibility that "sidestream smoke" harms some exposed nonsmokers (70). Additional evidence has since accumulated on the adverse effects of "passive smoking" on fetuses, small children, and some sensitive adults (26, 63, 84). Concerns about possible harm to respiratory functions of larger groups of passive smokers (39) has lent impetus to the "nonsmokers' rights movement," which finds collateral justification in the discomfort and irritation many passive smokers experience. Consequently, some kind of legislation or extensive administrative regulation aimed specifically at reducing nonsmokers' exposure to second-hand smoke had, as of 1984, been enacted in 38 states and the District of Columbia. Twenty-five states had established comprehensive packages known as "clean indoor air acts," often by aggregating and extending existing laws, sometimes starting from none (17).

In the judgment of the American Lung Association (but not based on controlled evaluation research), the more effective of these laws accomplish at least the following five tasks. They (a) specify legislative intent (such as protecting the right of nonsmokers to breathe clean air); (b) define in unambiguous terms the specific restrictions being imposed (spelling out inclusions and exclusions lost in broad categories like "public place," "small food and beverage establishment," and so on); (c) require the posting of plainly visible signs in all smoking-regulated areas; (d) delineate clear responsibility for publicizing and enforcing the regulations; (e) designate penalties for infractions (68). The second of the tasks is generally the hardest. Most statutes specify areas where smoking must be restricted. Six states simplify the task by prohibiting any indoor smoking in public places unless expressly permitted.

Advocates of comprehensive clean indoor air acts see them as multipurpose vehicles; they generate publicity and educate the public, serve as a wedge to further action, and tip the legal scales in favor of nonsmokers (51). Efforts to establish them are often strongly resisted, though, not only by tobacco interests (said to have invested $6 million in the defeat of an antismoking referendum in California) (55) but also by employers and owners of restaurants, retail stores, and other affected enterprises. They express concern that the laws will be controversial and damaging to business as well as difficult and costly to enforce, but anecdotal accounts indicate that these worries may be unfounded (54).

What, if any, effect the laws are having (whether toward their avowed goal of conserving nonsmokers' health or on overall cigarette consumption rates) has yet to be demonstrated. Difficulties in trying to disentangle their impact from that of all the other initiatives in the "antismoking campaign" include the problems of establishing time order and controlling for selection bias in studies comparing smoking behavior of different natural groupings. Warner concludes that the "campaign" has had an impact but that within this broad construct, changes in taxes are not only easier than the clean air acts to evaluate but probably also more effective in reducing cigarette consumption (77).

Nevertheless, many nonsmokers' groups are pressing local governments, boards of health, and other agencies to pass similar ordinances or regulations. Several cities and towns now require employers to restrict smoking at work. A 1983 San Francisco ordinance typifies these. It requires employers to try to accommodate the preferences of both smokers and nonsmokers but to prohibit smoking if accord cannot be reached or face a fine of $500 per day as long as the dispute continues (17). The Los Angeles city council passed a similar ordinance late in 1984, and at least 28 other California jurisdictions have done so, as well as municipal and county governments in Massachusetts, New York, Ohio, and probably others too (17).

SPECIAL RESTRICTIONS: THE WORKPLACE   The worksite is a lightning rod for the clean indoor air movement because nonsmokers encounter second-hand smoke there over extended periods of time and in concentrated doses, and have a "compelling reason" for being there (12). Also, it is felt that worksite interventions (not only in the industrial sector, but also in hospitals, government agencies, and other places of commerce) can build on interpersonal networks to change the social norms and can mobilize incentives; moreover, employers are believed to have a vested interest in making this occur because their smoking employees are costing them money (37). To the extent that this is true and employers elect to take these steps, they lie beyond the scope of this review. But lest this logic escape employers (as some believe it may) (73, 83), antismoking activists are carving out a new body of law to oblige employers to take action against smoking.

Williams & Mulkeen (85) review the emerging legal framework as weaving together strands from seven major areas of law. First, under federal constitutional law, nonsmokers have filed and lost several suits claiming that smoking in the workplace infringes their constitutional rights (embodied in the first, fifth, ninth, and fourteenth amendments) (62). Second, some interpret the "general duty clause" of the federal Occupational Safety and Health Act to imply an obligation to protect workers from second-hand smoke (35, 58), but OSHA has set no standards for cigarette smoke, and in their absence employees have recourse to common law through the courts. Third, the common law precedent for nonsmokers' rights to clean air on the job was set by Shimp v. New Jersey Bell Telephone Company, decided in December 1976 (56). Two subsequent cases went the other way for insufficient evidence that a health hazard was at issue (28, 58). Fourth, under handicap discrimination law embodied in the Rehabilitation Act of 1973, several courts have ordered employers to make "reasonable accommodations" to employees' hypersensitivity to sidestream cigarette smoke (16, 72). Smoking employees have apparently not sought this legal protection but presumably could (as alcoholics can), assuming that smoking is an addiction (49). Fifth and sixth, suits filed under unemployment and workers' compensation law have argued successfully for the award of benefits to employees forced to leave their jobs because of a "reasonable, good faith, and honest fear of harm to health or safety" (2, 20, 48). Seventh, under wrongful discharge laws, several courts have ruled that nonsmokers who in good faith file complaints requesting their employers to provide a reasonably smoke-free work environment are protected from dismissal (32, 85).

Limited evidence suggests that smoking restrictions at the worksite may influence smoking behavior (43, 71), but more research on this question is needed, especially studies that can build on opportunities to conduct well-controlled natural experiments that compare alternative approaches. Also badly needed is a thorough analysis of social desiderata weighing for and against aggressive action by employers. Should employability in general depend on lifestyle choices on *and off* the job (73)? Is legally enforceable discrimination against people electing not to modify their known risk factors different in kind from discrimination against homosexuals and others the law has increasingly protected? Even if restrictions are limited to particular combinations of smoking workers and hazardous jobs, where will the lines be drawn? If smokers can be denied jobs as asbestos workers and firefighters (and the courts have said they can), from what other occupations can they be excluded? To what other classes of "hypersensitive" workers can this principle be extended? Can fertile females be refused jobs as nurses or video display terminal operators, where there might be harm to a fetus that could be conceived (61)? How compelling must the evidence be to justify discrimination, and at what point should the onus shift to a duty on the part of the employer to make the workplace safe for all?

Supply Side: Production and Distribution Controls

As Pollin (49) and others (6) emphasize in the analogy they draw to heroin in Vietnam, the sheer availability of cigarettes is itself a problem. Hardly any consumer product is so easily purchased at any hour of the day or night by anyone with the money, irrespective of age. Ten states currently prohibit cigarette sales to minors but these tend to be neither enforced nor observed. Legal mechanisms could be used much as they are in laws controlling alcoholic beverages. We found no states with legislation controlling the placement or supervision of cigarette vending machines and, in the current climate, this may be more likely to occur through local ordinances and through policies established by companies and other organizations. Similarly, the occasional restraint on the distribution of free samples either generally or to minors is being enacted at the local level rather than by state legislatures.

At least eight countries are now regulating the content of cigarettes but the US has declined to do so (51). The National Cancer Institute diverted millions of its research dollars into the development of a less harmful cigarette, and manufacturers have reduced tar and nicotine levels in response to market signals. But evidence casting doubt on the reduced risk of these newer cigarettes includes the known or suspected carcinogenicity of several of the hundreds of chemical additives now used to restore lost flavor and to make the cigarettes burn more evenly, as well as the suggestion that the lighter cigarettes may be responsible for increased smoking (29). The Comprehensive Smoking Education Act of 1984 does grant the federal government authority for the first time to undertake toxicological tests of the health risks of additives. Also it requires all cigarette manufacturers, packagers, and importers to supply DHHS a list of all additives, but allows the information to be provided anonymously.

As did the earliest antismoking laws more than a century ago (12), recent legislation has focused on the flammability of cigarettes, which makes them the leading cause of fatalities in all fire mortality data (42). Bills calling for fire performance standards have been filed in 11 states but none has passed. A 1984 federal Cigarette Safety Act empanels a group of experts to conduct a 30-month study of the feasibility of developing a fire-safe cigarette. The sale of "smokeless tobacco," used as snuff and to chew, has become a target for regulation in some states, beginning with Massachusetts.

INDIRECT INTERVENTIONS OPERATING THROUGH THE MARKET

The nation's "oldest industry," established in 1604, has had rare political clout, backed by the economic influence of a $20-billion business that is geographically concentrated, generates substantial tax revenue at the federal, state, and local levels (roughly $6.8 billion in 1981–1982) (44), and sustains some 2.5 million jobs either directly in the industry (500,000) or in related enterprises (2 million) (64). Ambivalent government policies reflect these political realities.

Because the industry's power originates in the market, special appeal attaches to legal deterrents operating through economic incentives. They offer a way to influence the behavior of producers (by robbing this product of its strategic market appeal) and consumers (by making cigarettes prohibitively expensive), and also a way to remove the government from the paradoxical position of subsidizing the product it has declared its public health enemy number one (33). Also, as market approaches, they should be ideologically salable to the current political power structure, with its strong antipathy toward command and control regulation.

Demand-side interventions (those intended principally for buyers) include direct efforts, chiefly through taxation, to increase the costs of cigarettes, and measures through insurance underwriting to provide the consumer with a financial incentive not to smoke. An extreme case that touches the vital issue of livelihood occurs when an employer declines to hire or employ smokers, a policy that does not appear to contravene laws restraining the employer's power to hire and fire at will. Tax policy toward the tobacco industry has had a long history, during which a literature has accumulated on its impact; the other interventions in this group are embryonic and unstudied.

On the supply side (addressing growers, manufacturers, marketers, and distributors) two important trends merit note. At the federal level, Congress has been debating the elimination of its tobacco support program. At the grass roots, a plaintiffs' litigation movement is taking shape in several states and hopes in time to press "the biggest mass tort" in history against the manufacturers and advertisers of cigarettes (50).

Using Tax and Other Policies to Stifle Demand

The price a consumer sees on a pack of cigarettes at the point of sale includes a federal excise tax, another imposed in each of the 50 states, and, in over 300 counties and municipalities, an additional tax averaging 0.4 cents per pack (65). Nearly a third of the retail sales value of that pack of cigarettes enters the public treasury. Together with normal business and sales taxes on manufacturing, wholesaling, and retailing, these tobacco taxes represent about 0.4% of federal tax revenues and about 1% of state and local taxes (44).

Setting an appropriate level for taxes has always been a balancing act in which governments have sought to maximize their revenues by projecting the price elasticity of demand and finding a tax ceiling just short of the point where aggregate tax revenues would start to fall. Decades of scholarship have undergirded these deliberations, and much is now known about the effects of cigarette price increases on consumption behavior.

Application of these analytic techniques enabled Warner to build a strong case for the "tremendous potential of cigarette excise taxes as an incentive to improve health behavior" (77, p. 123). But harnessing this potential has been anything but simple, owing in part to governmental balancing to protect the tax base and in part to other kinds of balancing that tax policy engenders. A sales tax is inherently regressive, the more so when applied to a product used more by lower- than higher-income consumers. Keeping pace with inflation is a challenge. State and federal policy objectives are at times contradictory, and there is a danger, if the policy is too draconian or is applied inconsistently, of making the commodity so expensive and the margins of profit so high as to stimulate illicit dealing and a black market. These themes emerge as we look first at federal tax policy and then at activities at the state level.

DEVELOPMENTS IN FEDERAL TAX POLICY   In 1982, for the first time in 31 years, Congress raised the federal excise tax on cigarettes (from 8 to 16 cents a pack), but the Tax Reform Act of 1984 allowed it to revert back to the 8-cent level on October 1, 1985. Twelve bills were introduced in the ninety-ninth Congress to raise the excise tax to the 16-cent level or higher.

Harris estimated that the 1982 doubling of the cigarette tax would produce a 3% decline in the number of adult smokers and a 15% reduction among teenagers, moving 1.5 million adults and 700,000 adolescents out of the high-risk cohort of current smokers (31). Testimony in the *Congressional Record* (11) suggests that at least some policy makers saw federal taxation as an explicit mechanism for addressing the health problem from smoking. Formerly the health impact of taxation had been chiefly serendipitous, much like the influence on highway safety of the 55 mile per hour speed limit passed to conserve gasoline during the fuel crisis.

TAXES ON THE STATE LEVEL   Nonfederal tax policy has grown more consequential as state and local taxes have overtaken those levied nationally. While the federal tax stayed at 8 cents, state taxes (on average) moved from 2.8 to 13.4 cents per pack from 1951 to 1981 (65). As of 1968–1969, state and local governments have been collecting more than half of total tobacco taxes; the state-local share reached 62% of the total by 1981 (44). Even so, because of inflation, the cost of cigarettes has been decreasing in real terms (83).

State-imposed excise taxation of cigarettes began in Iowa in 1921, long before health hazards had emerged as a major concern. By 1969 all states had followed suit. The absence of an antismoking impulse was evident in the similarity of tax policies in the six tobacco-producing states to those of other jurisdictions until after 1953 when studies began to implicate cigarettes in illness (24).

The 1964 surgeon general's report (69) stimulated increases in state excise taxes, which began to decline again after 1973. Enthusiasm for them waned as bootlegging across state lines became apparent in levels of consumption recorded in low-tax states (Kentucky, North Carolina, and New Hampshire) that could otherwise not be explained (67). States with high taxes were said to be losing as much as $500,000 a year in tax revenues. A Contraband Cigarette Law was enacted in 1978, but excise tax rates still differ markedly from state to state (44). Warner has estimated that excise taxes did depress consumption to a significant degree. He concludes that although tax policy is a potent deterrent, states seem not to view taxation "as an appropriate and effective weapon against smoking" (77, p. 145), largely because of the bootlegging issue (78). However, some states are at least considering legislation to dedicate tobacco tax receipts to preventive or palliative measures. One such proposition, in Massachusetts, has been inspired by the estimate that one quarter of all the uncompensated care in hospitals across the state could be defrayed by the $51 million collected annually in tobacco taxes. These revenues, it is argued, could be used to improve the access to health care for the medically indigent at a time when public resources are increasingly stretched (S. Crane, personal communication).

MANDATING INSURANCE INCENTIVES   Mounting evidence that nonsmokers are significantly better underwriting risks for life, health, and disability insurance, and even for automobile collision coverage (4, 30), has led some carriers in the US and Great Britain to offer nonsmokers' discounts. For purposes here, these trends are relevant only if legally mandated (or stimulated). This could be done at the federal or state level through statute (nonsmokers' rights groups often instigate such bills) or through regulation of the insurance business or of employee benefits (1). Also the courts have a role to play, as in an August 1985 class action suit filed by the National Organization for Women against Mutual of Omaha contending that gender-based rate setting is discriminatory and ought to be replaced by pricing based on lifestyle (66). Nonsmoking policyholders, corporations, and government welfare programs could enter lawsuits against insurers, demanding a reallocation of social costs. For the most part, however, the creation of incentives through insurance underwriting seems more likely to evolve through a natural process of competitive pricing and positioning in the marketplace than by government fiat.

Either way, important questions need to be debated. For example, should health insurance rates be higher for policyholders who are obese, hypertensive, Type A personalities, overeaters of saturated fats or undereaters of fiber, frequent drinkers and/or drivers, or non-wearers of seatbelts? These and other such value-laden questions receive relatively little sustained attention in the private sector where they arise; insurance company executives tend to deal with more pragmatic concerns, such as whether verification of smoking status is feasible for health insurance underwriting.

When the focus shifts from privately to publicly funded third-party payment plans, decisions to restructure the incentives have to be made in public, through a legal mechanism and weighing of competing values. This possibility has only recently been discussed in a serious way and embodied in at least one legislative proposal. Filed by Senator Durenberger in January 1985, the bill would require smoking Medicare recipients to pay a higher premium. The proposition is one small piece in a complex political mosaic and seems likely to move slowly if at all. Targeting the elderly, it probably crosses the fine line in any incentive program between offering a constructive stimulus toward attainable behavior change and penalizing victims bereft of the power to respond in a meaningful way.

Interventions to Change Incentives on the Supply Side

On the supply side, government could seek to discourage tobacco production by increasing its normal business and sales taxes on the manufacturing, wholesaling, and retailing of such products. This possibility is little discussed, no doubt because attention has been riveted on supply-side policies with the opposite intent.

THE TOBACCO SUPPORT PROGRAM   For half a century, the government's price support system has "guarantee(d) the tobacco farmer a greater return on his investment than on almost any crop" (64, p. 155). In theory self supporting, because farmers repay federal loans after their tobacco is sold, the program has actually cost the American taxpayer hundreds of millions of dollars over the years in loan defaults, interest charges, and administrative costs. Further, it has placed the federal government in a contradictory position, characterized by one senator as "a tragic comedy of moral and fiscal irresponsibility" (64, p. 158).

Repeated efforts to dismantle the program have generally foundered. A "concerted attack" (64, p. 159) on it met with defeat in 1981, but was followed in 1982 by the No Net Cost Tobacco Program Act, requiring producers to contribute to a fund designed to cover any losses incurred in government price support activities. This was a compromise measure to deflect mounting criticism of the program. Even so, it became a target again in the Reagan administration's 1985 "market-oriented" farm bill, which included, among many proposals, ending the program outright. The tobacco lobby countered by calling its continuation "non-negotiable" and threatening that should it end, tobacco farmers would default on over $1 billion in outstanding loans (57).

PRODUCT LIABILITY AND PERSONAL INJURY   Of all the legal smoking deterrents reviewed here, developments in tort liability are the most protean and potentially radical (14, 15, 41, 50). Antismoking groups are orchestrating a grass roots campaign with the intent of moving the struggle into the courts and mobilizing the underlying purposes of product liability law, namely that (*a*) victims be compensated; (*b*) manufacturers be compelled to make their products safe or at least to warn consumers fully of the hazards; (*c*) prices of dangerous products be made to reflect their social costs; and (*d*) the public be informed of risks associated with consumer products (15). They predict that the eventual result will be a flood of product liability judgments and settlements that could build to perhaps $50 to $100 billion a year, and would deter smoking by elevating the price of a pack of cigarettes to $3 or more and stimulating a dramatic increase in media coverage of the ravages of smoking.

This revival of an approach that failed in the 1960s takes place now in a rapidly changing legal, social, and scientific context. Although many cases were filed in the 1950s and 1960s, and several went to trial, all were defeated (27). Since then, however, product liability law has increasingly seen the plaintiff's side, as evident in successful suits against manufacturers of dangerous toys, asbestos, diethylstilbesterol, the Dalkon Shield, and other products. Virtually all states have now adopted strict liability rules, allowing injured consumers to recover compensatory damages even if the defects in the product are not the manufacturer's fault.

The tobacco industry's defense in the earlier cases rested on the orthogonal arguments that smokers willingly assume the risk and that proof is lacking of the causal link between cigarettes and disease. The evolving legal doctrine of "comparative negligence" now leaves room for awards that would recognize a certain amount of responsibility on the part of consumers, while at the same time holding manufacturers to account for "superior knowledge" they ought to have and for an "implied warranty" that a product is safe.

But the warranty from the tobacco industry is more than implied; a strong theme in complaints being filed is that the manufacturers and advertisers of cigarettes "intentionally, willfully, and wantonly," through "false, fraudulent, and misleading advertising," "conspire" to "mislead the public" and "to neutralize" the government-mandated warnings regarding the adverse health effects of smoking (14).

In fact, this theme was prominent in the preliminary judgment that has inspired the current optimism among product liability proponents. In 1984, New Jersey Federal District Court Judge Sarokin refused to dismiss a case being brought against three of the country's largest cigarette manufacturers on behalf of the family of Rose Cipollone, who died of lung cancer. Sarokin ruled that the federally mandated warnings on cigarette packs are not a bar against suits because they are "legal minimums" that were "never intended to supplant moral maximums" (52). The plaintiff's claims, he said, "deserve their day in court" to determine, among other questions, whether "defendants have wrongfully attempted to neutralize the warning" thus violating "the very statute" they "brandish as a shield" (10).

In addition to the strict liability doctrine, and the emphasis on false advertising, the new cases rest on the argument that most smokers were enticed before they were adults to use a product no one told them would be addictive both physically and psychologically. The director of the National Institute on Drug Abuse has made strong statements supporting the addiction argument, contending that "more than 60%" of smokers "become addicted to nicotine as adolescents before the age of majority," that nicotine, our society's "most prevalent drug of abuse," is six to eight times more addictive than alcohol ("when measured by the percentage of users who lose control of their substance intake") (49).

Scores of product liability and personal injury suits on behalf of smokers stricken by lung and other diseases or serious cigarette-related burns (S. Teret, personal communication) are being brought by victims or their survivors against manufacturers, advertisers, distributors, and the Tobacco Institute. Suits have been filed in at least nine states, with new cases appearing all the time; these developments are being tracked by the Tobacco Products Liability Project organized in 1984 at the Northeastern University School of Law in Boston and by ASH in Washington. These groups hope to engage legal entrepreneurs, working on a contingency fee basis, in speculative investments to open up a large and potentially lucrative new area of tort law.

INDIRECT INTERVENTIONS OPERATING THROUGH PERSUASION

The tobacco interests' success in deflecting strong legal sanctions against cigarettes has thrown government back on public education as a preeminent reponse. Of relevance to this review are legally mandated or supported informational and educational thrusts: reports to Congress and the public, sponsorship of research and education, restraints on advertising.

Legislation Aimed at Educating the Public to Curb Demand

The 1964 surgeon general's report (69) established the US government in the business of generating and disseminating public information on the health effects of smoking. As one of its first official responses, in the Cigarette Labelling and Advertising Act of 1965, Congress directed the Public Health Service and the FTC to submit reports on these effects and to recommend government policies. Subsequent surgeons general have issued 16 such reports; they summarize the massive scientific literature (one estimate placed the number of published studies at 45,000) (50), assess the impact of interventions, identify areas needing further study, recommend legislation, educate the public, and strongly advise smokers to stop and nonsmokers not to start.

Also, the FTC has investigated the potential of package warnings (taken up below) and the status of public knowledge and attitudes about smoking. The Commission has made the case that although skeptics commonly question the value of educational approaches on grounds that "everyone already knows" smoking is harmful to health, research actually reveals serious gaps in that knowledge, and significantly more ignorance of the health risks among smokers than nonsmokers (45). Although they leave unanswered the question of how to educate the public, these and other findings suggest that a major educational challenge remains if the message is to reach the young and less educated, blue-collar workers, minority populations, and other groups who smoke the most or whose smoking puts them or people around them at special risk.

Over the past two decades Congress has passed a number of smoking bills with an educational intent. Some states have been active too. The majority (35 states) require their public schools to provide instruction on the health effects of smoking, generally as part of an alcohol and drug education curriculum. Federal block grants for public health education sometimes funnel limited monies to schools and community agencies to support work on smoking prevention or cessation. Rarely do these funds even cover the costs of the programs, however, and repeated efforts at the federal and state levels to claim tax funds for their support have been unsuccessful. The government's annual outlays for public education on the hazards of smoking are roughly equivalent to a single day's investment by the cigarette manufacturers on sophisticated advertising to counter the government's negative news (53). The industry's advertising practices therefore have particular significance for public health policy.

Advertising and Labeling Restrictions Directed at Suppliers

Cigarette advertising, by definition a high-visibility activity, has sparked much controversy. The law has played a prominent role in efforts to restrict the channels and content of advertising and to mandate warnings on cigarette packages. The story travels a long and convoluted path of compromises by health advocates in the face of the industry's overwhelming influence and power (64).

In keeping with its mandate to regulate unfair and deceptive business practices, the FTC focused in the 1950s and 1960s on the veracity of advertising claims. But the time consumed in formal inquiries usually permitted a given ad to be used long enough to achieve its optimal effect even if ultimately it was removed. Within a week of the publication of the 1964 surgeon general's report, the FTC began what turned out to be a protracted effort to require effective warnings on cigarette packages and advertisements. The first labeling bill, enacted in 1965, was called "a shocking piece of special interest legislation" (64, p. 174) because it traded a mild warning on packages but not on ads for three years of exemption from FTC and FCC regulation and from state and local controls.

In 1967 the FCC brought smoking under the "fairness doctrine" by designating it a controversial issue so that broadcasters had to donate air time to balance the tobacco industry's pro-smoking advertisements, which they did from 1968 to 1970, donating time for public service announcements equalling about one third of paid advertising and worth some $75 million (75). The FTC continued to recommend in annual reports to Congress that cigarette advertising be banned entirely from the airwaves, as in fact it was in 1970. Thus ended the equal time for antismoking ads, which had been "a highly effective deterrent to smoking" at least for the short term (75, p. 443). Rates of smoking had dropped

SMOKING DETERRENCE   143

precipitously during the fairness doctrine years and began to climb again after 1970.

In 1970 the FTC issued a proposed rule to require that advertisements include the tar and nicotine content of cigarettes, but the industry elected to comply voluntarily instead. The FTC continued to press for warning labels that would have more impact, through greater specificity in the wording, bigger size and more prominent placement, and a system of rotating warnings to keep the consumer's attention. These measures were embodied in the Comprehensive Smoking Education Act of 1984, which restored the FTC's authority to regulate the content and display of cigarette health warnings and provided for a system of four warnings to be rotated on a quarterly basis. More stringent controls on advertising are being proposed: limiting tobacco producers to "tombstone advertising," with only the product pictured in the ad; prohibiting sponsorship of sporting events; using tax monies to restore the antismoking messages to the broadcast media; requiring fuller disclosure of tar and nicotine content, additives, and the addictive properties of cigarettes or imposing a kind of "fairness doctrine" principle on print and billboard media (51). From a health standpoint, the last proposal has in its favor the evidence that the revenues magazines and newspapers receive in cigarette advertising deflect editorial attention from the dangers of smoking (59, 80). From a legal perspective, though, this abrogation of first amendment principles is unprecedented, highly unlikely, and probably unwise in the precedent it would set (L. Glantz, personal communication).

CROSSCUTTING THEMES AND CONCLUSIONS

Underlying this review of legal attempts to deter smoking are a few recurrent themes. Analysis of them helps to impose order on various approaches to the smoking problem, and, by inference, provides insight into the more global question of how the law can be used to advance public health.

1. *Jurisdictions are complex and overlapping.* The law functions on the federal, state, and local levels, through legislative, judicial, and executive branches. Some legal interventions are feasible at all levels (taxation is an example) while others (such as those involving the regulation of interstate business conduct) fall or are circumscribed within a narrower jurisdictional domain. States vary in their postures toward the tobacco issue. Policies fashioned even within the same jurisdiction are sometimes complementary but more often contradictory, as the case of price supports illustrates.

2. *Relevant legal principles are diffuse and complex.* The several legal entities embody the law in constitutions, statutes, regulations, and judicial opinions. Smoking policy springs from all these processes, and three major bodies of law have come chiefly into play: (*a*) federal statutory and administrative law, (*b*) state statutory and administrative law, and (*c*) common or case

law. The situation is therefore complex and unstable; some see potentially significant changes, especially in the torts arena, on the immediate horizon.

3. *It is unsafe to assume that a smoking law or regulation is necessarily "about" smokers' health.* Historically, smoking laws were passed to raise taxes, prevent fires, promote morality and occasionally also health. Not until the 1960s was there a resurgence of antismoking law, this time with a clear health theme. One indicator of this shift is that a scholarly tradition extending back to 1933 of estimating the price elasticity of demand for cigarettes took 50 years to diffuse from journals on economics and taxation into the health literature. More recently, the clean indoor air movement has shifted the focus again. When the health issue first emerged, the concern was to protect smokers, but much of the impetus behind recent legal developments—often harking back to the old morality theme—is to protect the rights and health of "innocent" nonsmoking bystanders. This refocusing has been catalyzed by grass-roots organizations that foment indignation to rally support. Ultimately, these various means to discordant ends may have similar effects on the consumption of cigarettes. Again, there are direct and indirect routes to the surgeon general's stated goal of a "smoke-free society by the year 2000" (34).

4. *Unintended consequences are ubiquitous.* Perhaps partly because of the multiple and ambiguous intentions behind them, legal interventions have repeatedly produced results that were entirely unanticipated and often unwelcome. This pattern began with one of the first federal incursions into the affairs of the tobacco manufacturers when the FTC broke up the industry in 1911 on antitrust grounds and indirectly created an oligopoly in which advertising became the "main mode of rivalry" among firms. Advertising has since been central to the industry's resilience (55) "in the face of overwhelming medical evidence that its product is lethal" (64, p. xxi).

Other examples have been touched upon: (*a*) The cigarette advertising ban silenced the public service messages and elevated per capita cigarette consumption (75). (*b*) The broadcast ad ban, moreover, concentrated the industry's investment in print media advertising, stifling editorial coverage of smoking hazards (59, 80). (*c*) The government's package labeling requirements lend support to the industry's position that smokers knowingly assume the risk, and indeed perhaps they discourage product liability suits. (*d*) Low tar and nicotine cigarettes may increase consumption by making the first few cigarettes more palatable, and causing veteran smokers to smoke more of the lighter cigarettes for a maintenance dose of nicotine. (*e*) Cigarette tax revenues have been said to trap governments in a fiscal "addiction" where they are essential links in a "smoke ring" protecting the industry (64), although their negligible proportion (1%) of total tax revenues hardly seems sufficient to substantiate this view (J. Pinney, personal communication). (*f*) State excise taxes did stimulate bootlegging across state borders, and—another geographical spillover effect—the industry is responding to the slow erosion of demand for cigarettes in developed nations by marketing assiduously in the third world (8).

Mindful of this pattern, antismoking activists are alert to the possibility that their legal strategies may recoil. An editorial in *The Nation's Health,* proposing an economic boycott of the many nontobacco products being sold by the now-diversified tobacco manufacturers (40), was followed in the next issue by a letter to the editor worrying that such a campaign could thrust the industry back on its tobacco products and intensify rather than vitiate the force of its resistance to antismoking initiatives (13). In a similar vein, Sapolsky argued that if the government removes its tobacco price supports, which have stifled innovation, the growers and producers will likely become more efficient, causing prices to fall and consumption to rise (55), and others predict that relaxed restrictions on foreign imports would have the same effect. The activists working to win a precedent-setting tort liability case say they are watching closely for evidence that manufacturers are preparing to take refuge under the banner of "product liability reform" or a Chapter 11 reorganization (M. Charney, personal communication).

5. *Passing a law or writing a policy still leaves it to be enforced.* Rules governing the punctilio of personal comportment are difficult to enforce. Serious surveillance and real penalties seem like overkill; slaps on the wrist have little sting. If moral indignation rises to a high pitch, ordinary citizens become vigilantes, demanding their no-smoking seats in overbooked airplanes and buses, plucking cigarettes from the lips of rule violators in enclosed places like elevators. Citizens' organizations like ASH and GASP have focused much of their energy on the enforcement of existing laws and regulations, often with success. Still, the passage from Shakespeare reputed to have been President Kennedy's favorite applies here. Glendower boasts "I can call spirits from the vasty deep" and Hotspur responds, "Why, so can I, or so can any man; but will they come when you do call for them?" (Henry IV, Part I).

6. *Research plays a strategic role in moving the law ahead.* Surveys of public opinion have helped government officials and other decision makers plumb latent public support for a stronger stand (several corporations have conducted opinion surveys before instituting new smoking policies). This is useful when opponents of such stands have superior resources with which to purchase a louder voice. Research also mobilizes public opinion: Evidence on the health effects of second-hand smoke and on the economic costs of smoking provided antismoking activists with a new philosophical and political case against cigarettes as an intrusion on nonsmokers' lives.

Evaluation research can help fine-tune legal strategies to deter cigarette smoking. With the exception of Warner's studies (74–78, 81, 82), this use of research has not been adequately exploited. As states and smaller entities (like corporations) become more active in promulgating smoking policies, opportunities multiply for focused natural experiments comparing the relative impact of alternative approaches. Part of the evaluative task is to monitor for unintended effects. This has been an important theme in studies of smoking policy. Research showing how smokers subvert the intent of low tar and nicotine cigarettes (7, 21, 36) raised important questions about the wisdom of promoting their development. Finally, research has served to expose erroneous claims of cigarette manufacturers. One example is the purpose and effect of advertising, often justified with the assertion that it does not recruit new smokers but merely creates "brand loyalty." Some evidence is beginning to suggest that this is not strictly true (8, 60, 79), and it should help clarify where legal controls are warranted.

7. *There is always a larger context and a wider framework.* The "antismoking campaign" is taking place against a backdrop of secular changes that have gradually affected the balance of power in the smoking controversy. They have eroded to some extent the enormous concentrated power that the manufacturers enjoyed, while the antismoking forces (formerly fragmented in small, turf-conscious groups) have begun to centralize their diffuse interests in governmental interagency committees and private political coalitions. Antismoking activists have been capitalizing on these secular changes by pursuing a conscious strategy of disseminating their struggle as widely as possible in state and local governments and throughout the courts, so the tobacco industry will have to spread its resources thinly in self-defense. These shifts in the diffusion and concentration of power (47, 86) make this an arena in which rational models explain certain things but need to be augmented by an understanding also of organizational and political force fields (3).

8. *Lives can be saved.* With all the qualifications, caveats, and complexities, it is still true that much of the damage from smoking is reversable within about five years, so getting smokers to quit yields dividends quickly (38). As a longer term strategy, children can be protected from having to struggle to quit. The legal approaches reviewed here can be part of a comprehensive, multipronged assault on cigarette smoking (8). There is a circularity and synergy among a variety of approaches. Changing the norms and public opinion creates the climate in which legislators, regulators, and the courts can enact and enforce tough laws. As a legal matter, for instance, a smoker is liable for the smoke around him only if he is aware that involuntary smoke is harmful and offensive to others (62), something he learns when smoking/health issues come into public view. Discussions leading to the enactment of new laws, in turn, create new awareness and mold public opinion.

Since the first surgeon general's report in 1964, at least 34 million Americans have given up cigarettes. Adult per capita consumption has fallen every year since 1973 (79). Some 55 million Americans still smoke, though—about a third of the adult population—and they smoke, on average, a record amount every day: more than 30 cigarettes each. Americans are legitimately chary of paternalistic and coercive assaults on personal liberties, because the state possesses police powers unavailable to private corporations, however superior their wealth. Nevertheless, a close examination of legal attempts to stem this epidemic compels us, on balance, to conclude that governments have intruded much less on the consumer's sovereignty to make a truly informed, autonomous, and uncoerced decision about the wisdom of smoking cigarettes than has the tobacco industry.

ACKNOWLEDGMENTS

We are indebted to Stephen Crane, PhD, Richard Daynard, JD, Leonard Glantz, JD, MPH, John Pinney, and Stephen Teret, JD, for incisive and helpful comments on the manuscript and to Susan Cornelius and Susan Kelleher for assistance with the research.

Dr. Walsh was supported in part by a grant from the Pew Memorial Trust, and Dr. Gordon was supported in part by a grant from the W. K. Kellogg Foundation to the Working Group on Health Promotion and Disease Prevention of the Harvard Division of Health Policy Research and Education.

Literature Cited

1. Action on Smoking and Health. 1985. ASH wins major health insurance victory for nonsmokers. *Smoking Health Rev.* (March):3
2. *Alexander v. California Unemployment Insurance Appeals Board.* 1981. 163 Cal. Rptr. 441, 104 Cal. App.3d 97
3. Allison, G. 1971. *Essence of Decision.* Boston: Little Brown
4. American Cancer Society. 1984. *World Smoking Health* 9(3):4
5. Bagdakian, B. H. 1983. *The Media Monopoly.* Boston: Beacon
6. Bennett, W. Cigarettes: Prevention or cure? *Harvard Med. Lett.* (March):3–5
7. Benowitz, N. L., Hall, S. M., Herning, R. I., Jacobs, P. III, Jones, R. T., Osman, A. L. 1983. Smokers of low yield cigarettes do not consume less nicotine. *N. Engl. J. Med.* 309:139–42
8. Breslow, L. 1982. Control of cigarette smoking from a public policy perspective. *Ann. Rev. Public Health* 3:129–51
9. CAB decision on smoking on airlines. 1984. *GASP Newslett.* (Winter):1
10. *Cipollone and Cipollone v. Liggett Group, Inc., Philip Morris Inc., Loews Corp., and Loew's Theatres, Inc.* 1984. Civil Action No. 83-2864. U.S. District Court for the District of New Jersey
11. *Congressional Record.* 1982. (July 21): S8814
12. Cristoffel, J. D., Stein, S. 1979. Using

the law to protect health: The frustrating case of smoking. *Mediolegal News* (Winter):5–20
13. Davis, R. M. 1985. Would boycott drive tobacco companies back to tobacco? *Nation's Health* (March):2
14. Daynard, R. A. 1984. *Preliminary legal outline: Cigarette company liability in Massachusetts.* Boston: Tobacco Products Liability Project, Northeastern Univ. School of Law. 10 pp.
15. Daynard, R. 1985. *Tobacco Products Liability Project: Its purpose and rationale.* Boston: Northeastern University School of Law, Feb. 27. 15 pp.
16. *Department of Fair Employment and Housing v. Fresno County.* 1982. Case no. FED 81-82, Calif. Fair Employment Practices Comm.
17. Doyle, N. 1984. State and municipalities regulate smoking in work, public places. *Business Health* 2(1):12
18. Editorial. 1985. Where there's smoke. *The Boston Globe* (Jan. 8):14
19. Deleted in proof
20. *Flaniken v. Office of Personal Management, U.S. Merit Systems Protection Board* (Dallas Field Office). 1980. 24 Atla. L. Rptr. 403
21. Folsom, A. R., Pechacek, T. F., de Gaudemaris, R., Luepker, R. V., Jacobs, D. R., Gillum, R. F. 1984. Consumption of 'low-yield' cigarettes: Its

148   WALSH & GORDON

frequency and relationship to serum thiocyanate. *Am. J. Public Health* 74:564–68
22. 49 C. F. R. 1061. 1979
23. 49 C. F. R. 1124.21. 1979
24. Friedman, K. M. 1975. *Public Policy and the Smoking-Health Controversy.* Lexington, Mass.: Lexington Books
25. 14 C. F. R. 252. 1979
26. Garfinkel, L. A. 1981. Time trends in lung cancer mortality among nonsmokers and a note on passive smoking. *J. Nat. Cancer Inst.* 66:1061–66
27. Garner, D. W. 1980. Cigarette dependency and civil liability: A modest proposal. *So. Cal. Law Rev.*, p. 1423
28. *Gordon v. Raven Systems and Research, Inc.* 1983. 462 A.2d 10 (D.C. App. 1983)
29. Gori, G., Bock, F. 1980. A safe cigarette? *Banbury Rep.* Cold Spring Harbor, NY.: Cold Spring Harbor Lab.
30. Grout, P., Cliff, K. S., Harman, J. L., Machin, D. 1983. Cigarette smoking, road traffic accidents, and seat belt usage. *Public Health* 97:95–101
31. Harris, J. E. 1982. Increasing the federal excise tax on cigarettes. *J. Health Econ.* 1:117–20
32. *Hentzel v. The Singer Company.* 1982. 188 Cal. Rptr. 159 (App. 1982)
33. Iglehart, J. K. 1984. Smoking and public policy. *N. Engl. J. Med.* 310(8):539–44
34. Koop, C. E. 1984. *A smoke-free society by the year 2000.* Presented at ann. meet. Am. Lung Assoc., Miami Beach, Florida, May 20, 1984. Condensed in *World Smoking and Health* 9(3):2–4
35. Kotin, P., Gault, L. A. 1980. Smoking in the workplace: A hazard ignored. *Am. J. Public Health* 70:575–76
36. Kozlowski, L. T., Frecker, R. C., Khouw, V., Pope, M. A. 1980. The misuse of 'less-hazardous' cigarettes and its detection: Hole-blocking of ventilated filters. *Am. J. of Public Health* 70:1202–3
37. Kristein, M. M. 1983. How much can business expect to profit from smoking cessation? *Prev. Med.* 12:358–81
38. Kuller, L., Meilahan, E., Townsend, M. Weinberg, G. 1982. Control of cigarette smoking from a medical perspective. *Ann. Rev. Public Health* 3:153–78
39. Lefcoe, N. M., Ashley, M. J., Pederson, L. L., Keays, J. J. 1983. The health risks of passive smoking. A growing case for control measures in enclosed environments. *Chest* 84(1):90–95
40. Madoff, M. A. 1985. Are you kidding? A boycott of tobacco companies? *Nation's Health* (Feb.):20
41. Margolick, D. 1985. Antismoking cli-
mate inspires suits by the dying. *New York Times* (March 15):B1
42. McGuire, A. 1983. Cigarette and fire deaths. *NY State J. Med.* 83(13):1296–98
43. Meade, T. W., Wald, N. J. 1977. Cigarette smoking patterns during the working day. *Br. J. Prev. Soc. Med.* 31:25–29
44. Miller, R. H. 1980. *Tobacco products situation and estimates of cigarette consumption.* Presented at 54th ann. meet. Natl. Tobacco Tax Assoc., Mystic, Conn., Oct. 5–7
45. Myers, M. L., Iscoe, C., Jennings, C., Lenox, W., Minsky, E., Sacks, A. 1981. *Staff Report on the Cigarette Advertising Investigation.* Washington DC: Fed. Trade Comm., Bur. of Consumer Protection
46. Nuehring, E. M., Markle, G. E. 1974. Nicotine and norms: The re-emergence of a deviant behavior. *Social Problems* 21:513–26
47. Olson, M. 1977. *The Logic of Collective Action.* Cambridge: Harvard Univ. Press
47a. Oster, G., Colditz, G. A., Kelly, N. 1984. The economic costs of smoking and benefits of quitting for individual smokers. *Prev. Med.* 13:377–89
48. *Parodi v. Merit Systems Protection Board.* 690 F.2d 731 (9th Cir. 1982)
49. Pollin, W. 1984. The role of the addictive process as a key step in causation of all tobacco-related diseases. *J. Am. Med. Assoc.* 252((20):2874
50. Ranii, D. 1985. New group takes aim at the tobacco industry. *Natl. Law J.* (Feb. 11):4
51. Roemer, R. 1982. *Legislative Action to Combat the World Smoking Epidemic.* Geneva: WHO
52. Rosen, B. S. 1984. Cigarette pack warnings no bar against suits. *Natl. Law J.* (Oct. 8):5–6
53. Saltus, R. 1985. Harvard dean seeks curbs on tobacco ads. *The Boston Globe* (April 27):1
54. Sandell, S. 1984. State cleans up indoor air. *Business and Health* 2(1):19–21
55. Sapolsky, H. M. 1980. The political obstacles to the control of cigarette smoking in the United States. *J. Health Polit. Policy Law* 5:277–90
56. *Shimp v. New Jersey Bell Telephone.* 1976. 145 N.J. Super. 516, 368 A.2d. 408
57. Sinclair, W. 1985. Proposal to end tobacco program has Congressional backers smoking. *Washington Post* (Febr. 5)
58. *Smith v. Western Electric Company.* 1982. 643 S.W.2d 10 (Mo. App. 1982)
59. Smith, R. C. 1978. The magazines' smoking habit. *Columbia Journal. Rev.* 16(5):29–31

60. Sports sponsorship by tobacco companies. 1984. *Lancet* (Dec. 22/29):1484
61. Stellman, J. M. 1977. *Women's Work, Women's Health.* New York: Pantheon
62. Swingle, M. 1980. The legal conflict between smokers and nonsmokers: The magestic vice versus the right to clean air. *Missouri Law Rev.* 45:444–75
63. Tager, I. B., Weiss, S. T., Munoz, A., et al. 1983. Longitudinal study of the effects of maternal smoking on pulmonary function in children. *N. Engl. J. Med.* 309(12):699–703
64. Taylor, P. 1984. *The Smoke Ring: Tobacco, Money and Multinational Politics.* New York: Pantheon
65. Toder, E. 1982. *Impact of the 1982 tax law change on state cigarette revenue.* Presented at the 56th ann. meet. of Natl. Tobacco Tax Assoc., Chicago, Ill., Aug. 31. (Available through the author, financial economist at the US Dept. Treasury)
66. United Press International. 1984. NOW challenges alleged bias in insurance pricing in $2M suit. *The Boston Globe* (Aug. 17):3
67. United States Advisory Commission on Intergovernmental Relations. 1977. *Cigarette bootlegging: A state and federal responsibility.*
68. United States Department of Health, Education, and Welfare, Public Health Service. 1977. *The Smoking Digest* 26:83
69. United States Public Health Service. 1964. Report of the Advisory Committee to the Surgeon General. *Smoking and Health.* Washington DC: US GPO. DHEW Publ. No. (PHS) 1103
70. United States Public Health Service. 1972. *The Health Consequences of Smoking: A Report of the Surgeon General.* Washington DC: US GPO. DHEW Publ. No. (HMS) 72–7516
71. Van Peenen, P. F. D., Blanchard, A. G., Wolkonsky, P. M. 1984. Smoking habits of refinery workers. *Am. J. Public Health* 74(12):1408–9
72. *Vickers v. Veterans Administration.* 1982. 549 F. Supp. 85 (WD WASH 1982)

73. Walsh, D. C. 1984. Corporate smoking policies: A review and an analysis. *J. Occup. Med.* 26:17–22
74. Warner, K. E. 1977. The effects of the anti-smoking campaign on cigarette consumption. *Am. J. Public Health* 67:645–50
75. Warner, K. E. 1979. Clearing the airwaves: The cigarette ad ban revisited. *Policy Analysis* 5:435–50
76. Warner, K. E. 1981. Cigarette smoking in the 1970's: The impact of the antismoking campaign on consumption. *Science* 211:729–31
77. Warner, K. E. 1981. State legislation on smoking and health: A comparison of two policies. *Policy Sci.* 13:139–52
78. Warner, K. E. 1982. Cigarette excise taxation and interstate smuggling: An assessment of recent activity. *Natl. Tax J.* 35:483–90
79. Warner, K. E. 1984. The effects of publicity and policy on smoking and health. *Business Health* 2(1):7–14
80. Warner, K. E. 1985. Cigarette advertising and media coverage of smoking and health. *N. Engl. J. Med.* 312(6):384–88
81. Warner, K. E., Murt, H. A. 1982. Impact of the antismoking campaign on smoking prevalence: A cohort analysis. *J. Public Health Policy* 3:374–90
82. Warner, K. E., Murt, H. A. 1983. Premature deaths avoided by the antismoking campaign. *Am. J. Public Health* 73:672–77
83. Warner, K. E., Murt, H. A. 1984. Economic incentives for health. *Ann. Rev. Public Health* 5:107–33
84. White, J. R., Froeb, H. F. 1980. Small-airways dysfunction in nonsmokers chronically exposed to tobacco smoke. *N. Engl. J. Med.* 302(13):720–23
85. Williams, T. H., Mulkeen, J. F. 1985. Smoking in the workplace: A growing controversy. New York: Am. Management Assoc.
86. Wilson, J. Q. 1980. *The Politics of Regulation.* New York: Basic

Ann. Rev. Public Health. 1986. 7:151–69

CARCINOGENESIS MODELING: From Molecular Biology to Epidemiology

Suresh H. Moolgavkar

Division of Public Health Sciences, The Fred Hutchinson Cancer Research Center, Seattle, Washington 98104

INTRODUCTION

The problem of cancer has received intense scrutiny on at least three different levels. On the most fundamental level, the complex and intricate dynamics of cellular growth and differentiation and their disruption during oncogenesis are being studied in laboratories around the world. This work has yielded some spectacular successes. Inappropriate activation of a normally occurring cellular gene, the oncogene, could well be the final common pathway in carcinogenesis.

On the next level up, experiments in animals have demonstrated that at least two broad classes of agents—initiators and promoters—facilitate carcinogenesis. Further, this work has elucidated major biochemical changes that occur in parallel with malignant transformation. For regulatory purposes, the animal bioassay is still the gold standard for measuring the carcinogenicity of agents.

Finally, epidemiologic studies in human populations have shown that the burden of cancer falls unequally on different populations, and on different subgroups within a single population. The reasons for these differences are not well understood except that hereditary, environmental, and life-style factors are all clearly important.

The purpose of this chapter is to discuss briefly some models for carcinogenesis that relate fundamental cellular processes to the epidemiology of cancer in human populations. Underlying all these models are the assumptions that carcinogenesis is a multistage process and that it is the end result of a sequence of rare, specific, and heritable (at the level of the cell) changes in a

0163-7525/86/0510-0151$02.00

single cell. Good evidence, some of which is reviewed in this chapter, supports each of these assumptions.

First I discuss one of the earliest, most successful multistage models for carcinogenesis, that of Armitage & Doll (1). A careful consideration of all the evidence suggests that no more than two rate-limiting steps need to be postulated in carcinogenesis. In the second, larger part of this chapter, I discuss a two-stage model and its implications for human cancer.

THE ARMITAGE-DOLL MODEL

Multistage models for carcinogenesis were first advanced in the 1950s (1, 12, 30) to explain the observation that, in many adult carcinomas, the logarithm of the age-specific incidence rates increases linearly with the logarithm of age. Fisher & Hollomon suggested that this observation could be explained if a critical number of six or seven cancer cells were required for subsequent independent tumor growth. However, Armitage & Doll pointed out that this hypothesis "also leads to the conclusion that cancer incidence should be proportional to the fifth or sixth power of the concentration of the effective carcinogen whereas experimental data suggest that, in general, tumor incidence and concentration of the carcinogen vary in arithmetical proportion. The hypothesis in its simple form is, therefore, untenable."[1] Nordling (30) and Armitage & Doll (1) proposed models in which carcinogenesis was the end result of several (six or seven for most cancers) stable changes in the cell. The Armitage-Doll model suggested further that these changes had to occur in a definite sequence.

Before discussing the Armitage-Doll model further, it is worth providing perspective by noting the time during which these models were proposed. The first initiation-promotion experiments had been performed by Berenblum & Shubik (4) only a few years earlier; the structure of the DNA molecule had only recently been reported by Watson & Crick; and the genetic code had yet to be deciphered.

The Armitage-Doll model postulates that a malignant tumor arises in a tissue when a single susceptible cell in that tissue undergoes malignant transformation via a finite sequence of intermediate stages. Schematically, the model may be represented as follows:

$$E_0 \xrightarrow{\lambda_0} E_1 \xrightarrow{\lambda_0} E_2 \to \cdots \xrightarrow{\lambda_{n-1}} E_n.$$

Here E_0 represents the normal cell, E_n represents the malignant cell, and λ_j

---

[1]There is now good evidence that malignant tumors are clonal, i.e. derived from a single cell that has been malignantly transformed (11).

represents the "rate of transition" from stage E_j to stage E_{j+1}. The reciprocal of λ_j, measured in years, can be thought of as the average sojourn time in stage E_j.

An intuitive derivation of the age-specific incidence predicted by this model then proceeds as follows. Suppose that the steps leading to malignancy can occur in any order. The probability that the jth event has occurred by time (age) t is approximately $\lambda_{j-1}t$, and thus the probability that all events have occurred by time t is approximately $\lambda_0\lambda_1\cdots\lambda_{n-1}t^n$. Since the events are required (by the model) to occur in a specific order and there are $n!$ possible orderings in which the events can occur, the probability that a cell is malignant by time t is approximately $\lambda_0\lambda_1\cdots\lambda_{n-1}t^n/n!$. The probability of malignancy is a measure of prevalence. In order to obtain the incidence, the above expression is differentiated with respect to t to yield $\lambda_0\lambda_1\cdots\lambda_{n-1}t^{n-1}/(n-1)!$. Thus, the age-specific incidence is proportional to a power of age, i.e. a plot of the logarithm of age-specific incidence versus the logarithm of age yields a straight line with slope $n-1$, where n is the number of stages required for malignant transformation.

It must be emphasized once again that the derivation given above depends upon a number of approximations. For a rigorous treatment of the Armitage-Doll model together with a discussion of the approximations made, see Moolgavkar (24). Suffice it to say here that if the average sojourn λ_j^{-1} in stage j is large compared to the human life span (i.e. λ_j^{-1} is of the order of 1000 years for each j), then the approximate age-specific incidence rate per 100,000 predicted by the Armitage-Doll model is $I(t) \times 100,000$, where

$$I(t) = N\lambda_0\lambda_1\cdots\lambda_{n-1}t^{n-1}/_{(n-1)!}, \qquad\qquad 1.$$

with N the total number of susceptible cells in the tissue.

In 1969, Cook, Doll & Fellingham (8) undertook a comprehensive test of the Relationship 1 for the age distribution of cancer. They tested this relationship in 31 types of cancer in 11 populations, and concluded that the constant n "might be a biological constant characteristic of the tissue in which the cancer is produced." However, these authors also concluded that in a large number of data sets, the age-specific incidence rates showed significant departures from the simple Relationship 1. Some possible reasons for these departures are discussed by the authors. A fuller discussion is to be found in a thoughtful article by Peto (32).

Epidemiologic data on exposure to specific carcinogens has been examined within the framework of the Armitage-Doll model by various authors (5, 9, 37). By studying the pattern of evolution of risk after exposure to a carcinogen begins and after exposure stops, it is possible to deduce whether an "early" or a "late" stage (or both) is affected by the carcinogen. However, epidemiologic data are unequal to the task of defining the exact stage or stages affected. Particularly relevant to the discussion to follow is that the only distinction that can be made is between "early" and "late" stages. This suggests that no more than two stages are necessary to "explain" the epidemiologic data. This is indeed true, and is discussed in the latter part of this paper.

That the Armitage-Doll model successfully describes the age-specific incidence curves of a large number of human tumors does not provide strong evidence in favor of its "correctness." Several different models fit the age-specific incidence data equally well. The ultimate vindication of a model must derive from biological considerations. In this regard, the Armitage-Doll is somewhat unsatisfactory. First, no more than two distinct rate-limiting steps have been experimentally demonstrated. Second, initiation-promotion experiments and a host of other considerations suggest that both mutations and active cell division are important in carcinogenesis: the Armitage-Doll model makes no explicit allowance for cell growth and differentiation. Third, the Armitage-Doll model provides no satisfactory explanation for hereditary tumors such as retinoblastoma and Wilms' tumor.

In the next section, I introduce a two-stage model for carcinogenesis and interpret it within the framework of recent results in laboratory cancer research. I discuss the epidemiology of human cancer in light of this model.

A TWO-STAGE MODEL FOR CARCINOGENESIS

Laboratory and human data reveal the existence of two distinct classes of cancer genes. The first class of genes, the oncogenes, were discovered by work on the acutely transforming retroviruses, such as the Rous Sarcoma Virus. Indeed, convincing evidence that the protein product of a single gene is sufficient for malignant transformation was first provided by experiments with this retrovirus. The gene responsible for transformation, the *src* gene, was subsequently found to have cellular homologues in all vertebrates tested. Thus, it would seem that normal cells contain genes, the oncogenes, the inappropriate expression of which can lead to malignant transformation. Evidence that malignant transformation can indeed result from the inappropriate expression of a cellular oncogene is again provided by study of an oncogenic retrovirus, the Avian Leukosis Virus. This virus, which causes bursal lymphomas in chickens, inserts a "promoter" sequence adjacent to a cellular oncogene, the *myc* gene, and turns it on (2).[2]

Evidence of quite another sort strongly suggests that another class of genes, distinct from oncogenes, plays an important role in human carcinogenesis. In many human cancers, pedigree analysis reveals that in some families tumors are transmitted in an autosomal-dominant fashion. Examples are two childhood

---

[2]The situation here may be somewhat more complicated in that activation of another gene, the *b-lym* gene, may also be necessary. See (22).

tumors, retinoblastoma and Wilms' tumor, and an adult tumor, carcinoma of the colon in familial polyposis. The gene locus for retinoblastoma is known to be on the long arm of chromosome 13 (band 13q14), tightly linked to the locus for the enzyme esterase D; the gene locus for Wilms' tumor is on the short arm of chromosome 11 (band 11p13), close to the locus for β-globin. Cytogenetic analysis reveals that in many instances of hereditary retinoblastoma and Wilms' tumor, the respective genes are deleted. Thus, in contrast to oncogenes, it is the inappropriate *inactivation* of these genes that leads to malignancy. Knudson (19) has coined the term *antioncogenes* for this class of genes.

A study of the hereditary human neoplasms reveals two further facts. First, inheritance of an inactive antioncogene is not sufficient to lead to malignant transformation. In these cancers, every cell in the affected tissue has the inactivated antioncogene; however, only a few of the cells go on to develop malignancy, indicating that at least one other event is necessary for transformation. Second, inheritance of an inactivated antioncogene is the strongest known risk factor for cancer in humans. For example, in non–gene carriers the lifetime risk of retinoblastoma is about 1 in 30,000. In contrast, the gene carrier develops three to four tumors on average. Thus, inheritance of the affected gene increases the risk some 100,000-fold (at the level of a cell). Similarly, it can be computed that inheritance of the gene for polyposis coli increases the risk for colon cancer some 5000-fold at age 45.

The Model

Epidemiologic data can distinguish only between an "early" and a "late" stage in carcinogenesis. Further, biological and human data indicate that more than one stage is necessary for carcinogenesis; however, more than two rate-limiting steps have never been convincingly demonstrated. A two-stage model is biologically attractive because it is consistent with the development of homozygosity at a genetic locus.[3]

The working hypothesis that oncogene activation is the final common pathway in malignant transformation may be incorporated into a two-stage model for carcinogenesis by using a genetic regulatory schema postulated by Comings (7). According to this schema, all cells contain genes capable of coding for transforming factors that can release the cell from normal growth constraints. These oncogenes are expressed during histogenesis and tissue renewal; their expression is controlled by diploid pairs of antioncogenes (regulatory genes). Malignant transformation of a cell occurs when the oncogenes are turned on to inappropriately high levels. For most human tumors, this occurs with inactiva-

[3]The word "stage" is used to mean different things by different authors. In this paper, a stage refers to a mutation (defined as an alteration of the genome inherited by daughter cells) that is necessary for malignant transformation.

tion of the appropriate pair of antioncogenes. However, oncogenes could be directly activated by chromosomal rearrangement to bring an oncogene adjacent to a promoter site, or by insertion of a viral promoter next to an oncogene (as happens, for example, with the Avian Leukosis Virus referred to above). Candidates for tumors in which chromosomal rearrangement turns on an oncogene are the lymphomas and leukemias, which are characterized by specific chromosomal rearrangements.

The model discussed here presupposes that human tumors most commonly arise by mutations of the antioncogenes. This model, which has been discussed in detail in previous publications (27, 29), thus requires the occurrence of two rare and irreversible events, namely mutations of the two homologous antioncogenes. The first mutation leads to partial abrogation of growth control, so that a stem cell that has sustained it has a small growth advantage over the surrounding cells. Such a cell may be thought of as an "initiated" cell, and over a period of time will give rise to a clone of initiated cells—a premalignant lesion. The second mutation leads to total abrogation of growth control, i.e. to malignant transformation.

The biological model requires that the two steps involved in carcinogenesis lead to the development of homozygosity at the antioncogene locus. The mathematical formulation of the model is somewhat more general: the two rate-limiting steps involved need not be mutations and the same locus on homologous chromosomes need not be involved. However, there is now some evidence that, at least for two tumors, retinoblastoma and Wilms' tumor, homozygosity at the antioncogene locus is necessary for malignant transformation. This evidence comes from the study of restriction fragment length polymorphisms on the respective chromosomes. Briefly the techniques used exploit the observation that the human DNA fragments that are generated by digestion with restriction enzymes show a great deal of polymorphism. The reader interested in more details should consult the appropriate papers (6, 10, 21).

Epidemiology of Human Cancer

AGE-SPECIFIC INCIDENCE   Many of the biologic and epidemiologic implications of the model follow immediately without any mathematical development (see below). However, if the model is to be tested quantitatively against human epidemiologic and animal experimental data, it must be translated into mathematical terms.

The model is schematically represented in Figure 1. The mathematical details can be found in papers by Moolgavkar & Venzon (29) and Moolgavkar & Knudson (27). The age-specific incidence rate per 100,000 individuals in the population is given by $I(t) \times 10^5$, where

$$I(t) \approx \mu_1 \, \mu_2 \int_0^t X(s) \, \exp\{(\alpha_2 - \beta_2)(t-s)\}ds. \qquad 2.$$

Here, as depicted in Figure 1, μ_1 and μ_2 are the transition rates per cell per year, and $X(s)$ represents the number of normal susceptible cells at time (age) s. This expression for the age-specific incidence is not as simple as that derived from the Armitage-Doll model. However, it should be noted that the growth of normal and intermediate cells enters explicitly into the expression for the age-specific incidence. It should also be noted that (a) the transition rates μ_1 and μ_2 are multiplicative factors and are important in determining the overall incidence rates of the cancer in question (however, they do not influence the shape of the incidence curve), and (b) the shape of the incidence curve is determined by the growth curve of the normal tissue and the cellular kinetics of intermediate cells. Moreover, it is the difference between "birth rate" and "death rate" (i.e. $\alpha_2-\beta_2$) that affects incidence, not the individual parameters. The result that the shape of the age-specific incidence curve depends upon the kinetics of growth and differentiation is biologically appealing.

The growth curves of human tissue show three main patterns:

1. Most tissues show a steady increase in size during childhood and adolescence. The growth curve of such tissues, e.g. the lung and the colon, can be reasonably well represented by a Gompertz curve. Once adult size is reached, the epithelia of these tissues continue to shed and replenish themselves.

2. Some tissues, such as the sex organs, show relatively little growth before puberty, followed by a spurt of growth during adolescence. The growth of such tissues may be represented by a logistic curve. In addition, these tissues are sensitive to changes in physiologic state. Thus, the breast in females grows during puberty and varies in size in response to hormonal influences during pregnancy and after menopause.

3. Certain tissues show a sudden burst of growth in early life followed by a greatly decreased rate of cell division in later life, as in lymphoid tissue, or by virtually no cell division in later life, as in neural tissue.

Reflecting these growth patterns, cancer incidence rates in human populations also show three main patterns.

1. A steady increase in incidence rates with age. Cancers that exhibit this behavior include those that Peto (32) calls the log-log cancers: cancers for which the age-specific incidence rates increase roughly with a power of age. These were the cancers for which the Armitage-Doll model was first proposed. They are comprised mainly of the common carcinomas, i.e. cancers that arise from epithelia. Examples are provided by carcinomas of the colon and the stomach. With the growth of the normal tissue, $X(s)$, represented by a Gompertz curve, Expression 2 is capable of generating incidence curves that describe well the age-specific incidence rates of the cancers in this group (27).

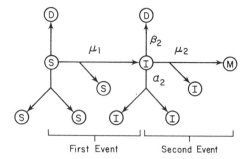

Figure 1   Two-stage model for carcinogenesis. S = normal stem cell, I = intermediate (one-hit) cell, D = differentiated (or dead) cell, M = malignant cell; μ_1 = rate at which first event occurs, μ_2 = rate at which second event occurs, α_2 = rate of division of intermediate cells, β_2 = rate of differentiation and death of intermediate cells. In a small time interval, a given stem cell (S) may divide with a certain probability to give rise to two daughter cells (S), or it may differentiate (or die) (D) and thus leave the pool of susceptible cells, or it may divide (with a small probability) into two cells, one of which is normal (S) and the other of which has suffered the first event to become an intermediate cell (I). The intermediate cell may in turn give rise to two intermediate daughters (I); die or differentiate (D); or give rise (with a small probability) to one intermediate cell (I) and one malignant cell (M). From Moolgavkar & Knudson (27).

2. Incidence rates that exhibit a peak sometime in life followed by a decline. Childhood cancers, such as retinoblastoma, Wilms' tumor, and acute lymphocytic leukemia, provide examples of this pattern. Among adult tumors, testicular carcinoma exhibits this behavior, with a peak incidence at about the age of 30–35 years. As discussed in Moolgavkar & Knudson (27), the two-stage model provides an excellent description of these incidence curves.

3. Exceptional incidence curves, such as those of cancers of the sex organs. As an example, carcinoma of the female breast is discussed in some detail below.

It should be reemphasized here that the Armitage-Doll model was introduced to explain the age-specific incidence curves of the log-log cancers, and is incapable of generating the other patterns of age-specific incidence rates. In contrast, when the growth curve of the tissue in question is taken into account, the two-stage model described here can generate all the age-specific incidence curves observed in human populations.

EPIDEMIOLOGY OF BREAST CANCER (26)   The epidemiology of breast cancer in females is discussed in some detail for the following two reasons. First, the pitfalls of drawing inferences from cross-sectional data are clearly illustrated by breast cancer. Second, breast cancer in females is one of the most intriguing tumors from the point of view of epidemiology.

When cross-sectional age-specific incidence rates of female breast cancer are observed, two distinct patterns emerge. In Western populations, in which risks are high and more or less stable, the age-specific incidence rates rise until menopause, level off, and then continue to rise, albeit more slowly. In Eastern populations, exemplified by the prefecture of Osaka in Japan, in which risks are low and increasing, the age-specific incidence curve rises until menopause, levels off, and then actually falls. This difference in post-menopausal pattern between Western and Eastern populations has been cited as evidence that breast cancer in females consists of premenopausal and postmenopausal components, with both components being present in Western populations, and the post-menopausal component being largely absent in Eastern populations. However, the fall in post-menopausal rates observed in cross-sectional data in Osaka, is due to a cohort-wise increase in risks. After adjustment for cohort effects, the age-specific incidence curve continues to rise after menopause, as it does in the West (28). Thus, the shapes of the age-specific incidence curves of female breast cancer are identical in Eastern and Western populations: The magnitude of the rates sets these populations apart.

The two-stage model described here, with appropriate modifications to incorporate the physiologic responses of the breast tissue to menarche and menopause, generates an age-specific incidence curve that describes well the age-specific incidence curves of breast cancer in six test populations: Connecticut, Denmark, Finland, Slovenia, Iceland, and Osaka (Figure 2). According to the model, hormones influence the epidemiology of breast cancer in females by their action on the kinetics of growth of nonmalignant breast tissue. The breast grows in response to hormonal stimuli at puberty, and it involutes when these stimuli are removed at menopause. These two major kinetic changes imposed on the breast by hormonal influences determine, according to the two-stage model, the basic shape of the age-specific incidence curve of carcinoma of the breast.

In a paper applying this model to female breast cancer, Moolgavkar et al (26) conjectured that a full-term pregnancy causes a certain fraction of normal and intermediate cells to undergo terminal differentiation. These cells are then no longer susceptible to malignant transformation. Direct experimental evidence that this might be the mechanism involved in the protective effect of a full-term of pregnancy was obtained in the rat by Russo & Russo (34). When the assumption that pregnancy causes terminal differentiation of a certain fraction of susceptible cells is incorporated, the model predicts a protective effect of pregnancy that is in good quantitative agreement (Figure 3) with the results of a large multinational study of MacMahon, et al (23).

For a discussion of other aspects of the epidemiology of female breast cancer within the framework of the model, see (26).

ACTION OF ENVIRONMENTAL AGENTS   According to the model, an environmental agent could modify the risk of cancer (*a*) by directly affecting the

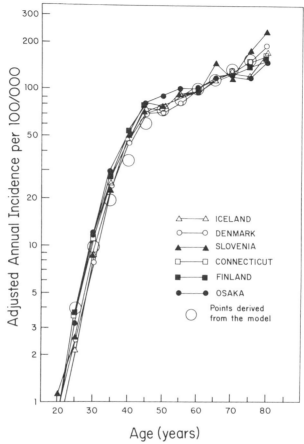

Figure 2   Fit of the model to age-specific breast cancer incidence data from various populations. All curves have been normalized so that the sum of the rates over all age groups is the same. From Moolgavkar et al (26).

transition rates μ_1 and μ_2; or (*b*) by affecting the kinetics of growth of normal or intermediate cells. The effects of acute and of chronic exposure to environmental agents are considered here, as are the effects of discontinuing chronic exposure.

First consider chronic exposure to an agent that affects only the transition rates (μ_1 or μ_2 or both)[4], and suppose that exposure to such an agent starts early in life. Then Expression 2 for age-specific incidence shows that the risk in persons exposed to a given dose relative to nonexposed individuals remains constant with duration of exposure (regardless of whether the first or second transition rate is affected), provided that exposure to that dose increases the transition rates to new constant levels. If, on the contrary, an agent increases the

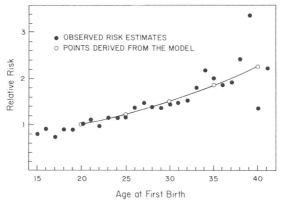

Figure 3   Risk of breast cancer for different ages at first full-term pregnancy relative to first full-term pregnancy at age 20 compared with predictions from the model. From Moolgavkar et al (26).

proliferation of intermediate cells by a constant amount, i.e. increases $\alpha_2-\beta_2$ without affecting μ_1 and μ_2, then the risk in persons exposed relative to those not exposed increases with duration of exposure (Figure 4). As is discussed below, within the framework of this model promoters increase $\alpha_2-\beta_2$. Even small changes in $\alpha_2-\beta_2$ lead to large changes in incidence. Thus, promoters are remarkably effective in facilitating carcinogenesis. Small changes in the growth kinetics of normal cells have little effect on cancer incidence.

Suppose now that chronic exposure to an environmental agent ceases (e.g. a long-time smoker gives up the habit). If the agent affects only the first transition rate, then stoppage of exposure leads to an incidence curve that lies in between the incidence curves in exposed and nonexposed individuals. In other words, even after exposure is stopped, the incidence rate never goes back to pre-exposure levels. The reason for this is intuitively clear: During exposure, there is a build-up of cells in the intermediate compartment. However, if the agent affects the second transition rate alone, discontinuance of the exposure leads to a quick reversion of the incidence rate to pre-exposure levels (Figure 5). Finally, if exposure to an agent that increases $\alpha_2-\beta_2$ is discontinued, the incidence rates will again lie between the incidence curves among exposed and nonexposed individuals (25).

---

[4]If μ_1 and μ_2 are mutation rates, there is little reason to believe that an agent could affect one without affecting the other. See discussion of initiation-promotion below. However, homozygosity at an antioncogene locus could be brought about either by two mutations or by a mutation followed by a recombination event. Thus, it is theoretically possible for an agent acting as a "recombinogen" to increase μ_2 without increasing μ_1. Within the framework of the model, such agents could be called "completers" (25). See also the discussion of the genetics of human cancer, below.

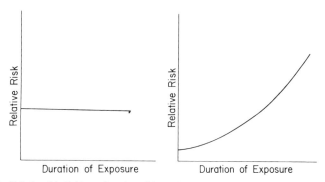

Figure 4   Relative risk *(left)* as a function of time when chronic exposure to an agent (from time 0) increases μ_1 or μ_2 (or both) to a new constant level and *(right)* as a function of time when chronic exposure to an agent increases $\alpha_2 - \beta_2$. From Moolgavkar (25).

Consider now short-term high-intensity exposure to an agent that affects mutation rates, such as the radiation exposure suffered by the atomic bomb survivors of Hiroshima and Nagasaki. Such exposure may remove a certain proportion of non-neoplastic cells from the susceptible pool either by killing them or by greatly diminishing their capacity to divide. However, the main effect of such an exposure is to cause a certain fraction of normal cells to sustain the first mutation and become intermediate cells. A certain fraction of intermediate cells will sustain the second mutation and become malignant. Since there are only a small number of intermediate cells at any given time, however, the latter effect has negligible impact on cancer incidence. The model predicts that relative risk will increase after exposure and then gradually decline with time to approach an asymptote. For more details see Moolgavkar & Knudson (27).

Acute exposure to an agent that affects cellular kinetics will have little effect on cancer incidence.

FAMILIAL HUMAN CANCER   It is well-known that the occurrence of cancers in relatives can increase individual risk. In some families, the risk is increased enormously, and pedigree analysis reveals that predisposition to cancer is inherited in an autosomal-dominant fashion. Such hereditary cancers form only a small fraction of all cancers. However, a large proportion of some embryonal cancers are hereditary. For example, Knudson has estimated that approximately 40% of all cases of retinoblastoma are inherited in an autosomal-dominant fashion. Currently, there are approximately 50 cancers in humans in which predisposition is known to be inherited in an autosomal-dominant fashion (20).

Within the framework of the model presented here, such hereditary cancers are caused by mutations at the same antioncogene loci as the sporadic forms of

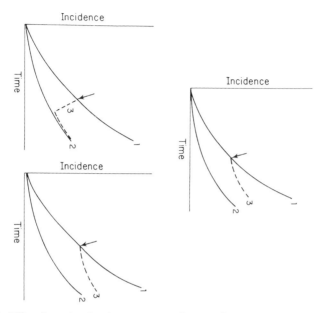

Figure 5   Effect of stopping chronic exposure to environmental agents: *(top)*, exposure to an agent that increases μ_1 (initiator); *(bottom left)*, exposure to an agent that increases μ_2; *(bottom right)* exposure to an agent that increases $\alpha_2 - \beta_2$ (promoter). In all three figures, (1) is the incidence curve in the exposed population, (2) is the incidence curve in the unexposed population, and (3) is the incidence curve after exposure is stopped at the time indicated by the *arrow*. From Moolgavkar (25).

the cancer. However, whereas in the sporadic cases both mutations occur in somatic cells, in the dominantly inherited cases the first mutation has occurred in a germ cell.[5] Thus, the affected individual is born with all the cells of the target organ in the intermediate stage (18). That this is indeed a plausible mechanism has been demonstrated for retinoblastoma and Wilms' tumor [see (20) for a brief review of the pertinent literature]. One inherited case of retinoblastoma, reported by Benedict et al (3) is interesting and easy to understand. As mentioned above, the gene (antioncogene) for retinoblastoma is located on the long arm of chromosome 13, tightly linked to the locus for

[5]The two-stage model proposes that the antioncogene acts *recessively* to cause cancer, i.e. antioncogenes on both members of a pair of homologous chromosomes must be mutated for malignant transformation. However, inheritance of one mutated gene leads to *dominant* inheritance of cancer predisposition. This is because all the cells of the affected tissue are in the intermediate stage, and the probability that one of them will sustain the second mutation and become malignant is close to 1. Thus, recessivity at the cellular level leads to dominance at the population level.

esterase D. The karyotyped lymphocytes showed no abnormality. However, measurement of esterase D activity showed that it was 50% of normal. Thus, the presumption was that *submicroscopic* deletion of the retinoblastoma and esterase D loci on one of the chromosomes 13 had occurred. When the tumor itself was karyotyped, one of the chromosomes 13 was missing, and esterase D activity was measured to be zero. Thus, the *normal* chromosome 13 had been deleted in the tumor, leading to homozygous deletion at the retinoblastoma locus. For a more detailed discussion, see (20).

The dominantly inherited conditions increase predisposition to single cancers or to a small number of specific cancers. Thus, individuals with the retinoblastoma gene are at high risk for osteogenic sarcoma in addition to retinoblastoma. In contrast, there are recessively inherited conditions, exemplified by xeroderma pigmentosum (XP) and Bloom's syndrome, that increase the risk for a wide variety of cancers. XP is characterized by defective repair of UV-induced DNA damage, and afflicted persons are remarkably sensitive to sunlight, the most lethal effect being skin cancers—basal cell and squamous cell carcinomas and melanomas. Within the context of the model, XP increases the risk of cancer by increasing both mutation rates in the presence of UV light.

Bloom's syndrome is characterized by chromosomal fragility leading to increased frequency of sister chromatid and homologous chromosome exchanges. Afflicted persons are predisposed to leukemia and to other cancers. Bloom's syndrome could facilitate the production of homozygosity in a cell with the first mutation by mitotic recombination. Indeed, recent work by Cavanee et al (6) indicates that mitotic recombination is an important mechanism for bringing about homozygosity in retinoblastoma. Thus, within the context of the model, Bloom's syndrome increases μ_2 without increasing μ_1.

Only single gene defects predisposing to malignancy have been discussed here. Undoubtedly other, less readily definable, factors run in families and predispose to cancer. For example, the ability to process and detoxify chemical carcinogens is clearly genetically determined and must affect the risk to individuals [see e.g. Omenn & Gelboin (31)]. Likewise, it seems reasonable that levels of hormones, such as the estrogens, are correlated in members of the same family. Finally, family members share similar lifestyles and thus share, to some extent, risk factors for cancer. Some familial clustering of cancer therefore may occur without a genetic basis.

Initiation and Promotion

The words "initiator" and "promoter" were originally defined within the context of chemical carcinogenesis in animals. The definitions were phenomenological: initiator and promoter had to be administered in the proper sequence (initiator followed by promoter) to produce tumors. The concepts of initiation and promotion have been picked up and used rather loosely by scientists in "other" disciplines. In epidemiology, an initiator is often thought of as an "early-stage" carcinogen, whereas a promoter is thought of as a "late-stage" carcinogen. In fact, little experimental evidence supports this point of view. While it seems to be true that promoters do not facilitate carcinogenesis in the absence of initiation, every initiator seems capable of causing malignant transformation even in the absence of promoters, as is discussed below.

Within the context of the model presented above, the words "initiator" and "promoter" can be given precise meaning. An initiator is any agent that increases μ_1, the probability of transition from a normal stem cell to a once-hit intermediate cell. A promoter is an agent that acts on intermediate cells to increase α_2, decrease β_2, or both. Application of a promoter leads to a proliferation of intermediate cells to give rise to intermediate lesions. The papillomas that arise in the skin-painting experiments and the enzyme-altered foci that have been described in hepatocarcinogenesis experiments can be considered to be examples of such intermediate lesions. Thus, promoters act on cells that have sustained a single critical event to cause their proliferation, i.e. they act as selective mitogens. Promoter-induced proliferation leads to an increase in the number of intermediate cells, which, in turn, increases the probability that one of these cells will sustain the second critical event and become malignant.

The scenario proposed above implies that initiation-promotion should yield mainly benign tumors (e.g. papillomas), and later only a few malignant tumors. This is indeed observed in initiation-promotion experiments (36). Further, a protocol in which initiation is followed by promotion until the appearance of intermediate lesions and then by a second application of initiator should lead to many more malignant tumors [Moolgavkar & Knudson (27), Potter (33)]. This has now been experimentally demonstrated (14).

The model for initiation-promotion presented above raises some fundamental questions. If both critical events in carcinogenesis are mutations, can there be agents that could be classified as "pure" initiators? Prolonged application of an initiator (a mutagen) should facilitate both critical events and should lead eventually to malignant transformation. For many years urethane was classified as a pure initiator in mouse skin (35). However, urethane is a toxic substance, and the experiments that concluded that urethane is a pure initiator faced technical difficulties with prolonged application. Recently, Iversen (16) has concluded that urethane alone is capable of causing carcinomas in mouse skin.

If, as is proposed here, the two critical events in carcinogenesis occur at the same site on homologous chromosomes, an intriguing possibility arises. Homozygosity at the critical site could be brought about not only by two mutations but by one mutation followed by mitotic recombination. Thus, within the context of the model, in addition to initiators, which increase both mutation rates μ_1 and μ_2, and promoters, which act as mitogens on the intermediate cells, it is possible to postulate a third class of agents, which could be called "completers," that facilitates carcinogenesis. Any agent that favors mitotic recombination would act as a completer. Such agents would increase μ_2 without increasing μ_1. As noted above, a recessive human condition, Bloom's syndrome, could facilitate carcinogenesis in this way. It has also been suggested by Kinsella & Radman (17), although not verified by others, that the classical promoters in mouse skin, the phorbol esters, facilitate mitotic recombination. If this is true, the phorbol esters have both promoting and completing properties.

Intermediate Lesions

If carcinogenesis is a two-stage process, it would clearly be of interest to identify and study the intermediate lesions, i.e. clones of cells that have sustained the first mutation. In chemical carcinogenesis experiments, papillomas of mouse skin and enzyme-altered foci in the rat liver were identified above as intermediate lesions.

Candidates for intermediate lesions may be identified in human cancers as well. Cancers that occur in both sporadic and dominantly inherited forms provide leads to the identification of intermediate lesions and also generate testable biologic hypotheses. Gene carriers often exhibit characteristic pathologic lesions in the tissue that is at high risk for cancer. These lesions may represent *identifiable* clusters of initiated cells. The same lesions in non–gene carriers may be interpreted as *clones* of initiated cells. As is discussed in Moolgavkar & Knudson (27), premalignant lesions would be predicted, on the basis of the model, to be clonal in sporadic cases and polyclonal in gene carriers. The malignant lesions would be clonal in both sporadic and hereditary cases.

A table of putative intermediate lesions can be found in (27). Since the publication of that paper, the predictions regarding clonality have been fulfilled for one tumor type. It was known that sporadic neurofibromas are clonal, whereas the neurofibromas in von Recklinghausen's disease (neurofibromatosis), a dominantly inherited condition, are polyclonal. The neurofibrosarcomas that arise from these lesions have recently been shown to be clonal (13).

The abundance of polyps of the colon in polyposis syndromes suggests that adenomatous polyps represent the intermediate stage in both hereditary and sporadic cases of colon cancer. It should perhaps be clarified that not all clones of initiated cells will be detectable as polyps: The polyps represent clones that have become large enough to be visible. A consequence of this is that many tumors of the colon arise in preexisting polyps, but at least some do not. The latter presumably arise from clones of initiated cells that are too small to be visible. As predicted by the model, it has recently been shown that polyps in Gardener's syndrome (a dominantly inherited polyposis syndrome) are polyclonal (15).

CONCLUDING REMARKS

Multistage models provide a convenient conceptual framework within which to view the process of carcinogenesis. Since there is no firm evidence for more than two discrete rate-limiting stages in carcinogenesis, parsimony dictates that a two-stage model be given serious consideration. Further, it is imperative that the kinetics of cell growth and differentiation be explicitly considered in any model. The role of tissue kinetics in multistage models is widely misunderstood. For example, as mentioned above, a promoter is usually modeled as a late-stage carcinogen. The transition rate λ_k is assumed to be a linear function of the dose of the carcinogen, $\lambda_k = a + bd$, where a and b are constants and d is dose. This is totally wrong for the following reason. Under the simplest possible model for cell growth, the cell divides with a certain rate constant α and differentiates or dies with a rate constant β. Then the expected total number of cells at time t is given by $N \exp[(\alpha - \beta)t]$ if N is the number of cells at time 0. Now a reasonable way to model the effect of a promoter is to assume that $(\alpha - \beta) = a + bd$. The implications of this formulation for dose-response are quite different from those derived from the assumption that the transition rate λ_k is a linear function of dose.

In the two-stage model described here, the two events are thought of as mutations. If this is indeed true, then one must expect to see a certain background rate of cancer that is consonant with background mutation rates. For example, the rates of Wilms' tumor are remarkably constant around the world.

The incidence rates of cancer generated by the model are sensitive to small changes in the kinetics of the intermediate cells. Thus, promoters have a profound effect on cancer incidence rates. The epidemiologic data are consistent with the hypothesis that estrogens act as promoters in the female breast, and that the main carcinogenic effect of cigarette smoke in the lung is promotion (27).

Finally, no model can be said to be "correct." The role of any model is to provide a framework for viewing known facts and to suggest experiments. This the two-stage model does successfully. The model is of necessity crude. For example, there is in vitro evidence that activation of two distinct oncogenes may be necessary for malignant transformation. Transfection experiments indicate that the human *ras* oncogene does not transform fibroblasts unless they have been immortalized by another gene such as the *myc* gene (22). The significance or relevance of this finding for human carcinogenesis is not clear. It suggests that the two-stage model may, in some instances, be interpretable as leading to partial abrogation of cellular control of each of two distinct oncogene loci.

The literature on the molecular biology of cancer is growing explosively. The nonspecialist cannot possibly keep abreast of it much less digest it, reconcile seeming inconsistencies, and incorporate latest developments into comprehensive models for human carcinogenesis. We are still struggling with the melody. Harmony and counterpoint must come later.

ACKNOWLEDGMENT

Supported by Public Health Services grant CA39949 and CA 30671.

Literature Cited

1. Armitage, P., Doll, R. 1954. The age distribution of cancer and a multistage theory of carcinogenesis. *Br. J. Cancer* 8:1–12
2. Astrin, S. M., Rothberg, P. G. 1983. Oncogenes and cancer. *Cancer Invest.* 1:355–64
3. Benedict, W. F., Murphree, A. L., Banerjee, A., Spina, C. A., Sparkes, M. C., et al. 1983. Patient with 13 chromosome deletion: Evidence that the retinoblastoma gene is a recessive cancer gene. *Science* 219:973–75
4. Berenblum, I., Shubik, P. 1947. A new, quantitative, approach to the study of the stages of chemical carcinogenesis in the mouse's skin. *Br. J. Cancer* 1:383–91
5. Brown, C. C., Chu, K. C. 1982. Approaches to epidemiologic analysis of prospective and retrospective studies: Example of lung cancer and exposure to arsenic. In *Environmental Epidemiology: Risk Assessment,* ed. R. L. Prentice, A. S. Whittemore. Philadelphia: SIAM
6. Cavanee, W. K., Dryja, T. P., Phillips, R. A., Benedict, W. F., Godbout, R., et al. 1983. Expression of recessive alleles by chromosomal mechanisms in retinoblastoma. *Nature* 305:779–84
7. Comings, D. E. 1973. A general theory of carcinogenesis. *Proc. Natl. Acad. Sci. USA* 70:3324–28
8. Cook, P. J., Doll, R., Fellingham, S. A. 1969. A mathematical model for the age distribution of cancer in man. *Int. J. Cancer* 4:93–112
9. Day, N. E., Brown, C. C. 1980. Multistage models and primary prevention of cancer. *J. Natl. Cancer Inst.* 64:977–89
10. Dryja, T. P., Cavenee, W., White, R., Rapaport, J. M., Peterson, R., et al. 1984. Expression of recessive alleles by chromosomal mechanisms in retinoblastoma. *N. Engl. J. Med.* 310:550–53
11. Fialkow, P. J. 1977. Clonal origin and stem cell evolution of human tumors. In *Genetics of Human Cancer,* ed. J. J. Mulvhill, R. W. Miller, J. F. Fraumeni Jr., pp. 439–53. New York: Raven
12. Fisher, J. C., Holloman, J. H. 1951. A hypothesis for the origin of cancer foci. *Cancer* 4:916–18

13. Friedman, J. M., Fialkow, P. J., Greene, C. L., et al. 1983. Probable clonal origin of neurofibrosarcoma in a patient with hereditary neurofibromatosis. *J. Natl. Cancer Inst.* 69:1289–92
14. Hennings, H., Shores, R., Wenk, M. L., Spangler, E. F., Tarone, R., et al. 1983. Malignant conversion of mouse skin tumours is increased by tumour initiators and unaffected by tumour promoters. *Nature* 304:67–69
15. Hsu, S. H., Luk, G. D., Krush, A. J., et al. 1983. Multiclonal origin of polyps in Gardner syndrome. *Science* 221:951–53
16. Iversen, O. H. 1984. Urethan (ethyl carbamate) alone carcinogenic for Mouse skin. *Carcinogenesis* 5:911–16
17. Kinsella, A. R., Radman, M. 1978. Tumor promoter induces sister chromatid exchanges: Relevance to mechanisma of carcinogenesis. *Proc. Natl. Acad. Sci. USA* 75:6149–53
18. Knudson, A. G. 1971. Mutation and cancer: Statistical study of retinoblastoma. *Proc. Natl. Acad. Sci. USA* 68:820–23
19. Knudson, A. G. 1983. Model hereditary cancers of man. *Cancer Invest.* 1:187–93
20. Knudson, A. G. 1985. Hereditary cancer, oncogenes, and antioncogenes. *Cancer Res.* 45:1437–43
21. Koufos, A., Hansen, M. F., Lampkin, B. C., Workman, M. L., Copeland, N. G., et al. 1984. Loss of alleles at loci on human chromosome 11 during genesis of Wilms' tumour. *Nature* 309:170–72
22. Land, H., Parada, L. F., Weinberg, R. A. 1983. Tumorigenic conversion of primary embryo fibroblasts requires at least two cooperating oncogenes. *Nature* 304:596–601
23. MacMahon, B., Cole, P., Lin, T. M., et al. 1970. Age at first birth and breast cancer risk. *Bull. WHO* 43:209–21
24. Moolgavkar, S. H. 1978. The multistage theory of carcinogenesis and the age distribution of cancer in man. *J. Natl. Cancer Inst.* 61:49–52
25. Moolgavkar, S. H. 1983. Model for human carcinogenesis: Actions of environmental agents. *Environ. Health Perspect.* 50:285–91

26. Moolgavkar, S. H., Day, N. E., Stevens, R. G. 1980. Two-stage model for carcinogenesis: Epidemiology of breast cancer in females. *J. Natl. Cancer Inst.* 65:559–69

27. Moolgavkar, S. H., Knudson, A. G. Jr. 1981. Mutation and cancer: A model for human carcinogenesis. *J. Natl. Cancer Inst.* 66:1037–52

28. Moolgavkar, S. H., Stevens, R. G., Lee, J. A. 1979. Effect of age on incidence of breast cancer in females. *J. Natl. Cancer Inst.* 62:493–501

29. Moolgavkar, S. H., Venzon, D. J. 1979. Two-event models for carcinogenesis: Incidence curves for childhood and adult tumors. *Math. Biosci.* 47:55–77

30. Nordling, C. O. 1953. A new theory on the cancer inducing mechanism. *Br. J. Cancer* 7:68–72

31. Omenn, G. S., Gelboin, H. V., eds. 1984. *Genetic variability in responses to chemical exposure.* Banbury Rep. 16. Cold Spring Harbor, NY: Cold Spring Harbor Lab.

32. Peto, R. 1977. Epidemiology, multistage models, and short-term mutagenecity tests. In *Origins of Human Cancer, Book C: Human Risk Assessment,* ed. H. H. Hiatt, J. D. Watson, J. A. Winsten, pp. 1403–28. Cold Spring Harbor, NY: Cold Spring Harbor Lab.

33. Potter, V. R. 1980. Initiation and promotion in cancer formation: The importance of studies on intercellular communication. *Yale J. Biol. Med.* 53:367–84

34. Russo, J., Russo, I. H. 1980. Susceptibility of the mammary gland to carcinogenesis. II. Pregnancy interruption as a risk factor in tumor incidence. *Am. J. Pathol.* 100:497–512

35. Salaman, M. H., Roe, J. F. 1953. Incomplete carcinogens: Ethyl cabamate (urethane) as an initiator of skin tumour formation in the mouse. *Br. J. Cancer* 7:472–81

36. Stenback, F., Garcia, H., Shubik, P. 1974. Present status of the concept of promoting action and co-carcinogenesis in skin. In *Physiopathology of Cancer,* Vol. 1: *Biology and Biochemistry,* ed. P. Shubik, pp. 155–225. Basel: Karger

37. Thomas, D. C. 1982. Temporal effects and interactions in cancer: Implications of carcinogenic models. In *Environmental Epidemiology: Risk Assessment,* ed. R. L. Prentice, A. S. Whittemore. Philadelphia: SIAM

Ann. Rev. Public Health. 1986. 7:171–92
Copyright © 1986 by Annual Reviews Inc. All rights reserved

ASBESTOS AS A PUBLIC HEALTH RISK: Disease and Policy

Hans Weill*

Tulane University School of Medicine, Department of Medicine, Pulmonary Diseases Section, New Orleans, Louisiana 70112

Janet M. Hughes

Tulane University School of Medicine, Pulmonary Diseases Section, and School of Public Health, Department of Biostatistics and Epidemiology, New Orleans, Louisiana 70112

Optimal societal benefit from public policy decision making concerning environmental and occupational health issues can be obtained only when these decisions are fully and appropriately based on existing scientific knowledge. Regarding asbestos and its use in our society, this important goal has been elusive for a number of reasons. First, scientists have been unwilling or unable to communicate technical issues to decision makers, in part due to their complexity, but also because the forum for this interaction has often been adversarial in nature. Second, the public and their policymakers have sometimes mistrusted science and technology; particularly recently, technological progress is often viewed as detrimental to society, particularly in environmental matters. And third, scientists' opinions have, at times, been based more on personal choice than on professional expertise. These, and possibly other factors, have made for an uneasy union between scientists and policymakers in areas in which communication is essential if society is to deal effectively with many of these complex expectations.

Nevertheless, communication between these two sectors is improving. Scientists, recognizing the importance of these concerns (and that decisions must often be made, with or without scientific input), are becoming increasingly willing to participate in dialogues concerning public policy issues. The public,

*Work partially performed while a Fellow in Science and Public Policy, The Brookings Institution, Washington D.C.

171

0163-7525/86/0510-0171$02.00

made more aware of the inevitable uncertainties and limitations of science, apparently understands that sometimes the available information simply does not provide the needed answers. Policymakers are increasingly sensitive to the vulnerability of their decisions when competent and balanced input from the scientific community is absent.

The two primary policy issues concerning asbestos-associated health risks are risk reduction and compensation of asbestos-exposed workers who have developed an asbestos-associated disease. Risk reduction depends on the use of population studies to relate type and amount of exposure to the relevant disease outcomes. These dose-response relationships are used to estimate the potential risks associated with specified exposure situations; the risk estimates provide a basis for choosing between available courses of action. The issue of worker compensation depends on the development of sound, medically based criteria for the ascertainment of compensible health effects, together with a reliable, equitable system for channeling this compensation to the eligible worker. Rational approaches to both policy areas can be accomplished on the basis of existing scientific knowledge. Impediments to these approaches, when they have occurred, have been motivated by nonscientific concerns, frequently based on economic considerations.

BACKGROUND ON THE ISSUES

Concerns regarding the serious health consequences of asbestos exposure have been marked during the past decade and have resulted in a wide range of regulations, a number of legislative initiatives, and a unique judicial burden of litigation. In addition to the thousands of workers whose health has been affected by exposure to asbestos, the economic consequences of these health effects to the asbestos industry (and presumably in some instances, the public) have been reflected by a substantially contracted market and by corporate bankruptcy. Health risks from asbestos exposure have been claimed not only for workers but also for millions of industrial users of these products (e.g. shipbuilding and construction), family members of exposed workers, individuals living in the vicinity of industrial asbestos emissions, residents of communities with asbestos fibers in the water supply, and even to occupants of buildings containing asbestos ceiling materials, most notably, public schools.

Public policy has been made in response to the increasing awareness of real or perceived risks associated with asbestos exposure, often without adequate recourse to the available knowledge or to the broad range of experts on this subject. Not surprisingly, many of these policy decisions have been very costly and, in the case of injured workers, have not always resulted in adequate or equitable compensation. More than 20,000 law suits await disposition in the courts. A protracted struggle continues among insurance companies and between manufacturers and their insurance carriers regarding allocation of liability. Public concern is leading to widespread replacement of intact asbestos-containing ceilings in public buildings, estimated to cost eventually billions of dollars.

How and why did we get to this point? Has policy in the United States been less rational than in other industrialized nations? Is it now likely that careful and informed choices between available and socially acceptable current policy options will lead to resolution of the many outstanding issues? And finally, have lessons been learned to avoid similar consequences in the future?

Development of Knowledge Regarding Asbestos Health Effects

Approximately two decades following the commercial introduction of asbestos, shortly after the turn of the century, the first case of lung fibrosis, later called asbestosis, was recognized and reported to the British government. By the 1930s, asbestosis risk was clearly recognized in asbestos textile manufacturing. This risk was shown to be dose-related in a US Public Health Service study in the late 1930s (11), leading to the first suggestion of a dust level putatively associated with no risk of disease (threshold limit value, TLV).[1] Asbestosis risk in users of asbestos products was regarded as minimal as a result of a 1946 report on New England shipyard workers (19). However, 20 years later, studies of insulators showed substantial risk of lung fibrosis (46). Case reports in the 1930s first suggested that an increased number of lung cancers seemed to occur in workers with asbestosis. An autopsy study in the UK supporting this association was published in the late 1940s (32) and, in 1955, the first epidemiologic study of workers in asbestos manufacturing convincingly showed an increased lung cancer risk (10). In 1967, a study of US asbestos products manufacturing workers showed this risk to be dose related (12). Excess lung cancer risk was established to be associated with insulators in the early 1960s (47) and with mining and milling in the early 1970s (31).

Mesothelioma, a rare and highly malignant tumor of the pleural and peritoneal surfaces, was first related to asbestos exposure in a 1960 report from South Africa, in which workers and others exposed to crocidolite asbestos in and near the mines in the Northwest Cape were found to develop this cancer with alarming frequency (50). Subsequently, mesothelioma risk was confirmed in manufacturing and end-product use of asbestos around the world. The importance of nonoccupational exposures in the causation of this tumor became

---

[1]Abbreviations used: ACGIH, American Conference of Governmental Industrial Hygienists; CPSC, Consumer Product Safety Commission; EPA, Environmental Protection Agency; ETS, emergency temporary standard; ILO, International Labour Office; mppcf, million particles per cubic foot; NRC, National Research Council; PEL, permissible exposure level; TLV, threshold limit value.

increasingly apparent. Exposures were often short, with a long latency period (time from first exposure to manifestation of the tumor) of generally two to four decades.

Clearly, knowledge of the types of disease and the circumstances of causal asbestos exposure did not appear suddenly, but evolved over several decades. Awareness was influenced by both the increased smoking prevalence and more intense asbestos exposures during World War II. The state of knowledge in the past is of more than academic interest today. Who knew or should have known what, and what should have been done about it are often hotly debated under the rubric of "state of the art" in courts hearing product liability cases. In fact, the data base concerning asbestos, with its attendant knowledge, evolved over many decades. This evolutionary nature is frequently neglected in the public debate over this public health risk.

Assessing the Risk

The data available for relating amount of asbestos exposure to excess risk of cancer come from studies of workers exposed to asbestos in industry, usually many years ago. Therefore, cancer risk at today's lower industrial exposure levels or at the very much lower environmental levels is primarily estimated by extrapolation from past, relatively high exposure levels. Estimation of potential risk by extrapolation rather than by direct observation necessarily results in considerable uncertainty of the risk estimates, especially when extrapolation is performed over several orders of magnitude of exposure, such as for environmental exposures. Mathematical models have been developed for extrapolating the risks of lung cancer and mesothelioma—cancers well established as being associated with asbestos exposure. Evidence of an increased risk of cancers of other sites has been inconsistent, causing many researchers and review groups, including the Ontario Royal Commission (43) and the British Government's advisory panel (21), to conclude that the evidence for an association is not convincing.

Unlike for cancer risk, there is direct evidence of asbestosis resulting from the industrial exposure levels of recent years (2). These cases generally have been mild in severity, not resulting in serious disability. There is no evidence that this disease can occur as a result of environmental exposures.

Modeling of lung cancer risk is based on the observation in several industrial studies that the number of excess lung cancers is approximately proportional to cumulative asbestos exposure. The proportionality factor, or slope of the dose-response relationship, however, varies considerably in the seven cohorts (Figure 1). Some of this variability is apparently explained by the industrial process: textile workers exhibit the steepest slope, asbestos cement and other manufacturing workers have intermediate slopes, and miners and friction product workers, the shallowest. A similar conclusion regarding differences in risk by industrial process has been reached by other reviewers (6a). Consistent with the observed risk trend is that exposures in textile processing are likely to be more to individual fibers than in other manufacturing, with the least separation of fibers occurring in mining and milling. These findings are also consistent with expected differences in the physical dimension distribution of the asbestos fibers in these settings; e.g. airborne fibers in textile manufacturing tend to be longer and thinner than those during mining and asbestos cement manufacturing. Moreover, animal experiments have demonstrated long, thin fibers to be more pathogenic that short, coarse fibers (42, 49). Based on the epidemiologic studies, an approximate slope (or range of slopes, to reflect the inevitable uncertainties of a particular value) may be selected as the most appropriate for an exposure situation of interest.

The linear, no-threshold model for lung cancer risk assumes that any asbestos exposure, no matter how small or how brief, will result in some increased risk. Thus, the model necessarily results in an estimate of lung cancer cases attributable to any specified asbestos exposure. There is general agreement that the model possibly overestimates the potential risk from low cumulative asbestos exposure levels but, in all probability, does not underestimate it.

Mesothelioma occurs less frequently than excess lung cancer among most asbestos-exposed populations, and few studies have any quantitative dose information in relation to mesothelioma risk. Consequently, although mesothelioma has been unquestionably associated with asbestos exposure, there is only limited information upon which to base a dose-response relationship.

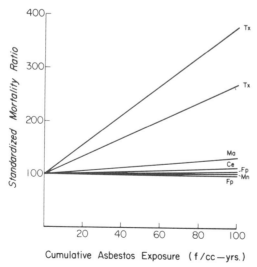

Figure 1 Estimated lung cancer dose-response relationships from seven epidemiologic studies (Refs. 26, 27, 22, 51, 28, 30, 1, respectively, from top). Tx = textile; Ma = manufacturing; Ce = asbestos cement; Fp = friction products; Mn = mining.

Strong qualitative evidence supports a differential in mesothelioma risk for the different asbestos minerals. Chrysotile, a serpentine mineral, appears to pose less risk than the amphibole fibers, of which amosite seems less hazardous than crocidolite. In terms of usage, chrysotile constitutes the great majority of the asbestos used commercially, with amosite now used rarely and crocidolite still utilized in some countries but not others. In fact, most industrialized countries have recognized this differential risk by setting different control limits for these minerals; US regulatory agencies have not made such a distinction. The evidence of a difference in mesothelioma risk by asbestos type has recently been summarized (8). Combined results of epidemiologic studies show that mesothelioma cases constitute 12% of the excess lung cancers in populations exposed only to chrysotile, compared to 22% for amosite and 165% for crocidolite, whereas cohorts exposed to a mixture of fibers exhibit an intermediate value of 66%. These findings suggest that chrysotile may pose approximately one fifth the risk of a mixed fiber exposure (12% vs 66%). Case-control studies (29, 37) have found similar results, and tissue analysis studies of persons exposed to a mixture of fibers have found higher levels of amphibole fibers but similar chrysotile fibers in the lungs of cases compared with controls (24, 25). Recent reports of the amphibole tremolite in the lungs of Quebec chrysotile miners (4) suggest that these exposures were not to chrysotile alone and could be interpreted as strengthening the evidence of a difference in mesothelioma risk between chrysotile and the amphiboles.

This evidence of a difference in mesothelioma risk by fiber type cannot be considered wholly conclusive without demonstration of a different risk after controlling for extent of total asbestos fiber exposure, thus demonstrating a "fiber-for-fiber" difference. Because of the limited exposure information from the past, such detailed comparisons are not possible, nor are they likely to be available in the future because of the marked decrease in worldwide amphibole use. However, since the number of excess lung cancers is related to the amount of asbestos exposure (as well as population size), the expression of total mesothelioma cases as a percentage of excess lung cancers can be expected to at least partially adjust for cumulative exposure level.

Mesothelioma incidence rates have been demonstrated to be a power function of time since initial exposure (40), and this fact has been used to derive a mesothelioma model that expresses incidence as a function of time since initial (and cessation of) exposure, as well as the concentration and duration of exposure. Although the available data are not sufficiently detailed to allow validation of the model's assumptions concerning the effect of exposure duration and concentration of incidence rates, these assumptions are consistent with the mathematical theory of carcinogenicity. As with the lung cancer model, the mesothelioma model assumes that any amount of asbestos exposure necessarily increases mesothelioma risk and therefore results in an estimated potential risk for any specified asbestos exposure.

The details of the mesothelioma model have been reported elsewhere (5). As with the slope of the lung cancer model, it is necessary to estimate a multiplicative parameter of the mesothelioma model from epidemiologic studies. For each study, the value of the model parameter depends on the amount of asbestos exposure in the study population; however, most of the studies reporting sufficiently detailed mesothelioma information have limited exposure data available. Moreover, because of the qualitative evidence of a differential risk by fiber type, this parameter also depends on the type of fiber exposure. There are four epidemiologic studies of populations exposed to a mixture of fibers (chrysotile and amphiboles) from which a parameter estimate may be obtained (18, 22a, 39, 48). [There are two populations with exposure to chrysotile (7, 38), but these have only a total of two mesothelioma cases; there is one population reportedly exposed to amosite only (44)]. Since the evidence suggests that chrysotile may pose one fifth or less the risk of a mixed-fiber exposure, the parameter for chrysotile exposure can be assumed to be one fifth the value for mixed fibers.

An Application of Risk Assessment

Based on these models, several groups of researchers have calculated the potential asbestos-associated risk under various assumptions of exposure concentration and duration. In order to compare these calculations adjusted to common assumptions, we consider here the exposure of students attending schools containing friable asbestos products. The Ontario Royal Commission (43), after a complete review of the available data, concluded that the best available estimate of the average asbestos concentration inside buildings containing asbestos is .001 fibers per milliliter of air (f/ml), with peaks of .01 f/ml occurring occasionally. For comparison purposes, we assume an average of .001 f/ml, with students exposed to this concentration 35 hours per week, 36 weeks per year. For students enrolled in these schools for an average of five years, beginning at age ten years, the adjusted risk estimates based on five reports appear in Table 1.

These reports agreed fundamentally in general methodology and risk models [the National Research Council (NRC) did not use lifetable methods for mesothelioma risk, but their reported value has been adjusted in Table 1]. Consequently, there is reasonably good agreement of the risk estimates. The differences are primarily due to differences in the choice of values for the model parameters (although there are also differences due to the assumed background risk of lung cancer). Similarly, the range of risks reported by two groups [Environmental Protection Agency (EPA) and Consumer Product Safety Commission (CPSC)] are a result of a range of the parameter values, chosen to reflect wide variability in exposure situations rather than a particular exposure. The range for the potential risk can be narrowed for a specified fiber type and exposure situation, such as exposure in schools. For example, a steep lung

Table 1   Estimated lifetime risk[a] from asbestos exposure in schools per one million students exposed to .001 f/ml of mixed fibers for five school years beginning at age 10, based on six reports

| Report | Lung cancer | | Mesothelioma | Total |
	Slope[b]	Estimate	Estimate[c]	
EPA (16)	.3–3.0	.5–4.6	1.7–17.3	2.2–21.9
CPSC (5)	.3–3.0	.3–2.8	1.6–16.0	1.9–18.8
NRC[d] (35)	2.0	2.7	10.0	12.7
RCA (43)	NA[e]	NA	NA	12.0 (6.0)[f]
HSE (21)	.04–5.3	.1–8.8		NA
Authors (22a)	.5–1.5	.5–1.6	1.8–5.4	2.3–7.0

[a]Estimated total deaths over a lifetime attributable to asbestos exposure.

[b]Slope of the dose-response line, increase in Standardized Mortality Ratio per unit increase in cumulative asbestos exposure (f/ml-yr).

[c]Because of minor differences in the mesothelioma models, the parameter values for these models are not strictly comparable and therefore are not reported here.

[d]Published mesothelioma estimate did not use lifetable methods; published lung cancer risk did not adjust for continuous exposure, as claimed; both estimates adjusted here by authors.

[e]Not available.

[f]Estimate, derived by Julian Peto, depends on whether insulators are assumed to have been exposed to an average of 15 f/ml (estimate 12.0) or 30 f/ml (6.0).

cancer slope possibly appropriate for asbestos textiles would not be appropriate for exposure to construction and acoustical products inside a building. Thus, the upper values of the lung cancer estimates by the EPA and CPSC (based on a slope of 3.0), as well as the estimate by the NRC (a slope of 2.0), would probably be too high for building exposures. Similarly, the highest estimates of mesothelioma risk are likely to be overestimates, especially if products in schools are composed of chrysotile only, which is generally the case for ceiling plaster, one of the primary products of concern.

Additionally, since parameter values are based on epidemiologic studies, the choice of these studies is critically important in the ultimate calculation of potential risk. In some cases, studies with little or no exposure data and with no demonstration of the validity of exposure estimates have been used in estimating dose-response relationships. This is a particularly important issue in modeling mesothelioma risk, since the highest parameter values used in the EPA and CPSC reports, as well as the single, high value used in the NRC report, resulted from the inclusion of two studies whose exposure estimates have been questioned. [The first (17) because of the finding of decreasing lung cancer risk with increasing estimated asbestos exposure, and the second (44, reportedly amosite exposure only) because no exposure measurements were made at the study plant site.]

As Table 1 indicates, several agencies or governments concerned with the issues of potential risk from asbestos exposure have obtained scientific input into the decision-making process; subsequent policy decisions will un-doubtedly reflect this input. The derivation of potential risk estimates, howev-er, has not always proceeded optimally. The evolution of EPA's risk estimates for school asbestos exposures was a particularly lengthy process, with consider-able changes over a series of draft reports. For example, an estimate of "100 to 8000 premature deaths" attributable to prevalent asbestos concentrations in the schools was reduced (13) to "a total of 40 to 400" in the following draft (14), and no estimates were given in the next (15). [All estimates were based on the same exposure assumptions.]

Important aspects of risk estimation (e.g. model selection, parameter estima-tion, critical review of epidemiological studies, details of the risk calculations) are best resolved through wide, balanced, and experienced input before draft reports are issued. This approach is not only more timely than obtaining and incorporating reviews for a series of drafts, but also avoids the likelihood of preliminary risk estimates being used by others as a basis for decision making, even when they have been superseded by subsequent versions. More careful and wider input into risk estimates before the release of draft reports would certainly have resulted in greater confidence in EPA by scientists and a more rational approach to the issue of asbestos in the schools by school boards.

In contrast to EPA, the CPSC convened a panel of experts, including several experienced in asbestos risk assessment, to provide input for that agency's approach to rule making for consumer products containing asbestos. This panel's single draft report, released for public comment, as well as its final report, therefore represented a wide range of perspectives, including compro-mise when possible and delineation of the issues, when not.

The specific issue of potential risk to students from friable asbestos products in schools has received considerable public attention in the US. Indeed, if these products pose a significant cancer hazard, this is a critically important societal concern and drastic measures are needed. EPA's sequence of draft reports, with initially very high estimates of potential risk, contributed to the public's uncertainty and, in some cases, panic. Estimates in the latest EPA report (16) are appropriate for continuous asbestos exposure (24 hours a day for a full year) rather than for a school exposure; no instructions are provided for converting these estimates to the school situation. Public concerns have been compounded by EPA's requirement (backed by fines for noncompliance) that all schools test for the presence of asbestos-containing products; if found, the schools are required to notify teachers and parents. However, to date, EPA has provided no guidelines for the schools to use in determining subsequent action concerning asbestos products. Inevitably, many parents and school boards have concluded that these products pose a high cancer risk and have taken action based on that assumption. Some schools have probably removed asbestos-containing prod-ucts (primarily ceilings) that were in excellent condition, emitting very few or no fibers, and possibly with lower exposure levels than in the general environment of the community. Indeed, some experts have claimed that removal of products in good condition could pose greater risk than proper maintenance because of the likelihood of elevated exposure levels during and following removal. EPA, far from assisting the public and school officials in rationally addressing a possible problem of asbestos products in the schools, has worsened the situation by calling attention to the presence of asbestos and its carcinogenicity, but providing neither estimates of how great the associated risks might be nor guidelines for rational action. Consequently, not only have some schools probably taken unnecessary (and possibly detrimental because of the possibility of increased exposure levels) action, others have likely failed to take needed action.

A reasonable approach to the issue of asbestos products in schools and other buildings would include a monitoring system in conjunction with a program of proper maintenance and repair. Risk estimates in relation to estimated exposure levels may be compared to other risks in our society, and the costs and benefits of possible risk reduction methods contrasted. These considerations may be used as guidelines in determining appropriate modes of action. For example, estimates of lifetime risk resulting from five school years of exposure to .001 f/cc of mixed asbestos range from 1.9 to 21.9 cancers per million exposed (Table 1). Assuming an average life expectancy of 75 years (60 years beyond school exposure), these estimates would indicate an average annual rate of .03–.37 deaths per million (1.9/60–21.9/60). Since this potential risk is below many other estimated risks (Table 2), policy makers may decide that this constitutes an acceptable risk and recommend no action if average exposure levels remain at .001 f/cc or lower. However, since risk is dose-related, similar calculations at higher exposure levels may estimate potential risks that are deemed unacceptable, and corrective action may be called for.

SETTING OF WORKPLACE STANDARDS

Attempts in the US to set limits for the exposure of workers to asbestos-containing dust began in 1946 when the American Conference of Governmental Industrial Hygienists (ACGIH) proposed a threshold limit value (TLV) of five million particles per cubic foot of air (mppcf). At that time and for many years following, the intent of limiting asbestos exposure was primarily the prevention of asbestosis. The subsequent history of occupational standards for asbestos in the US is summarized in Table 3.

The ACGIH is a nongovernmental organization whose recommended standards, while providing valuable guidance, do not carry enforcement implications. Federal activity began in 1969 when the US Department of Labor, under the Walsh-Healey Act, set an asbestos standard for government con-

Table 2   Published estimates of risk from various causes (US)

Cause	Annual rate (deaths per million)	Reference
VOLUNTARY RISKS		
Long-term smoking	1200	52
Bicycling, ages 10–14 (1978)	14	33
High school football (1970–1980)	10	20
Eating 4 tbsp peanut butter/day (aflatoxin)	8	6
Aircraft accidents (1979)	6	36a
Living in a brick building rather than wood (radiation)	5	6
Whooping cough vaccination (1970–1980)	1–6	49a
Asbestos in schools (prevalent conditions)	.02–.37	Table 1
INVOLUNTARY RISKS		
Home accidents (ages 1–14)	60	8a
Motor vehicle accident[a]—pedestrian (ages 5–14)	32	34
Drowning (ages 5–14)	27	34
Fires (ages 5–14)	16	34
Inhalation/ingestion of foreign objects	15	6
Falls (ages 5–14)	4	34
Tornadoes (Midwest)	2	9
Floods	2	9

[a]In 1975, there were approximately 200 persons (90 pupils, 10 drivers, 100 others) killed in school bus accidents (36).

tractors of 2 mppcf or, in terms of the modern unit of measurement, 12 f/ml. Responsibility for workplace standards passed to the Occupational Safety and Health Administration (OSHA) when it was created by Congress in 1970.

Until 1972, only two studies of textile workers, published in 1938 (11) and 1968 (3), quantitatively related asbestos dust exposure to asbestosis risk; these therefore provided the scientific basis for standards until the 1970s. Cancer risk had not been quantified in relation to asbestos exposure, but it was generally assumed that limiting exposure to reduce asbestosis risk would also reduce risk of malignancy.

OSHA established the first permanent standard of 5 f/ml in 1972, with an automatic reduction to 2 f/ml in 1976. In 1975, OSHA published a notice of intent to lower the permissible exposure level (PEL) for asbestos to 0.5 fibers. For the first time the focus was on asbestos as a carcinogen, although only limited quantitative dose-response data were available for cancer risk. The basis for the proposed standard was that since no threshold had been demonstrated for carcinogens, the exposure limit should be set at the lowest technologically and economically feasible level.

Surprisingly, after publishing its notice of proposed rule making in 1975, neither public hearings nor other public actions concerning its proposal were

Table 3 History of the US occupational standard for asbestos

Agency[a]	Year	TLV/PEL[b]	Scientific Basis	Notes
ACGIH	1946	5 mppcf	1938 Dreesen textile study (11)	
ACGIH	1968	2 mppcf/12 f/ml	1968 BOHS[c] textile study (3)	
	1970			Proposed effective
Dept. of Labor	1969	12 f/ml	1968 BOHS[c] textile study (3)	Walsh-Healey Act
OSHA	1971	12/f/ml	1968 BOHS[c] textile study (3)	Initial adoption after creation of OSHA
OSHA	1971	5 f/ml	BOHS textile study (1968) and un-quantified cancer risk	ETS[d]
OSHA	1972	5 f/ml	Quantitative cancer risk assessment	Permanent
OSHA	1975	.5 f/ml	Quantitative cancer risk assessment	Proposed, no further action
OSHA	1976	2 f/ml	Quantitative cancer risk assessment	Permanent, automatic reduction from 1972 rule
OSHA	1983	.5 f/ml	Quantitative cancer risk assessment	ETS, overturned by court
OSHA	1984	.2–.5 f/ml	Quantitative cancer risk assessment	Proposed

[a] ACGIH—American Conference of Governmental Industrial Hygienists. OSHA—Occupational Safety and Health Administration.
[b] TLV—Threshold Limit Value. PEL—Permissible Exposure Limit.
[c] BOHS—British Occupational Hygiene Society.
[d] ETS—Emergency Temporary Standard.

conducted by OSHA. In fact, OSHA activity concerning an asbestos standard could at best be described as "low level," with only some contracts outside the agency to investigate exposure and construction industry issues. Inexplicably, this dormant interval occurred during the tenure of a national administration— more specifically, OSHA leadership, known for its zealous regulation of other workplace hazards. One cannot help but wonder why asbestos, which had become the best studied of occupational carcinogens, had lost priority in the OSHA agenda.

The establishment of an exposure standard on the basis of technological feasibility was rejected by the Supreme Court in 1980 in a case involving the benzene standard, in which the Court ruled that it was necessary for the agency to demonstrate that a more stringent standard would result in health benefit. In light of this decision, quantitative risk assessment with low-dose extrapolation became the primary justification for any proposed new OSHA standard. By the late 1970s, dose-response relationships for lung cancer risk in various segments of the asbestos industry had been published, although not for end-product users (e.g. insulators, shipyard workers). Ultimately, an OSHA in-house preliminary asbestos risk assessment was prepared in 1981, although the complete document was made available to the public only as a result of litigation concerning another standard (ethylene oxide) in 1983. In mid-1983, based on its 1981 risk assessment and another prepared by an outside contractor, OSHA initiated new rule making with regard to asbestos and sought balanced external peer review of the risk analyses and the proposed asbestos standard. Representatives of EPA and CPSC were also asked to comment, since these agencies had themselves produced asbestos exposure risk assessments.

While substantial agreement was reached among the consultants and OSHA staff concerning calculated risks of malignant disease at varying levels of asbestos exposure, differences remained. One dealt with the interpretation of the evidence regarding asbestos causation of nonpulmonary cancers (e.g. gastrointestinal, laryngeal, ovarian, renal). Observations of excesses of these cancers in published mortality studies are inconstant and generally not strongly dose-related. Nevertheless, OSHA included these cancers in the risk analysis. However, since it was assumed that these malignancies add only 10% of the excess lung cancers to total tumor excess, this decision had little effect on the total estimated risk and the proposed standard.

An issue of greater consequence is whether the different asbestos fiber types have differing levels of pathogenic potency. As stated above, the preponderance of epidemiologic evidence indicates that the amphibole mineral fibers (amosite and crocidolite) are more hazardous than chrysotile asbestos in regard to mesothelioma risk. For this reason, most asbestos regulations in industrialized countries deal differentially with the separate types of fibers. Moreover, in the US, the ACGIH recommended in 1980 that different standards be established for these fiber types: .2 f/ml for crocidolite, .5 for amosite, and 2.0 for chrysotile. Nevertheless, OSHA and the other US regulatory agencies have not been convinced by the increasingly strong evidence on this issue. Most asbestos-containing products are, or can be, made using only chrysotile asbestos, which constitutes more than 95% of asbestos use. More rigid control (or banning) of amphibole fiber exposures would likely influence the asbestos PEL, since it no longer would need to allow for the possible widespread use of mixed fibers.

A possible explanation for OSHA's failure to differentiate between the fiber types in setting standards lies in the position on this issue of OSHA's two main constituencies, labor and management. Neither supports differential regulation by fiber type, but for different reasons. One of the remaining asbestos industry's major products is asbestos cement pressure pipe, which contains crocidolite and is difficult in some applications to replace, although this has been accomplished in several countries. Labor has interpreted a differential regulatory approach as weakening the chrysotile standard rather than as more rigid control of amphiboles.

In 1983, OSHA, rather than follow the normal rule-making process for a permanent standard, issued an emergency temporary standard (ETS), mandating an immediate lowering of the asbestos PEL to 0.5 fibers. As expected, the ETS was challenged in the courts on the basis that OSHA had not shown that a health emergency existed. There were two issues to be considered: first, whether the proposed lowering of the PEL was supported by the scientific evidence; and second, if so, should this have been effected through an ETS? Under the law, the normal rule-making procedure allows time for written submissions and a public hearing. The ETS circumvents these procedures, but is effective for only six months, after which OSHA must initiate the normal rule-making process. In issuing an ETS, OSHA is obliged to demonstrate that the existing standard poses a grave danger and that the ETS is necessary to protect workers from that danger. OSHA argued that the normal procedures were inadequate and that the ETS was necessary because delaying a reduction in the PEL for six months would constitute a serious hazard. The agency produced a numerical estimate of potential deaths resulting from this exposure. A claim that a six months' delay posed a serious hazard was in marked contrast to OSHA's general inactivity concerning asbestos during the previous eight years. Moreover, most of the epidemiologic studies used for risk assessment had been available for several years.

A panel of three judges, after hearing arguments from both sides, found that the ETS was not justified, and OSHA proceeded with a permanent rule-making process. Public hearings on the OSHA proposal (which proposes to lower the PEL to 0.2 or 0.5 f/ml) were held in 1984. A permanent rule has, at the time of this writing, not yet been promulgated. OSHA's decision to issue the ETS and defend it against the expected challenges, rather than proceeding directly with permanent rule making, ultimately resulted in a delay of a lowered standard.

Compensating the Injured Worker

During the past century, societies have increasingly considered it their responsibility to provide special recompense to individuals who have been injured or become ill as the result of the conditions of their work. In Germany, a system for compensating injured workers dates back to 1894; in the United Kingdom, the Workmen's Compensation Act was passed in 1897. In principle, the worker exchanges the right to bring civil suit (tort) against his employer for such injuries in return for "no-fault" administrative determination of a compensible condition, a process falling under the rubric of workmen's compensation. Currently in the United States, this "trade-off" is failing to result in a reasonable approach to the discharge of this social responsibility.

Rather than accepting the compensation provided by this system (widely perceived to be capricious and generally inadequate), workers are increasingly bringing legal action against suppliers of products used in the workplace (product liability suits alleging a defective product) and claiming negligence of employers. For the claimant, awards received from these actions are unpredictable, and estimates indicate that only about one third of the amount expended in the litigation system actually goes to the claimant. For the defendant, the uncertainty of the awards constitutes a substantial financial problem, with uninsured punitive awards (that portion beyond compensatory damages, intended as a deterrent) sometimes extremely costly. Equity is elusive, since medical expert witnesses are often called to testify because of their predictable opinion rather than their objectivity or competence. Substantial problems with the use of expert witnesses have been recognized by legal scholars and comprise an important consideration in proposals for tort reform.

Contributing to the unevenness in the compensation system is that these systems are primarily administered by the individual states. Exceptions are programs for workers covered by federal plans: longshoremen, harbor workers, federal employees, and coal miners.

Workers' compensation is intended to provide financial support to individuals for lost income and medical costs resulting from injuries or disease; awards are not intended simply for exposure to a potentially toxic substance. In determining compensation, the relevant medical issues are diagnosis, causation, and extent of impairment. While these issues are usually straightforward in work-related traumatic injuries such as accidents, substantial difficulties arise in the occupational diseases, many of which have long exposure and latency periods before they become manifest and which frequently exist in the general, unexposed population. These are major problems in the asbestos-associated diseases.

Diagnosis of a disease for purposes of compensation is no different than diagnosis for other purposes and must be based solely on medical evidence. If this is misunderstood or ignored, the process will ultimately fail.

The greatest difficulties arise in dealing with the second issue, assessment of causation (assuming a diagnosis has been established). It is here that most disagreement occurs and the scientific evidence is most incomplete. Causal associations must frequently be evaluated on the basis of probabilities, often taking into account both workplace and other exposures, as well as known relationships between the amount of these exposures and risk of the adverse health effect observed (or alleged) in the claimant. While a causal association between exposure and disease in an individual is seldom certain, in the legal system causality is often inferred if it is deemed "more probable than not" that the specified exposure was the cause of an observed condition.

The issue of degree of impairment should be the least troublesome in determining compensation for the asbestos-related diseases. In the functionally important benign disorders, diffuse lung fibrosis and extensive pleural thickening, pulmonary function tests are used to quantify the extent of functional impairment. These procedures are widely available, well standardized, noninvasive, and painless, and they provide highly useful information regarding the type and severity of lung impairment. In the malignant diseases, lung cancer and mesothelioma, impairment determination is not likely to be a major issue because of their poor prognosis for long-term survival.

The greatest proportion of disease claims continues to be for asbestosis. Reasons for this include the substantial prevalence of this condition among workers exposed to the asbestos levels of the past and the high prevalence of chronic airways obstructive diseases in the general population, resulting in a potential for misdiagnosis. By contrast, mesothelioma is relatively infrequent, and lung cancer, because of its high background incidence and strong association with smoking, is particularly difficult to attribute to asbestos exposure in the individual case. While other cancers have been found to occur in excess in some studies of asbestos-exposed populations, these findings are not sufficiently consistent to be causally associated with asbestos exposure for purposes of compensation.

In an effort to make the compensation of asbestos-associated diseases more efficient and equitable, and to remove the burden of litigation from the courts, various alternate approaches have been or are being proposed. One initiative, under the leadership of Dean Harry Wellington of the Yale Law School, has involved representatives of the insurance companies, the asbestos industry, and plaintiffs attorneys. The objective has been to establish national claims facilities for individual case determinations. Initial efforts have been directed at the financing of the plan, a subject beyond the scope of this review.

Another approach, proposed as part of the Manville Corporation reorganization plan and developed under their Chapter 11 bankruptcy proceedings, is presently under consideration by the Court. It has to date not received enthusiastic support by attorneys for the plaintiffs, and its medical criteria are presently being debated by pulmonary medicine specialists who have been asked to review it. For reasons that are not clear, Manville has declined to participate in the Wellington plan.

Congressional concerns have been reflected by the introduction of the Occupational Disease Compensation Act of 1983 by Congressman George Miller, which deals primarily with asbestos-related diseases. Opposition to the bill focused on the exclusion of government participation in funding and on the free use of "presumptions" in determining asbestos-exposure attributability. The bill included no provision for expert medical guidance or case-by-case determination of disease. A new bill, the Asbestos Workers' Recovery Act (H.R. 1626), introduced in 1985 by Congressman Austin Murphy and 49 cosponsors, has attempted to address the cited objections to the earlier bill, but falls far short of adequately dealing with the medical issues regarding a rational approach to compensation of these diseases.

Whether the ultimate solution to the compensation of asbestos-related disease is through a private or governmental process, its success will depend on competent individual case assessment based on uniform, sound medical guidelines. These guidelines should be established by a national panel of experts, with case assessment carried out by regional compensation medical panels. Such systems have been established in countries around the world, including Britain and Canada; while not perfect, they have in general provided equitable, reliable compensation and have been accepted by workers. They should serve as an encouraging example to our policy makers.

Under any compensation system, after appropriate workplace asbestos exposure has been established for a claimant, the primary issue for asbestosis and mesothelioma is diagnosis, whereas for lung cancer it is causation. The basis for a diagnosis of asbestosis is most often the chest radiograph, although other clinical and laboratory features are well recognized and may be supportive when present. The X-ray reading can be standardized by use of the international classification method of the International Labour Office (ILO, 23), although substantial interobserver variability can occur, particularly at the low levels of disease most commonly encountered recently. However, film-reading approaches have been devised that improve validity and reliability and should be used. The diagnosis of mesothelioma, while often suggested clinically and on X ray, invariably depends on examination of tissue obtained by surgical biopsy or post-mortem examination. The histopathologic diagnosis is not easy; an expert panel (available in a number of countries, including the US) should be utilized to resolve difficult cases. With both asbestosis and mesothelioma, dispassionate ascertainment has become a reasonable expectation; the relevance to compensation is obvious.

The situation with lung cancer is far more complex. Diagnosis is generally not a problem, but attributing the cause often is. Multiple causes of lung cancer have been identified; two are almost always present in asbestos-related claims: asbestos and cigarette smoking. While arbitrary decisions can be made to ascribe cause to either the smoking or the asbestos exposure, the fact is that, by far, most of the cases in a population exposed to both factors must be attributed to both. Since, like lung cancer, asbestosis has been shown to be dose-related, the presence of asbestosis (or other fibrotic effect) has been used as an indicator of significant asbestos exposure; in this approach, malignancies in the presence of asbestosis are judged to be "asbestos-attributable."

Some have suggested semiquantitative estimates of the two exposures to provide probabilities for each risk factor, with partial apportionment of cause (and award) rather than an "all or nothing" decision. Such an approach would depend on data relating risk to estimates of exposure to each carcinogen. These data are substantial for smoking-related risk of lung cancer and, while less complete for asbestos, are sufficient for development of reasonable risk ratios under varying durations and conditions of exposure. For example, for a 60-year-old man who has smoked one to two packs of cigarettes per day for 40 years and who worked in an asbestos manufacturing plant for 25 years, the lung cancer relative risks might be 10 for smoking and 3 for his asbestos exposure. The comparison for these ratios can lead to a proportional compensation award for the asbestos contribution to his lung cancer risk, e.g. perhaps one fourth (approximately 3/13). Although it does not deal with the problem of interaction (most tumors "due" to both factors), the concept is presented as a reasonable solution to the current dilemma. Additional refinements of such a system might include provision for the presence of asbestosis automatically triggering a full award and the requirement of a minimum proportion for the asbestos contribution for any award. The choice of the best alternative should clearly be a decision for the suggested panel of experts.

ADVOCACY, ECONOMICS, AND SCIENCE

Attempts to deal with concerns of health risks associated with asbestos exposure have been based on a mixture of scientific knowledge with social judgments and activism. The latter are often intended to play on emotions, particularly fear, and are too often influenced by economic considerations. Public information and perceptions have often come from individuals and institutions in which the separation of science and advocacy has not been distinct. These sources have generally not labeled their scientific and nonscientific judgments as such, and understandably, a confused public frequently imputes the scientific credentials of such scientist-advocates to all of their public utterances.

An example is taken from the transcript of an EPA public hearing on the school asbestos issue, held in Washington DC on May 7, 1984 (45). The testimony quoted was given by the only biomedical scientist appearing, a physician widely recognized as an expert in the asbestos-associated diseases.

> How has this happened? I really do not know. I was just speaking to the president of the Buffalo Teachers Association, when he was telling of his peregrinations through upstate New York to the school boards, the health department, the state department, EPA and each step has been frustrating and (asbestos) exposures continue in Buffalo. And the only explanation I have and I do not know if it is a good one is that we are dealing with some gigantic Kitty Genovese Syndrome. Remember 20 years ago in . . ., a young woman, Kitty Genovese, . . ., for a half-hour was being stabbed by a killer and eventually he killed her . . . and all through this time there were 38 people in the apartment houses above at their windows, staring down at what was happening and nobody even called the police. Nobody did anything to help her. Nobody got involved.
>
> And it is similar to what is happening now. We are gazing at children being exposed to asbestos . . . We do not really need any additional research very much about what can happen. We know what can and will happen. Because ultimately . . . what you will do, what Mr. Alm will do, what Mr. Ruckelshaus [note: the deputy administrator and administrator of EPA at the time] has to do is to decide who is going to live and who is going to die.

The implication of the preceding testimony of an overwhelming risk to school children is not supported by the scientific evidence (Table 1). The public would have been better served by quantitative assessment of risk from prevailing levels of school asbestos exposure so that these risks may be placed in proper perspective.

It is inevitable that society will often be required to consider the economic cost of preventing disease and making restitution to its injured members. This is appropriate and necessary; however, personal or corporate self-interest is involved and has often led to blurring of the distinction between the economic issues and medical/scientific information. If the most credible risk analysis indicated that the level of risk considered "reasonable" or "acceptable" by those taking these risks required that workplace exposures be limited to a certain concentration level, then the appropriate dust control measures would be necessary, regardless of their economic costs. The role of science in this process is to provide the best possible calculations of potential risk; it cannot assist in making the economic decisions, nor should its methods and estimates be modified to reflect economic concerns.

If an insurer contracts with a manufacturer to cover employees with work-related injuries, can one ignore the science that clearly indicates that fibrogenesis and carcinogenesis are long-latency diseases and that cellular alterations may begin long before the disease is detected? Does the injury exist (and is therefore covered) only when the disease is diagnosed (manifestation theory) or is this a long process of reaction to the injurious exposure (exposure theory), with relevant coverage over the many years of exposure? Expert scientific testimony has been obtained to support both views, but this issue seems to be more an economic dispute, with attempts by the interested parties to use science to resolve it.

Attempts by former asbestos-exposed workers, or their representatives, to obtain compensation awards have frequently been pursued when the sole condition has been pleural plaques (no documented effect on respiratory health) or chronic airways obstruction (not a demonstrated effect of asbestos exposure when the condition is clinically significant). The economic incentives to the claimant (and attorney) are clear, but so is the state of medical science in regard to these conditions, which indicates that occupationally induced disease is not present under these circumstances, so compensation should not be an issue.

With respect to the topical subject of asbestos in the schools, assuming an appropriate analysis results in risk estimates that are widely believed to compare favorably with the great number of voluntary and involuntary risks that we all face daily, is it a reasonable use of the resources of financially limited school boards to engage in wholesale replacement of asbestos-containing ceilings, at a national cost of many billions of dollars? Many would conclude not, although this approach is increasingly being chosen. The accurate and dispassionate communication of these risks to parents and local decision makers by credible scientists is clearly a needed effort.

Asbestos risks share with other occupational and environmental issues the interface of social objectives, costs and benefits (both economic and noneconomic), and a scientific data base. That these factors all be taken into account in policy decision making should be encouraged. Attempting to revise rather than to use the science in order to meet predetermined social or economic objectives is inefficient and unreasonable. It does not lead to the most rational allocation of our national resources and often places disease or economic burdens on those least able to deal with either. Moreover, the inefficient use of science has amply been demonstrated to delay the policy-making process to the detriment of both risk reduction and compensation of affected individuals.

ACKNOWLEDGMENT

Supported in part by Specialized Center of Research (SCOR) Grant Number HL-15092, from the National Heart, Lung and Blood Institute. The authors express their appreciation to John C. Gilson for his valuable suggestions in the preparation of this manuscript.

Literature Cited

1. Berry, G., Newhouse, M. L. 1983. Mortality of workers manufacturing friction materials using asbestos. *Br. J. Indust. Med.* 40:1–7
2. British Occupational Hygiene Society. 1983. A study of the health experience in two U.K. asbestos factories. *Ann. Occup. Hyg.* 27:1–25
3. British Occupational Hygiene Society, Committee on Hygiene Standards. 1968. Hygiene standards for chrysotile asbestos dust. *Ann. Occup. Hyg.* 11:47–69
4. Churg, A., Wiggs, B., Depaoli, L., Kampe, B., Stevens, B. 1984. Lung asbestos content in chrysotile workers with mesothelioma. *Am. Rev. Respir. Dis.* 130:1042–45
5. Consumer Product Safety Commission.

1983. 1983. *Report of the Chronic Hazard Advisory Panel on Asbestos.* Washington DC

6. Crouch, E., Wilson, R. 1982. *Risk/ Benefit Analysis.* Cambridge, Mass.: Ballinger

6a. Davis, D. L., Mandulla, B. 1985. Airborne asbestos and public health. *Ann. Rev. Public Health* 6:195–221

7. Dement, J. M., Harris, R. L., Symons, M. J., Shy, C. 1982. Estimates of dose-response for respiratory cancer among chrysotile asbestos textile workers. In *Inhaled Particles V*, ed. W. H. Walton, pp. 869–83. Oxford: Pergamon

8. Dept. of National Health and Welfare, Canada. 1985. *Report of the committee of experts concerning the scientific basis for occupational standards for asbestos.*

8a. Dershewitz, R. A., Christophersen, E. R. 1984. Childhood household safety. *Am. J. Diseases Children* 138:85–88

9. Dinman B. 1980. The reality and acceptance of risk. *J. Am. Med. Assoc.* 11:1226–28

10. Doll, R. 1955. Mortality from lung cancer in asbestos workers. *Br. J. Indust. Med.* 12:81–86

11. Dreessen, W. C., Dalla Nalle, J. W., Edwards, T. I., Miller, J. W., Sayers, R. R., Easom, H. F., Trice, M. F. 1938. A study of asbestosis in the asbestos textile industry. *Public Health Bull.*, No. 241

12. Enterline, P. E., Kendrick, M. A. 1967. Asbestos-dust exposures at various levels and mortality. *Arch. Environ. Health* 15:181–86

13. Environmental Protection Agency. 1980. *Technical support document for regulatory action against friable asbestos-containing materials in school buildings.* Preliminary draft. Washington DC: EPA

14. Environmental Protection Agency. 1981. *Support document for final rule on friable asbestos-containing materials in school buildings. Health effects and magnitude of exposure.* Preliminary draft. Washington DC: EPA

15. Environmental Protection Agency. 1982. *Support document for final rule on friable asbestos-containing materials in school buildings. Health effects and magnitude of exposure.* Preliminary draft. Washington DC: EPA

16. Environmental Protection Agency. 1985. *Asbestos health assessment update.* (Prepared by W. Nicholson.) Washington DC: EPA

17. Finkelstein, M. M. 1983. Mortality among long-term employees of an Ontario asbestos-cement factory. *Br. J. Indust. Med.* 40:138–44

18. Finkelstein, M. M. 1984. Mortality among employees of an Ontario asbestos-cement factory. *Am. Rev. Respir. Dis.* 129:754–61

19. Fleischer, W., Viles, F., Gade, R., Drinker, P. 1946. A health survey of pipe covering operations in constructing naval vessels. *J. Indust. Hyg. Toxicol.* 28:9–16

20. Gerberich, S. G., Priest, J. D., Boen, J. R., Straub, C. P., Maxwell, R. E. 1983. Concussion incidences and severity in secondary school varsity football players. *Am. J. Public Health* 73:1370–75

21. Health and Safety Executive (UK). 1983. *Asbestos: The control limit for asbestos.* London: Health and Safety Commission, HMSO. (Prepared by A. D. Acheson, M. J. Gardner)

22. Henderson, V. I., Enterline, P. E. 1979. Asbestos exposure: Factors associated with excess cancer and respiratory disease mortality. *Ann. NY Acad. Sci.* 330:117–26

22a. Hughes, J. M., Weill, H. 1986. Asbestos exposure—Quantitative assessment of risk. *Am. Rev. Resp. Dis.* In press

23. International Labour Office. 1980. *Guidelines for the Use of ILO International Classification of Radiographs of Pneumoconioses.* Geneva: ILO. [*Occup. Safety and Health Ser.* No. 22 (Rev.)]

24. Jones, J. S. P., Roberts, G. H., Pooley, F. D., Clark, N. J., Smith, P. G., Owen, W. G., Wagner, J. C., Berry, G., Pollock, D. J. 1980. The pathology and mineral content of lungs in cases of mesothelioma in the United Kingdom in 1976. In *Biological Effects of Mineral Fibres*, ed. J. C. Wagner, W. Davis, 1:187–99. Lyon: Int. Agency for Res. on Cancer (IARC Sci. Publ. No. 30)

25. McDonald, A. D. 1980. Mineral fibre content of lung in mesothelioma tumours: Preliminary report. See Ref. 24, pp. 681–85

26. McDonald, A. D., Fry, J. S., Woolley, A. J., McDonald, J. C. 1983. Dust exposure and mortality in an American chrysotile textile plant. *Br. J. Indust. Med.* 40:361–67

27. McDonald, A. D., Fry, J. S., Woolley, A. J., McDonald, J. C. 1983. Dust exposure and mortality in an American factory using chrysotile, amosite, and crocidolite in mainly textile manufacture. *Br. J. Indust. Med.* 40:368–74

28. McDonald, A. D., Fry, J. S., Woolley, A. J., McDonald, J. C. 1984. Dust exposure and mortality in an American chrysotile asbestos friction products plant. *Br. J. Indust. Med.* 41:151–57

29. McDonald, A. D., McDonald, J. C.

1980. Malignant mesotheliomas in North America. *Cancer* 46:1650–56

30. McDonald, J. C., Liddell, F. D. K., Gibbs, G. W., Eyssen, G. E., McDonald, A. D. 1980. Dust exposure and mortality in chrysotile mining. *Br. J. Indust. Med.* 37:11–24

31. McDonald, J. C., McDonald, A. D., Gibbs, G. W., Siemiatycki, J., Rossiter, C. E. 1971. Mortality in the chrysotile asbestos mines and mills of Quebec. *Arch. Environ. Health* 22:677–86

32. Merewether, E. R. A. 1949. Asbestosis and carcinoma of the lung. In *Annual Report of the Chief Inspector of Factories for the Year 1947*, pp. 79–87. London: Her Majesty's Stationery Office

33. Metropolitan Life Insurance Company. 1981. *Stat. Bull.* 62(4):5

34. Metropolitan Life Insurance Company. 1981. *Stat. Bull.* 62(3):11–13

35. National Research Council, Committee on Nonoccupational Health Risks. 1984. *Asbestiform Fibers—Nonoccupational Health Risks.* Washington DC: Nat. Acad. Press

36. National Safety Council. 1976. *Accident Facts.* Chicago: NSC

36a. National Safety Council. 1980. *Accident Facts.* Chicago: NSC

37. Newhouse, M. L., Berry, G., Skidmore, J. W. 1982. A mortality study of workers manufacturing friction materials with chrysotile asbestos. *Ann. Occup. Hyg.* 26:899–909

38. Nicholson, W. J., Selikoff, I. J., Seidman, H., Lilis, R., Formby, P. 1979. Long-term mortality experience of chrysotile miners and millers in Thetford mines, Quebec. *Ann. NY Acad. Sci.* 330:11–21

39. Peto, J. 1980. The incidence of pleural mesothelioma in chrysotile asbestos textile workers. See Ref. 24, p. 703

40. Peto, J., Seidman, H., Selikoff, I. J. 1982. Mesothelioma mortality in asbestos workers: Implications for models of carcinogenesis and risk assessment. *Br. J. Cancer* 45:124–35

41. Deleted in proof

42. Pott, F. 1978. Some aspects of dosimetry of the carcinogenic potency of asbestos and other fibrous dusts. *Staub-Reinhalt Luft* 38:486–90

43. Royal Commission on Matters of Health and Safety, Canada. 1984. *Report on matters of health and safety arising from the use of asbestos in Ontario.* Toronto: Ontario Ministry of Govern. Serv.

44. Seidman, H., Selikoff, I. J., Hammond, E. C. 1979. Short-term asbestos work exposure and long-term observation. *Ann. NY Acad. Sci.* 330:61–89

45. Selikoff, I. J. 1984. *EPA Response to SEIU Asbestos Petition,* Washington, D.C., May 7, 1984, pp. 11–12. Washington DC: Acme Reporting Co.

46. Selikoff, I. J., Churg, J., Hammond, E. C. 1965. The occurrence of asbestosis among insulation workers in the US. *Ann. NY Acad. Sci.* 132:139–55

47. Selikoff, I. J., Churg, J., Hammond, E. C. 1964. Asbestos exposure and neoplasia. *J. Am. Med. Assoc.* 188:22–26

48. Selikoff, I. J., Hammond, E. C., Seidman, H. 1979. Mortality experience of insulation workers in the United States and Canada, 1943–1976. *Ann. NY Acad. Sci.* 330:91–116

49. Stanton, M. F., Layard, M., Tegeris, A., Miller, E., May, M., Morgan, E., Smith, A. 1981. Relation of particle dimension to carcinogenicity in amphibole asbestos and other fibrous minerals. *J. Natl. Cancer Inst.* 67:965–75

49a. Sun, M. 1985. Whooping cough vaccine research revs up. *Science* 227:1184–86

50. Wagner, J. C., Sleggs, C. A., Marchand, P. 1960. Diffuse pleural mesothelioma and asbestos exposure in the North Western Cape Province. *Br. J. Indust. Med.* 17:260–71

51. Weill, H., Hughes, J., Waggenspack, C. 1979. Influence of dose and fiber type on respiratory malignancy risk in asbestos cement manufacturing. *Am. Rev. Respir. Dis.* 120:345–54

52. Wilson, R. 1980. Risk/benefit analysis for toxic chemicals. *Ecotoxicol. Environ. Safety* 4:370–83

Ann. Rev. Public Health. 1986. 7:193–215

MILD HYPERTENSION: The Question of Treatment

Darwin R. Labarthe

The Epidemiology Research Center, University of Texas Health Science Center at Houston, School of Public Health, Houston, Texas 77225

INTRODUCTION

"Mild" hypertension is a major public health problem, not only in the US, but in many other areas of the world. It is a predictor and an important causal factor for a large proportion of premature mortality and morbidity as well, due principally to cardiovascular complications. Its prevalence is such that millions of adults, in the US alone, are currently or potentially affected by policies and practices concerning its treatment to prevent these complications. The feasibility of reducing the risks of complications, as reported from controlled clinical trials, appears to be accepted generally, though not universally. Guidelines to accomplish this on a national and even international scale have been published, and they have been adopted widely in some countries. Thus, in the US for example, the proportion of persons detected and classified as hypertensive who are under treatment with effective blood pressure reduction has increased markedly since the early 1970s. Still, in some demographic groups with especially high prevalence, hypertension (predominantly "mild") remains largely uncontrolled (89). From the public health point of view, we are thus confronted with a problem of great importance, the availability of an effective response, and the evident need to bring further efforts to bear, if progress is to continue toward reduction of avoidable risks in the population at large.

Treatment of "mild" hypertension is not a matter free of controversy, however. The recent literature reflects differences of judgment in several areas, including: (*a*) the true benefit of blood pressure reduction in relation to particular levels of pressure at the start of treatment; (*b*) the nature and extent of adverse consequences of treatment, chiefly from antihypertensive drugs; and (*c*) the proper role of "nonpharmacologic therapy." The importance of these

193

0163-7525/86/0510-0193$02.00

issues for public health may be indicated most clearly by the questions these areas of difference imply, respectively:

1. Does the potential benefit warrant treatment at all?
2. Does this condition justify use of drugs for a large segment of the population, individually over periods of several years or longer?
3. Can any nonpharmacologic therapy replace antihypertensive drugs, or are they ineffective and thus wasteful of resources without benefit in reducing risks?

The purpose of this review is to examine these issues, and others related to them, on the basis of publications appearing especially within the past several years, that is, since the availability of results from the trials noted above.

Essential aspects of this review are discussions of: (a) definition of "mild" hypertension; (b) evidence of the effects of treatment provided by the most relevant clinical trials; and (c) the evolution of treatment guidelines in the US, as reflected by the successive reports of the National High Blood Pressure Education Program. In each area, the supporting references should be consulted for details. The next section addresses issues raised in several published commentaries on the treatment of "mild" hypertension, and some concluding observations follow.

DEFINITION OF "MILD" HYPERTENSION

Usage of the term "mild" hypertension varies. Because it might be construed as denoting only minor health implications, the US Joint National Committee on Detection, Evaluation, and Treatment of Hypertension in 1980 denoted the categories "mild," "moderate," and "severe" by "stratum I," "stratum II," and "stratum III," respectively (69). Unfortunately, this forward step was not reflected in the 1984 report of the next Joint National Committee (43). In any case, the term "mild" continues to be used and will be used (with reservation) in the remainder of this review.

Considerations underlying the concept of mild hypertension and the impact of the blood pressure levels chosen to define it are discussed in detail elsewhere (48). Inconsistency of usage and differences in measurement procedures require close examination of any report to avoid misinterpretation of study results.

On single-occasion screening, for example, some 15% of adult men and 13% of adult women in the US would be classified as mild hypertensives, in the conventional range from 90 to 104 mm Hg diastolic. However, perhaps only 50% of such persons would still be found in this range of pressure on re-examination within several days. Thus multiple screening removes a large proportion of those identified in single-stage screening. However, in the two-stage screening for the Hypertension Detection and Follow-up Program (HDFP), the 90 to 104 mm Hg range at *second* screening included 57% of those initially in the 105–114 mm Hg range, and 31.4% of those initially above 114 mm Hg. Thus, those classified as mild hypertensives in the HDFP represented a range of *initial* screening blood pressures and related risks well above those of the casual, single-occasion 90 to 104 mm Hg levels (48). After two-stage screening, 71% of the HDFP study population, or a substantial majority of those with confirmed high blood pressure, were mild hypertensives.

The preponderance of premature deaths in persons with high blood pressure (90 mm Hg and greater) is also found in the stratum (after two-stage screening) with pressures in the 90 to 104 mm Hg range (35, 36). These and analogous data from diverse studies of both observational and experimental designs support the view that mild hypertension is a very significant part of the public health problem of high blood pressure (71).

THE EVIDENCE PROVIDED BY CLINICAL TRIALS

The Veterans Administration Study

The first major stimulus to treatment of persons with diastolic pressures from 90 to 104 mm Hg was the 1970 report from the Veterans Administration Cooperative Study Group on Antihypertensive Agents (VA Study). In this highly selected group of 380 men, reductions of 20 to 50% in rates of occurrence of study endpoints were observed in the active versus the placebo treatment group, depending upon age and cardiovascular status at entry (86–88). Soon after, a series of six new trials of therapy in mild hypertension were initiated in the US, the UK, Australia, Belgium, and France. In general, this new generation of trials had in common a minimum diastolic blood pressure in the range 88 to 95 mm Hg as a criterion for entry (49, 76). Five trials have been completed and their results published since the VA Study report of 1970: those from the HDFP in 1979, 1982, and 1984 (33–41); the United States Public Health Service, or USPHS, Study, 1977 (80); the Australian National Blood Pressure Study, or ANBPS, 1980 (6–8); the Oslo Study, 1980 (30); and the British Medical Research Council, or MRC, trial, 1985 (59).

The US Public Health Service Study

The first of these five to be completed after the VA study was the USPHS Study (80). Organized and initiated in the mid-1960s, this was a placebo-controlled, random-allocation trial of drug therapy in 389 persons 21–55 years of age at entry, followed for periods of seven to ten years. Subjects found at screening to have demonstrable target organ damage or other specified conditions were excluded. Qualifying blood pressures were in the range from 90 to 115 mm Hg diastolic on repeated prerandomization visits. Fatal endpoints were few in this study, two in each group, although the combination of all study endpoints (first blood pressure-related morbid events) affected 29.0% of actively treated participants vs 45.9% of those on placebo. Power to detect differences in fatal or other major events was quite low. The author of the published report suggested that the low event rates in this group might warrant substitution of "hygienic intervention" for drug therapy in persons similar to those studied, and that it might be appropriate to defer drug therapy until electrocardiographic abnormalities or a progressive rise in blood pressure were observed.

The Hypertension Detection and Follow-up Program

The second trial to be completed for reporting of all follow-up experience was the HDFP, with the main mortality findings published in 1979 (35, 36). The HDFP was a trial of systematic management of hypertensives in study clinics (Stepped Care) in comparison with care received from other sources available in the same 14 community settings (Referred Care). Participants were identified from special household censuses in defined geographic areas (excepting one employed group) so as to represent unselected hypertensives in the population at large. Designed to test a reduction in total mortality, with five years of follow-up for each participant, the HDFP enrolled 10,940 persons aged 30 to 69 years at entry, including black and white men and women, each sex-race group constituting a substantial proportion of the study population. Diastolic blood pressures in the range from 90 to 104 mm Hg at the second screen accounted for 71.5% of the whole group, or 7825 persons.

For this stratum of participants, mortality was reduced by 20.3% for Stepped Care vs the Referred Care group. Further treatment comparisons within this stratum indicated relative reductions of five-year mortality by 21.9% among participants entering at 90 to 94 mm Hg diastolic pressure, 23.1% for those at 95 to 99 mm Hg, and 13.8% for those at 100 to 104 mm Hg. Further analyses based upon the presence or absence of end-organ damage or antihypertensive therapy at entry to the trial also indicated substantial trends favoring the Stepped Care group as well (39). The greatest relative benefit for the Stepped Care vs the Referred Care group, within the stratum from 90 to 104 mm Hg, was for participants free of both end-organ damage and antihypertensive therapy at entry—28.6%. The authors of the detailed report on the 90 to 104 mm Hg stratum emphasized that, while benefit accrued to those already demonstrating end-organ damage at entry, their treatment did not reduce mortality to the level experienced by those who entered the program free of these abnormalities. This finding was taken to support recommendations to treat even uncomplicated mild hypertension. The most recent reports suggest favorable results for the Stepped Care group in this stratum for other endpoints as well—incidence or reversal of left ventricular hypertrophy or cardiomegaly, incidence of angina pectoris, and possibly incidence of nonfatal myocardial infarction. However, as noted by the authors of these reports, interpretation of these results requires very careful attention to the particular design features of the HDFP (40, 41).

The Australian National Blood Pressure Study

The next trial completed, with overall results published in 1980, was the Australian Therapeutic Trial in Mild Hypertension, or Australian National Blood Pressure Study (ANBPS) (7). This, like the VA and USPHS studies, was a placebo-controlled trial. It included 3427 persons aged 30 to 69 years identified as volunteers in three communities, randomized after exclusion of persons with diastolic pressures outside the range from 95 to 109 mm Hg (or systolic pressure of 200 mm Hg or greater) and those with any evidence of target-organ damage. The study was terminated ahead of schedule due to the judgment that endpoint rates were sufficiently favorable to active treatment to make continuation inappropriate. Analyses were presented for both "intention to treat" and actual treatment, and in both instances indicated significant reduction of both cardiovascular deaths and all trial endpoints combined, for the group randomized to active treatment. Rates of all endpoints combined were lower with active treatment in each substratum of participants by diastolic pressures at entry (95–99, 100–104, and 105–109 mm Hg). The results were taken to show that even persons with "modest" elevation of blood pressure can benefit with reduced morbidity and mortality as a result of antihypertensive drug therapy.

A subsequent analysis addressed separately the experience of the 1943 participants in the placebo group and the course of blood pressure changes and other events during their follow-up (8). The relation of entering blood pressure levels both to endpoint event rates and to blood pressure levels at three years of follow-up were examined in detail. The fact that these outcomes could not be predicted from any of the variables recorded at entry was emphasized. The authors suggested that in persons whose initial diastolic pressures averaged over two visits are 95 mm Hg or greater, but whose readings on a third occasion result in an overall average below 95 mm Hg, a limited period of weight reduction and possibly other nonpharmacological intervention should be encouraged.

The Oslo Study

The trial conducted in Oslo was reported also in 1980 (30). Participants were 785 men aged 40 to 49, who were free of target organ damage and had systolic pressures between 150 and 199 mm Hg and diastolic pressures below 110 mm Hg at entry. Subjects were randomly allocated to either active treatment or nontreatment, without placebo. In the study population as a whole, after five years of follow-up, the total number of endpoint events favored the treated group, but this difference was not statistically significant. Power to detect differences was low in this trial, as in the USPHS Study. The complications and events under study were classified as "pressure-related" or other (e.g. coronary heart disease-related events). The former occurred almost exclusively in the control group, while the coronary events occurred somewhat more often in the actively treated group. When comparisons were made between treated and control groups with different entry diastolic blood pressure ranges, the treated subjects at entry pressures above 100 mm Hg had a reduced five-year rate of cardiovascular events relative to untreated persons (7.6 vs 16.4%, $p = 0.06$). The authors cautioned that conclusions as to mortality reduction should not be drawn from this trial.

The World Health Organization/International Society of Hypertension Review

These four studies were critically reviewed by the WHO/ISH Mild Hypertension Liaison Committee in a report published early in 1982 (96). The main features of each study were presented, including its design, operation, principal results, and the Committee's conclusions and comments. Overall, two of the studies were judged as too small to give firm results on "hard" endpoints (the USPHS and Oslo studies). The remaining studies were both found to give evidence that treatment of persons with mild hypertension, even those free of other manifestations, can reduce morbidity (ANBPS) and mortality (HDFP and ANBPS).

The Medical Research Council Trial

The last large-scale trial in treatment of mild hypertension to be reported was the Medical Research Council (MRC) trial in Britain (59). The MRC trial, reported in 1985, included 17,354 men and women aged 35–64 years at recruitment, which began in 1973 and ended in February 1982. Eligibility was based on mean diastolic pressures in the 90–109 mm Hg range, with systolic pressure below 200. Exclusions for specific medical conditions eliminated more than half of the persons eligible by blood pressure criteria alone. Treatment allocation was to active therapy with bendrofluazide or propranolol or their corresponding placebos. Average follow-up was approximately five years.

The endpoint on which the evaluation of the trial was designed was the incidence of fatal or nonfatal stroke, which was reduced 45% in the combined actively treated groups. The category of all cardiovascular events was also significantly reduced by active treatment, although overall rates did not differ significantly for coronary events or for deaths, whether cardiovascular, noncardiovascular, or all causes combined. Further analyses addressed the rates of events in relation to treatment regimen, smoking status, and sex.

One additional trial, that of the European Working Party on Hypertension in the Elderly, has recently been concluded but addresses the elderly population specifically. Like the Systolic Hypertension in the Elderly Program, this trial is beyond the scope of the present review. We may turn, then, against the background of the studies described, to consider recommendations for treatment of mild hypertension over the past decade or more.

RECOMMENDATIONS FOR TREATMENT OF MILD HYPERTENSION

Through the 1970s and extending into the mid-1980s, while the foregoing trials were in progress and their results were appearing, public policy on treatment of hypertension was evolving. In the US, for example, the National High Blood Pressure Education Program sought to develop and disseminate recommendations for the public and for health professionals in dealing with high blood pressure. The principal landmarks in that program have been the successive reports released in 1973, 1977, 1980, and 1984 containing these recommendations (68, 61, 69, 43). Other agencies and organizations have also issued reports or guidelines for high blood pressure control, and for the primary prevention of hypertension, including the US Department of Health and Human Services (85, 13) and the World Health Organization (94, 95, 97, 98).

Task Force I

First, in the US, the "Task Force I" report of 1973 identified the diastolic and systolic blood pressure levels of 95 mm Hg or greater and 160 mm Hg or greater as requiring rescreening before high blood pressure could be confirmed (68). Notably, at least three visits were suggested, with three blood pressure readings per visit and the second and third of these diastolic readings to be averaged across all three visits. The resulting value for diastolic pressure was to indicate the further measures needed: treatment, at or above 105 mm Hg; periodic screening (annually), below 95 mm Hg; and, for persons at pressures from 95 to 104 mm Hg, observation with individualization of the judgment concerning treatment. This latter recommendation was further elaborated to suggest repeated observation, combined with management not involving specific drugs, unless otherwise decided by the physician in the individual case.

The Joint National Committee—1977

The first successor to Task Force I under the auspices of the National High Blood Pressure Education Program was its Joint Committee on Detection, Evaluation, and Treatment of High Blood Pressure, whose report was published in January, 1977 (61). In comparison with the Task Force I report, a more explicit statement of considerations in the decision to treat in the 90 to 104 mm Hg range of diastolic pressures (no longer 95 to 104) was given. It was recommended that the presence of other risk factors lends some weight toward treatment, although use of drugs to control blood pressure was to be a later decision: "For some patients, weight control and a reduced salt intake may lower blood pressure, but if this proves ineffective after three to six months, specific drug therapy may be necessary in addition to diet" (61).

The Joint National Committee—1980

A new Joint National Committee (whose membership only partly coincided with that of its predecessor) was charged in 1978 to review, revise, and augment the 1977 report, under the aegis of the National High Blood Pressure Coordinating Committee (69). With respect to therapy, the Committee statement on mild hypertension is especially noteworthy:

> The findings of the Hypertension Detection and Follow-up Program suggest that *long term reduction of blood pressure decreases overall mortality at all levels of hypertension* [emphasis in the original]. This is of special importance with regard to mild hypertension because of its high prevalence in the population. Although reduction in overall mortality has not yet been demonstrated in patients below age 50 with mild hypertension, treatment of these patients reduces the incidence of such hypertensive complications as stroke, congestive heart failure, left ventricular hypertrophy, and progressive rise of blood pressure [citation of the USPHS Study in the original]. *It is therefore reasonable to reduce blood pressure even in uncomplicated mild hypertension by pharmacologic or non-pharmacologic therapy* [emphasis added].

A further qualification for young persons with uncomplicated mild hypertension suggested special consideration of the disadvantages of long-term therapy in relation to low short-term risks of the condition. In general, however, the stated goal of therapy was to maintain the diastolic pressure below 90 mm Hg, and lower as safety and tolerance permit.

The Joint National Committee—1984

The most recent report in this series, published in May 1984, differs from its predecessors in several respects (43). As before, the new Committee membership had only partial overlap with its predecessor. Most relevant in the context of this review are this Committee's statements about the rationale for treatment in the range of diastolic pressures from 90–94 mm Hg and about the status of nonpharmacologic approaches as an alternative to the use of antihypertensive drugs. The position of the current Committee on these and closely-related questions is indicated in the following excerpts:

> Controversy remains about whether all patients with diastolic blood pressures between 90 and 94 mm Hg should receive pharmacotherapy if nonpharmacologic measures do not control blood pressure adequately. . . . Although it is prudent to be concerned and cautious about the theoretic implications of long-term adverse drug effects, this should not be a reason to withhold antihypertensive [drug] treatment from patients 50 years of age and older. . . . The benefits of drug therapy seem to outweigh any known risks from such therapy for those

with a diastolic blood pressure persistently elevated above 95 mm Hg and for those with lesser elevation who are at high risk. . . . For those with diastolic blood pressures in the 90- to 94-mm Hg range who are otherwise at low risk, nonpharmacologic therapy should be pursued aggressively while blood pressures are carefully monitored. . . . Data from HDFP suggest that if the diastolic blood pressure remains above 90 mm Hg, despite non-pharmacologic therapy, antihypertensive drugs should be started. Other authorities, however, would delay specific drug therapy in this group if blood pressures are not consistently above 94 mm Hg and if there is no evidence of target organ disease or other risk factors for cardiovascular disease. . . . Physicians who elect not to use drug therapy for patients with diastolic blood pressures in the 90- to 94-mm Hg range should follow up these patients' conditions as closely as if they were on pharmacologic therapy, because many will progress to higher levels of diastolic blood pressure that all agree should be treated with anti-hypertensive agents.

With respect to the goal of therapy, the current report offers two explicit statements:

The goal of treating patients with hypertension is to prevent the morbidity and mortality attributable to high blood pressure. This means the reduction of elevated blood pressure to the extent that excess cardiovascular risk is eliminated. [and]

The initial goal of antihypertensive therapy is to achieve and maintain diastolic blood pressures at lower than 90 mm Hg if feasible. A reasonable further goal is the lowest diastolic blood pressure consistent with safety and tolerance.

Summary of These and Other Guidelines

To summarize this series of recommendations, as they have evolved to the mid-1980s, the most important changes relevant to mild hypertension have been: first, a reduction in the high blood pressure threshold to 90 from the earlier 95 mm Hg diastolic; second, a consideration of other risk factors constituting added justification for treatment in this range; and third, the recommendation to initiate treatment with drugs at 95 mm Hg for all ages and, by implication, at 90 mm Hg for persons aged 50 or older. Goals of blood pressure reduction are expressed both quantitatively and in relation to reduction of risk.

Importantly, nonpharmacologic management and the need for additional evidence concerning its role in blood pressure control came to be recognized prominently in the 1980 report (69); the current Committee recommendations place further confidence in these (with reservations concerning the effectiveness of behavior modification techniques) and note their potential application in primary prevention of hypertension (43).

The 1984 report of the Joint National Committee, strictly interpreted, retracts some aspects of the previous recommendations: First, it expresses the view that drug therapy need not be initiated even if nonpharmacologic therapy fails to bring the diastolic pressure below 90 mm Hg, so long as the pressure does not rise to 95 mm Hg or higher. Second, it may be read to suggest lesser concern in persons under 50 years of age. However, it opens the consideration of primary prevention, discusses special age groups and other issues not previously addressed in such detail, and identifies elimination of excess cardiovascular risk as the goal of therapy. It is certainly a clearer statement with respect to the 90–94 mm Hg range of diastolic pressures than is the WHO/ISH statement of guidelines for mild hypertension, with which it is otherwise in general agreement (97). Neither of these reports is altogether clear in its recommendations for blood pressure measurement. Because the number and timing of measurements may influence markedly the selection of persons for treatment, both reports leave some concern as to their actual implementation.

COMMENTARIES ON THE PROBLEM OF MILD HYPERTENSION

The Benefit of Blood Pressure Reduction

The evolution of treatment recommendations discussed above indicated especially major change in 1980 (69). This revision was directly attributable to the HDFP experience, which was especially applicable to the diastolic levels below 95 mm Hg, with 2941 participants in this substratum. The HDFP was also especially informative about the 95 to 104 mm Hg substratum, with 4884 participants, all observed for five-year mortality (39). Not surprisingly, then, the majority of commentaries that have addressed any particular trial concern the design, conduct, and results of the HDFP.

STEPPED CARE INTERVENTION AND ITS EFFECTS   The most frequently recurring issue concerning interpretation of the results of the HDFP has been the nature of Stepped Care management, which entailed frequent medical contacts with possible effects beyond those of antihypertensive therapy alone. This possibility has led to attribution, by some commentators, of the reduced mortality associated with Stepped Care to general medical care and, by implication, only partially to antihypertensive therapy, if at all (1, 3, 17, 23, 28, 31, 44, 45, 50, 51, 56, 57, 73, 75). Several points can be offered with respect to this suggested interpretation. First, the 1979 reports on the HDFP did acknowledge the possibility of some enhancement of benefit from more frequent medical contact in Stepped Care, which as stated in those reports "cannot be dismissed completely" (35). A problem then is to identify those aspects of care which might explain the reduced mortality, other than blood pressure reduction itself. However, specifically reported information on major cardiovascular risk factors—hypercholesterolemia, cigarette smoking, and overweight—indicated no difference between treatment groups at the conclusion of the trial. This is not surprising, since only minimal ancillary advice or treatment of any kind apart from management of hypertension was authorized by the study protocol. Nor has any commentator suggested what aspects of general medical care could plausibly account for the substantial relative reduction in mortality that was observed. Further, the Referred Care approach was itself very likely to have included more regular clinical contact than that received by the general population, although not to the degree experienced by the Stepped Care group.

Second, more recent analyses of the HDFP data support strongly the attribution of the benefit of Stepped Care to its paramount component, antihypertensive therapy. Fatal and nonfatal strokes were from 32 to 45% less frequent among Stepped Care participants from Stratum I to Stratum III, respectively, than in Referred Care. In addition, analyses to test the contributions of blood pressure treatment to mortality differentials over the course of the study confirm that most of the between-group difference can be accounted for in statistical terms by the blood pressure treatment (29, 39). Thus to invoke another explanation of benefit beyond that of antihypertensive therapy is not necessary.

Third, another issue related to nonspecific therapy is that the reduced mortality associated with Stepped Care extended to deaths assigned to noncardiovascular as well as cardiovascular causes, as determined from coded death certificates (3, 17, 28, 44, 45, 84). That survival was prolonged in general could plausibly have resulted from improved cardiovascular status, more directly evident in the reduced rates of specific blood pressure-related cardiovascular events. This interpretation is also consistent with the long-known predictive relation of blood pressure levels to all-cause mortality. These considerations do not strongly suggest an alternative to antihypertensive therapy as an explanation of the mechanism of action of the Stepped Care program of management.

DEMOGRAPHIC SUBGROUPS OF THE HYPERTENSIVE POPULATION   The fact that treatment in Referred Care was not homogeneous across subgroups of the study population has also posed difficulty for some commentators (3, 4, 19, 25, 28, 51, 56, 75). The issue is whether equal effects are to be expected in such a trial as the HDFP when specific subgroups of the population are examined. If so, such differences could be of some importance, and an understanding of this aspect of the study is therefore desirable. Referred Care was the designation for the reference or comparison group, against which Stepped Care was to be evaluated. Unlike a placebo comparison, the reference group might easily be actively treated. The determinants of treatment status for individuals in the Referred Care group were the prevailing beliefs and practices that could easily vary by blood pressure level, age, sex, race, and other attributes. Thus subgroups of the HDFP study population defined by any attribute of interest—such as blood pressure at entry, sex, race, or age—might therefore represent quite different types and intensities of management in Referred Care.

Accordingly, any comparisons between the Stepped Care and Referred Care assignees must be made independently within particular subgroups, and results for one such subgroup need not resemble those for another. For example, as some commentators have observed, relatively small blood pressure differentials between groups in any particular comparison (such as for white women, in the HDFP) would be expected to be accompanied by a relatively small mortality differential (63, 78).

A further question about the benefit of treatment in demographic subgroups (those defined by sex, race, or age, singly or in combination) arises from the general lack of statistically significant differences in such subgroup analyses (2, 3, 11, 28, 31, 44, 51, 63). This issue arises, despite the obvious limitation of statistical power for subgroup analysis, because some commentators express reluctance to recommend treatment on the basis of available evidence without demonstration of statistically significant effects in any given specific subgroup. The results of HDFP reflect the combined experience of black and white men and women aged 30–69 years at entry; even with nearly 11,000 participants, separate tests of the intervention effects by subgroups are not justified by the design. Accordingly, interpretation of study results in such subgroups and their generalization to the population at large will necessarily remain based on trends in the data rather than on independent statistical tests in specific strata, unless or until such data become available from future studies.

LEVELS OF PRESSURE AT WHICH BENEFIT APPEARS   Another issue is, at what levels of blood pressure, in relation to those in the general population, were benefits of treatment observed in these trials (31, 53, 63)? This question concerns the possible differences in participant selection, with respect to initial blood pressure levels, among the several major treatment trials: To whom do the respective results apply? This issue has already been discussed and the need for careful reading of published reports noted. The large number of participants in the HDFP with pressures from 90–94 mm Hg at randomization, and the results for that substratum, have been noted above. The initial home-screening criterion of an average of diastolic readings of 95 mm Hg or greater made eligible for the HDFP some persons whose usual diastolic pressures would have been well below those in the corresponding stratum of the VA trial. Accordingly, reductions in endpoint rates in the HDFP were observed at initial levels below those reported for the VA trial.

A related question has been the entry levels of pressure for which treatment appeared effective in the ANBPS (46, 57, 75). As the full follow-up analysis shows, benefit was not limited to those with diastolic pressures of 100 mm Hg or greater alone. An endpoint rate reduction equivalent to that for the 100–104 mm Hg stratum was observed for those entering at 95–99 mm Hg: 15.6 vs 22.3 events/1000 person-years (30.0% reduction) at 95–99 mm Hg, and 17.5 vs 24.5

events/1000 person-years (28.6% reduction) at 100–104 mm Hg, respectively (7).

THE SCOPE OF BENEFITS OF TREATMENT   An extension of this discussion leads to the broader question of benefit and, as posed by some, the following kind of argument (3, 4, 17, 56): First, the absolute rates of events in untreated mild hypertension are very low ("The majority of untreated patients have survived the trials"). Second, not all who are on treatment are spared these events ("Some patients, though treated, do not benefit"). Third, benefit accrues exclusively to those patients who would have experienced an event but who, having been on treatment, avoided it. Fourth, treatment is therefore unjustified for the vast majority of those with mild hypertension. Fifth, and finally, it is presently unknown how to identify, in advance, the few true potential beneficiaries of treatment; therefore, treatment should not be recommended at all.

This argument is difficult to sustain on many grounds, including the following:

1. Rates of undesirable effects (including development or progression of cardiac, renal, cerebrovascular or ocular complications) are underestimated by references to "hard" endpoints alone, and broader classifications of unwanted hypertensive complications suggest several-fold higher rates in some trials, such as the USPHS Trial and the HDFP (80, 39).

2. Few if any medical or public health interventions are universally effective; inadequacy or delay in treatment and inattention to additional risk factors appear likely to reduce the benefit otherwise attainable through treatment of mild hypertension. However, a criterion of 100% effectiveness will not likely be achieved under the best imaginable circumstances, since blood pressure levels and the other recognized risk factors are not the only determinants of any of the events or conditions of concern. In other terms, the attributable risk of particular blood pressure-related events, which varies by blood pressure levels and other attributes, is less than 100% in all instances; therefore elimination of blood pressure-related risks will not suffice to prevent all such events, e.g. strokes.

3. Whether reduction of risk constitutes a "benefit" is perhaps an issue judged differently according to the philosophical approach taken. From one point of view, it is in the interest of the individual to reduce his or her chances of adversity, even though absolute protection is not conferred. It is erroneous to think of risk as characterizing treatment alone, and if treatment risks are less than those of remaining untreated, the individual choice may be for the lesser risk, even though it is not zero. Treatment might therefore be seen as fully justified if it clearly improved the balance of the risks. From this point of view, the true beneficiaries of treatment would represent a much broader spectrum of the mild hypertensives than some would imply. It should be clear, in any case,

that considerations of the potential costs and benefits of alternative treatment policies would be influenced greatly by the assumptions made in the foregoing respects.

The last concern to be raised in the present context is the failure to observe consistently in trials of antihypertensive therapy a specific reduction in morbidity and mortality from coronary heart disease (14, 15, 17, 19, 24, 62, 74). However, the most recent data from the HDFP are consistent with a coronary disease reduction, and the ANBPS is suggestive of the same (7, 18). If a reduction in coronary heart disease incidence is required to justify treatment in mild hypertension, the basis for this reservation is diminished.

Adverse Consequences of Treatment

A prominent theme in the collected commentaries on management of mild hypertension has been a strong reluctance to treat all persons in the 90 to 104 mm Hg diastolic range with drugs to achieve sustained blood pressure control at levels below 90 mm Hg. The specific concerns emphasized repeatedly relate to undesirable features attributed to drugs and to the scale of the treatment problem, as inferred from projected estimates of the prevalence of diastolic blood pressures in this range. Proposals stimulated by these concerns include: (a) restriction of treatment eligibility to a lower limit of diastolic pressures, set as 95 or 100 mm Hg (44, 51, 63); (b) extension of pretreatment observation for several months or longer, in order to identify those persons whose pressures remain below the suggested criterion level for initiating treatment (3, 17, 28, 44, 45, 51, 63); and (c) elimination of drug therapy altogether from consideration in treatment at these levels (presumably up to 105 mm Hg) (44).

Problems with the use of drugs loom large in the view of several commentators, who cite excessive side effects and toxicity, including major metabolic derangements and possible sudden cardiac death as risks of drug treatment, to be weighed against the immediate risks (implied as being very small) of untreated mild hypertension (1, 3, 28, 45). The extent of severe toxicity which is assumed as the basis for this concern deserves more explicit presentation and discussion, in order that adverse effects of therapy may be assessed with the same care as are its beneficial effects—and, in addition, the adverse effects of withholding treatment. Alderman, for example, attributes to drug therapy "an increased incidence of sudden death" in the Oslo study; but in that trial only 19 deaths in all occurred; and, of those, ten and nine were in the treatment and placebo groups, respectively; there were altogether 25 and 34 "cardiovascular events" in these respective groups (3). The authors of that study report observed, "No serious drug-induced disease occurred during the observation period" (30). This latter interpretation accords with that of the HDFP investigators, who reported as follows: "In the judgment of the [Toxicity and Endpoint Evaluation] Committee, no deaths were attributed to drug toxicity in the SC [Stepped Care] group. Few hospitalizations occurred because of suspected drug toxicity. Moreover, toxicity problems with the SC regimen rarely prevented achievement of BP control, since alternative medications could be utilized" (35).

In this connection, Freis has stated, "It is interesting to speculate on the frequency and severity of the side effects that would result if this advice [to lower diastolic pressure to below 85 mm Hg] were implemented" (17). This was the protocol requirement for the great majority of Stratum I participants in the HDFP, and the comments from the HDFP report cited above partially address this important question. Fuller reports from the completed studies could be of great value in this respect. For example, the recent report of the MRC trial gives some evidence on this question (59). But the data reported combined the presence of side effects with the physician's decision to withdraw therapy—a decision made with knowledge of treatment status and therefore expected most often in the active treatment groups. Overall, the authors concluded that side effects in the MRC trial were "mostly but not all minor."

These brief references are not presented as a final disposition of the matter of drug toxicity and its relevance to antihypertensive therapy. The possibility of adverse effects of interventions of any kind must always be a conscious concern, even when the interventions in question involve drugs that have been in use for many years by millions of persons. The drug trials do not offer sufficient evidence, in themselves, of either very long-term or latent effects, owing to their limited population sizes and their durations. The unexpected or unanticipated suggestion of an adverse effect must be regarded seriously and evaluated with care. Such, for example, is the interpretation that excessive mortality may have occurred in the Special Intervention group of participants in the Multiple Risk Factor Intervention Trial (MRFIT), who were hypertensive and had some types of electrocardiographic abnormalities at entry (67). In this instance, the possibility of an adverse drug effect, consideration of which arose in extensive post hoc subgroup analyses, cannot be ruled out, and is a matter for continuing investigation (55). However, preliminary reports of special analyses of the HDFP experience indicate no support to such a risk in approximately similar patients observed in that trial (10, 21).

The range of viewpoints with respect to the choice of drugs, and in particular the use of diuretics versus alternative drugs as the first step in drug therapy, implies wide differences of opinion on the matter of the relative safety and acceptability of the thiazide and thiazide-like diuretics (6, 9, 14, 16, 43, 46, 52, 58, 65, 66). Significantly, the Joint National Committee Report of May 1984 recommends use of a thiazide-type diuretic (or a beta-blocker) "at less than a full dose" as Step One of therapy, with progression to a "full dose if necessary and desirable" (43). While the several commentaries cited state preferences for one or another approach to therapy, the views expressed are supported without

quantitation of either efficacy or safety of any of the drugs considered—
whether diuretic, beta-blocker, alpha-blocker, or other. This underscores the
difficulty of reaching a reasoned resolution of the counter-claims, not only for
one drug relative to another, but for the larger question of drug therapy versus
nonpharmacologic approaches, to be discussed below.

The scale of the mild hypertension problem has been cited repeatedly in
discussions of treatment. It is ironic that this aspect has been taken both to
support the withholding or deferral of therapy, lest too many persons be treated,
and to emphasize the potential public health impact on morbidity and mortality
if the prevailing treatment recommendations are followed, since the available
intervention can reach so large a population at risk (12, 17, 27, 28, 44, 45, 51).
Several concerns appear to hinge on this issue of scale, such as the societal
implications as to costs and allocation of health care resources; the perception of
an implied need for an extraordinary effort (presumably on the part of providers) to achieve blood pressure control for a large population at risk; and
inconvenience and anxiety (on the part of those with high blood pressure), the
latter especially being intensified by the often-cited presumption of a need for
lifelong treatment from the time at which it is initiated. [Studies of the course of
blood pressure change after interruption of treatment continue but remain
inconclusive (54, 90).] Although the problems of scale are undeniably serious,
they relate to both the question of treatment and the prevalence and risks of the
underlying condition. Therefore, it is especially important to measure the
prevalence and risks with some care. This has been emphasized in the recent
report of the Working Group on Risks and High Blood Pressure (93). Instead,
crude estimates of prevalence of hypertension on single-occasion screening are
those most often cited. For reasons discussed above, these may inflate the
correct estimates by a factor of two or more.

The effect of repeated observation upon the identification of persons with
sustained "treatable" blood pressure levels is also important in discussions of
prevalence (93). Existing recommendations provide for multiple occasions of
examination and therefore substantial "fall-out" of persons whose diastolic
pressures do not remain above 90 mm Hg (43). Thus the inclusion for treatment
of a large proportion of persons whose blood pressure levels will decline
without intervention can be prevented. Further evidence of the effects of
repeated measurement is found in the reports of serial blood pressure readings,
through screening and early follow-up, as for the ANBPS control group. With
or without placebo tablets, the major mean decrement in blood pressure occurred between first screening and the fourth examination, at four months'
follow-up (8). A similar result was reported from the MRC trial (59). Whether
the number of occasions at which blood pressure was measured or the lapse of
time was the more relevant factor in the fall in blood pressure is unclear from
these data. This question could be answered with alternative serial screening

strategies in defined populations. In any case, the suggestion that long periods (many months, or years) are needed to distinguish between sustained and relatively short-term elevations of blood pressure appears to be incorrect (3, 28, 44, 45, 63).

A further suggestion has been that initiation of treatment should be deferred until after a definite *increase* in blood pressure, beyond the upper limit of mild hypertension, is observed (17). This more extreme proposal may have been abandoned following publication of the HDFP data on Stratum I, the mild hypertensives (39). In that report, the relative benefit of Stepped vs Referred Care was shown to be greater for persons without either target organ damage or current antihypertensive therapy at entry than for those already demonstrating target organ damage before treatment was initiated.

Proposals to withhold or defer treatment arise in part from the difficulty addressed on several occasions by Alderman, that of the prognostic "heterogeneity" of the mild hypertensive stratum (3, 4, 56). He has stressed that some persons on no treatment will nonetheless experience a fall in blood pressure, while others may remain hypertensive with or without complications, and still others, even though on treatment, will experience the complications whose prevention was the purpose of treatment. From these results of follow-up, Alderman has identified differences in the course of hypertension that would be desirable to predict, so that treatment could be offered only to those who would surely benefit and not offered to those who surely would not. However, the limited prognostic value of available baseline data, within the mild hypertension group, has been noted, except that risks are increased with the presence of several well-recognized concomitant risk factors (3, 4, 28, 56, 77). [These have been incorporated in the Joint National Committee reports as added indicators both of risk and of the need for treatment in the 90 to 104 mm Hg stratum (43, 61).] It is also relevant that excess risks characterize this stratum relative to the risks at diastolic pressures *below* 90 mm Hg (93). Thus, gradation of risks within the range of mild hypertension does not necessarily imply that treatment of the lesser-risk subgroups is without justification. Whether prolonged withholding of all known approaches to blood pressure control could be defended for any subgroup appears seriously doubtful on the present evidence, however.

Nonpharmacologic Therapy

The last general issue concerning the question of treatment has been anticipated in much of the preceding discussion: An undercurrent in many commentaries, which is strongly expressed in some, is the unwelcome prospect of the use of drugs to deal with the massive problem of mild hypertension (22, 26, 50, 60, 70, 72, 82). Even if the scale is much reduced in a proper assessment, it remains very large. The problems raised by several commentators in connection with widespread use of antihypertensive drugs have been noted, and many of the other difficulties seem related to these. Suggestions have been raised frequently to place much greater, even total, reliance on "nondrug" or "nonpharmacologic" approaches to the control of mild hypertension. The extent to which the available nonpharmacologic approaches have been shown efficacious and in other ways practical as a major strategy of blood pressure control has been addressed less thoroughly. However, the impression develops, in review of the entire body of material cited, that if the role of drugs were superceded by nonpharmacologic approaches, many of the arguments against treatment would be withdrawn. Whether a recommendation to substitute nonpharmacologic approaches for drug treatment reflects a belief in their efficacy or, instead, a rejection of the need for blood pressure reduction in mild hypertension is presently unclear (19).

Perceptions have differed widely as to the strength of the evidence that sustained effective blood pressure control can be achieved through the nonpharmacologic methods being advocated (weight reduction, dietary sodium restriction, biofeedback, and others) (91, 92, 5, 42, 47, 32). Little attention has apparently been given to such issues as cost, resource allocation, logistical aspects, and patient acceptance for these approaches, relative either to drugs or to one another. The fullest discussion of alternatives to drug therapy is perhaps that of Guttmacher and others (27). They have taken the further step to characterize the problem of high blood pressure as essentially one of social causation, therefore most amenable to social interventions to reduce stress and burdens of the social existence of many persons. In their view, the medical approach is inappropriate and in effect diverts the attention of society from the optimum remedy and indeed the root of the high blood pressure problem. This viewpoint leads to the ultimate solution to high blood pressure: primary prevention.

It is not possible within this review to assess the current status of each of the nonpharmacologic approaches to high blood pressure control in detail. Several additional comments about such approaches do seem appropriate, however. First, the spectrum of these approaches may be thought of quite broadly to include assistance in adherence to prescribed drug regimens, modification of dietary habits, and psychophysiological interventions such as biofeedback, relaxation techniques, and others (79). Second, to the extent that any or all of these approaches may serve to enhance sustained, effective blood pressure control at goal levels, even with continued use of drugs, there is an evident climate of receptivity to their use; this is reflected in the conclusions reported by some of the mild hypertension trials, in the recommendations at each juncture from the National High Blood Pressure Education Program Coordinating Committee, and in many of the commentaries reviewed. Third, if such approaches would provide an actual alternative to reliance on drugs while affording maintenance of adequate blood pressure control, their use would predictably be even more enthusiastically welcomed. Fourth, demonstration of efficacy of these nonpharmacologic approaches in the primary prevention of high blood pressure might well provide an important means by which this broader objective could be pursued on a meaningful scale. Thus, at several levels, nonpharmacologic or behavioral strategies may have very significant potential for application in the field of high blood pressure control and prevention.

CONCLUSIONS

The question of treatment of mild hypertension is complex, as many sub-ordinate questions can be raised that are interrelated, and to which inconsistent answers are offered in the literature. Even where directly relevant data are provided from completed studies of prevalence, risk, and treatment benefit, differences of interpretation are common. In areas where data are not available, the judgments expressed are more difficult to resolve, since their bases are less accessible to objective evaluation.

The available data, as illustrated here, lead this reviewer to conclude that treatment of mild hypertension to achieve diastolic pressures below 90 mm Hg is the appropriate public health policy based on current evidence. Indefinite deferral of effective treatment is to prolong risks of target organ damage whose prognosis cannot be reversed by later treatment. At present, the knowledge of this risk outweighs the unsupported impression that widespread use of Step 1 drugs necessarily entails equal or greater risks due to unwanted drug effects. This view, shared by the author, is generally consonant with those elaborated more fully by Gifford, by Moser, and by the Joint National Committee on which they both served (20, 64, 43).

This judgment does not overlook the difficult questions that remain in-completely answered (31, 63, 78, 83). The question of the safety of anti-hypertensive drugs can be addressed more fully from the data collected in the completed trials, but the limited duration of follow-up and size of study populations may leave open the question of rare, serious adverse effects. Even then, there remain difficulties in the process of synthesizing evidence on the benefits and risks of both treating and withholding treatment. Whether newer drugs, or effective alternatives to drugs, may diminish these concerns remains to be seen. Attention to nonpharmacologic approaches has increased and deserves to expand greatly in the interest of both treatment and primary prevention.

Under the auspices of the WHO and other organizations, discussions in the recent past have emphasized the world-wide concern with hypertension and its treatment and prevention (81, 98). A constructive step toward future investiga-tion of this problem would perhaps be to convene the proponents of the main points of disagreement in the literature reviewed here, with the following charge: to review each issue so as to resolve it if possible on the available evidence, and where not possible, to develop the appropriate research agenda. The importance of the problem warrants such an attempt, and the emergence of promising avenues of investigation on the most critical questions would be an invaluable contribution.

ACKNOWLEDGMENTS

The author wishes to acknowledge the assistance of Ms. Sally Shirts and Ms. Nancy Martin in the collection of materials and preparation of the manuscript. This review is substantially revised and updated following an earlier presentation to the NATO Symposium on Behavioral Epidemiology and Disease Prevention, Bellagio, Italy, April, 1983.

Literature Cited

1. Abeles, J. H., Snider, A. H. 1980. *Drug industry: Mild hypertension therapy.* Industry follow-up report. New York: Kidder, Peabody & Co., Inc. 7 pp.
2. Abernathy, J. D. 1980. Letter. The pressure to treat. *Lancet* 2:364–65
3. Alderman, M. H. 1980. Mild hypertension: New light on an old clinical controversy. *Am. J. Med.* 69:653–55
4. Alderman, M. H., Madhavan, S. 1981. Management of the hypertensive patient: A continuing dilemma. *Hypertension* 3:192–97
5. Andrews, G., MacMahon, S., Austin, A. 1982. Response to letter. *Br. Med. J.* 285:1046–47
6. Australian Therapeutic Trial in Mild Hypertension Management Committee. 1979. Initial results of the Australian Therapeutic Trial in mild hypertension. *Clin. Sci.* 57:449s–52s
7. Australian Therapeutic Trial in Mild Hypertension Management Committee. 1980. The Australian Therapeutic Trial in Mild Hypertension. *Lancet* 1:1261–67
8. Australian Therapeutic Trial in Mild Hypertension Management Committee. 1982. Untreated mild hypertension. *Lancet* 1:185–91
9. Birkenhager, W. H., de Leeuw, P. W. 1983. Session III: Therapeutic profile of trimazosin in hypertension. Opening remarks: Mismatch of essential hypertension's pathophysiology and current antihypertensive drugs: A perspective for alpha-1-adrenergic blockade. *Am. Heart J.* 106:1235–36
10. Borhani, N. O. 1984. Editorial. Treating mild hypertension. *Ann. Intern. Med.* 100:312–13

11. Borhani, N. O., Langford, H., Hawkins, C. M., Curb, J. D., for the Hypertension Detection and Follow-up Program Cooperative Group. 1983. Response to letter. *N. Engl. J. Med.* 308:524–25
12. British Medical Journal. 1980. Editorial. Millions of mild hypertensives. *Brit. Med. J.* 281:1024–25
13. Centers for Disease Control. 1983. Perspectives in disease prevention and health promotion. Implementing the 1990 prevention objectives: Summary of CDC's seminar. *Morbid. Mortal. Weekly Rep.* 32:21–24
14. Dollery, C. T. 1983. Hypertension and new antihypertensive drugs: Clinical perspectives. *Fed. Proc.* 42:207–10
15. Doyle, A. E. 1983. Hypertension: The realities. *Aust. N.Z. J. Med.* 13:185–86
16. Franklin, S. S. 1983. Geriatric hypertension. *Med. Clinics North Am.* 67:395–417
17. Freis, E. D. 1982. Should mild hypertension be treated? *N. Engl. J. Med.* 307:306–9
18. Freis, E. D. 1982. Response to letter. *N. Engl. J. Med.* 307:1524–25
19. Freis, E. D. 1983. Mild Hypertension: Which patients to treat. *Postgrad. Med.* 73:180–89
20. Gifford, R. W. 1982. Mild hypertension: Should it be treated? *Postgrad. Med.* 71:19–23
21. Gifford, R. W., Borhani, N. O., Krishan, I., Moser, M., Levy, R. I., et al. 1983. Commentary. The dilemma of 'mild' hypertension. Another viewpoint of treatment. *J. Am. Med. Assoc.* 250:3171–73
22. Gill, J. S., Beevers, D. G. 1983. Hy-

pertension and wellbeing. *Br. Med. J.* 287:1490–91

23. Gove, S., Hulley, S. B. 1983. Letter. Treatment for "mild" hypertension. *N. Engl. J. Med.* 308:524

24. Green, K. G. 1982. The role of hypertension and downward changes of blood pressure in the genesis of coronary atherosclerosis and acute myocardial ischemic attacks. *Am. Heart J.* 103:579–82

25. Grell, G. A. 1980. Letter. Race and hypertensive complications. *Lancet* 2: 744–45

26. Gross, F. 1983. Session IV. Hypertension: Control and treatment of hypertension. *Postgrad. Med. J.* 59(Suppl. 3): 117–26

27. Guttmacher, S., Teitelman, M., Chapin, G., Garbowski, G., Schnall, P. 1981. Ethics and preventive medicine: The case of borderline hypertension. *Hastings Center Rep.* 11:12–20

28. Gutzwiller, F. 1982. Letter. *N. Engl. J. Med.* 307:1524

29. Hardy, R. J., Hawkins, C. M. 1983. The impact of selected indices and antihypertensive treatment on all-cause mortality. *Am. J. Epidemiol.* 117:566–74

30. Helgeland, A. 1980. Treatment of mild hypertension: A five-year controlled drug trial. *Am. J. Med.* 69:725–32

31. Henderson, W. G., Tosch, T. J. 1980. Letter. Hypertension detection and follow-up. *J. Am. Med. Assoc.* 244:1317–18A

32. Hovell, M. F. 1982. The experimental evidence for weight-loss treatment of essential hypertension: A critical review. *Am. J. Public Health* 72:359–68

33. Hypertension Detection and Follow-up Program Cooperative Group. 1978. Mild hypertensives in the Hypertension Detection and Follow-up Program. *Ann. NY Acad. Sci.* 304:254–66

34. Hypertension Detection and Follow-up Program Cooperative Group. 1978. Patient participation in a hypertension control program. *J. Am. Med. Assoc.* 239:1507–14

35. Hypertension Detection and Follow-up Program Cooperative Group. 1979. Five-year findings of the Hypertension Detection and Follow-up Program. I. Reduction in mortality of persons with high blood pressure, including mild hypertension. *J. Am. Med. Assoc.* 242:2562–71

36. Hypertension Detection and Follow-up Program Cooperative Group. 1979. Five-year findings of the Hypertension Detection and Follow-up Program. II. Mortality by sex-race and age. *J. Am. Med. Assoc.* 242:2572–77

37. Hypertension Detection and Follow-up Program Cooperative Group. 1980. Letter. Hypertension detection and follow-up. *J. Am. Med. Assoc.* 244:1318

38. Hypertension Detection and Follow-up Program Cooperative Group. 1980. Five-year findings of the Hypertension Detection and Follow-up Program. III. Reduction in stroke incidence among persons with high blood pressure. *J. Am. Med. Assoc.* 247:633–38

39. Hypertension Detection and Follow-up Program Cooperative Group. 1982. The effect of treatment on mortality in "mild" hypertension. Results of the Hypertension Detection and Follow-up Program. *N. Engl. J. Med.* 307:976–80

40. Hypertension Detection and Follow-up Program Cooperative Group. 1984. Effect of stepped care treatment on the incidence of myocardial infarction and angina pectoris. Five-year findings of the Hypertension Detection and Follow-up Program. *Hypertension* 6(supp. I):I-198–I-206

41. Hypertension Detection and Follow-up Program Cooperative Group. 1985. Five-year findings of the Hypertension Detection and Follow-up Program: Prevention and reversal of left ventricular hypertrophy with antihypertensive drug therapy. *Hypertension* 7:705–112

42. Johnston, D., Steptoe, A. 1982. Letter. Non-drug treatments of hypertension. *Br. Med. J.* 285:1046

43. Joint National Committee on Detection, Evaluation, and Treatment of High Blood Pressure. 1984. The 1984 Report of the Joint National Committee on Detection, Evaluation, and Treatment of High Blood Pressure. *Ann. Intern. Med.* 144:1045–57

44. Kaplan, N. M. 1981. Whom to treat: The dilemma of mild hypertension. *Am. Heart J.* 101:867–70

45. Kaplan, N. M. 1983. The clinical use of diuretics in the treatment of hypertension. *Clin. Exp. Hyper. Theory Pract.* A5:167–76

46. Kaplan, N. M. 1984. Therapy of mild hypertension: An overview. *Am. J. Cardiol.* 53:2A–8A

47. Kobayashi, Y., Kajiwara, N. 1983. Treatment of borderline hypertension: Moderate salt restriction in the treatment of borderline hypertension. *Jpn. Circ. J.* 47:268–75

48. Labarthe, D. R. 1978. Problems in definition of mild hypertension. *Ann. NY Acad. Sci.* 304:3–14

49. Labarthe, D. R. 1983. Evaluation of the treatment of hypertension. *Isr. J. Med.* 19:471–78

50. Lancet. 1980. Editorial. The pressure to treat. *Lancet* 1:1283–84
51. Lancet. 1980. Editorial. Lowering blood pressure without drugs. *Lancet* 2:459–61
52. Lancet. 1982. Editorial. Diuretic or beta-blocker as first-line treatment for mild hypertension? *Lancet* 2:1316–17
53. Levine, S. R. 1981. Letter. "True" diastolic blood pressure. *N. Engl. J. Med.* 304:362–63
54. Levinson, P. D., Khatri, I. M., Freis, E. D. 1982. Persistence of normal blood pressure after withdrawal of drug treatment in mild hypertension. *Arch. Int. Med.* 142:2265–68
55. Lundberg, G. D. 1982. MRFIT and the goals of the Journal. *J. Am. Med. Assoc.* 248:1501
56. Madhavan, S., Alderman, M. H. 1981. The potential effect of blood pressure reduction on cardiovascular disease. A cautionary note. *Arch. Intern. Med.* 141:1583–86
57. McAlister, N. H. 1983. Should we treat 'mild' hypertension? *J. Am. Med. Assoc.* 249:379–82
58. McCarron, D. A. 1984. Diuretic therapy for mild hypertension: The "real" cost of treatment. *Am. J. Cardiol.* 53:9A–11A
59. Medical Research Council Working Party. 1985. MRC trial of treatment of mild hypertension: Principal results. *Br. Med. J.* 291:97–104
60. Menard, J., Chatellier, G., Degoulet, P., Plouin, P.-F., Corvol, P. 1983. How much can blood pressure be lowered? *Hypertension* 5(supp. 3):3-21–3-25
61. Moser, M. 1977. Report of the Joint National Committee on Detection, Evaluation and Treatment of High Blood Pressure. A cooperative study. *J. Am. Med. Assoc.* 237:255–61
62. Moser, M. 1980. Letter. Antihypertensive drugs and coronary heart disease. *Lancet* 2:745
63. Moser, M. 1981. "Less severe" hypertension: Should it be treated? *Am. Heart J.* 101:465–72
64. Moser, M. 1983. A decade of progress in the management of hypertension. *Hypertension* 5:808–13
65. Moser, M. 1983. Hypertension: America's major solvable public health problem. *Am. Pharmacy* 5:36–39
66. Moser, M. 1983. Stepped-care treatment of hypertension: The rationale for an empirical approach. *Postgrad. Med.* 73:199–210
67. Multiple Risk Factor Intervention Trial Research Group. 1982. Multiple Risk Factor Intervention Trial. Risk factor changes and mortality results. *J. Am. Med. Assoc.* 248:1465–77
68. National Institutes of Health. National High Blood Pressure Education Program. 1975. Report to the Hypertension Information and Education Advisory Committee. Task Force I. Data Base. US Dept. Health, Education and Welfare, Public Health Serv., Natl. Inst. Health. Washington DC: DHEW Publ. No. (NIH) 75–593
69. National Institutes of Health. Joint Committee on Detection, Evaluation and Treatment of High Blood Pressure. 1980. The 1980 Report of the Joint National Committee on Detection, Evaluation and Treatment of High Blood Pressure. US Dept. Health and Human Services, Public Health Serv., Natl. Inst. Health. Washington DC: NIH Publ. No. 81–1088
70. Pacy, P., Dodson, P. 1984. Letter. Hypertension and wellbeing. *Br. Med. J.* 288:327
71. Paul, O. 1980. The risks of mild hypertension. *Pharmacol. Ther.* 9:219–26
72. Paul, O. 1983. Editorial. Hypertension and its treatment. *J. Am. Med. Assoc.* 250:939–40
73. Peart, W. S., Miall, W. E. 1980. Letter. MRC Mild Hypertension Trial. *Lancet* 1:104–5
74. Pickering, T. G. 1983. Editorial. Treatment of mild hypertension and the reduction of cardiovascular mortality: The 'of or by' dilemma. *J. Am. Med. Assoc.* 249:399–400
75. Ram, C. V. S. 1983. Editorial. Should mild hypertension be treated? *Ann. Intern. Med.* 99:403–5
76. Reader, R. 1978. Therapeutic trials in mild hypertension ongoing throughout the world. *Ann. NY Acad. Sci.* 304:309–17
77. Reader, R. 1980. Letter. Australian hypertension trial. *Lancet* 2:744
78. Relman, A. S. 1980. Mild hypertension. No more benign neglect. *N. Engl. J. Med.* 302:293–94
79. Shapiro, A. P., Schwartz, G. E., Redmond, D. P., Ferguson, D. C. E., Weiss, S. M. 1978. Non-pharmacologic treatment of hypertension. *Ann. NY Acad. Sci.* 304:222–35
80. Smith, W. McF. 1977. Treatment of mild hypertension. Results of a ten-year intervention trial. *Circ. Res.* 40(Supp. I):I-98–I-105
81. Strasser, T. 1982. Research policies in mild hypertension and the role of the WHO/ISH Liaison Committee. *Clin. Sci.* 63:427s–30s

82. Taylor, R. B. 1980. Letter. Hypertension detection and follow-up. *J. Am. Med. Assoc.* 244:1317

83. Thomson, G. E., Alderman, M. H., Wassertheil-Smoller, S., Rafter, J. G., Samet, R. 1981. High blood pressure diagnosis and treatment: Consensus recommendations vs. actual practice. *Am. J. Public Health* 71:413–16

84. Traub, Y. M. 1980. Letter. Hypertension detection and follow-up. *J. Am. Med. Assoc.* 244:1317

85. US Dept. of Health and Human Services. 1980. *Promoting Health/Preventing Disease. Objectives for the Nation.* US Dept. Health and Human Serv., Public Health Serv. Washington DC: US GPO

86. Veterans Administration Cooperative Study Group on Antihypertensive Agents. 1967. Effects of treatment on morbidity in hypertension. I. Results in patients with diastolic blood pressures averaging 115 through 129 mm Hg. *J. Am. Med. Assoc.* 202:116–22

87. Veterans Administration Cooperative Study Group on Antihypertensive Agents. 1970. Effects of treatment on morbidity in hypertension. Results in patients with diastolic pressures averaging 90 through 114 mm Hg. *J. Am. Med. Assoc.* 213:1143–52

88. Veterans Administration Cooperative Study Group on Antihypertensive Agents. 1972. Effects of treatment on morbidity in hypertension. III. Influence of age, diastolic pressure and prior cardiovascular disease; further analysis of side effects. *Circulation* 45:991–1004

89. Wassertheil-Smoller, S., Apostilides, A., Miller, M., Oberman, A., Thom, T. 1979. Recent status of detection, treatment and control of hypertension in the community. *J. Commun. Health* 5:82–93

90. Wassertheil-Smoller, S., Langford, H., Blaufox, M. D., Oberman, A., Babcock, C., et al. 1982. Rate of hypertension return after withdrawal of prolonged antihypertensive therapy. *Clin. Sci.* 63:423s–25s

91. Watt, G. C. M., Edwards, C., Hart, J. T., Hart, M., Walton, P., Foy, C. J. W. 1983. Dietary sodium restriction for mild hypertension in general practice. *Br. Med. J.* 286:432–36

92. Watt, G. C. M., Hart, J. T., Foy, C. 1983. Letter. Dietary sodium restriction for mild hypertension in general practice. *Br. Med. J.* 286:1146–47

93. Working Group on Risk and High Blood Pressure. 1985. An epidemiological approach to describing risk associated with blood pressure levels. *Hypertension* 7:641–51

94. World Health Organization. 1978. Report of a W.H.O. Expert Committee. *Arterial Hypertension. Tech. Rep. Ser.* No. 628. Geneva: WHO

95. World Health Organization. 1982. Report of a W.H.O. Expert Committee. *Prevention of Coronary Heart Disease. Tech. Rep. Ser.* No. 678. Geneva: WHO

96. World Health Organization Mild Hypertension Liaison Committee. 1982. Trials of the treatment of mild hypertension. An interim analysis. *Lancet* 1:149–56

97. World Health Organization/International Society of Hypertension. 1983. Guidelines for treatment of mild hypertension. *Bull. WHO* 61:53–56

98. World Health Organization. 1983. *Report of the Scientific Group on Primary Prevention of Hypertension. Tech. Rep. Ser.* No. 686. Geneva: WHO

Ann. Rev. Public Health. 1986. 7:217–35

INTERNATIONAL DRUG REGULATION

Philip R. Lee and Jessica Herzstein

Institute for Health Policy Studies, School of Medicine, University of California at San Francisco, San Francisco, California 94143

INTRODUCTION

Drug regulation is almost universal in the industrialized nations of the world and is becoming increasingly common in third world countries. It is increasingly based on the premise that regulation is needed to ensure that new drugs will be safe and effective, labeled accurately, and marketed responsibly. In short, the potential benefits and hazards of modern drugs are too important to be left to the marketplace and the unregulated functioning of the pharmaceutical industry.

The concept that drugs and the pharmaceutical industry should be regulated is a relatively recent development, whereas control by society of the use of medicines and those who dispense and prescribe them is very old. Indeed, Penn (27) cited examples of such regulation that date back 3000 years. In the Middle Ages, regulation of apothecaries was practiced in Europe and in Moslem countries (19b). Gradually the focus shifted from apothecaries to the drugs themselves. Official lists of drugs were introduced in cities in Italy and Germany in the sixteenth century, and by the nineteenth century pharmacopoeias had achieved legal or quasilegal status in most European countries (10).

Almost two centuries ago, two developments set the stage for evolution of the modern pharmaceutical industry and subsequent development of international drug regulation: (*a*) in the United States and Europe patent laws were instituted to provide market protection for patented inventions, including drugs, for a period of years after marketing, and (*b*) pure morphine was isolated from crude opium by a German pharmacist in 1805 to mark the first step in the science of drug development. Increased regulation and scientific advances have progressed together, although not always harmoniously, ever since. Patent

0163-7525/86/0510-0217$02.00

laws in the United States and Europe provided a means for industrial competition, with an emphasis on patented products and advertising directly to the public. Competition among drug firms during the next 150 years was based primarily on price, rather than product innovation, because of price-conscious consumers who at that time purchased drugs directly without the need for a physician's prescription (39). It was not until enactment of the Food, Drug and Cosmetic Act in the United States in 1938 and subsequent regulations that physicians assumed a central role as agent for the consumer.

Scientific advances related to drugs continued slowly and intermittently through the nineteenth and early twentieth centuries. In the 1930s, developments in research and clinical practice dramatically changed the role drugs played in the practice of medicine and consequently the role of the drug industry in medical care.

DRUG REGULATION IN EUROPE AND THE UNITED STATES

The first specific legislation to control drugs was enacted in England a little more than a century ago. Switzerland followed suit and established a federal office, the Interkantonale Kontrollstelle für Heilmittel (IKS), charged with drug regulation, in 1900. In the United States, Congress debated the issue for more than 30 years before enacting the Pure Food and Drug Act of 1906. The emphasis in the early debates and in the early laws was on protecting consumers against grossly fraudulent advertising and the marketing of impure and adulterated foods and drugs (31, 2). Although most European countries developed some form of drug regulation in the early decades of the twentieth century, several had only limited systems as late as 1960 (10).

Norway and Sweden were among the first countries to develop drug regulations related to safety and efficacy. Norway's legislation dates from 1928 (15), while Sweden first developed a drug regulatory system with tight controls over approval and marketing in 1934. A Board on Pharmaceutical Specialties was established to advise the state. Subsequently, a list of 2500 to 3000 registered pharmaceuticals represented the only ones permitted to be marketed. Evaluations were based on efficacy, safety, accuracy of promotion, and reasonable pricing (9).

The spectacular technological advance represented by sulfanilamide led to a major reform of drug legislation in the United States. The Roosevelt administration had tried without success to prod Congress to enact new drug regulations in the early 1930s. After the death of more than 100 people, including many children, following the use of elixir of sulfanilamide, legislation was quickly enacted. In 1938, Congress passed the Food, Drug, and Cosmetic Act, which dramatically changed drug regulation in the United States and provided the basis for changes that followed in Europe and then throughout the world (31).

The 1938 law prohibited the marketing of a new drug unless the manufacturer submitted an application to the Food and Drug Administration (FDA). The 1938 law required that a manufacturer convince the FDA that a drug was safe; whether the drug was effective was left to the physician and was regarded as outside the purview of FDA. Each manufacturer who wished to market a new drug was required to submit an application to the FDA containing reports of investigators. If the FDA did not reject the drug within a specified period it was deemed approved and could be marketed.

In addition to the premarket testing of drugs and the approval required by the FDA before marketing, major provisions of the 1938 law included: (*a*) strengthening regulations against false and misleading advertising; (*b*) requiring that appropriate warnings be part of a drug's label; and (*c*) establishing enforcement procedures and penalties for violations. Among the critically important regulations promulgated by the FDA to implement the law's labeling requirements was one that permitted an exception to the warning label if the drug was to be used only by or on the prescription of a physician, dentist, or veterinarian (39, p. 46). This regulation dramatically altered the relationship between physician and patient. Physicians became, in effect, drug purchasing agents for their patients. Advertising, instead of being directed at the public, was directed primarily at physicians. This policy was reflected in drug regulations throughout the world during the next 40 years.

France followed Norway, Sweden, and the United States in developing laws regulating drug safety and the drug industry. A new drug regulatory law in France, promulgated in 1941, required ministerial authorization of new drugs for marketing. A committee of experts evaluated new drugs on the basis of therapeutic promise and evidence that the drugs would not endanger physical or mental well-being (44). In 1959, French reforms were undertaken to protect the interests of industry (a 20-year patent) and the health of consumers (technical analysis of new drugs by a panel of experts). Approval for marketing became known as "autorisation de mise sur le marche" (AMM) and required renewal every five years.

The period between 1938 and 1962 witnessed a transformation of the pharmaceutical industry in the United States and Europe. Powerful new drugs, such as antibiotics and tranquilizers, revolutionized pharmacology and medical care. To be part of this revolution, a firm had to invest in research and development and become vertically integrated. The revolution resulted in high profits and a change in industry structure with increasing concentration and gradual emergence of multinational and transnational firms (2, 31, 39).

The most significant development affecting drug regulation in Europe and the United States was the thalidomide tragedy in Europe in the late 1950s and early 1960s. Important changes in drug regulation stemming from this incident were made initially in the United States, Norway, Sweden, and the United Kingdom. Amendments to the Food, Drug, and Cosmetic Act in 1962 and later rulings by the federal courts, including the United States Supreme Court, provided the basis for modern drug regulation in the United States. The principal features of the 1938 Food, Drug, and Cosmetic Act were retained and strengthened in 1962. Both safety and efficacy had to be demonstrated after the 1962 legislation (17, 25).

Few European countries followed the lead of Norway, Sweden, and the United States in drug regulation in the late 1930s, but virtually all of them developed regulations as a result of the thalidomide tragedy. The policy of industry regulation had become worldwide by the 1980s.

While regulations covering pharmaceuticals did exist in the United Kingdom in the pre-thalidomide era, they were uncoordinated and dealt mostly with quality control. In January 1964, the Committee on Safety of Drugs (CSD), a committee of experts responsible for reviewing data on new drugs, was created. This initiated a voluntary system of controls, which consisted of an agreement by two major trade organizations, the Association of the British Pharmaceutical Industry (ABPI) and the Proprietary Association of Great Britain (PAGB), to take the advice of the CSD before initiating large-scale clinical trials or marketing new drugs. Though safety became a major concern after 1961, the CSD was also concerned with efficacy of new drugs (9, p. 32).

The Medicines Act of 1968, implemented in 1971, provided the first statutory basis for regulation of the manufacture, marketing, labeling, and importing of medicines for human use in the United Kingdom. It established strict control over safety, efficacy, and quality (1). The Act is administered by the Medicines Division of the Department of Health and Social Security (DHSS). Having gained statutory powers, the CSD became the Committee on Safety of Medicines (CSM). The CSM has a scientific secretariat to process applications for licenses and prepare summaries for CSM subcommittees.

A review of the British Medicines Act has emphasized several points distinguishing it from FDA regulations in the United States.

1. The informality of the British regulatory system contrasts with the more formal relationship between government and industry in the United States. In the United Kingdom, frequent direct communication between industry and government is the rule at all stages of regulation.
2. Early Phase I studies are permitted on normal healthy volunteers without notification of or approval by any regulatory body.
3. Efficacy has not been considered as important as safety in drug approval (9, p. 34).
4. Although the overall approval process has been praised for its swift decisions, excessive delays have been reported in granting of the clinical trial certificate.
5. The results of the process have not always been effective in preventing entry into the market of drugs that later prove to be unsafe.

Although West Germany is the second largest producer of drugs in the world, its drug regulatory system has been called "underdeveloped" (9, p. 74). Drug regulations adopted before World War II were still in use in 1961 despite rapid growth in the economy and major advances in drug development. A new drug law in 1961 and further amendments failed to bring the system up to par with those in other European countries. In 1971, however, new guidelines on drug approval were issued. In West Germany until 1971 any combination drug product could be marketed after approval of its individual chemical components. About 30,000 drugs are marketed in West Germany, including many nonsensical combination products. West German law prohibits withdrawing these products from the market, and they are widely used by physicians, often without full knowledge of the identity of constituent chemicals. Laws governing drug regulation were further modified by the German Drug Act of 1976, which did not become effective until January 1978. The new law strengthened regulations related to manufacturing practices, clinical investigations, and protection of human subjects during clinical trials, but did not involve drugs registered before 1971. Since the law governs primarily the licensing of drugs prior to marketing, it has had little effect on marketing and prescribing practices (13).

In Switzerland, the IKS is authorized to assess new therapeutic agents prior to marketing and to notify the cantons (local government units responsible for health care) of its appraisal regarding composition, advertising, and price, as well as its decision concerning approval or denial of authorization for sale (20). Specific requirements for registration, including data on safety and efficacy, are included in regulations formulated in 1955, 1963, and 1972. Since 1973, the IKS has also been empowered to control the manufacturing of pharmaceutical agents. The Swiss system of drug approval is notable for its simplicity and lack of detailed specifications and requirements. A Swiss university pharmacologist has noted that the high level of cooperation between the IKS and the industry is a remarkable feature (9, pp. 51, 52).

Sweden, Norway, and Denmark regulate drugs more strictly than do most other countries. In Sweden, the approved list of drugs contains only about 2500 to 3000 drugs, permitting easy and in-depth review by control authorities. Drugs are registered for an unlimited period of time and then reviewed as questions of efficacy or adverse reactions dictate. The number of drugs on the market is kept small through strict approval requirements. Drugs with highly specified use (e.g. agents for tropical diseases) and drugs not approved for mass marketing may receive licenses for distribution to a limited group of people. Licensing may also permit limited marketing as part of ongoing clinical trials with cautious monitoring of adverse drug reactions. A license may confine drug use to hospitals. Since 1964, the Department of Drugs must be notified of all anticipated clinical trials, which may proceed if no objection has been raised after two weeks.

Norway and Denmark have drug approval systems comparable to those of Sweden. Relative need plays a role in the decision to register a drug in Norway (15). Assessment of need is difficult, and indeed this criterion may rarely be applied (9, p. 92). Norway had approximately 1800 pharmaceutical products and Denmark 1500 in 1976. Norway had a regulatory system that assessed efficacy of new drugs as early as 1928, and it represents the exception to the observation that general acceptance of the need for proof of efficacy did not occur within the regulatory community until the growth of clinical pharmacology in the 1960s and 1970s (10).

Drug regulation in the United States, as in Europe, has evolved gradually since the dramatic changes of the early 1960s. There have been no major legislative changes in drug regulation in the United States since 1962, but a variety of administrative decisions have significantly modified regulations.

A number of drug regulatory reform proposals were considered by the United States Congress in the late 1970s, and a number of actions were taken administratively by the FDA, including informing subjects in clinical trials of the risks; expediting the review of "breakthrough" drugs; improving the scientific competence of FDA staff; and improving systems of postmarketing surveillance (25, p. 421).

Reforms within the FDA structure have been extensively researched and debated. In 1979, the Commissioner of Food and Drugs initiated a revision of the regulations concerning the Investigational New Drug (IND) and New Drug Application (NDA) requests. The NDA rewrite was eventually published in the *Federal Register* on February 22, 1985. A majority of the regulations became effective in May 1985. The IND procedure rewrite is now in the final phases of review. The 1985 revisions are the most extensive drug regulation reforms in the nation since the Kefauver-Harris Amendment.

In most cases involving an NDA the new regulations require concise data tabulations rather than lengthy case report forms, although the latter must be readily available for review if requested. One objective is to shorten the time required for review of NDAs in the FDA. The mean processing time of an NDA application has been over two years (10). The new rule allows the FDA 180 days from receipt of an application to issuance of a letter stating "approval," "approvable," or "not approvable." An additional regulation permits approval of a drug for marketing in the United States even if the clinical research was conducted entirely in foreign countries, provided that the studies meet certain criteria. There are a number of other modifications in the regulations, including ones concerning application format, safety update reports while the application is under review, clarification of the three action letters, improved communication between the agency and the applicant during the review process, and provisions for dispute resolution and extended postmarketing surveillance (24, 29).

DRUG REGULATION IN THIRD WORLD COUNTRIES

Except for those in China, India, Mexico, Brazil, and Egypt, the pharmaceutical sector in most third world countries is dependent for drugs mainly upon multinational corporations based in Europe, Japan, and the United States. The private sector is usually in the dominant position with respect to drug marketing and distribution. The relative share in dollar value of pharmaceuticals distributed through the private sector ranges from a low of 35% in Guyana to a high of 95% in Argentina (K. Balasubramaniam 1984, personal communication).

Although regulation of the marketplace of prescription and nonprescription drugs in the third world resembles that in industrial countries on paper, in practice the effects are far different. A number of recent studies (23, 47, 30, 32) have demonstrated that drugs are promoted in the third world with grossly exaggerated claims of therapeutic scope; adverse drug reactions are either minimized in importance or ignored in labeling and advertising; most prescription drugs are customarily dispensed without prescription, often by untrained clerks; drugs exported to third world countries include those that are no longer approved for use in the exporting country (drug dumping); and widespread bribery affects physicians, national drug policies (e.g. no list of essential drugs is implemented), and procurement of drugs nationally and locally and by hospitals and pharmacies.

Many problems in this area, especially since the mid-1970s, have been identified by a number of independent but mutually confirmatory studies that can best be described as investigative reporting. Some of these have been broad investigations covering entire continents (8, 22, 23, 30, 32). Others have focused on problems associated with individual drugs (16, 36). These reports, widely covered by press, radio, and television, have provided ammunition with which such consumerist organizations as the International Organization of Consumer Unions (IOCU) and Health Action International (HAI) and such key individuals as Sidney Wolfe in the United States; Charles Medawar, Andrew Herxheimer, and Dianna Melrose in the United Kingdom; Virginia Beardshaw in the Netherlands; and the late Olle Hansson in Sweden have induced regulatory agencies and even some pharmaceutical companies to alter their policies. It seems likely that consumer pressures on national and international agencies and on the drug industry will continue, and that they will continue to be effective.

To address these problems, K. Balasubramaniam (personal communication) has proposed an integrated pharmaceutical policy for the third world, including (a) product selection and nomenclature; (b) drug legislation and regulation; and (c) drug procurement. These are policy issues of concern to third world countries, to industrialized nations, to the pharmaceutical industry, and to the United Nations and the World Health Organization.

THE ROLE OF THE WORLD HEALTH ORGANIZATION AND OTHER UNITED NATIONS AGENCIES

The World Health Organization (WHO) and other United Nations (UN) agencies have made a variety of efforts to improve drug regulation during the past 30 years, particularly in the past 10 years. The response of WHO and other UN agencies in recent years has, in part, been the result of an increasingly active consumer movement, led by the IOCU and HAI, as well as growing concern on the part of third world countries.

WHO has participated in organizing regional and global meetings of regulatory agencies to improve the exchange of information and to establish common principles of drug regulation. Although progress has been made, it is more in the exchange of information and informal contacts than in the harmonization of policies, even among the industrial nations of Western Europe.

A basic strategy recommended by WHO is limiting procurement of drugs to those that meet the broadest range of health needs most economically and that comply with defined standards of quality and safety. This effort was formally initiated in 1977 when a WHO panel recommended a list of 214 drug products, 182 classified as "essential" and 32 as "complementary." This list has become known as the WHO list of essential drugs (41), and it forms the basis of drug import policies in a growing number of third world countries.

In one of the most important actions taken in recent years on the rational use of drugs, the World Health Assembly on May 17, 1984 adopted Resolution 37.33, which urged member states to take a number of steps to improve the exchange of information, strengthen the capability of member countries to select needed drugs, and improve drug policies. In addition, the resolution requested the director general of WHO to arrange a meeting in 1985 of experts and concerned parties, including representatives of governments, pharmaceutical industries, patients, and consumer organizations to discuss the means and methods to ensure rational drug use, especially through improved knowledge and flow of information, and to discuss related marketing practices, especially in developing countries.

The UN General Assembly, the UN Secretariat, and other UN agencies have also been involved in issues related to drug safety and regulation. In accordance with a resolution adopted by the UN General Assembly in 1982, the UN Secretariat published the monograph entitled *Consolidated List of Products Whose Consumption and/or Sale Have Been Banned, Withdrawn, Severely Restricted, or Not Approved by Government* in July 1984 (40). Among the products included were many that have been identified as unsafe or ineffective by other investigators. These include chloramphenicol, aminopyrine, phenacetin, phenyl butazone, oxyphenbutazone, clioquinol, and a variety of related quinolines. In addition, the UN Center for Transnational Corporations has been examining a variety of issues relating to international drug regulation.

THE IMPETUS FOR CONTROLS

The current impetus behind regulation of drug marketing is four-fold: (*a*) to insure that medicinal therapy is safe and effective; (*b*) to provide health professionals and the public with sufficient, unbiased information about marketed drugs; (*c*) to insure an adequate supply of drugs; and (*d*) to protect the drug industry from unfair competition.

International drug regulation includes three broad areas: (*a*) development; (*b*) manufacture; and (*c*) marketing. Regulations relating to drug development may include animal studies, studies on normal human beings, and clinical trials for the assessment of safety and efficacy before marketing. Regulations related to manufacturing may include good manufacturing practices, quality control, and packaging. Marketing regulation may cover labeling, advertising, distributing, prescription or nonprescription status of a drug, inclusion in public insurance or health service programs, price, and import and export control.

To ensure the safety and effectiveness of drugs before marketing, regulators, particularly in industrialized nations, increasingly demand scientific evidence demonstrating safety and efficacy that is based on laboratory, animal, and clinical testing. However, premarket testing, no matter how well designed and executed, cannot detect all potential adverse effects, particularly those rare events that require either the use of the drug by many thousands of patients or its use over an extended period of time. In addition, those who regulate the entry of drugs into the marketplace cannot control their use and misuse after marketing. Drug regulatory decisions are made without an absolute standard for determining safety and effectiveness and with limited knowledge of the effects of the drug in question and of how it will be used.

Increasingly, concern for stricter regulation stresses problems associated with adverse drug reactions and inadequacies in current premarket testing and postmarketing surveillance that fail to detect adverse drug reactions before the damage is done. The recent withdrawal from markets in the United States and Europe of several drugs that had been widely promoted has emphasized the problem. In 1980, the antihypertensive drug, Selacryn, was withdrawn by Smith Kline and French after significant liver toxicity became apparent. In 1982, Eli Lilly withdrew the heavily promoted anti-inflammatory agent, Oraflex, but not until it had been implicated in nearly 100 deaths. Criminal charges were brought successfully against Eli Lilly executives for withholding damaging information on this drug from the FDA. In 1983, Johnson and Johnson withdrew Zomax, another nonsteroidal anti-inflammatory agent, after the occurrence of fatal anaphylactoid reactions in five people who used the drug. In this last case, the problem was limited largely to the United States. In the same year Merck withdrew Osmosin, a slow-release variant of indomethacin, which was associated with at least 12 deaths in the United States. Phenylbutazone and oxyphenbutazone, as well as pyrithroxine and oxametacin, could also be added to this list (12).

While a goal of public policy on drugs is to minimize risks, it is an accepted fact that the use of medications must involve certain risks. Not all risks can be eliminated through conscientious manufacturing, rigorous clinical testing, and wise prescribing. The dream of lifesaving drugs that possess no significant human toxicity is no longer considered realistic.

The central issue is this: to what extent are government controls over the pharmaceutical industry necessary to achieve the basic goals of regulation? Various types of controls have the potential for both positive and negative impact on the public's health, as well as upon the development of new drugs and the health of the industry. In most industrial countries, standards for many industrial products take into account safety and quality. Labeling the product, banning it, or removing it from the market are the methods used most commonly in enforcing regulations over consumer products. Regulations may require the label to portray accurately important properties of the product. While in many countries a product may be removed from the market if it proves unsafe, in other countries such regulations do not exist or they are unenforced.

Drug use can be controlled by requiring a prescription for dispensing certain pharmaceutical products. Countries such as Sweden and Czechoslovakia impose an additional level of control by restricting the prescription of selected drugs to certain physician specialties or hospitals (42). In addition to standards reflecting safety and quality (including effectiveness), a few countries, including Norway and Iceland, require that a new drug product be medically needed, and its approval for marketing is based on its relative efficacy as related to that of similar products.

Criteria for premarketing approval that extend beyond efficacy and safety have resulted in reduced numbers of drugs on the market. For example, in Norway, Sweden, and Denmark the requirement for assessment of relative need has resulted in very limited national formularies. Policies such as those in Sweden that actually limit distribution of certain highly toxic or specialized drugs to physicians or medical centers with specified qualifications were proposed and debated at length in the United States in 1978–1980.

Additional and significant restrictions in drug availability are created in many countries by cost-conscious third party payment plans, including government health insurance (France) and health service plans (United Kingdom) that limit payment for drugs or require consumer cost-sharing. Reimbursement by an insurance plan for a limited number of pharmaceuticals and a limited number of indications means, in effect, that not all marketed drugs are available to all patient populations.

While there has been a trend toward increasing government controls over pharmaceuticals throughout the world, there is little agreement on the public health and economic benefits or adverse consequences of modern drug regulation. There is as yet little consensus on what constitutes too much or too little regulation. The aim of drug legislation was originally the prevention of fraud, and now it is closer to the protection of the uneducated consumer (10) or the "public health interest" (42). Some analysts believe that the right to individual choice has been removed from the consumer and placed in the hands of the physician, the technical expert, and the bureaucrat (10, 39). These analysts urge greater emphasis on physician and patient choices about drugs and fewer regulatory controls by the FDA.

THE CONTROVERSY REGARDING GOVERNMENT CONTROLS

Drug regulations may have negative effects over and above their intended effects. There has been a great deal of debate but too few objective data on the benefits and costs of drug regulation.

During the past 20 years there have been a number of studies of the impact of drug regulation. Although his work was controversial, Peltzman's pioneering studies (26) utilized the tools of economics, including cost-benefit analysis, to assess the effects of drug regulation in the United States. He concluded that the missed benefits were far more costly to society than the gains from keeping ineffective drugs off the market.

More recently, important studies have been conducted by the European office of the World Health Organization under the direction of Graham Dukes. The WHO group has provided a well-founded methodological approach to studying the effects of drug regulation.

Dukes has reviewed in depth the regulatory issues (10) and noted the controversy over intensifying and relaxing government drug regulations. The pharmaceutical industry has developed much of the argument against what it considers to be excessive regulation, and has attempted to gain physician support through popularizing the concept that regulations restrict a physician's freedom to prescribe.

Three arguments to support the relaxing of drug regulation policy have been described by Dukes:

1. From the public health perspective, over-regulation tends both to delay the marketing of medically needed drugs and to hinder research and therefore the development of new drug products.
2. Industry risks facing a declining return on its investment and succumbing to economic pressures to diversify into other more profitable markets and possibly discontinue pharmaceutical production.
3. The national economy risks increased unemployment and reduced exports.

The last is particularly at issue in an increasingly competitive world market when the United States has a relatively strict regulatory system for drug approval.

A major issue in the controversies on costs and benefits of drug regulation has been the impact of regulation on innovation in the pharmaceutical industry. The argument has been made by Wardell & Lasagna (43), Bailey (4), Peltzman (26), Grabowski (14), and a National Academy of Engineering Panel (28) that drug regulations in the United States since 1962 have had a significant negative impact on drug innovation. This view has been clearly stated by a former regulator: "The issue isn't whether . . . regulation cuts down on innovation. Indeed it does. It must. There's hardly any way that regulation can stimulate innovation" (J. R. Crout, cited in Ref. 19a).

It is also argued that there are unacceptably long delays in drug approval by the FDA, creating a "drug lag," a term used to describe the delayed entry of new drug products into the United States or any other given country when compared, for example, to the United Kingdom, Switzerland, or the Federal Republic of Germany. Although a drug lag can be demonstrated, it varies from drug to drug and country to country, and many factors other than regulatory decisions affect it. Studies purporting to demonstrate the adverse effects of drug lag have been criticized on methodological grounds by Ashford (3) and Dukes (10). Its impact is difficult to assess, but its deleterious effect on public health appears to have been exaggerated.

When the costs of introducing a new drug are raised (by regulatory and nonregulatory factors), one result will be a decrease in the number of new drugs marketed. The number of drugs introduced onto the United States market showed a significant decrease from the late 1950s to the 1960s and 1970s (39, Table 2). To what extent the FDA is responsible for that declining rate of introduction of new drugs and whether or not drug regulation inhibits research are disputed (10). Dukes argues that the standards enforced by regulatory agencies are those the industries would choose to maintain on their own. Yet he notes that the track records of the marketing policies of pharmaceutical companies before and after introduction of effective regulations argues against the practicality of voluntary regulations (11).

In a careful and detailed study, Wiggins (45) examined the effects of increased regulatory stringency on new drug introduction. As in previous studies, he used the FDA processing time of an NDA as the index of regulatory stringency. The index increased rapidly during the 1960s to a high in the early 1970s. This correlates with the introduction of stricter regulatory guidelines in 1962. Wiggins concluded that increased regulatory stringency in the 1960s caused a doubling of the cost of new drug development and approval for marketing. His findings are supported by other investigators (39, p. 142).

However, as others have noted, the decline in new drug introductions began even before the stricter 1962 regulatory guidelines. Indeed, the reduced rate of introduction of tranquilizers may have accounted for most of the overall reduction in new drug introductions in the 1960s. Approval of new tranquilizers was affected by both regulatory and nonregulatory factors, including the thalidomide tragedy.

One argument that has received much attention contends that nonregulatory factors have had a significant impact on drug innovation. The research depletion hypothesis contends that the therapeutic revolution, which produced new antibiotics in the 1930s and 1940s, ended by 1960. Industry then concentrated on new formulations and new indications for existing molecules. The drug amendment that passed in 1962 complicates the analysis, but it was not responsible for a decline in the introduction of new clinical entities (NCEs). There is little evidence for this hypothesis, though it is regarded as a plausible explanation.

Although social regulation of the drug industry has been the predominant method used, other forms of regulation may affect the pharmaceutical industry, particularly economic regulation (e.g. tax policies).

Governmental efforts to lessen the financial burden of drug use on consumers have taken several forms. In countries such as the United Kingdom, drugs have been a benefit under a national health service or national health insurance program. Some countries, including West Germany, Holland, and the United Kingdom, have anticipated savings from use of a limited drugs list which allows reimbursement by the government only for specified drugs but not for all drugs on the market. A consumer who wants a drug that is not on the list usually must pay for it directly out of pocket. In the United Kingdom, however, a national formulary was not adopted until April 1, 1985. Before that time, a price negotiation was required between government and industry with respect to drugs to be purchased through the National Health Service. Prescribing patterns of practitioners were audited regularly to identify aberrant behavior and reduce the use of drugs.

Cost constraints have created the impetus for third-party payment plans (including those of federal and state governments in the United States) to limit the number of drugs for which the consumer or provider will be reimbursed. Though in many areas the list includes drugs simply on the basis of price differential among chemically equivalent compounds, some unique chemical entities may not be included. This has established an economic barrier for some consumers who no longer have access to the drug of choice for a particular condition.

Both social and economic regulation of the pharmaceutical industry have become increasingly difficult because of the transnational and multinational character of the pharmaceutical industry. One third of the assets of United

States–based pharmaceutical firms are now located in other countries (21). Pfizer, the fourth largest United States-based pharmaceutical manufacturer, has 63 plants in 34 countries. As early as 1968, United States–based companies had 332 manufacturing subsidiaries abroad: 110 in Latin America, 106 in Europe, 31 in Africa and the Middle East, and 60 in Asia and other areas (7). The great dispersion of manufacturing and marketing resources of multinational pharmaceutical manufacturers permitted a variety of practices by the firms to avoid taxes and maximize profits. These include manufacturing in low tax countries, selling drugs at inflated prices to countries with high taxes, and transfer pricing and other practices that have effectively avoided many forms of economic regulation (7, 5).

Another area of controversy relates to the use of generic-name drug products. The pharmaceutical industry is undergoing a transition from the "glory days" of strong sales, high profits, and high productivity to a period of markedly increased competition among fewer new products for consumer markets and stricter national regulatory systems (46). A major new force in the pharmaceutical business is the development of the generic drug market. Generic-name drugs—compounds chemically equivalent to marketed brand-name drugs—have been gaining in popularity with consumers as patents expire on an increasing number of popular brand-name products. Increased sales of generic drugs have resulted mainly from limited drug or price lists of health plans (including the British National Health Service and Medicaid), recent expiration of patents of drugs with a large share of the market, and growing numbers of elderly patients seeking relief from high medical expenses.

Issues of concern with generic-name drugs include the fact that bioequivalence may vary between formulations and the existence of fierce competition between low-overhead generic companies and research-intensive companies. Typically, 7% of a generic manufacturer's sales are spent on research and development, as compared to 20% for innovative pharmaceutical companies, which have significantly smaller profit margins (10). In the United States, the Waxman-Hatch bill, passed in November 1984, combined a provision for marketing generic drugs with extension of drug patents. This has been termed "compromise legislation," the patent extension designed to maintain an incentive for basic research and thus spur innovation (37, 38).

INTERNATIONAL COOPERATION

Developing international cooperation among drug regulatory agencies and introducing uniformity in some policy areas are important long-term objectives of WHO and other UN agencies. The pharmaceutical industry once supported adopting standardized regional or international systems of laws controlling drugs. Since the pharmaceutical industry is multinational or transnational, and since the scientific and medical knowledge on which it is based is also international, development of a globally consistent approach is appealing. The potential benefits of harmonization of drug regulatory practices include: improved public health, less bureaucracy and decreased government spending, lower drug development costs for the pharmaceutical industry, and, perhaps, elimination of drug lag.

One important issue that must be addressed in developing international policies is the export of unapproved drug products. Traditionally, pharmaceutical firms in industrial nations have exported unapproved, inefficacious, and unsafe drugs to third world countries where appropriate regulatory decisions cannot be made or enforced because of limited resources and experience. Another issue is the parallel importing of drugs from a market where prices are low, perhaps subsidized, in order to make a profit in a market where the retail price is much higher.

There is evidence of progress toward greater international cooperation. The European Economic Community (EEC) has encouraged the development of similar legislation and common guidelines affecting drug policy. However, the EEC aim of attaining mutual recognition of regulatory decisions has proved unacceptable because of a wide divergence in regulatory policies and public health concepts among member states. The goal of EEC involvement in drug policy is primarily the liberalization of trade within the community (6). International harmonization of regulatory practices nonetheless is in the early stages of planning by the Nordic Council on Medicines and the Council for Mutual Economic Assistance (CMEA). WHO has organized international meetings of regulatory agencies to explore the practical gains to be derived from international cooperation, including harmonization in the drug approval process (25, p. 441). That drug regulation is not an entirely objective or scientific process today limits the scope of policy unification. Differences among drug markets are now much greater, even in related countries, than are people's medical needs.

Postmarketing surveillance is an area of growing importance in international drug regulation. Although most industrial countries, including the United States, provide their drug regulatory agencies with limited authority to monitor the use of drugs after marketing, pressures to do so are increasing. Postmarketing surveillance might provide information on efficacy and toxicity of drugs used for unapproved indications. Monitoring is not, however, a replacement for controlled clinical trials in the evaluation of premarket safety and effectiveness of drugs. To determine efficacy for new but unapproved indications may require clinical studies that are nonexperimental and controlled trials (34, 35). Data from well-designed postmarketing studies would permit comparison of efficacy and toxicity of drugs used for the same indication. Strom has argued in favor of an increased emphasis on postmarketing studies of efficacy. Premarket evaluation of efficacy is incomplete and may not involve the most efficacious use of a new drug. Postmarketing studies can achieve at least partial evaluation of secondary drug effects, variables affecting drug efficacy, and relative efficacy.

Strom also notes (35, p. 9) a discrepancy between the drug information needed for clinical decision making and that needed for the regulatory decision process. Postmarketing studies can address the special need for clinically relevant data, which Phase II and III studies do not provide (e.g. studies in a heterogeneous population, drug interaction information, and data on use in children and pregnant women).

Postmarketing studies also permit discovery of rare adverse reactions (one in every 1000 or more patient years of treatment) and allow assessment of efficacy as compared with similar drugs on the market. Testing involving laboratory animals and clinical trials is often insufficient to do this (18). The need for surveillance is not limited to newly marketed drugs, as evidenced by discovery of vaginal adenocarcinoma in female offspring of women who used DES during pregnancy.

The features of national and international postmarketing surveillance systems, including voluntary reporting, cohort studies, and the WHO system, have recently been detailed and analyzed with future trends in mind (18). Developing countries must rely on governments with established regulatory systems to share their experiences. In 1968, WHO initiated an international program for drug monitoring based on the concept that a large international study population could generate warning signs to be investigated earlier than would be possible in individual countries (18, p. 5). Various methods have been utilized to record international drug experience, including: (a) regulations requiring manufacturers to forward information on adverse events; (b) direct physician reporting to national monitoring centers; and (c) studies by independent intensive monitoring units (40).

Stewart et al (33) have described eight objectives for drug monitoring: (a) early detection of previously unknown adverse drug reactions; (b) assessment of risk-benefit ratios for certain drugs; (c) provision of information including epidemiologic data for regulatory and educational purposes; (d) estimation of the impact of drug use and drug-induced illness; (e) provision of data relevant to adverse drug reactions; (f) information to increase public awareness of drug reactions; (g) development of drug utilization review and peer review systems; and (h) acquisition of information useful in improving drug regulatory and monitoring schemes. In addition, the cost of monitoring must be reasonable. The benefits will depend on the nature and scope of the postmarketing surveillance systems adopted. It is likely that this area will be marked by rapid advances in industrial countries because of increased availability of computer-based drug information systems in hospitals and ambulatory care settings.

CONCLUSION

Drugs are among the most heavily regulated products in society. Although the initial impetus for regulations derived from an intent to protect manufacturers through patents and the use of brand names, it later shifted to protecting consumers against fraud by manufacturers. During the past 50 years, rapid scientific and technological advances have transformed the pharmaceutical industry and have brought with them both remarkable therapeutic advances and an increasing number of potentially hazardous drugs. With this has come increased emphasis on the public health aspects of drug regulation.

The primary impetus for increasing regulation has been a series of drug-related disasters, including elixir of sulfanilamide (1937), thalidomide (1961), and clioquinol (1970s). As a result, government agencies in country after country have been empowered to extend or deny authorization to manufacturers for marketing new drugs. These regulations require premarket testing and approval. Although requirements to prove safety and efficacy did not become widespread until the 1970s, they are now worldwide, at least in industrial nations. These standards had their origins in earlier laws regulating the marketing of drugs. In addition to premarket testing and approval by government before marketing, strict controls have been placed on labeling, dispensing, and manufacturing practices.

A debate has raged for two decades about the costs and the benefits of drug regulation. Despite the contention that excessive regulation stifles new drug innovation and delays access to much-needed drugs, there is strong political and public support here and abroad that controls and monitoring by national governments are necessary in today's world. The question, however, is not whether or not regulation should exist, but rather how the benefits can be achieved while the burdens of regulation are minimized. There is need for a stronger scientific base for drug regulatory policies and a need to understand the complex relationship between social and economic regulation.

Opportunities for international cooperation exist; however, planning is in the early stages, and there is little agreement about how to proceed. The multinational nature of the pharmaceutical industry and the absence of effective controls in the third world indicate that there are practical gains to be derived from increased international unification and standardization of drug policies, but at present this remains a long-term objective.

ACKNOWLEDGMENTS

Funding for research and analysis in this chapter was provided by the Samuel Rubin Foundation and the University of California, San Francisco.

Literature Cited

1. Andrews, P., Thompson, G., Ward, C. 1984. A regulatory view of the Medicines Act in the United Kingdom. *J. Clin. Pharmacol.* 24:6–18
2. Asbury, C. 1985. *Orphan Drugs.* Cambridge, Mass.: Ballinger
3. Ashford, N. A., Butler, S. E., Zolt, E. M. 1977. Regulation and innovation in the pharmaceutical industry. Unpublished manuscript. 32 pp.
4. Bailey, M. N. 1972. Research and development costs and returns: The U.S. pharmaceutical industry. *J. Polit. Econ.* 80:70–85
5. Barnet, R. J., Muller, R. E. 1974. *Global Reach: The Power of the Multinational Corporations.* New York: Simon & Schuster
6. Blum, Richard, et al., eds. 1981. *Pharmaceuticals and Health Policy.* London: Croom Helm
7. Bodenheimer, T. S. 1984. The transnational pharmaceutical industry and the health of the world's people. In *Issues in the Political Economy of Health Care,* ed. J. B. McKinley, pp. 187–216. New York: Tavistock
8. Braithwaite, J. 1984. *Corporate Crime in the Pharmaceutical Industry.* London: Routledge & Kegan Paul
9. Burrell, C. 1980. Drug assessment in uproar. In *Risk and Regulation in Medicine,* ed. A. W. Harcus. London: Assoc. Med. Advisors in the Pharmaceutical Industry
10. Dukes, M. N. G. 1985. *The Effects of Drug Regulation: A Survey Based on the European Studies of Drug Regulation.* Lancaster, England/Boston: MTP Press
11. Dukes, M. N. G. 1984. The seven pillars of foolishness. In *Side Effects of Drugs Annual 8,* ed. M. N. G. Dukes, J. Ehs, pp. xvii–xxiii. Amsterdam: Elsevier
12. *The Economist.* 1985. Business brief: An anti-depressant for America's drug industry. Jan. 12, 1985, pp. 70–71
13. Federal Ministry for Youth, Family Affairs, and Health. 1976. *Law on the Reform of Drug Legislation in the Federal Republic of Germany of 24 August, 1976.* Bonn: Federal Republic of Germany
14. Grabowski, H. G. 1976. *Drug Regulation and Innovation: Empirical Evidence and Policy Options.* Washington, DC: American Enterprise Inst.
15. Halse, M., Lunde, P. K. M. 1978. Norway. In *Controlling the Use of Therapeutic Drugs,* ed. W. M. Wardell, Part 2, pp. 187–210. Washington, DC: American Enterprise Inst.

16. Hansson, O. 1979. *Arzneimittel-Multis and der SMON-Skandal.* Berlin: Arznei-mittel-Informations-Dienst GmbH
17. Hutt, P. 1980. The legal requirement that drugs be proved safe and effective before their use. In *Controversies in Therapeutics,* ed. L. Lasagna, pp. 495–506. Philadelphia: Saunders
18. Inman, W. H. W., ed. 1980. *Monitoring for Drug Safety.* Lancaster, England: MTP Press
19a. Lasagna, L. 1976. Drug discovery and introduction: Regulation and overregulation. *Clin. Pharmacol. Ther.* 20:507–11
19b. Levey, M. 1963. Fourteenth-century Muslim medicine and the hisba. *Med. History* 7:176–82
20. Mattison, N., Thomas, E., Trimble, A. G., Wardell, W. M. 1984. The development of self-originated new drugs by Swiss pharmaceutical firms, 1960–1980. *Regul. Toxicol. Pharmacol.* 4:157–73
21. McGraine, N., Murray, M. 1978. The pharmaceutical industry: A further study of corporate power. *Int. J. Health Serv.* 8:573–88
22. Medawar, C. 1979. *Insult or Injury.* London: Social Audit
23. Melrose, D. 1981. *The Great Health Robbery: Baby Milk and Medicines in Yemen.* Oxford: OXFAM
24. New regulations to speed drug approvals, improve safety monitoring. 1985. *FDA Drug Bull.* 15:2–3
25. Nightengale, S. 1981. Drug regulation and policy formulation. *Health Soc.* 59:41:.-44
26. Peltzman, S. 1974. *Regulation of Pharmaceutical Innovation: 1962 Amendments.* Washington DC: American Enterprise Inst. for Policy Res.
27. Penn, R. G. 1979. The state control of medicines: The first 3000 years. *Br. J. Clin. Pharm.* 8:293–305
28. Pharmaceutical Panel, Committee on Technology and International Economic Issues, National Academy of Engineering. 1983. *The Competitive Status of the U.S. Pharmaceutical Industry: The Influence of Technology in Determining International Competitive Advantage.* Washington DC: Natl. Acad. Press
29. Pharmaceutical sector in the Third World: A strategy. 1985. *Fed. Reg. Part II* 50:7452–7518
30. Silverman, M. 1980. *The Drugging of the Americas.* Berkeley: Univ. Calif. Press
31. Silverman, M., Lee, P. R. 1974. *Pills,*

Profits and Politics. Berkeley: Univ. Calif. Press

32. Silverman, M., Lee, P. R., Lydecker, M. 1982. *Prescriptions for Death: The Drugging of the Third World.* Berkeley: Univ. Calif. Press

33. Stewart, R., Cliff, L., Philp, J., eds. 1977. *Drug Monitoring: A Requirement for Responsible Use.* Baltimore: Williams & Wilkins

34. Strom, B., Miettinen, O., Melmon, K. 1984. Post-marketing studies of drug efficacy: How? *Am. J. Med.* 77:703–8

35. Strom, B., Miettinen, O., Melmon, K. 1985. Post-marketing studies of drug efficacy: Why? *Am. J. Med.* 78:475–86

36. *Suffer the Children.* Sunday Times of London. 1979. New York: Viking Press

37. Sun, M. 1984. The price for more generic drugs. *Science* 224:369

38. Sun, M. 1985. Generics, Roche joust for Valium market. *Science* 228:472–73

39. Temin, P. 1980. *Taking Your Medicine: Drug Regulation in the United States.* Cambridge, Mass.: Harvard Univ. Press

40. United Nations. *Consolidated List of Products Whose Consumption and/or Sale Have Been Banned, Withdrawn, Severely Restricted, or Not Approved by Governments.* 1984. New York: UN

41. WHO Expert Committee. 1977. *WHO Techn. Rep. Ser.* 615. Geneva: World Health Organization

42. Wardell, W. W. 1973. Introduction of new drugs in the U.S. and Great Britain: An international comparison. *Clin. Pharmacol. Ther.* 14:773–90

43. Wardell, W. W., Lasagna, L. 1975. *Regulation and Drug Development.* Washington DC: American Enterprise Inst.

44. Weintraub, M. 1982. The French drug approval process. *J. Clin. Pharmacol.* 22:213–22

45. Wiggins, S. N. 1979. *Product Quality Regulation and Innovation in the Pharmaceutical Industry.* Cambridge: Massachusetts Inst. Technol. Unpublished

46. Williams, W. 1985. Glory days end for pharmaceuticals. *New York Times* Feb. 24, 1985

47. Yudkin, J. S. 1980. The economics of pharmaceutical supply in Tanzania. *Int. J. Health Serv.* 10:455

Ann. Rev. Public Health. 1986. 7:237–66

MONITORING FOR CONGENITAL MALFORMATIONS

Neil A. Holtzman

Department of Pediatrics, The Johns Hopkins University School of Medicine, Baltimore, Maryland 21205

Muin J. Khoury

Department of Epidemiology, The Johns Hopkins University, School of Hygiene and Public Health, Baltimore, Maryland 21205

Prior to 1960, few reports paid attention to associations between congenital malformations (CMs) and environmental agents (81). Monitoring—routine determination of the occurrence of CMs for the purpose of detecting trends and clusters—was performed in only a few localities. The thalidomide disaster of 1959–1961 rapidly stimulated the development of such systems. Between 1963 and 1976, birth defects monitoring started nationwide in seven countries (12, 21, 29, 36, 45, 117a, 128, 145) and in parts of 12 others (34), including the United States (27, 110, 121, 122). In 1974, the International Clearinghouse for Birth Defects Monitoring was created (34, 86); by 1982, 22 programs, collecting data from 26 countries, were participating (63).

During the 1970s, problems of toxic waste dumps and accidents such as those at Three Mile Island and Seveso raised concern about the possible teratogenicity of environmental agents other than drugs. Between 1981 and 1985, 11 states in the US passed laws either requiring reporting or giving state agencies access to medical records (L. Edmonds, Centers for Disease Control, personal communication; 44). Many of these laws specifically mention environmental hazards and permit the establishment of "registers" in which the identity of those with CMs is recorded, thereby facilitating follow-up investigation. In 1979, the EUROCAT project was started to establish registers of CMs within each country in the European Economic Community (93, 144). Identification of births with CMs is not a required feature of monitoring, but it is of registers.

237

A few monitoring systems, such as the one conducted by the Centers for Disease Control (CDC) in Metropolitan Atlanta (27), also record names. Issues of confidentiality and privacy do not arise in monitoring *per se* and are not considered here in assessing systems.

Monitoring systems have described upward trends in the incidence of patent ductus arteriosus, ventricular septal defects (4, 92), hypospadias (23), renal agenesis (61), gastroschisis (62, 71), and congenital hip dislocation (145), as well as a downward trend for neural tube defects (83, 150). Greater than expected changes in maternal age-specific rates of Down syndrome have also been noted (58, 61, 63). No associations with etiologic agents have been demonstrated. Improvements in diagnostic techniques, correlations with autopsy rates, and, in the case of Down syndrome in infants of older pregnant women, prenatal diagnosis and induced abortion provide partial explanations.

Short-lived increased incidences or localized clusters have also been observed. A sharp increase in reduction deformities of the femur reported from the Rhone-Alpes program (61) seems to have subsided spontaneously (62); it was not seen elsewhere. Data in the CDC's Birth Defects Monitoring Program suggested higher rates of central nervous system defects in some counties with vinyl chloride industrial plants. Further study failed to establish an association with parental exposure (26). Data from US monitoring systems were used to correlate sales of spray adhesives with birth defect rates; no correlation was found (32b). Other studies also failed to confirm an association reported earlier (cited in 114). Monitoring has also failed to reveal that birth defect rates were higher in counties with nuclear power or reprocessing plants (122).

In only one instance has a monitoring system contributed to demonstrating the teratogenicity of a new drug. The Rhone-Alpes program reported a higher than expected proportion of open spina bifida cases in the offspring of women with epilepsy; nine of the ten women had taken valproic acid (13). A number of other reports followed (38, 100a, 124, 138).

In view of this sparse yield, the value of monitoring systems can be questioned. Did other changes in the wake of the thalidomide tragedy prevent subsequent disasters of such magnitude? Are the existing systems capable of detecting weaker associations? If not, what are the reasons? Are there other adverse reproductive outcomes that should be measured on a population-wide basis, perhaps by other methods? These are the questions that we attempt to answer.

RESPONSES TO THE THALIDOMIDE TRAGEDY

Between 1959 and 1961 approximately 7000 cases of reduced or absent limbs (phocomelia), sometimes with gastro-intestinal and cardiac malformations, followed maternal use of thalidomide in the first trimester of pregnancy (96).

This tragedy sensitized manufacturers, governments, professionals, and the public to the problem of birth defects, as well as the possible teratogenicity of drugs.

Increased Awareness of Congenital Malformations and Teratogenicity

Stimulated in part by the thalidomide tragedy (141, p. 22), the teratogenic effects of drugs already in use came under close scrutiny. The teratogenicity in humans of antithyroid medications, folic acid antagonists, androgenic hormones, coumarin anticoagulants, synthetic estrogens, and vitamin A have been established (76, 91, 129). Ototoxic antibiotics, cancer chemotherapeutic agents, some anticonvulsants, lithium carbonate, and D-penicillamine are probably teratogenic in humans (125).

Other agents consumed by pregnant women for many years have only recently been studied for teratogenicity. Maternal ingestion of alcohol early in pregnancy leads to multiple problems in the offspring, including microcephaly and mental retardation. Teratogenicity of cigarette smoking has not been clearly established, but low birth weight does result (45, 89, 142).

Teratogenicity of maternal rubella infections was established in 1941, and more recently cytomegalovirus and *toxoplasma gondii* have been demonstrated to cause CMs; the teratogenicity of other infectious agents has not been unequivocally established (76).

A number of reviews considering possible associations between CMs and exposures resulting from occupations, industrial agents, or pollutants have appeared recently (76, 85, 86, 90, 100, 111). Methyl mercury is clearly teratogenic (see reviews) and exposure to organic solvents may be (48). The catalog compiled by Shepard (133) should be consulted for the evidence for teratogenicity of specific agents. Despite the advances, the causes of most malformations remain unknown (76).

The public and physicians have been alerted to possibilities of harm from environmental exposure, and both patients and practicing physicians have instigated studies of harmful effects (111). It was a single case report of an association between maternal valproic acid treatment and spina bifida that "prompted" the monitoring system to describe its cases (125). Studies in Sweden and Germany indicate that drug consumption during pregnancy has decreased in recent years (129).

Government and Industry Response

Ten days after Lenz (97) communicated his findings of an association between intrauterine exposure to thalidomide and phocomelia to the German manufacturer, the drug was withdrawn. The British manufacturer followed suit a day later (137a). Other countries were slower to act (118).

Lenz subsequently commented that the original animal and clinical reports on thalidomide were on such a "low level" that in his opinion they "should not have been accepted for publication by the editor of a medical journal who should be aware of his responsibilities" (96).

In the United States, where the drug had not been approved for marketing, the tragedy played a key role in the passage of the 1962 amendments to the Food, Drug, and Cosmetic Act. The amendments for the first time gave the Food and Drug Administration (FDA) jurisdiction over the testing of all new drugs before they were approved for marketing, as well as the authority to remove drugs that were unsafe (139, pp. 120–26). In 1966 it issued "Guidelines for Reproduction Studies for Safety Evaluation of Drugs for Human Use," which described procedures for testing the teratogenicity of new drugs prior to human use (149).

The investigational requirements, as well as those for labeling of drugs approved for marketing, have recently been described by Kelsey (78). She also points out that once a drug is approved for marketing, the manufacturer must make periodic reports to the FDA of all accounts of adverse reactions it receives. In addition, the *FDA Drug Bulletin,* which is mailed to more than one million health professionals, includes a form for reporting adverse drug effects. These latter mechanisms were responsible for the prompt reporting of spontaneous abortions and CMs in association with the use of isotretinoin within one year following its marketing in the United States as an oral agent for treating acne in 1982 (127). These cases occurred despite the warning of teratogenicity in the package insert. With only 21 infants with CMs reported from throughout the United States by 1984 (91), the human teratogenicity of isotretinoin could not have been detected so promptly by birth defects monitoring. Other countries have also adopted more stringent drug testing regulations (139, 149).

Thus, through regulation, the chances that new drugs with the teratogenic potential of thalidomide will reach the market have been reduced; even if they should reach the market, post-marketing requirements reduce the likelihood of another major epidemic.

BIRTH DEFECTS MONITORING SYSTEMS

Rapid reporting, inclusiveness of CMs, and complete coverage of the population are criteria against which to measure monitoring systems. Unfortunately, all three cannot be completely satisfied simultaneously.

Criteria for Monitoring CMs for Environmental Hazards

TIMING   Almost one and a half years elapsed between the first births of infants with phocomelia and awareness that an epidemic was at hand (97, 98, 137a). In this period, at least 153 affected infants had been born (98). Once the epidemic was recognized, less than six months elapsed before the etiological agent was identified. Kallen & Winberg (73) estimated that had the Swedish system been in place in 1960, it would have sounded an alarm about thalidomide after the first seven infants had been born with the syndrome over a four-month period.

Early recognition requires prompt reporting of CMs to the monitoring agency, as well as rapid analysis of the data by the agency. To accomplish this, many systems limit reporting to CMs detectable in the first seven to ten days after birth (12, 27, 62, 107, 128, 135b). Less published information is available on the maximum time allowed to transmit this information to the monitoring agency. It is usually between two and six months after birth (12, 27, 29, 107). Once the agency receives the information, rapid analysis is also important. In the CDC's Atlanta program the data are analyzed each month (27), in Sweden every two months (29), and in Italy by three months (107). An early age of cutoff is not without its problems. Some CMs do not become manifest in the first week. In actuality, CMs that are not diagnosed prior to discharge, which may be as early as 24 or 48 hours, will not be reported. In Sweden, only 61% of CMs that were ultimately detected were reported by six months of age (29). A large prospective study in the United States found that about twice as many severe CMs were detected by one year as by six days, and about four times as many by five years. The investigators point out that their finding of an association between "moderate" CMs, particularly strabismus, and smoking depended on ascertainment after one year of age (19). In the US Collaborative Perinatal Project, only 37.4% of all malformations present at one-year were detected at birth (116). Many of the new laws in the United States set one year as the cutoff point for reporting.

Another problem with early reporting is that the diagnosis of certain CMs cannot be made with certainty. To reduce this problem, some systems insist that only definitely diagnosed CMs be reported; others permit the report to be amended. Nevertheless, false positives may be retained. A study in Birmingham, UK found an overall false positive rate of reporting to the national program of 17% (87).

INCLUSIVENESS OF CMs   In many systems, physicians or hospitals are asked to report all CMs. Some systems request a written description and drawings or photographs. Coding is generally left up to the staff of the monitoring system. The code must be specific enough to distinguish within categories of defects. Kallen et al (72) point out that the epidemic of thalidomide embryopathy might have been missed by monitoring systems that simply coded the limb defects as "skeletal malformations."

Sentinel defects   The new monitoring laws in Maryland, Washington, and West Virginia emphasize reporting of 12 "sentinel" defects that are usually detectable within the first week after birth (anencephaly, spina bifida, hydrocephaly, cleft lip or palate, esophageal atresia, rectal and anal atresia, hypospadias, reduction deformities of upper or lower limb, congenital hip dislocation, and Down syndrome). Although all CMs are reported to the systems participating in the International Clearinghouse, only the sentinel defects are routinely forwarded to the Clearinghouse. In New Zealand, although all CMs are reported, only the sentinel defects are monitored (35, 36). The National Center for Health Statistics is considering including a short list of CMs on the standard birth certificates, which can be checked off when present (S. Ventura, personal communication). This might facilitate collection of data on the occurrence of at least the CMs on the checklists among all US births. Currently, no data on CMs is reported to the National Center for Health Statistics on the computer tapes it receives from most states.

Despite the practical arguments for limiting the CMs reported, especially when detection is limited to the period of newborn hospitalization, the possibility exists that exposure to a new environmental teratogen would result in other CMs. Thus, at the other extreme, arguments can be made for monitoring minor CMs.

Minor CMs   These include antimongoloid palpebral slant, ocular hypertelorism, preauricular pits, simian creases, and hallucal or mammillary (e.g. supernumerary nipples) abnormalities. Two arguments can be made for monitoring them:

1. Minor CMs, which can be detected in the newborn period, may indicate the presence of major CMs that will not be manifest until later. In Hungary, 11,508 neonates were carefully examined and scored for the presence of the above minor abnormalities. The only minor CMs that appeared significantly associated with later-diagnosed, hidden major defects were ocular hypertelorism and mamillary abnormality. However, the scoring was such that infants with these abnormalities may also have had intrauterine growth retardation, a positive family history of CMs or other adverse pregnancy outcome, or other minor abnormalities. Their predictive value as isolated findings cannot be determined from the report (Table V, 109).

2. Minor CMs could signal the presence of environmental exposures. In a study of children of epileptic mothers, Rating et al (123) found that mothers exposed to antiepileptic drugs in utero ($n = 84$) had significantly more minor CMs than those of epileptic mothers receiving no anticonvulsants or than epileptic fathers. In a study of over 7000 births, Holmes et al (49) did not find an increase of minor CMs in 39 infants exposed to phenytoin in utero. The power of the study was adequate to detect an increase as large as that reported by Rating.

With immense difficulties in standardizing the reporting of minor CMs, and of training physicians and other health providers to look for and recognize them, the equivocal findings suggest the need for more investigation of the value of monitoring minor CMs before any recommendation for including them can be made.

Stillbirths   The inclusion of CMs in stillbirths in monitoring has been debated (22, 55, 56). Although stillbirths have higher rates of CMs than live births (22, 55, 135b), they constitute no more than 1% of all births (22, 59, p. 9). Moreover, they are neither consistently autopsied nor reported. Without autopsy, internal manifestations in a stillbirth will be missed. Finally, states and countries differ in their definitions of fetal deaths. Some base it on gestational age (e.g. deaths after 20 or 28 weeks); others on weight (e.g. fetuses over 500 or 1000 g) (55).

The programs participating in the International Clearinghouse differ in their definitions and whether or not they count stillbirths (63). For anencephaly, hydrocephaly, and spina bifida, these differences make comparisons of rates difficult to interpret. In Budapest, for instance, the rate of anencephaly in stillbirths is over 200 times higher than live births; consequently the rate in total (still plus live) births is 6.5 times higher than in live births. Hydrocephaly is 49 times higher in still than live births and the rate in total births is 3.5 times higher than in live births. For spina bifida cystica, a two-fold difference in rates was found. The rates for other CMs are not altered much by the inclusion or exclusion of still births (calculated from Table 1, Ref. 22).

Despite their relatively small number, the larger rate of at least some abnormalities in stillborns makes them valuable for monitoring, provided that all fetal deaths are autopsied and reported to the monitoring system. We agree with Hook's suggestion (55) that fetal deaths should be reported separately from live births.

Multiple CMs   There is general agreement that when a CM appears with others, each CM should not be reported as an isolated occurrence (22, 56, 70). A CM that appears as part of a syndrome may have different causes than when it appears alone (82, 83). If monitoring agencies simply record occurrences of a CM, without regard to whether it was part of a syndrome, they may miss syndromes that may be the only evidence of the introduction of a teratogen into the environment.

POPULATION BASE   The reporting of all affected births within the geographical area will provide the most rapid indication of a change in rate of occurrence. In a few systems (63), reports are obtained only from certain hospitals. Bias will be introduced if the hospitals' births are not representative of all births in the area (70, 99). For instance, an association between a CM and some new pesticide, or other agent used in agriculture, might be missed if urban hospitals are the source of data. If hospitals to which high risk pregnancies or sick newborns are referred are over-represented, bias will result because of the association of these complications with CMs. In some systems, hospitals are selected because of interest of physicians. Although this does not resolve the bias problem (and may contribute to it), it may improve diagnosis and reporting. In the International Clearinghouse, however, CM rates do not differ between hospital-based and population-based systems (70).

Methods for Obtaining Information

Since births must be recorded in most countries, the birth certificate is the source of information on CMs in a number of systems. In many places, however, the birth certificate may not require sufficient detail. It also may be filed before the infant is carefully examined. Moreover, there is frequently a time lag before data processing (121). To circumvent these problems, some monitoring systems are either special forms or hospital discharge records. In Atlanta (121), personnel of the monitoring program review the hospital records. The laws in California and Arizona also provide for this method. A few systems use more than one of these sources, and others as well, such as chromosome laboratories and genetics, cardiac, and other specialty clinics. When multiple sources are used, identifiers are needed so that the same infant is not counted more than once. Multiple sources improve completeness, but they also extend the time before all sources can report.

Studies have compared the completeness of different modes of reporting. In Birmingham, UK, substantially more CMs were reported to the local system, which used the birth certificate and other sources, than were reported to the national system, which depended entirely on a special notification form. The differences were present even when reports to both systems were limited to the first week after birth (87). A study from northern Ireland found that only 60.7% of neural tube defects, ascertained from multiple sources, were in the national system (117a). In Sweden, reporting of CMs on the medical birth record was started in 1973; a special report of congenital malformations was required beginning in 1964. A comparison of the two systems in 1973–1974 indicated that neither had complete ascertainment of CMs; only 64% of ten types of CMs were reported to both, while 13% were reported only on the special form and 22% only on the birth record. Some specific defects were better ascertained by the special form, others by the birth record (29). The authors suggested that the introduction of the second system may have reduced reporting to the first. Deficiencies of reporting on birth certificates in a number of states in the US have also been described (122). Down syndrome appeared as a CM on birth certificates of less than 40% of infants determined to have the abnormality by chromosome analysis in California (43), New York (57), and Ohio (60).

Detecting Significant Rate Changes

Monitoring systems usually conduct periodic analyses [e.g. every month in the Atlanta system (27)] of incoming data. One of three statistical methods that depend on rate changes are used to detect significant increases: the Poisson distribution, CUSUM, or sets techniques. Alternatively, cluster analysis can be performed (16, 17).

THE POISSON DISTRIBUTION   The number of newly registered cases of a specific CM is periodically tested against an expected number derived from a baseline rate, usually obtained from previous monitoring periods, and the number of births in the current period. This expected number is assumed to be a Poisson variable. An alarm is signaled if the observed number exceeds a critical value, usually 2.4 standard deviations above the expected number. The method relies on the assumption that most CMs are quite rare. It is used by several monitoring systems, including the Centers for Disease Control systems in the US (27).

CUMULATIVE SUM (CUSUM) TECHNIQUE   A constant value, computed using baseline rates from earlier periods, is subtracted from the observed number of cases in a defined time period (e.g. one month). With only random fluctuations, positive and negative differences will be observed around an expected value of 0. If the sum of the differences for successive periods exceeds an upper limit, computed on the basis of baseline rates, an alarm is signaled. This procedure has been shown to be very efficient in reducing the time interval until detection of a true increase, and may cause fewer alarms than the other methods (10, 16). It requires the use of computers, which may limit its applicability. The CUSUM technique is used in the UK monitoring system (145).

SETS METHOD   The time interval between births of consecutive infants with a specific CM born in individual hospitals or in the area as a whole is measured (18). An alarm is signaled when the time interval between cases is less than that calculated on the basis of known incidence data. The technique is simple to apply and is as efficient as the Poisson distribution in signaling alarms. Once the critical interval is established, monitoring can be performed each time a new case is reported. The other techniques require an accumulation of cases over a defined time before analysis.

CLUSTER ANALYSIS   For these methods (88, 105, 146), information is not usually required on the size of population monitored or the rate of malformation. For example, Knox's method (88) tests for space-time clustering by classification of all possible case pairs on the basis of geographical distance between each member of a pair and the interval between their respective occurrences. Care must be taken that the space vector is chosen, not on the basis of the mothers' residences at birth, but during the critical period of their respective pregnancies. The time vector should be based on estimated times of conception rather than birth (28). The method was applied to determine possible clusters of cleft lip and palate (88), neural tube defects (140), and Down syndrome (94), all with negative results.

PROBLEMS IN MONITORING

False Alarms (Type I Error)

False alarms present a common problem in birth defects monitoring. These type I errors are inevitable when a large number of statistical tests are performed; the expected number of alarms due to chance alone are quite large (27). This problem may be reduced by ranking the increases on the basis of their p-values or the ratio of observed-to-expected numbers of cases. Alternatively, the Bonferoni technique can be used to alter the significance level for rejection of the null hypothesis by dividing the critical p-value by the number of comparisons carried out. However, the stringency of this method could lead to missing true effects (99).

The problem of disentangling a true increase in the occurrence of a CM from a false alarm has been addressed by several authors (17, 27, 70, 120). When faced with an increase, several possibilities must be considered in addition to type I errors before investigating a true increase. First, changes in number of births registered, or CMs reported or ascertained, have to be considered. For example, the increase in the incidence of preauricular tags in the Swedish birth defects registry between 1965 and 1972 probably was due to increased reporting (74). Second, an apparent increase may be due to changing demographic factors, or changes in fertility (70). For example, because Down syndrome is highly dependent on maternal age, a change in the maternal age distribution will result in a change in the overall incidence of Down syndrome (2).

Investigation of a true increase usually requires follow-up studies. Before undertaking them, biologic plausibility, as well as attempts to eliminate the factors discussed above, should be considered. For example, an increase in the number of cases with a specific combination of defects is more likely due to a common exposure when embryological development of the various affected organs is consistent with a single exposure and when geographic aggregation and time clustering of cases is noted than when these conditions are not satisfied.

Statistical Power (Type II Error)

Failure to detect genuine increases in the occurrence of CMs (type II error) has recently received attention (72). An epidemic may go unnoticed regardless of the statistical methods used. Important factors that influence detection are the frequency of the malformation, the size of the population monitored, the relative risk of the exposure, and the proportion of the at risk population (parents) exposed at the critical time.

Table 1 shows the minimal ratio of observed to expected cases that would signal an alarm (alpha = .05, beta = .20) in populations of defined size for defects of varying baseline frequency. For a relatively common malformation, such as cleft lip, with an incidence of about .001, an observed:expected ratio of less than 1.3 would be overlooked if 75,000 infants are monitored. If only 10,000 are monitored, only ratios of 2 or more would signal an alarm. Still higher ratios are needed to signal an alarm for less common defects. Of the 22 systems that belong to the International Clearinghouse, six monitor between 25,000 and 50,000 births per year, and seven between 50,000 and 100,000 (62). They would be incapable of detecting ratios of less than two for CMs with baseline frequencies of less than .0001.

Table 2 shows the number of cases of a CM of specified baseline frequency (.001) that would be observed in a population of specified size (50,000) when varying proportions of the population are exposed to teratogens of varying relative risk. With relative risks of 3 or less the epidemic will be missed if less than 10% of the population at risk is exposed to the teratogen. Although the relative risk conferred by thalidomide was over 100 (95), the relative risks of other teratogens are much lower. For instance, the relative risk of hydantoins for the most commonly found abnormality associated with it (distal digital hypoplasia) is only 7.3 (95% confidence intervals = 2.5 − 21.5) (calculated from Ref. 80a). Exposures of more than 10% of the at risk population to proven

Table 1 Effect of number of births monitored and baseline frequency of malformation on the minimal ratio of observed to expected cases that will signal an alarm[a]

Number of births	Frequency of malformation	Expected number of cases	Observed number of cases needed to signal increase	Minimal ratio of observed to expected cases
10,000	.00001	0.1	3	30.0
	.0001	1.0	6	6.0
	.001	10.0	20	2.0
25,000	.00001	0.25	3	12.0
	.0001	2.5	8	3.2
	.001	25.0	39	1.6
50,000	.00001	0.5	5	10.0
	.0001	5.0	13	2.6
	.001	50.0	70	1.4
75,000	.00001	0.75	5	6.7
	.0001	7.5	16	2.1
	.001	75.0	100	1.3

[a]Based on Poisson distribution for α = .05 (one-sided) and β = .20).

teratogens are unusual. Only about 2% of pregnant women were exposed to thalidomide (95), and fewer than 0.1% to isotretinoin (E. Lammer, personal communication). It seems likely, therefore, that weak teratogens to which only a small fraction of the at-risk population are exposed will be missed by monitoring (M. Khoury and N. Holtzman, in preparation).

In using monitoring systems, one cannot be confident that all cases classified under one diagnostic rubric are clinically homogeneous. Poor reporting, excessive inclusiveness of the code used, or failure to distinguish single from multiple abnormalities will result in heterogeneity and a consequent loss in statistical power. For instance, neural tube defects that occur singly probably have different etiologies than those that occur in conjunction with other malformations in the same infant (multiples) (83, 84). If they are lumped together in monitoring, the detectability of a teratogen that causes an increase in multiples, which account for about 20% of all cases, is likely to be lessened (M. Khoury, N. Holtzman, in preparation).

Statistical power is of paramount importance in follow-up studies as well as in monitoring. Investigators mounting case-control studies of birth defects are increasingly using larger sample sizes to attain adequate power to detect risk factor differences. In the recently completed study of the possible teratogenic risk of service in Vietnam and agent orange exposure, information was obtained on past military service and exposure to agent orange on the fathers of about 4000 babies with CMs and the fathers of about 2500 normal infants. The study was designed to yield a 70 to 90% chance of detecting a relative risk of 1.2 for *all* defects. However, the power to detect increased risks for specific defects was much smaller. The very few significant associations that were found among the many sought could well be due to chance (30).

Table 2 Effect of proportion of population exposed to a teratogen, and relative risk on number of cases observed[a]

Proportion of population exposed to the teratogen	Relative risk of teratogen					
	1.25	1.5	2.0	3.0	4.0	10.0
			Number of cases observed			
.10	51	53	55	60	70[b]	95[b]
.20	53	55	60	70[b]	90[b]	140[b]
.50	57	63	75[b]	100[b]	150[b]	275[b]
.80	60	70[b]	90[b]	130[b]	210[b]	410[b]
1.0	63	75[b]	100[b]	150[b]	250[b]	500[b]

[a]Based on Poisson distribution for an expected number of cases = 50 (e.g. if 50,000 births are monitored and the baseline frequency of the defect is .001). For $\alpha = .05$ (one-sided) and $\beta = .20$, detectable teratogens are those that give 70 or more observed cases.
[b]Significant increase [$\alpha = .05$ (one-sided) and $\beta = .20$].

Variations in Susceptibility; Genetic-Environmental Interactions

With the exception of thalidomide it is unlikely that most teratogens cause birth defects or other adverse outcomes in the offspring of *all* parents exposed to teratogenic doses at critical times. Environmental factors including nutrition and exposure to other agents undoubtedly influence susceptibility to the harmful effects of a specific agent. Although genetic differences in susceptibility have been known for years in animals (37), only recently have genetically determined factors been identified in humans.

Manchester and his colleagues (103, 104) found that women who smoked in pregnancy and had high placental monooxygenase activity were significantly less likely to have infants with CMs than smokers with low activity. One explanation is that the organs of fetuses who have inherited an allele for high activity of the enzyme in their placentas are protected from the teratogenic effects of cigarette smoke. If this effect is confirmed it may explain why studies have failed to find an association between smoking and CMs; they did not take differences in susceptibility into account.

Strickler et al (136) presented evidence that an inherited deficiency in the ability to detoxify arene oxide metabolites of phenytoins explains the occurrence of major CMs in offspring of mothers receiving these anticonvulsants during pregnancy. Fourteen of 24 children exposed in vitro had at least one major CM. Twelve of the 14 with major CMs had detoxification defects ($p =$ .002, Fisher's exact). For each subject with a defect, one parent also had evidence of the same defect. Use of this test should make it possible to tease apart the roles of maternal epilepsy and phenytoin anticonvulsants in the etiology of CMs.

Recent recombinant DNA (5) and chromosome morphology studies (66) suggest the presence of genetic factors that increase the likelihood of the common, non-dysjunction type of Down syndrome. The ability to document the presence of predisposing genetic factors, increasingly possible with recombinant DNA technology (52), will enhance the ability to detect potential teratogens. If the genetic factor is incapable of causing the CM by itself, the relative risk of a CM following parental exposure to a potential teratogen will be higher when a genetic predisposition is present than when it is absent. Higher relative risks require a smaller increase in the number of infants with the resultant CMs in order to detect a significant effect.

Perhaps the failure of most efforts to detect associations between environmental agents results from the model imposed by our ignorance of the complexities of etiology. In essence, the model assumes that single agents, after adjusting for non-interacting confounding factors that can be measured, are capable of causing CMs. The likelihood of genetic-environmental interactions has been ignored, largely because of the seeming impossibility at getting at the genetic factors. As the examples cited above indicate, this is no longer the case.

Obtaining Information on Exposures

Obtaining information on exposures is not an inherent feature of monitoring, and programs differ markedly in the extent to which they do so. This information can be obtained at the ecological level by determining whether differences in incidence rates in time or geographical area have been accompanied by differences in exposure to specific environmental agents (26, 114). More direct evidence can be obtained at the individual level, but many difficulties arise. Evidence of exposure that is collected prior to the birth of the infant with a CM avoids problems of bias, but may be sparse, or difficult for monitoring systems to obtain. Evidence collected afterwards requires contact with the mother, something that is not possible in all monitoring systems. Access to the parents, or at least to other records pertaining to them, is possible through registers, if parents consent. When information on exposure is available, controls are needed to determine the magnitude of risk of CM conferred by the exposure.

COLLECTION OF INFORMATION OBTAINED PRIOR TO DIAGNOSIS OF THE CM   Information in the mother's prenatal record can be transcribed to the notification form used for monitoring (either the birth certificate or the special form). In Finland, the maternity record is included with the notification (46). Birth certificates in most states (44) and countries do not contain information about occupation of both parents. In general, special forms ask for more information about exposures, but to simplify reporting not much is requested. In addition to occupational and residential information, data regarding exposure to drugs, cigarettes, alcohol and non–work-related chemicals would be helpful. Frequently, the information is easier to obtain directly from the mother rather than the records.

Record linkage   The monitoring agency itself can tap into information about the mother's exposures provided that the report it receives contains adequate identifiers on the mother. This can be a unique identifying number, or her name. If she is married, her maiden name should be included as well. In systems using special notification forms, inclusion of the name of the infant, or a unique identifier used on all the infant's records, permits linkage to the mother through the birth certificate, provided the monitoring agency has access to it. Registers and a few other systems obtain infant identifiers (7, 12, 13a, 29, 36, 135b), but linkage to mothers' records is not always possible.

In addition to the mother's medical records, linkage permits the use of central repositories of prescriptions (67, 134) to determine drug intake before and during pregnancy. Such data does not, however, demonstrate that the drug was taken, or with what regularity. An association between spermicide use prior to pregnancy and CMs (68) that was derived by using prescription records as the source of data has been criticized on this score (14).

Acheson (1) has proposed the creation of registers of women who have worked in industry during pregnancy. Linkage with them would permit the monitoring agency to determine occupational exposures of mothers of infants with CMs. In Maryland, the names of all employers of both parents for the year preceding the birth of the CM infant are required on the notification form. The state also maintains a toxic substances registry containing this information. The two systems are linked (N. Holtzman, unpublished).

Occupational and other information relevant to exposures can be obtained from the census (1, 11). In Norway, a study of CMs occurring between 10 months before and 38 months after the 1970 census was able to link 98.8% of all births to the census data. The study found a small but significant relative risk of CMs in first borns of mothers who worked, adjusted for age, educational level, and residence. The highest relative risks were found for nurses and technicians (11). Census data has the disadvantage of providing information only at the time of the census.

COLLECTION OF INFORMATION OBTAINED AFTER DIAGNOSIS OF THE CM   In some systems, information is collected from the mother prior to her discharge from the hospital. This may be by direct interview or abstracting information from the infant's medical record. In a few others, the mothers of at least some CM infants receive questionnaires, and may be interviewed after their infants are discharged from hospital (35, 121, 128). In northeast France (Bas-Rhin, including Strasbourg), every family of an infant with a CM has a genetic study as well as genetic counseling (135b).

When a cluster is observed, interviews may be the only means of establishing a possible exposure. Mothers of affected infants do not always recall exposures. This was evident in attempts to establish exposures in the epidemic of phocomelia that was eventually traced to thalidomide; many mothers, as well as their physicians, denied use of the drug (135, 137a). Sometimes it was necessary to inquire about stressful episodes early in pregnancy that might have led to use of the drug before a positive response was forthcoming (96, 137a). Once thalidomide was suspected, the outcomes of 13 pregnancies still in progress, in which the mother had used the drug during the critical time, were determined prospectively. All 13 infants were affected, thus providing strong support for the hypothesis formulated from the retrospective data.

CASE-CONTROL STUDIES   A number of systems request the reporting of control infants to the monitoring agency for the birth of each infant with a CM, or at least for infants with certain categories of CMs (15, 121, 128, 135b).

Frequently, this is the previous or next birth, although other restrictions may be used as well, for instance residence (128). Information on exposures is then collected by the same methods on both case and control families. The laws in Maryland and Washington also permit the collection of controls. Analysis of case-control studies is beyond the scope of this review, but brief consideration of bias and confounding are in order.

Bias   Participation in case-control studies will be voluntary, even when both groups have been identified by monitoring. Once an exposure is suspected, it is possible that women of affected offspring who have been exposed to the agent are more likely to participate then nonexposed (100).

In reviewing an earlier study, Lippman & Mackenzie (101) point out that while postdelivery information obtained from mothers is inconsistent with that obtained in midpregnancy—thus raising the question of reliability of recall—the inconsistency was not different for mothers of dead or malformed children than for mothers of healthy children. They plan to study this matter further. Sometimes it is possible to verify the information provided by the mother. The early reports of an association between in utero X-ray exposure and childhood cancer were criticized because of possible recall bias. The same results were obtained, however, when the mothers' pregnancy records were used to establish exposure (99). Situations of underreporting by mothers of affected children may also arise. For instance, guilt about an exposure such as alcohol ingestion may lead to denial (99).

Confounding   Before CMs are attributed to maternal drug exposure, consideration must be given to the reason that the drug was used. The role of anticonvulsant drugs in causing CMs has been disputed (33, 79, 80); the underlying disease, as is the case for diabetes (20), may be responsible, as well as differences in genetic susceptibility, as discussed above. It has been suggested that factors responsible for reducing fertility (23) or increasing the chance of spontaneous abortion (106), rather than drugs used to overcome these problems, are responsible for harmful outcomes, including CMs.

Problems of confounding are not unique to retrospectively collected information. In Finland, an association between influenza and CMs was found using the maternity records. In this matched pair study, the records of mothers of affected infants also showed increased analgesic use. The authors concluded, "We cannot see how (the two factors) can be distinguished in an epidemiologic study" (128). Human randomized trials to test teratogenicity are obviously out of the question. Sometimes, as Doll has pointed out, removal of a suspected agent "as an experiment in prevention . . . is not a bad last resort. . . . Proof in the strict logical sense may not have been obtained but does this matter if the disease has disappeared?" (quote in full in Ref. 99).

ARE CONGENITAL MALFORMATIONS THE BEST MEASURE OF TERATOGENICITY?

Congenital malformations in liveborns or stillborns constitute a small proportion of all of the possible adverse outcomes of teratogenic agents. Infertility, spontaneous abortions, intrauterine growth retardation, low birth weight, altered sex ratio at birth, developmental disabilities, childhood cancer, and late onset diseases that result from new mutations are others. A number of studies have shown correlations between one or more of these factors and CMs (90, 128, 131, 133, 135b, 152). A chromosome abnormality in the sperm of men exposed to 1,2-dibromo-3-chloropropane (DBCP), which might result in certain CMs in surviving fetuses, was postulated to selectively cause fetal death of male offspring (39). In addition to impairing male fertility, DBCP has been associated with a significant excess of female livebirths among the offspring of exposed males; spontaneous abortions may also be elevated (39). Smoking has also been associated with impaired fertility, as well as spontaneous abortions (discussed further below), low birth weight (8, 142), and strabismus (19).

The ability of environmental agents to cause more than one adverse outcome is biologically plausible. The specific outcome could depend on the time of parental exposure, the dose, and other environmental and genetic factors (75, 122, 126). The structural and functional properties of the agent, which influence its reactivity (e.g. as a mutagen) or its ability to compete with or bind to endogenous molecules, or alter its chemical reactivity (e.g. mutagenicity) (108), will also influence the specific effect. Exposure to agents very early in pregnancy, when many cells are still totipotential, usually has an "all or none" effect, resulting in early loss of the embryo or complete repair (90). Mutagens that reach germ cells in prospective parents could lead to chromosome abnormalities in the offspring; if they "hit" certain somatic cells of the fetus during the stage of organogenesis, malformations might result; at a later stage, childhood cancers could result (90). Genetic factors in the parents, which could be transmitted to the fetus, could predispose to these events. Kellogg (77) suggests that prenatal exposure of the fetus to drugs that bind to central nervous system receptors may not be expressed until childhood or later.

There are a number of objections to using these other outcomes as indicators of the introduction of teratogens into the environment. Those that do not occur until some time after birth will be further removed from the time of the exposure, so that more individuals will be exposed until a causative agent is incriminated. Moreover, determining exposures will be more difficult. Outcomes such as developmental delay, low birth weight, and infants small for their gestational age are known to be influenced by many factors in addition to potential teratogens. In the remainder of this section we consider the use of early postconceptional outcomes—spontaneous and induced abortions—for monitoring.

Monitoring of Spontaneous Abortions

SPONTANEOUS ABORTION RATES   With the use of human chorionic gonadotropin (hCG) assays, the occurrence of fertilization can be determined accurately by 14 days after ovulation. Consequently, the survival of fertilized ova in
apparently healthy young women wishing to conceive can be followed. Using
this technique, or direct examination of fertilized ova, clinically unrecognized
pregnancy loss has been reported in between 32 and 55% of all conceptions (25,
148, 152). A lower estimate of 8% was reported by Whittaker et al (147). In the
two most recent studies (25, 147), *recognized* spontaneous abortions occurred
in 12% of all conceptions. Over 90% of all fetal loss occurs before 20 weeks of
gestation (148). This may represent a loss of over 60% of all conceptions, and
certainly no lower than 20%.

Theoretically, a sample of fecund women could be followed by hCG assays
or recording menstrual irregularities. Those in whom fertilization occurred
could be followed to determine outcomes. Deviations from baseline rates of
spontaneous abortions could be determined by the methods already described.
Because of the high spontaneous abortion rate, the numbers needed to detect a
significant increase would be much lower than those shown in Tables 1 and 2
(148).

PATHOLOGICAL OUTCOMES   Judging from the high proportion of pathology
in spontaneously aborted embryos and fetuses, abortion is not truly "spontaneous" but a powerful selection mechanism against serious malformations.
Zakharov (152) has summarized the rates of chromosome abnormalities in
human spontaneous abortions found by different investigators. In spontaneous
abortions occurring at 8 to 15 weeks, an interval during which most abortions
would be recognized by the woman, approximately half of all abortuses have
chromosome abnormalities. From a review of surveys of chromosome
abnormalities in live births, Hook (54) estimated that only 0.6% had any
cytogenetic abnormality. Considering that at least 20% of all conceptions abort
before 20 weeks, the use of chromosome abnormalities is statistically much
more powerful than chromosome monitoring of newborns (50) or than birth
defects monitoring. Most of the chromosome abnormalities observed in abortuses are lethal; a few of them, particularly trisomies of certain chromosomes,
and monosomy of the x chromosome, are seen occasionally in liveborns, but
occur more frequently in spontaneous abortuses (42, 64).

Not all chromosome abnormalities will reflect recent exposure of one of the
parents to a potential teratogen. The majority of trisomies, the most frequent
chromosome abnormalities found in abortuses (64), originate in the first meiot-
ic division of the ovum, which takes place in the fetal ovary. Others, such as
triploidy, which are never observed in liveborns, may have more recent origins
(54).

The Central Laboratory for Human Embryology at the University of Washington reported the pathological findings in a relatively unselected series of 748 spontaneous abortuses received from the Group Health Cooperative of Puget Sound. Only about 5% of material of gestational age less than two months could be considered "normal." The rate of neural tube defects in their study (13.4/1000 abortuses) was at least 10 times higher than the rate in newborns; the rate of Turner's syndrome (5.4/1000) was 100 times higher (31). This is consistent with the high rate of the x-chromosome monosomy in chromosome studies of abortuses (41, 69). Among chromosomally normal abortuses, Jacobs (64) noted that as many as 40% were reported to have ABO incompatabilities, a much higher proportion than in newborns.

Thus, certain chromosome abnormalities, other malformations, and ABO incompatability have much higher rates in conceptuses who do not survive the early months of pregnancy than in those that do. The factors that are responsible for the survival of some with a specific defect, and the fetal loss of others, is unknown. Experimental studies indicate that some teratogens cause an increase in embryonic or early fetal death and an increase in CMs in liveborns (75). If this is so, then the introduction of a teratogen could much more profoundly increase spontaneous abortions than CMs in liveborns. Consequently, by monitoring only liveborns, a greater time would elapse before the effect would be detected than if abortions were monitored as well; a greater number would need to be monitored to detect an effect.

For other teratogens the relationship between spontaneous abortions and CMs in liveborns or stillborns is inverse, at least in animal studies (75). Roberts & Lowe (126) found that women who delivered in the districts of South Wales that had high rates of neural tube defects had lower abortion rates than in the districts with low rates of this defect. They concluded, "the environmental factors at work in South Wales are not directly teratogenic but in some way change the uterine environment so that more abnormal fetuses remain in the uterus until the twenty-eighth week of pregnancy." If their hypothesis is correct, then vitamins may reduce the occurrence of neural tube defects in live and stillborns by increasing spontaneous abortions. Data in a recent report (130) showing the effectiveness of periconceptional vitamins in women who previously had babies with neural tube defects suggest that spontaneous abortions occur with greater frequency in women who are fully supplemented with vitamins than in women who are unsupplemented.

Ayme & Lippman (5a, 6) presented data to support their hypothesis that the greater risk of having liveborns with Down syndrome as maternal age increases could be due to an inverse relation of spontaneous abortion of affected fetuses with maternal age. Hassold & Jacobs (42) have summarized the data and arguments against the hypothesis, concluding that the increase in liveborns with Down syndrome in older women "is almost certainly due to factors acting at or before conception, not subsequent to it."

In view of the possibility of an inverse relationship between abortuses and CMs in liveborns, it is not necessarily the case that monitoring of abortuses will increase statistical power of detection of teratogens that have adverse outcomes on liveborns. It would be a mistake to abandon monitoring of CMs in liveborns (and stillborns) in favor of abortion monitoring. However, useful information about etiology, and, perhaps, an earlier warning of teratogenicity when there is a direct relationship between abortions and CMs, can be gained by monitoring both events, keeping the results separate.

Several of the same problems already addressed for CMs would be even greater in abortion monitoring. Inclusion of abortions below the gestational age at which most abortions reach medical attention could bias the results and make it impossible to establish rates (50, 59, 118). (The use of hCG testing of a random sample of fecund women in order to detect pregnancies is one way around this.) In countries in which abortion is illegal or not readily available, the inclusion of induced abortions would cause problems. If, in addition to rates, fetal CMs or chromosome abnormalities were sought, careful physical examination, autopsy, and karyotyping would be needed. Poor preservation of abortion material and scarcity of resources (including fetal pathologists) could make this difficult. In view of the dependence of chromosome abnormalities on gestational age, age-specific rates would be appropriate. Bias in determining antecedent exposures also enters in the study of abortions, although the time since antecedent events is less than with CMs in liveborns. Bias would not enter into studies in which exposures in the parents of one type of abortus were compared to those in another type, e.g. chromosomal compared to other abnormalities (142). Other factors known to influence spontaneous abortion, such as maternal age and smoking (142), could confound associations with environmental agents.

Monitoring of spontaneous abortions has been most extensively conducted in New York by the group at Columbia University. Warburton (142) reviewed the findings of this group and others. Independent associations between cigarette smoking and alcohol consumption during pregnancy and abortion of chromosomally normal embryos have been established. For smoking, a dose-response relationship with abortion was observed. Smoking prior to pregnancy increases the risk of trisomy in older pregnant women. In other studies cited by Warburton, maternal and paternal irradiation histories have been associated with chromosomally abnormal abortions. The effect of occupational exposures on abortion has been reviewed by Lindbohm et al (100).

Monitoring of Induced Abortions

Over one quarter of all recognized pregnancies were terminated by induced abortion in the United States in 1982 (47). As might be expected, the frequency of chromosome abnormalities and CMs in induced abortuses is higher than in liveborns (137, 143); some fetuses electively aborted would have spontaneous-ly aborted at a later time. Thus, for certain abnormalities monitoring of certain abortions could provide more statistical power and a shorter lag time than monitoring CMs in liveborns.

In addition to the problems discussed above for spontaneous abortions, the use of induced abortions has still others. They do not represent a random sample of all pregnancies, and consequently of potential exposures. The ability to examine fetal material will depend on the method used or the place of abortion; in the US in 1982, 82% of abortions were performed in nonhospital facilities (47). Tanimura (137) has summarized the relative merits of monitoring spontaneous and induced abortions and newborns.

The growing use of induced abortion following prenatal diagnosis of chro-mosomal or other CMs, particularly neural tube defects, must be taken into consideration in monitoring. The sharp decline in liveborns with Down syn-drome in some countries in women over 35 years, noted by the International Clearinghouse in its 1982 report (63), was attributed to prenatal diagnosis and elective termination. The use of maternal serum alpha-fetoprotein to screen for neural tube defects at 16–18 weeks gestation, followed often by termination when the diagnosis is confirmed, could contribute to the decline in liveborns with these conditions. Considerable power would be lost by not including fetuses electively aborted as a result of adverse prenatal diagnosis. As some of those discovered by prenatal diagnosis would not survive to term (53), fetuses with chromosome abnormalities detected prenatally should be counted sepa-rately from liveborns (55).

Prenatal diagnosis will become more important with technological discover-ies. Ultrasound makes it possible to detect some structural abnormalities early enough to permit pregnancy termination (51). The introduction of chorionic villus sampling (65, 113), which can be performed as early as the ninth week of gestation, may increase the use of prenatal diagnosis (51). Foreseeably, pre-natal diagnosis on fetal cells in the maternal circulation, which would be without risk to the fetus, and the use of recombinant DNA techniques to detect alterations in chromosome number much more inexpensively than current methods could permit detection of this large class of chromosome abnormalities in all pregnancies (52). This would be a powerful monitoring tool.

PROSPECTIVE MONITORING

In view of incompleteness and possible bias when information on exposures is collected after the occurrence of a CM, prospective collection is an attractive alternative. The use of hCG assays to follow pregnancy outcomes from shortly after conception in exposed versus unexposed women is mentioned above. Two innovations in health care in recent years make other forms of prospective monitoring feasible: health maintenance organizations (HMOs) and computerization of medical records.

HMOs often provide care to women before, during, and after their pregnancies, possibly to their mates, and to their offspring as well. Frequently, they computerize records and have the capability of linking those of different family members to each other as well as to prescription records. At least three organizations that have been providing prepaid care for many years have used their record systems to examine associations between prospectively collected maternal characteristics and pregnancy outcomes (19, 68, 131, 132). Although fewer than 10% of the population is currently enrolled in HMOs, the proportion is expected to grow rapidly (135a), making them a more representative source of information for monitoring. The quality and completeness of information on exposures, particularly occupational ones, in HMOs remains to be established.

Individuals could carry with them information about their exposures as well as pertinent medical information. In Canada, parents are given a Child Health Record that contains information on major illnesses and malformations. Its purpose is to enhance communication between parents and health professionals by providing continuity of records (9). Laser scanning permits the storage of extensive information on small cards that individuals could carry. Such cards could be updated to contain information on occupational, drug, and other exposures. The card would be the property of the individual, who would know what it contained and could decide when to provide others with access to it.

Other types of prospective studies have been reported, but they are of a special nature and do not lend themselves to continuous monitoring of CMs. In the US, the Collaborative Perinatal Project systematically and carefully followed about 56,000 pregnant women from the first months of their pregnancies, and their offspring, in order to relate "events which affect parents before and during pregnancy to the outcome of pregnancy" (116). Several studies on prenatal factors associated with CMs have emanated from the Project (19a, 19b, 40, 102, 115, 116). A follow-up study determined chromosome abnormalities when the study group was 7 or 8 years old and related their occurrence to prospectively recorded antenatal factors. More than 20% of mothers of children with de novo chromosome abnormalities had received abdominal and pelvic X rays in the year prior to conception, compared to only 6% of the entire study group (102).

Studies in which women with specific diseases are enrolled prior to pregnancy in order to determine factors influencing the occurrence of CMs have been described. A recent prospective study failed to clarify the relation between maternal epilepsy and anticonvulsant therapy during pregnancy on the one hand and CMs on the other (80, 33). A prospective study on the outcome of diabetic pregnancies is currently in progress (112).

Pregnancy outcomes have also been determined following known intrauterine exposures to potential teratogens as a result of environmental disasters (111). Microcephaly and mental retardation occurred with increased frequency in children exposed early in gestation to the atomic bomb explosions at Hiroshima and Nagasaki. Studies of children who were born more than nine months after the explosions have so far failed to reveal evidence of increased mutation rates, although such effects cannot be excluded (117). A birth defects registry established after the accidental release of dioxin at Seveso, in which intrauterine exposures could be established, did not show an increase in CMs. A peak of spontaneous abortions occurred six to nine months after the accident (32).

SUMMARY AND CONCLUSIONS

Many countries instituted birth defects monitoring systems in the wake of the thalidomide tragedy. Having these systems in place will shorten the time before an alarm is signaled, should a teratogen of the potency of thalidomide be introduced. However, with stronger laws and regulations for testing drugs for adverse reproductive outcomes, a tragedy on the scale of thalidomide *from ingestion of prescribed drugs by pregnant women* is unlikely. Prospective parents could be exposed at the critical times to *new* physical, infectious, or nondrug chemical agents teratogenically as potent as thalidomide. (Teratogenic agents whose widespread use antedates monitoring will not cause rate changes or clusters detectable by monitoring.) What seems more likely is that the introduction of "weakly" teratogenic agents, or the inadvertent use of new drugs that are teratogenic, like isotretinoin, will be responsible for increases in birth defects. In neither of these situations are large numbers of cases likely to accumulate in short periods of time, particularly in the relatively small catchment areas (fewer than 50 to 100,000 births per year) of many monitoring programs. In addition to having to cope with this problem of rare outcomes, many monitoring systems have not been able to obtain complete ascertainment of CMs, at least not from single, rapidly reporting sources.

Two remedies to these inadequacies are possible:

1. Expand the catchment area. All births in the US, for instance, could be monitored if information on specific CMs was included on birth certificates, which were then transmitted to a central agency that could analyse the data rapidly. Alternatively, if different monitoring systems had comparable methods of ascertainment and diagnostic classifications, their data could be pooled with greater reliability than is currently possible.

2. CMs in newborns are only one indicator of teratogenicity. At least 20% of all conceptions end in spontaneous abortions. A much higher proportion of abortuses have chromosome abnormalities, congenital malformations, or both, than newborns. The time necessary for such outcomes to manifest after the

introduction of a new teratogen could be considerably shorter than the time before significant increases of CMs occurred in liveborns and stillborns. Monitoring the spontaneous abortion rate or chromosomal and other abnormalities in abortuses would be an important adjunct to monitoring newborns. However, since some teratogens may only cause CMs in newborns, the current approach to monitoring should not be abandoned. Moreover, the problems of ascertainment encountered in monitoring newborns are greater still in monitoring abortuses.

Monitoring systems are inadequate on an additional count. They seldom receive much information on exposures to potential teratogens. Although more could be included in reporting, two other solutions should be considered. The first involves linkage with records of the parents that gives more information of exposures. These might be medical, prescription, or work records. The adequacy or even the existence of such records is problematic. With increased enrollment in HMOs and computerization of records, this type of prospective monitoring is not inconceivable in the future. If these records could be linked by code numbers, identity need never be disclosed. The second solution requires identifying infants with CMs so parents can be interviewed about past exposures. Controls would also have to be identified for more definitive studies. Aside from problems of bias in collecting information of exposures retrospectively, consent to release of names and confidentiality if they are released are issues that must be faced.

The proportion of infant deaths due to CMs is increasing. In the US, CMs are the leading cause of infant mortality (3, 119). CMs result in substantial impairments for many of those who survive (24). The causes of most of them remain unknown. Evidence that individuals differ in their susceptibility to harm from environmental exposures is slowly accumulating. Appreciation of the complex etiology of CMs may well lead to better epidemiologic and molecular approaches to their prevention.

Literature Cited

1. Acheson, E. D. 1979. Record linkage and the identification of long-term environmental hazards. *Proc. R. Soc. London Ser. B.* 205:165–78
2. Adams, M. M., Erickson, J. D., Layde, P. M., Oakley, G. P. 1981. Down's syndrome—recent trends in the United States. *J. Am. Med. Assoc.* 246:758–760
3. Advance Report of Final Mortality Statistics, 1982. 1984. *Monthly Vital Stat. Rep.* 33 (9) (suppl.). Nat. Cent. Health Stat., US Dept. Health and Human Serv. Publ. No. (PHS) 85-1120. Hyattsville, Md.: PHS
4. Anderson, C. E., Edmonds, L. D.,

Erickson, J. D. 1978. Patent ductus arteriosus and ventricular septal defect: Trends in reported frequency. *Am. J. Epidemiol.* 107:281–89
5. Antonarakis, S. E., Kittur, S. D., Metaxotou, C., Watkins, P. C., Patel, A. S. 1985. Analysis of DNA haplotypes suggests a genetic predisposition to trisomy 21 associated with DNA sequences on chromosome 21. *Proc. Natl. Acad. Sci. USA* 82:3360–64
5a. Ayme, S., Lippman-Hand, A. 1982. Maternal-age effect in aneuploidy: Does altered embryonic selection play a role? *Am. J. Human Genet.* 34:558–65

6. Ayme S., Lippman, A. 1985. Previous child with trisomy 21 and abortion rate. In *Prevention of Physical and Mental Congenital Defects. Part C: Basic and Medical Science, Education, and Future Strategies,* ed. M. Marois, pp. 15–20. New York: Liss

7. Baird, P. A., MacDonald, E. C. 1981. An epidemiologic study of congenital malformations of the anterior abdominal wall in more than half a million consecutive live births. *Am. J. Human Genet.* 33:470–78

8. Baird, D. D., Wilcox, A. J. 1985. Cigarette smoking associated with delayed conception. *J. Am. Med. Assoc.* 253: 2979–83

9. Bannister, P. 1985. The child health record and its uses for epidemiologic purposes. In *Prevention of Physical and Mental Congenital Defects. Part B: Epidemiology, Early Detection and Therapy, and Environmental Factors,* ed. M. Marois, pp. 33–38. New York: Liss

10. Barbujani, G., Calzolari, E. 1984. Comparison of two statistical techniques for the surveillance of birth defects through a Monte Carlo simulation. *Stat. Med.* 3:239–47

11. Bjerkedal, T. 1985. Occupation and outcome of pregnancy: A population-based study in Norway. See Ref 9, pp. 265–68

12. Bjerkedal, T., Bakketeig, L. S. 1975. Surveillance of congenital malformations and other conditions of the newborn. *Int. J. Epidemiol.* 4:31–36

13. Bjerkedal, T., Czeizel, A., Goujard, J., Kallen, B., Mastroiacova, P., et al. 1982. Valproic Acid and Spina Bifida. *Lancet* 2:1096

13a. Bower, C., Stanley, F. J. 1983. Western Australian congenital malformations register. *Med. J. Aust.* 2:189–91

14. Bracken, M. B. 1985. Spermicidal contraceptives and poor reproductive outcomes: The epidemiologic evidence against an association. *Am. J. Obstet. Gynecol.* 151:552–56

15. Castilla, E. 1983. Valproic acid and spina bifida. *Lancet* 2:683

16. Chen, R. 1979. Statistical techniques in birth defects surveillance systems. In *Epidemiologic Methods for Detection of Teratogens,* ed. M. A. Klingberg, J. A. C. Weatherall, pp. 184–89. Basel/Munchen: Karger. 203 pp.

17. Chen, R. 1985. Detection and investigation of subtle epidemics. See. Ref. 9, pp. 39–43

18. Chen, R., Mantel, N., Convelly, R. R., Isacson, P. 1982. A monitoring system

for chronic diseases. *Meth. Inform. Med.* 21:86–90

19. Christianson, R. E., van den Berg, B. J., Milkovich, L., Oechsli, F. W. 1981. Incidence of congenital anomalies among white and black live births with long-term follow-up. *Am. J. Public Health* 71: 1333–41

19a. Chung, C. S., Myrianthopoulos, N. C. 1975. Factors affecting risk of congenital malformations. II. Effect of maternal diabetes on congenital malformations. *Birth Def.* 11:23–38

19b. Chung, C. S., Myrianthopoulos, N. C. 1975. Factors affecting risk of congenital malformations. I. Analysis of epidemiologic factors in congenital malformations. Report from the Collaborative Perinatal Project. *Birth Def.* 11:1–22

20. Connell, F. A., Vadheim, C., Emanuel, I. 1985. Diabetes in pregnancy: A population-based study of incidence, referral for care, and perinatal mortality. *Am. J. Obstet. Gynecol.* 151:598–603

21. Czeizel, A. 1973. The Hungarian congenital malformation register. *Acta Univ. Carol (med. monogr.) Praha* 56:53–57

22. Czeizel, A. 1984. Re: "incidence and prevalence as measures of the frequency of birth defects." *Am. J. Epidemiol* 119:141–42

23. Czeizel, A. 1985. Increasing trends in congenital malformations of male external genitalia. *Lancet* 1:462–63

24. Czeizel, A., Sankaranarayanan, K. 1984. The load of genetic and partially genetic disorders in man. I. Congenital anomalies: Estimates of detriment in terms of years of life lost and years of impaired life. *Mutat. Res.* 128:73–103

25. Edmonds, D. K., Lindsay, K. S., Miller, J. F., Williamson, E., Wood, P. J. 1982. Early embryonic mortality in women. *Fertil. Steril.* 38:447–53

26. Edmonds, L. D., Anderson, C. E., Flynt, J. W. Jr., James, L. M. 1978. Congenital central nervous system malformations and vinyl chloride monomer exposure: A community study. *Teratology* 17:137–42

27. Edmonds, L. D., Layde, P. M., James, L. M., Flynt, J. W., Erickson, J. D., Oakley, G. P. Jr. 1981. Congenital malformations surveillance: Two American systems. *Int. J. Epidemiol.* 10:247–52

28. Elwood, J. M., Elwood, J. H. 1980. *Epidemiology of Anencephalus and Spina Bifida,* pp. 175–78. New York/Toronto: Oxford Univ. Press

29. Ericson, A., Kallen, B., Winberg, J. 1977. Surveillance of malformations at birth: A comparison of two record sys-

tems run in parallel. *Int. J. Epidemiol.* 6:35–41

30. Erickson, J. D., Mulinare, J., McClain, P. W., Fitch, T. G., James, L. M., et al. 1984. *Vietnam veterans' risk for fathering babies with birth defects.* Atlanta: US Dept. Health and Human Serv., Public Health Serv., Centers for Disease Control. 370 pp.

31. Fantel, A. G., Shepard, T. H., Vadheim-Roth, C., Stephens, T. D., Coleman, C. 1980. Embryonic and fetal phenotypes: Prevalence and other associated factors in a large study of spontaneous abortion. In *Human Embryonic and Fetal Death,* ed. I. H. Porter, E. B. Hook, pp. 71–87. New York: Academic. 371 pp.

32. Fara, G. M., Del Corno, G. 1985. Pregnancy outcome in the Seveso area after TCDD contamination. See Ref. 9, pp. 279–86

32b. Ferguson, S. W., Roberts, M. 1973. Spray adhesives, birth defects, and chromosomal damage. *Morbid. Mortal. Weekly Rep. Rev.* 22(44)

33. Finnell, R. H., Chernoff, G. F. 1984. Editorial comment: Genetic background: The elusive component in the fetal hydantoin syndrome. *Am. J. Med. Genet.* 19:459–62

34. Flynt, J. W., Hay, S. 1979. International clearinghouse for birth defects monitoring. See Ref. 16, pp. 44–52

35. Foster, F. H. 1982. Congenital anomaly monitoring in New Zealand, 1979–81. *NZ Med. J.* 95:780–81

36. Foster, F. H. 1979. Congenital anomaly monitoring system in New Zealand. *NZ Med. J.* 90:509–10

37. Fraser, F. C. 1977. Interactions and multiple causes. In *Handbook of Teratology I,* ed. J. G. Wilson, F. C. Fraser, pp. 445–63. New York/London: Plenum. 476 pp.

38. Garden, A. S., Benzie, R. J., Hutton, E. M., Care, D. J. 1985. Valproic acid therapy and neural tube defects. *Can. Med. Assoc. J.* 132:933–34

39. Goldsmith, J. R., Potashnik, G., Israeli, R. 1984. Reproductive outcomes in families of DBCP-exposed men. *Arch. Env. Health* 39:85–89

40. Hanson, J. W. 1976. Risks to the offspring of women treated with hydantoin anticonvulsants, with emphasis on the fetal hydantoin syndrome. *J. Pediatr.* 89:662–68

41. Hassold, T., Chen, N., Funkhouser, J., Jooss, T., Manuel, B., et al. 1980. A cytogenetic study of 1000 spontaneous abortions. *Ann. Hum. Genet. London* 44:151–63

42. Hassold, T. J., Jacobs, P. A. 1984. Trisomy in man. *Ann. Rev. Genet.* 18:69–98

43. Harlap, S., Shiono, P. H., Ramcharan, S., Golbus, M., Bachman, R., et al. 1985. Chromosomal abnormalities in the Kaiser-Permanente Birth Defects Study, with special reference to contraceptive use around the time of conception. *Teratology* 31:381–87

44. Hatch, M., Stefanchik-Scott, V., Stein, Z. A. 1983. *Surveillance of reproductive health in the U.S.: A survey of activity within and outside industry.* Washington DC: Am. Petroleum Inst. 148 pp.

45. Hemminki, K., Mutanen, P., Saloniemi, I. 1983. Smoking and the occurrence of congenital malformations and spontaneous abortions: Multivariate analysis. *Am. J. Obstet. Gynecol.* 145:61–66

46. Hemminki, K., Mutanen, P., Saloniemi, I., Luoma, K. 1981. Congenital malformations and maternal occupation in Finland: Multivariate analysis. *J. Epidemiol. Commun. Health* 35:5–10

47. Henshaw, S. K., Forrest, J. D., Blaine, E. 1984. Abortion services in the United States, 1981 and 1982. *Fam. Plan. Perspect.* 16:119–27

48. Holmberg, P. C. 1985. Congenital defects and environmental factors during pregnancy: Nationwide surveillance. See Ref. 9, pp. 287–90

49. Holmes, L. B., Cann, C., Cook, C. 1985. Examination of infants for both minor and major malformations to evaluate for possible teratogenic exposures. See. Ref. 9, pp. 59–64

50. Holtzman, N. A., Leonard, C. O., Farfel, M. R. 1981. Issues in antenatal and neonatal screening and surveillance for hereditary and congenital disorders. *Ann. Rev. Public Health* 2:219–51

51. Holtzman, N. A. 1986. Screening for congenital abnormalities. *Int. J. Tech. Assess.* In press

52. Holtzman, N. A. 1985. The application of recombinant DNA technology to genetic testing: Promise or peril. Baltimore: Johns Hopkins Univ. Press. Publication pending

53. Hook, E. B. 1978. Spontaneous deaths of fetuses with chromosomal abnormalities diagnosed prenatally. *N. Engl. J. Med.* 299:1036–38

54. Hook, E. B. 1981. Prevalence of chromosome abnormalities during human gestation and implications for studies of environmental mutagens. *Lancet* 2:169–72

55. Hook, E. B. 1982. Incidence and prevalence as measures of the frequency of

birth defects. *Am. J. Epidemiol.* 116: 743–47

56. Hook, E. B. 1984. Re: "incidence and prevalence as measures of the frequency of birth defects—the author replies." *Am. J. Epidemiol.* 119:142–44

57. Hook, E. B., Chambers, G. M. 1977. Estimated rates of Down syndrome in live births by one year, maternal age intervals for mothers aged 20–49 in a New York State study—implications of the risk figures for genetic counseling and cost-benefit analysis of prenatal diagnosis programs. *Birth Defects* 13(3a):123–41

58. Hook, E. B., Cross, P. K. 1981. Temporal increase in the rate of Down syndrome livebirths to older mothers in New York State. *J. Med. Genet.* 18: 29–30

59. Hook, E. B., Porter, I. H. 1980. Terminological conventions, methodological considerations, temporal trends, specific genes, environmental hazards, and some other factors pertaining to embryonic and fetal death. See Ref. 31, pp. 1–17

60. Huether, C. A., Gummere, G. R., Hook, E. B., Dignan, P. S., Volodkevich, H., et al. 1981. Down's Syndrome: Percentage reporting on birth certificates and single year maternal age risk rates for Ohio 1970–79; comparison with Upstate New York data. *Am. J. Public Health* 71:1367–62

61. International Clearinghouse for Birth Defects Monitoring Systems. 1982. *1980 Annual Report.* Stockholm: Garnisonstryckeriet. 44 pp.

62. International Clearinghouse for Birth Defects Monitoring Systems. 1983. *1981 Annual Report.* Stockholm: Garnisonstryckeriet. 46 pp.

63. International Clearinghouse for Birth Defects Monitoring Systems. 1984. *1982 Annual Report.* Stockholm: Garnisonstryckeriet. 56 pp.

64. Jacobs, P. A. 1978. Population surveillance: A cytogenetic approach. In *Genetic Epidemiology,* ed. N. E. Morton, C. S. Chung, pp. 463–82. New York/San Francisco/London: Academic

65. Jackson, L. D. 1985. First-trimester diagnosis of fetal genetic disorders. *Hosp. Pract.* March 15:39–47

66. Jackson-Cook, C. K., Flannery, D. B., Corey, L. A., Nance, W. E., Brown, J. A. 1985. Nucleolar organizer region variants as a risk factor for Down syndrome. *Am. J. Hum. Genet.* 37:1049–61

67. Jick, H., Holmes, L. B., Hunter, J. R., Madsen, S., Stergachis, A. 1981. First

trimester drug use and congenital disorders. *J. Am. Med. Assoc.* 246:343–46

68. Jick, H., Walker, A. M., Rothman, K. J., Hunter, J. R., Holmes, L. B., et al. 1981. Vaginal spermicides and congenital disorders. *J. Am. Med. Assoc.* 245:1329–32

69. Kajii, T., Ferrier, A., Niikawa N., Takahara, H., Ohama, K., Avirachan, S. 1980. Anatomic and chromosomal anomalies in 639 spontaneous abortuses. *Hum. Genet.* 55:87–98

70. Kallen, B., Hay, S., Klingberg, M. 1984. Birth defects monitoring systems: Accomplishments and goals. In *Issues and Reviews in Teratology,* ed. H. Kalter, 2:1–22. New York/London: Plenum

71. Kallen, B., Lindham, S. 1982. A women's birth cohort effect on malformation rates. *Int. J. Epidemiol.* 11:398–401

72. Kallen, B., Rahmani, T. M. Z., Winberg, J. 1984. Infants with congenital limb reduction registered in the Swedish register of congenital malformations. *Teratology* 29:73–85

73. Kallen, B., Winberg, J. 1968. A Swedish register of congenital malformations. *Pediatrics* 41:765–76

74. Kallen, B., Winberg, J. 1979. Dealing with suspicions of malformation frequency increase. *Acta Ped. Scand. Suppl.* 275:66–74

75. Kalter, H. 1980. The relation between congenital malformations and prenatal mortality in experimental animals. See Ref. 31, pp. 29–44

76. Kalter, H., Warkany, J. 1983. Congenital malformations: Etiologic factors and their role in prevention. *N. Engl. J. Med.* 308:424–31, 491–97

77. Kellogg, C. K. 1985. Drugs and chemicals that act on the central nervous system: Interpretation of experimental evidence. See Ref. 6, pp. 147–54

78. Kelsey, F. O. 1985. Drug labeling for teratogenicity: Requirements of the U.S. Food and Drug Administration. See Ref. 6, pp. 155–60

79. Kelly, T. E. 1984. Teratogenicity of anticonvulsant drugs. I: Review of the literature. *Am. J. Med. Genet.* 19:413–34

80a. Kelly, T. E., Rein, M., Edwards, P. 1984. Teratogenicity of anticonvulsant drugs. IV: The association of clefting and epilepsy. *Am. J. Med. Genet.* 19:51–58

80. Kelly, T. E., Edwards, P., Rein, M., Miller, J. Q., Dreifuss, F. E. 1984. Teratogenicity of anticonvulsant drugs. II: A prospective study. *Am. J. Med. Genet.* 19:435–43

81. Kennedy, W. P. 1967. Epidemiologic

aspects of the problem of congenital malformations. *Birth Def. Orig. Art. Ser.* 3(2):1–18

82. Khoury, M. J., Cordero, J. F., Greenberg, F., James, L. M., Erickson, J. D. 1983. A population study of the VACTERL association: Evidence for its etiologic heterogeneity. *Pediatrics* 71:815–20

83. Khoury, M. J., Erickson, J. D., James, L. M. 1982. Etiologic heterogeneity of neural tube defects: Clues from epidemiology. *Am. J. Epidemiol.* 115:538–48

84. Khoury, M. J., Erickson, J. D., James, L. M. 1982. Etiologic heterogeneity of neural tube defects. II. Clues from family studies. *Am. J. Hum. Genet.* 34:980–87

85. Kirsch-Volders, M., ed. 1984. *Mutagenicity, Carcinogenicity, and Teratogenicity of Industrial Pollutants.* New York/London: Plenum. 336 pp.

86. Klingberg, M. A., Papier, C. M., Hart, J. 1983. Birth defects monitoring. *Am. J. Indust. Med.* 4:309–28

87. Knox, E. G., Armstrong, E. H., Lancashire, R. 1984. The quality of notification of congenital malformations. *J. Epidemiol. Commun. Health* 38:296–305

88. Knox, G. 1963. Detection of low intensity epidemicity: Application to cleft lip and palate. *Br. J. Prev. Soc. Med.* 17:121–27

89. Kurzel, R. B. 1984. Substance abuse in pregnancy. In *The Problem-Oriented Medical Record for High-Risk Obstetrics,* ed. C. L. Cetrulo, A. J. Sbarra, 1:11–28, New York: Plenum. 486 pp.

90. Kurzel, R. B., Cetrulo, C. L. 1985. Chemical terateogenesis and reproductive failure. *Obstet. Gynecol. Surv.* 40:397–423

91. Lammer, E. J., Chen, D. T., Hoar, R. M., Agnish, N. D., Benke, P. J., Braun, J. T., et al. 1985. Retinoic acid retinopathy. *N. Engl. J. Med.* 313:837–41

92. Layde, P. M., Erickson, J. D., Dooley, K., Edmonds, L. D. 1980. Is there an epidemic of ventricular septal defects in the U.S.A.? *Lancet* 1:407

93. Lechat, M. F., De Wals, P., Weatherall, J. A. C. 1985. European Economic Community's concerted action on congenital anomalies: The Eurocat project. See Ref. 9, pp. 11–16

94. Leck, I. 1966. Incidence and epidemicity of Down syndrome. *Lancet* 2:457–60

95. Leck, I. 1979. Teratogenic risks of disease and therapy. See Ref. 16, pp. 23–43

96. Lenz, W. 1966. Malformations caused by drugs in pregnancy. *Am. J. Dis. Child.* 112:99–106

97. Lenz, W. 1985. Thalidomide embryopathy in Germany, 1959–1961. See Ref. 6, pp. 77–84

98. Lenz, W., Knapp, K. 1962. Thalidomide embryopathy. *Arch. Environ. Health.* 5:100–5

99. Levin, S. M. 1983. Problems and pitfalls in conducting epidemiological reseach in the area of reproductive toxicology. *Am. J. Indust. Med.* 4:349–64

100. Lindbohm, M. L., Taskinen, H., Hemminki, K. 1985. Reproductive health of working women. *Public Health Rev.* In press

100a. Lindhout, D., Meinardi, H. 1984. Spina bifida and in-utero exposure to valproate. *Lancet* 2:396

101. Lippman, A., Mackenzie, S. G. 1985. What is "recall bias" and does it exist? See Ref. 6, pp. 205–10

102. Lubs, H. A., Patil, S. R., Kimberling, W. J., Brown, J., Cohen, M. M., et al. 1979. Chromosomal abnormalities ascertained in the collaborative perinatal survey of 7- and 8-year old children. *Birth Defects* 15:191–202

103. Manchester, D., Jacoby, E. 1984. Decreased placental monooxygenase activities associated with birth defects. *Teratology* 30:31–37

104. Manchester, D. K., Parker, N. B., Bowman, C. M. 1984. Maternal smoking increases xenobiotic metabolism in placenta but not umbilical vein endothelium. *Pediatr. Res.* 18:1071–75

105. Mantel, N. 1967. The detection of disease clustering and generalized regression approach. *Cancer Res.* 27:209–20

106. Mantel, N. 1985. Some problems with investigations and epidemiologic studies relating to pregnancy. See Ref. 9, pp. 45–48

107. Mastroiacovo, P. 1985. The Italian birth defects monitoring system: Baseline rates based on 283,453 births and comparison with other registries. See Ref. 9, pp. 17–22

108. Mattison, D. R. 1983. The mechanisms of action of reproductive toxins. *Am. J. Indust. Med.* 4:65–79

109. Mehes, K. 1985. Minor malformations in the neonate: Utility in screening infants at risk of hidden major defects. See Ref. 6, pp. 45–50

110. Milham, S. Jr. 1971. Experience with malformation surveillance. In *Monitoring, Birth Defects and Environment,* pp. 137–42. New York/London: Academic

111. Miller, R. W. 1981. Areawide chemical contamination: Lessons from case histories. *J. Am. Med. Assoc.* 245:1548–51

112. Mills, J. L., Rishl, A. R., Knopp, R. H., Ober, C. L., Jovanovic, L. G., Polk, B.

F., the NICHD-Diabetes in Early Pregnancy Study. 1983. Malformations in infants of diabetic mothers: Problems in study design. *Prev. Med.* 12:274–86

113. Modell, B. 1985. Chorionic villus sampling. *Lancet* 1:737–40

114. Murphy, J. C., Collins, T. F. X., Black, T. N., Osterberg, R. E. 1975. Evaluation of the teratogenic potential of a spray adhesive in hamsters. *Teratology* 11: 243–46

115. Myrianthopoulos, N. C. 1978. Congenital malformations: The contribution of twin studies. *Birth Defects* 14:151–65

116. Myrianthopoulos, N. C., Chung, C. S. 1974. Congenital malformations in singletons: Epidemiologic survey. *Birth Defects:* 10(11):1–58

117. Neel, J. V., Beebe, G. W., Miller, R. W. 1985. Delayed biomedical effects of the bombs. *Bull. Atomic Scientists* 41:72–75

117a. Nevin, N. C., McDonald, J. R., Walby, A. L. 1978. A comparison of neural tube defects identified by two independent routine recording systems for congenital malformations in Northern Ireland. *Int. J. Epidemiol.* 7:319–21

118. Oakley, G. F. Jr. 1975. The use of human abortuses in the search for teratogens. In *Methods for Detection of Environmental Agents that Produce Congenital Defects, 1975,* ed. T.H. Shepard, J. R. Miller, M. Marois, pp. 189–96. Amsterdam: North Holland. 263 pp.

119. Oakley, G. P. Jr. 1981. Incidence and epidemiology of birth defects. In *Genetic Issues in Pediatric and Obstetric Practice,* ed. M. M. Kaback, pp. 25–43. Chicago/London: Year Book Medical. 604 pp.

120. Oakley, G. P. 1984. Population and case-control surveillance in the search for search environmental causes of birth defects. *Publ. Health Rep.* 99:465–68

121. Oakley, G. P. 1985. Birth defects epidemiology and surveillance. In *Prevention of Physical and Mental Congenital Defects, Part A: The Scope of the Problem,* ed. M. Marois, pp. 71–90. New York: Liss

122. Polednak, A. P., Janerich, D. T. 1983. Uses of available record systems in epidemiologic studies of reproductive toxicology. *Am. J. Indust. Med.* 4:329–48

123. Rating, D., Koch, S., Jager-Roman, E., Jacob, S., Helge, H. 1985. The influence of antiepileptic drugs on minor anomalies in the offspring of epileptic parents. See Ref. 6, pp. 57–60

124. Robert, E., Guibaud, P. 1982. Maternal valproic acid and congenital neural tube defects. *Lancet* 2:937

125. Roberts, E., Rosa, F. 1983. Valproate and birth defects. *Lancet* 2:1142

126. Roberts, C. J., Lowe, C. R. 1975. Where have all the conceptions gone? *Lancet* 1:498–99

127. Rosa, F. W. 1983. Teratogenicity of isotretinoin. *Lancet* 2:513

128. Saxen, L., Klemetti, A., Haro, A. S. 1974. A matched-pair register for studies of selected congenital defects. *Am. J. Epidemiol.* 100:297–306

129. Schardein, J. L. 1985. Current status of drugs as teratogens in man. See Ref. 6, pp. 181–90

130. Seller, M.J., Nevin, N. C. 1984. Periconceptional vitamin supplementation and the prevention of neural tube defects in south-east England and Northern Ireland. *J. Med. Genet.* 21:325–30

131. Shapiro, S., Abramowicz, M. 1969. Pregnancy outcome correlates identified through medical record-based information. *Am. J. Public Health* 59:1629–50

132. Shapiro, S., Ross, L. J., Levine, H. S. 1965. Relationship of selected prenatal factors to pregnancy outcome and congenital anomalies. *Am. J. Public Health* 55:268–82

133. Shepard, T. H. 1983. *Catalog of Teratogenic Agents.* Baltimore/London: Johns Hopkins Univ. Press. 529 pp. 4th ed.

134. Skegg, D. C. G., Doll, R. 1981. Record linkage for drug monitoring. *J. Epidemiol. Commun. Health.* 35:25–31

135. Speirs, A. L., Aberd, M. D. 1962. Thalidomide and congenital abnormalities. *Lancet* 1:303–5

135a. Starfield, B. H. 1985. Primary care in the United States. *Int. J. Health Serv.* In press

135b. Stoll, C. 1985. The Northeastern France birth defects monitoring system. See. Ref. 9, pp. 157–82

136. Strickler, S., Dansky, L., Miller, M. A., Seni, M.-H. Andermann, E., Spielberg, S. P. 1985. Genetic predisposition to phenytoin-induced birth defects. *Lancet* 2:746–49

137. Tanimura, T. 1975. The use of induced abortuses for monitoring. See. Ref. 118, pp. 197–201

137a. Taussig, H. B. 1962. A study of the German outbreak of phocomelia. *J. Am. Med. Assoc.* 180:1106–14

138. Tein, I., MacGregor, D. L. 1985. Possible valproate teratogenicity. *Arch. Neurol.* 42:291–3

139. Temin, P. 1980. *Taking Your Medicine.* Cambridge, Mass.:/London: Harvard Univ. Press. 274 pp.

140. Trichopoulos, E., Desmond, L., Yen, S., McMahon, B. 1971. A study of time-

place clustering in anencephaly and spina bidifida. *Am. J. Epidemiol.* 94:26–30

141. United Nations Environ. Programme, Int. Labour Organization, World Health Organization. 1984. *Environmental Health Criteria 30: Principles for Evaluating Health Risks to Progeny Associated with Exposure to Chemical During Pregnancy.* Geneva: WHO. 177 pp.

142. Warburton, D. 1985. Effects of common environmental exposures on spontaneous abortion of defined karyotype. See Ref. 6, pp. 31–36

143. Watanabe, G. 1979. Environmental determinants of birth defects prevalence. See Ref. 16, pp. 91–100

144. Weatherall, J. A. C., De Wals, P., Lechat, M. F. 1984. Evaluation of information systems for the surveillance of congenital malformations. *Int. J. Epidemiol.* 13:193–95

145. Weatherall, J. A. C., Haskey, J. C. 1976. Surveillance of malformations. *Br. Med. Bull.* 32:39–44

146. Weinstock, M. A. 1981. Generalized scan statistic for detection of clusters. *Int. J. Epidemiol.* 10:289–94

147. Whittaker, P. G., Taylor, A., Lind, T. 1981. Unsuspected pregnancy loss in healthy women. *Lancet* 1:1126

148. Wilcox, A. J. 1983. Surveillance of pregnancy loss in human populations. *Am. J. Indust. Med.* 4:285–91

149. Wilson, J. G. 1979. The evolution of teratological testing. *Teratology* 20:205–12

150. Windham, G. C., Edmonds, L. D., 1982. Current trends in the incidence of neural tube defects. *Pediatrics* 70:33–37

151. Windham, G. C., Bjerkedal, T., Langmark, F. 1985. A population-based study of cancer incidence in twins and in children with congenital malformations or low birth weight, Norway, 1967–1980. *Am. J. Epidemiol.* 121:49–56

152. Zakharov, A. F. 1985. Reproductive loss in man: Total and chromosomally determined. See Ref. 6, pp. 9–14

Ann. Rev. Public Health. 1986. 7:267–91

DIET AND CHEMOPREVENTION IN NCI'S RESEARCH STRATEGY TO ACHIEVE NATIONAL CANCER CONTROL OBJECTIVES[1]

Peter Greenwald and Edward Sondik

Division of Cancer Prevention and Control, National Cancer Institute, Bethesda, Maryland 20892

Barbara S. Lynch

Department of Health Education, University of Maryland, College Park, Maryland 20742

INTRODUCTION

Because it is the second major cause of death by disease and particularly because it is at least partially preventable, cancer is one of the most important public health problems of the century. Therefore, the National Cancer Institute, as the chief research center and as leader of the National Cancer Program, has spent several years in a systematic process to analyze research leads, identify the most promising research strategies, and set quantifiable objectives for reducing cancer mortality by the year 2000. The process involved a convergence of existing epidemiologic, laboratory, and clinical data and resulted in (*a*) a Research Flow Design for planning and funding studies, and (*b*) a set of cancer control objectives for prevention, screening, treatment, and surveillance. The goal is to reduce the 1985 cancer mortality rate by 50% by the year 2000. One area of research newly emphasized by NCI—chemoprevention—has the potential for making an important impact on nutrition-related cancer incidence. Chemoprevention is the utilization of defined chemicals, such as provitamins (B carotene), vitamins (A, C, and E), synthetic analogues, or other substances (for example, the trace metal selenium), for the purpose of reducing cancer incidence. In this article, we highlight the cancer control objectives for the nation, with emphasis on the prevention objectives and their public health impact; describe the research strategy designed to provide the information needed to achieve those objectives; discuss the role of chemoprevention in the research strategy; and review the chemoprevention data and current studies.

CANCER CONTROL OBJECTIVES

The current knowledge base about cancer and the network of cancer control resources are the basis for the aggressive effort NCI has launched to control cancer. The major gains made during the past decade in understanding cancer etiology, in developing diagnostic techniques, and in developing more effective treatment led NCI to the conclusion that a 50% reduction in cancer mortality is a reasonable goal for the year 2000 if the nation focuses on full application of state-of-the-art knowledge.

Prevention Objectives

In the 1950s and 1960s, it became increasingly apparent that most cancer is caused or promoted by lifestyle and environmental factors, although genetic or susceptibility factors may be involved since the majority of people similarly exposed to environmental factors do not develop cancer. Research data support the estimate that lifestyle and environmental factors are contributory to the development of roughly 90% of cancer incidence and, therefore, support the conclusion that in principle much cancer is preventable. However, this estimate cannot be translated into a 90% reduction in cancer mortality by the year 2000 for a number of reasons. Even if all of the population stopped smoking immediately, smoking-related cancer would continue to occur because of the accumulated effects of previous smoking (27). Further, it is unrealistic to expect total cessation of smoking, and so more modest goals for smoking cessation were set. Also, dietary changes that may minimize the risk of cancer may be too extreme for adoption by the entire population. Based on considerations such as these, an estimate of a 25% reduction in incidence and mortality by prevention activities was used in goal for the year 2000. The objectives for cancer prevention, screening, and treatment are summarized in Table 1.

Table 1   Cancer control objectives: summary

Control factor	Rationale	Year 2000 objective
PREVENTION		
Smoking	The causal relationship between smoking and cancer has been scientifically established.	Reduce the percentage of adults who smoke from 34 (in 1983) to 15% or less.
		Reduce the percentage of youths who smoke by age 20 from 36 (in 1983) to 15% or less.
Diet	Research indicates that high-fat and low-fiber consumption may increase the risk for various cancers. In 1983 NAS reviewed research on diet and cancer and recommended a reduction in fat; more recent studies lead NCI to recommend an increase in fiber. Research is underway to verify the causal relationships and to test the impact on cancer incidence.	Reduce average consumption of fat from 40 to 25% or less of total calories.

Increase average consumption of fiber from 8–12 g per day to 20–30 g per day. |
SCREENING		
Breast	The effectiveness of breast screening in reducing mortality has been scientifically established.	Increase the percentage of women ages 50–70 who have annual physical breast exam and mammography from 45% for physical exam alone and 15% for mammography to 80% for each.
Cervical	The effectiveness of cervical screening in reducing mortality has been scientifically established.	Increase the percentage of women who have a Pap smear every 3 years to 90 from 79% (ages 20–39) and to 80 from 57% (ages 40–70).
TREATMENT		
Transfer of research results to practice	NCI review of clinical trial and SEER data indicates that, for certain cancer sites, mortality in SEER is greater than mortality experienced in clinical trials.	Increase adoption of state-of-the-art treatment.

Cancer prevention is the lowering of cancer incidence by the avoidance or the minimization of exposure to those lifestyle and environmental factors which increase the occurrence and progression of cancer and the maximization of exposure to or use of protective factors. *Lifestyle factors* are behaviors over which the individual has some control, especially tobacco use, diet, occupational exposure to carcinogens, exposures to carcinogens in medical procedures, sexual behavior patterns, and general personal hygiene. *Environmental factors* are naturally occurring or man-made causes of cancer that contaminate water, air, and ground. These factors are largely beyond the individual's control, and thus require broad social actions or systems changes to achieve effective control.

Dietary Objectives

The dietary objectives for cancer prevention are as follows, with their rationale explained below (56):

I. Year 2000 dietary objectives:
Risk factor reduction:
1. By 2000, the per capita daily consumption of fat will decrease from 40 to 25% or less of total calories.
2. By 2000, the per capita consumption of fiber from grains, fruits, and vegetables will increase to 20–30 g per day, from 8–12 g per day.

II. Year 1990 dietary objectives:
Risk factor reduction:
1. By 1990, the per capita consumption of fiber from grains, fruits, and vegetables will increase to 15 g or more per day. (In 1976–1980, the per capita consumption of fiber from these sources was 8–12 g.)
2. By 1990, the per capita consumption of fat will decrease to 30% or less of total calories. (In 1976–1980, the per capita consumption of fat was 40% of total calories.)
Increased public/professional awareness:
1. By 1990, the proportion of the population that is able to identify the principal dietary factors known or strongly suspected to be related to cancer should exceed 75%.
2. By 1990, 70% of the adult population should be able to identify foods that are low in fat and high in dietary fiber.
3. By 1990, the proportion of adults who are aware of the added risk of head and neck cancer for people with excessive alcohol consumption should exceed 75%.
Improved services/protection:
1. By 1990, the labels of all packaged foods should contain useful calorie and nutrient information to enable consumers to select diets that promote and protect good health; similar information should be displayed where non-packaged foods are obtained or purchased.
2. By 1990, all states should include nutrition education as part of required comprehensive school health education at elementary and secondary levels.

(In 1979, only ten states mandated nutrition as a core content area in school health education.)

3. By 1990, virtually all routine health contracts with health professionals should include some element of nutrition education and counseling.

4. By 1990, all managers of institutional food service operations should understand and actively promote dietary patterns that accord with current knowledge of the relationship between diet and good health.

Poor dietary practices, including inadequate intake of fiber and important micronutrients, are probably as significant as tobacco smoking in causing cancer. The consensus of scientists is that as much as 25 to 35% of cancer mortality is related to dietary factors (16). This estimate is based on a large number of studies, although uncertainty surrounds the exact magnitude of the association and the biological mechanisms involved. A variety of studies indicate that excessive fat intake, inadequate consumption of dietary fiber, obesity, and inadequate consumption of foods containing certain micronutrients (vitamins and minerals) are associated with higher rates of certain cancers. Dietary components are associated with cancers of the gastrointestinal tract (esophagus, stomach, colon, rectum, and liver) and some sex hormone–specific sites (breast, prostate, ovaries, and endometrium). Dietary components also may have an impact on the cancers of the respiratory system and the urinary bladder. Four types of epidemiologic studies show a role of dietary components in cancer incidence: (a) international correlation studies comparing dietary intakes to cancer rates, (b) studies of migration from areas with low cancer rates to (or from) areas with high cancer rates, (c) comparison of certain low-risk US populations (Seventh Day Adventists, Mormons) to the general US population, and (d) case-control and cohort studies comparing dietary patterns in cancer patients to controls in the study population. These epidemiologic studies are supported by experimental observation in laboratory animals and other test systems.

DIETARY FAT AND FIBER   High intake of fat is associated with cancers of the breast, colon, rectum, uterus (endometrium), prostate, and possibly several other sites. High intake of dietary fiber, on the other hand, is associated with lower risk for colon and rectal cancers. Since dietary fat and fiber tend to vary inversely in human diets, it often is not possible to estimate precisely the relative contribution of fat or the protection of fiber in the risk for colon and rectal cancers. A few studies suggest a separate contribution from each, and the protective effects from reducing fat consumption and increasing fiber intake may be additive, but other studies suggest interaction. Furthermore, foods high in fiber are often high in some of the micronutrients which seem to protect against cancer.

MICRONUTRIENTS   Data from experimental studies and epidemiologic analyses of dietary patterns indicate that some vitamins and minerals might protect against certain types of cancer. Among the vitamins, vitamin A and its precursor, beta-carotene, appear to be particularly valuable, and vitamins E and C may be protective to a lesser degree. Among minerals, selenium may have benefits. These observations are being studied in human chemoprevention trials.

TRENDS IN FOOD CONSUMPTION   Trends in food consumption during the twentieth century have not been favorable from the point of view of cancer control, although recently this may have begun to change. While fiber consumption has declined, fat intake has increased, and obesity is a serious problem.

For dietary fiber, the per capita daily consumption level has declined by about 20% since 1909 to a current level of about 8 to 12 grams per person per day. At the same time, the proportion of calories in the diet contributed by carbohydrates fell from 56 to 46%; the number of these calories contributed by sugar has increased while those contributed by starches and plant foods rich in fiber have decreased. Also, decreases have occurred in per capita consumption of fruits, vegetables, dried beans, peas, nuts, flour, and cereal products (although exact analyses are lacking). Until 1972, grain product consumption had decreased by about 40%. Fortunately, this trend appears to be changing; since 1972, grain product consumption has increased by about 9%. Fruit and vegetable consumption has fluctuated greatly during this century. Processed fruit consumption, mainly of processed citrus fruit juice, has increased tenfold, consumption of processed vegetables has increased four-fold, while use of fresh fruits and vegetables has decreased 36% and 23%, respectively (72).

The per capita consumption of dietary fat has increased 31% since 1909, raising the proportion of total calories provided by fats from 32 to 41%. The increase in per capita fat consumption is explained largely by a two-fold increase in the use of fats and oils, mainly vegetable oils used in commercial processing of foods, especially in "fast foods," snacks, and convenience foods.

POTENTIAL IMPACT OF DIETARY OBJECTIVES   It is not yet possible to quantify the precise contribution of diet to overall cancer risk or to estimate with absolute confidence the reduction in cancer mortality to be expected from dietary modifications. However, a growing body of international and migrant population data suggests that diet is directly related to 25 to 30% of cancer deaths (16).

While precise relationships of the impact of dietary change on cancer mortality are not possible, these data can be useful to estimate potential reduction. For example, a number of studies show a correlation between dietary fat intake and breast cancer mortality (2, 11, 73). These international studies show an almost straight line relationship between per capita fat consumption and breast cancer mortality to the extent that countries with the lowest per capita fat consumption also have the lowest breast cancer mortality rates. Similarly, a survey of 4600 Hawaiians from five ethnic groups found correlation between breast cancer incidence and age-adjusted mean daily intake of total fats, animal fats, and saturated or unsaturated fats (37). Evidence can be drawn from case-control studies as well. An NCI Study compared the dietary fat intake of 577 breast cancer patients to that of 826 controls and found that persons in the highest quartile for beef and pork consumption had 2.7 times the breast cancer risk of those in the lowest quartile (45). In still another study, elevated high ratios for total fat and selected types of fat were found for both premenopausal and postmenopausal women. One association held for fat but not total calories (54). Based on these studies it is reasonable to estimate a potential 25% reduction of breast cancer mortality from reducing average per capita of dietary fat from 40 to 25% of calories. Today, some 36,000 women per year die of breast cancer; this reduction could save as many as 9000 lives annually.

Another diet component, dietary fiber, may have major benefits in reducing colon cancer risks. The productive effect of fiber-containing foods has been repeatedly observed by many investigators in different geographic locales, with different populations and using different methods of study. Together these studies make a convincing case for the protective effects of fiber-rich foods. Although research is still needed to outline the biologic actions of the different types of dietary fiber and their effects on fecal mutagen activity and the kinetics, morphology, and physiology of colonic epithelium, the existing evidence of a protective effect is strong. For example, an international comparison of 20 countries found that fiber was negatively and significantly correlated with colon cancer mortality (43). A study in Denmark concluded that changes in fiber intake are inversely related to changes in the prevalence of colon cancer (28). Still other epidemiologic studies have shown that a Finnish population at low risk for colon cancer has more fiber in the diet than do higher risk people in New York or Copenhagen (48, 60). Colon cancer patients in Israel also had less fiber in the diet than did other Israelis (55). In the United States, colon cancer patients in the Bay Area of San Francisco were less likely to have eaten fiber and more likely to have eaten fat than were controls (13), and the Mormon and Seventh-Day Adventist groups have high fiber diets and are low colon cancer risks (46, 58).

Although none of these studies allows precise estimates of the effect of increasing dietary fiber, the data suggest that if dietary fiber is increased to a per capita figure of 20–30 grams per day, a 50% reduction in cancer of the colon and rectum is possible. These fat and fiber dietary objectives could also result in mortality reduction in other cancers, including cancers of the prostate, endometrium, gall bladder, stomach, esophagus, pancreas, ovaries, liver, lung, and bladder.

The dietary prevention objectives strike a balance between acting now upon existing knowledge and waiting for the results of research underway or projected. If the research results support the hypotheses about the relationships between dietary components and cancer, waiting to change dietary behavior until those results are available could mean the unnecessary loss of lives. To begin efforts to change diets now seems prudent in light of existing knowledge and the recommendations of the National Research Council.

RESEARCH STRATEGY

The optimism about achieving the cancer control objectives for the nation derives partly from NCI's confidence in the research strategy it developed in the early 1980s. Two historical lessons in cancer research (25), one negative and one positive, provided an impetus for NCI's Division of Cancer Prevention and Control (DCPC) to undertake a process to establish a policy for directing and funding cancer research. The negative example is the inadequate progress on the route to preventing smoking-related lung cancer. Although research had established for at least two decades that the most effective means of preventing lung cancer was to eliminate cigarette smoking, only recently has a concentrated effort been made to develop policies to achieve that goal. Had a strategy been developed 20 years ago for ascertaining when a research base is adequate to support policymaking and information dissemination, the result might have been fewer deaths from lung cancer today. The positive example is the clinical progress made in cancer therapy since the 1950s. A research strategy evolved, based on clinical trials as a means of evaluating the efficacy of treatments. Then, in 1955, the National Cooperative Chemotherapy Program was organized, ensuring participation of the best researchers in the nation, high standards, and compatibility of studies. As results became available, they were quickly communicated and adopted. New leads for further advances were systematically brought into the process.

Now the rigor and systematic approach applied to clinical treatment research is being applied to cancer prevention research. NCI's new policy for prevention research is based on three assumptions:

1. that the scientific method of inquiry is an essential part of cancer control;
2. that the pursuit of excellence in science and the potential for reducing incidence, morbidity, and mortality in numerically important ways are prime considerations in setting priorities for action;
3. that the planning and conduct of activities are built on existing strengths of the National Cancer Program.

The policy is also based on a clear, consistent definition of cancer prevention. Cancer prevention has as a major foundation etiologic research. Cancer prevention is defined as *applied research* to *systematically* test or introduce a specific *intervention* aimed at having a *measurable impact* on an important cancer problem. The purpose of the intervention is to reduce cancer incidence (and thus also morbidity and mortality) rates in populations.

The Strategy: Research Phases for Cancer Control

The NCI now requires that development of cancer control interventions follow an orderly sequence of research phases (Figure 1). The sequence begins with new knowledge discovered through research and related to the existing knowledge base. The new knowledge, through applied research, becomes new technology, which is validated through clinical trials in defined populations and in other ways to determine its safety and efficacy for widespread dissemination through demonstration projects. Once the prevention intervention has been proven, the professional community is educated in its proper use and the public is informed about its nature and availability.

The cancer control phases are designed to enable NCI to assess the rigor of proposed interventions in a systematic manner. Each phase carefully, incrementally advances the research concept, thus allowing only those interventions evaluated and proven to be effective to be brought to widespread implementation. Phase I develops the hypothesis; Phases II–IV test the hypothesis in comparative or controlled studies.

Phase I, *Hypothesis Development,* is the identification and assessment of research leads based on a synthesis of available scientific evidence from basic laboratory, epidemiologic, and clinical studies. This phase of the research process results in hypotheses for cancer control strategies to be tested for efficacy in reducing incidence, morbidity, or mortality through the next four phases.

In Phase II, *Methods Development,* methodological research is the focus. Research in this phase characterizes the factors and outcomes that must be monitored in intervention studies to ensure that accurate and valid procedures are available before the actual study is begun. Because the spectrum of cancer

PHASE I	PHASE II	PHASE III	PHASE IV	PHASE V
HYPOTHESIS DEVELOPMENT	METHODS DEVELOPMENT	CONTROLLED INTERVENTION TRIALS	DEFINED POPULATION STUDIES	DEMONSTRATION AND IMPLEMENTATION

Figure 1   Sequence of cancer control research.

control intervention is so broad, Phase II includes a wide array of possible research, including pilot tests to investigate the feasibility or acceptability of using a proposed intervention in a specific population subgroup; population compliance studies; development, pilot testing, and validation of data collection forms; testing of translations of materials from other languages; and tests of the applicability of methods used with other diseases or disciplines. Interventions must be assessed in terms of their possible effectiveness and cost, as well as their risks to the subjects. Of particular concern is, for example, the assessment of whether long-term dietary habits can be changed and monitored accurately.

In Phase III, *Controlled Intervention Trials,* hypotheses developed in Phase I are tested, using the methods validated in Phase II. The Phase III studies test the efficacy of an intervention in a group of individuals. The group is generally more homogeneous than the actual target population and may be chosen for considerations that facilitate research management rather than as a representative sample of a population. The study group is compared with a control group to whom no intervention is applied; or, different interventions are compared to one another and/or to a control group.

In Phase IV, *Defined Population Studies,* a preventive intervention efficacious in Phase III is applied in a carefully controlled study of a defined population. A Phase IV study is conducted in a large, distinct, and well-characterized population chosen in such a way that the study subjects are representative of, and therefore the results can be extrapolated to, the ultimate target population. The defined population may be characterized in terms of demographics, such as geographic location, occupation, education, socioeconomic status; vital statistics, such as incidence, morbidity, and mortality; personal or lifestyle factors, such as diet and smoking; genetic and biological characteristics; or other factors associated with disease. Usually the population will include all persons who have certain demographic characteristics and live within a specific geographic area. These characteristics allow for calculating risk factor rates (for example, smoking); incidence, morbidity, and/or mortality rates; and the changes that are estimated to result from the intervention. Phase IV studies further validate the methods developed in Phase II and the efficacy determined in Phase III, and they resolve new issues about the extrapolation of interventions to the larger population represented. At times, it may be efficient to merge Phase III and IV studies.

In Phase V, *Demonstration and Implementation,* studies introduce the proven intervention (from Phase IV) to a community at large and measure the public health impact. To ensure that the intervention is applied uniformly with the validated methods, a system of evaluation and quality control must be in place. These studies may be part of other public health programs, but evaluation and quality control procedures are still required.

Phase V programs are conducted only after careful research studies in each of the preceding phases produce results that justify demonstration and implementation. Therefore, at the completion of Phase V, a proven intervention with the demonstrated public health benefit of reducing cancer incidence, morbidity, or mortality would have been introduced in a population with known characteristics, and a process for monitoring the impact of the program would be in place.

Essential Research Concepts

Two research concepts are essential to the strategy of prevention research. First, human trials must be conducted to test the cause-and-effect relationship of an hypothesis. Second, the sum of research data must meet the epidemiologic criteria of causality before human trials may be conducted or follow the laboratory convergence plan (noted below) for analogues and synthetic agents.

RATIONALE FOR HUMAN TRIALS   Human trials often are the most rigorous way to test a hypothesis that an intervention will have a specified effect. Because of their prospective nature and controlled designs, trials provide a specificity not possible in epidemiologic studies (14); they provide direct evidence of whether animal studies are applicable to people, and whether people will comply with the intervention over the duration of the trial.

Descriptive epidemiologic studies often suggest useful hypotheses, and analytical epidemiologic studies add to the evidence. Still, in the dietary research area, it generally is not possible to separate out all of the possible confounding factors. For example, persons eating a diet rich in vegetables will be ingesting appropriate amounts of beta-carotene, vitamin A, and vitamin C; they also may be eating less fat than other people. Thus, it is difficult to assess the effect of single nutrients in this type of study. Dose levels and specific interactions also can be tested specifically in a clinical trial.

Behavioral research also can be done in clinical prevention trials. From the point of view of the specific trial, it is essential that a high percentage of study subjects participate in order to test whether the intervention has a biological effect. From the point of view of later applications, knowledge, attitudes, beliefs, and ability to modify behavior will influence the utility of the intervention for a larger population.

Prevention trials also may help to assess the time required for an intervention to achieve its effect, adverse side effects, or impacts on other diseases. For example, lowering dietary fat is likely to have benefits for both cancer and heart disease. For the purpose of reducing the individual risk for a spectrum of diseases, it is useful to be able to examine multiple trial end points.

The first benefits of present cancer prevention intervention trials will not become clear until the end of the 1980s. Current trials may show negative or uncertain results because they are in early stages and many design problems must be worked out. For example, the early trials have less information upon which to base selection of the intervention agent or study population than will later trials. Furthermore, these commonly are testing natural micronutrients. Any new synthetic agents for chemoprevention must be tested and shown to be safe. In laboratory studies, some of the synthetic agents are the most potent inhibitors of carcinogenesis, but these must undergo laboratory studies of safety and efficacy before they are brought into human trials. As more is learned about which human populations are most likely to benefit from the trials, it should be possible to design the studies to be more precisely aimed at the populations likely to benefit. Thus, as with early treatment trials, a broadly based effort is needed initially, with attention given to focusing the trials as further data become available.

THE CHEMOPREVENTION RESEARCH APPROACH

Chemoprevention was initiated as a major research program at NCI as a result of the recommendations on numerous working groups that met between 1978 and 1981 to investigate the feasibility of a research effort in clinical and experimental chemoprevention. As mentioned in preceding sections, chemoprevention is an approach to understanding the role of specific chemicals in the etiology and prevention of cancer. It is different from diet and cancer research in that the diet research focuses on changes in macronutrients or food classes (for example, fat or fiber) that may be added to or subtracted from the diet. Chemoprevention involves administering specific amounts of specific natural and synthetic chemicals (for example, vitamins). The purpose is to identify agents that will prevent, halt, or reverse carcinogenesis. Potential chemopreventive agents and their sources are as follows:

I. Naturally occurring substances and sources:
1. Beta-carotene—dark-green vegetables, yellow-orange vegetables;
2. Carotenoids—yellow-orange fruits;
3. Vitamin A—liver, dairy products, egg yolks;
4. Vitamin C—citrus fruits, tomatoes, certain vegetables;
5. Vitamin E—vegetable oils, whole grains, liver, beans, fruits, vegetables;
6. Vitamin B_{12}—liver, milk, eggs, lean meats, cheese;
7. Folate—leafy green vegetables, liver;
8. Selenium—seafoods, organ meats, some cereal products.

II. Synthetic agents:
1. Vitamin A retinoids, BHT;
2. BHA, protease inhibitors;

3. Prostaglandin synthesis inhibitors;
4. Indoles;
5. Uric acid.

The chemoprevention research plan involves a series of flows and arrays of three research components: laboratory, epidemiology, and human intervention (Figure 2). The research flow is sequential, and movement from phase to phase and array to array is controlled by a review at specific decision points. For example, when a research lead has met all criteria in the laboratory and epidemiologic arrays, a decision point is reached and the strength of the lead is evaluated. If it is strong enough, the lead could move into the human intervention array, in which human trials occur. The five phases of the human prevention array are equivalent to the five phases of the prevention research strategy. Phase I is information gathering. Previous studies in animals or humans are reviewed for information on effectiveness and side effects, parameters of exposure to the agent, available data bases, and end points and outcomes.

Phase II studies establish intake levels and safety for humans. For chemoprevention, this will involve pharmacologic studies. The issues of acceptability are pursued and related to the intake level and the dose of the intervention.

Phase III involves the conduct of human trials for efficacy and safety. (The terminology is analogous to Phase III of clinical treatment trials that conform to FDA regulations in the development of a new drug.) Randomized, controlled

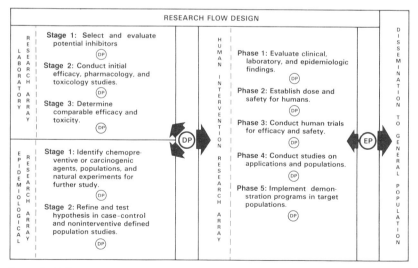

Figure 2   NCI chemoprevention program. DP = decision point; EP = evaluation point.

trials provide the most direct evidence of the preventive benefit of chemopreventive agents. In addition, the human trial, as it is formulated, will help define strategies for acceptance of a chemopreventive agent. Finally, trials will provide information on adverse effects and will allow consideration of risk-benefit relationships. The specific issues in Phase III relate to selection of the appropriate study population and the development of a protocol, taking into account the information on efficacy and safety. During the trial, ongoing analyses are made to ensure that if side effects occur, they are detected immediately and remedial action is taken. The analyses also focus on terminating the study early if the benefits are established at any point during the study.

The long-range goal often is application of the research leads to the population at large; therefore, Phase IV research is conducted not only on the effects of the intervention but also on the methods of intervention for large-scale application of preventive measures. Research on the method of intervention may be needed before initiating Phase IV. For example, the agent might be tested as a food additive in Phase IV rather than as a pill, as is usual in Phase III. The amount of chemopreventive agent that may be required for defined population studies, the availability of monitoring systems, the methods for assessing the outcomes of large population studies, and practical considerations regarding wide-scale use of the agent (such as cost/benefit) are the kinds of factors that must be considered during Phase IV and before conducting the population-wide studies appropriate in Phase V.

If an agent has shown efficacy in Phase III, and if the methods for applying this lead to large populations are successful (Phase IV), then, in Phase V, sufficient amounts of the agent must be produced, protocols must be developed, demonstration programs must be conducted, and both the acceptability and the adverse affects of this intervention must be monitored. Phase V studies will document the success of the intervention in the general population.

Research Leads

In this section we review the data for research leads in chemoprevention that were strong enough to enter the human intervention array. NCI's Chemoprevention Program is currently sponsoring 24 human intervention trials.

VITAMIN A, BETA-CAROTENE, RETINOIDS   To date, most of NCI's chemoprevention research has been to test the relationship among cancer and dietary vitamin A, beta-carotene, and retinoids. Retinoids include natural forms of vitamin A as well as synthetic derivatives that do not occur in nature. Beta-carotene is a precursor of vitamin A; it may be converted to vitamin A in the digestive tract and stored in the liver.

Whether the reduced cancer risk associated with beta-carotene is because of its conversion to vitamin A or because of its own effects is unknown. Beta-carotene is capable of quenching singlet oxygen and peroxides that are formed in the body, and carcinogens such as radiation may have their effect through singlet oxygen and peroxides. Retinoids are thought to interfere with the later stages of cancer development, but several mechanisms have been suggested. In skin cancer in mice, retinoic acid may inhibit the production of a key enzyme, ornithine decarboxylase, that enhances tumor promotion (8). Also, retinoids, by influencing the cell's protein synthesis, may directly compete for control of cell growth with agents that promote cancer (17, 67). Also, retinoids can block the effects of transforming growth factors that can cause cells to become cancerous (65).

Substantial laboratory and epidemiologic data have led to the current research of the relationship between vitamin A and cancer. The association between vitamin A and cancer was suggested in the 1920s when it appeared that a diet deficient in vitamin A might be the cause of stomach cancer in rats (18). A subsequent study found the stomach condition to be precancer rather than true cancer, but the link between vitamin A and cancer development was established (35).

An historically important study in chemoprevention was done by Lasnitzki in 1955; she developed a method for growing mouse prostate cells on a glass, transforming these cells to cancer cells by adding a carcinogen (methylchloranthene), and inhibiting the transformation by adding vitamin A (41). A later stage of cancer cell development was also inhibited by adding vitamin A. Subsequently, other research showed that retinoic acid inhibits the development of bladder tumors (4), mammary tumors (68, 69, 70), and skin cancer in mice (8). Animal studies clearly established the important principles that the effectiveness of a retinoid as a chemopreventive agent varies with the particular retinoid, the dose of the retinoid, the cancer-producing agent or carcinogen, the type of cancer, and the animal being studied (29, 44).

Natural retinoids have toxic effects in humans and animals, particularly at high doses. Researchers are trying to develop synthetic retinoids that are as effective as natural retinoids in inhibiting tumor growth, are less toxic, and are more site-specific. In addition, epidemiologic data support the vitamin A hypothesis. About 20 studies in various parts of the world suggest an inverse association between eating foods containing vitamin A or beta-carotene and various types of human cancer; risk is thereby reduced 30–50%. Graham, Mettlin, and colleagues have conducted nine retrospective dietary studies of vitamin A and cancer risk (20, 21, 23, 24, 49–53). Overall, they found a significantly increased cancer risk with decreasing vitamin A intake. The relative risks were modest; in most cases, the risk for the lowest intake group was approximately double that of the highest intake group. The authors speculated that vitamin A may have a protective effect against cancer in such organs as the lung, bladder, mouth, esophagus, larynx, breast, and uterine cervix, but may have an adverse effect in the prostate (21, 22). However, other studies of diet and prostate cancer have shown a protective effect for increasing vitamin A intake (5, 65). The Boston Collaborative Drug Surveillance Program has found that in over 800 cases of all types of cancer, there was a slight protective effect for men, but not for women, associated with use of vitamin A pills (66).

Two studies from Hawaii differ in their findings. A study correlating cancer incidence rates of the five major racial groups in Hawaii with their dietary intake of various nutrients, including vitamin A, found no relationship between vitamin A intake and cancer rate. Yet, using a case-control design comparing patients in these racial groups with noncancer controls, the same investigators showed that low vitamin A intake is associated with increased risk for cancers of the lung and lower urinary tract. The relative risks were small, but the amount of vitamin A did appear to affect the size of the risk. The vitamin A effect appeared to be smaller in men than in women (37, 38).

Several case-control epidemiologic studies show lower vegetable consumption or lower estimates of vitamin A intake among lung cancer patients than among controls. This relationship is supported by three cohort studies in which a negative association occurred between lung cancer and an index of vitamin A. The first study was by Bjelke, of 8278 Norwegian men (7). This study was updated and expanded; its findings were confirmed (40). Hirayama made a similar observation in a study of 265,118 Japanese adults during a ten-year period. He suggested that exsmokers might particularly benefit from daily vegetable consumption (30). Shekelle et al (64) found dietary beta-carotene to be inversely related to lung cancer in 2107 American men. Researchers have found a decreased risk for lung cancer in Singapore Chinese with a high carotene intake (47). Other scientists have reported that increased vitamin A, but not beta-carotene, protects against lung cancer in men but not women (26).

One of the first retrospective dietary studies showed that in both Norwegian and American patients with digestive tract cancers, decreased vitamin A intake was associated with an increased risk of colon cancer (6). The vitamin A intake of the cancer patients was lower than that of the noncancer controls with whom they were compared. In Japan, precancer of the stomach (gastric metaplasia), diagnosed by biopsy, was significantly associated with decreased consumption of vitamin A—lower than that in a control group who did not have cancer (57).

A study of diet and cancer of the mouth and throat revealed differences in adult food intake between women with cancer and normal women without cancer from the southern United States (76). The authors suggested that the protective effect seen for high consumption of fruits and vegetables is consistent with recent findings associating high intake of vitamins A and C with reduced risk of oral and throat cancers (50). Black men in Washington DC have a higher risk for cancer of the esophagus that is associated with low vitamin A intake; however, the low vitamin A intake is just one part of an overall poor nutrition (78).

Several prospective blood serum studies and more than ten retrospective studies have associated serum retinol levels with cancer risk. These studies compared the serum retinol levels of cancer patients with those of a matched population without cancer. With one exception, the retrospective studies found low vitamin A levels in the cancer patients. The one study that did not reach this conclusion did not use a comparison group without cancer (39).

Prospective studies in 1980 and 1981 reported an inverse correlation between cancer risk and total blood retinol in frozen, stored sera. Wald et al (71) followed 16,000 men from whom serum samples had been collected and stored. After 3–5 years of follow-up, 86 of the men had developed cancer. Kark et al (34) followed 3102 individuals from Evans County, Georgia, for 12–14 years. Serum vitamin A (retinol) levels were measured in the stored sera of 85 cancer patients and 174 matched controls. These also showed an inverse correlation between blood levels and cancers of various types. Later studies could not confirm these results. Willett et al (73) measured retinol-binding protein, vitamin E, and total carotenoids in serum collected in 1973 from 111 partici- pants in the Hypertension Detection and Follow-up Program who were free of cancer at the time, but diagnosed as having cancer during the subsequent 5 years. When compared to matched controls, no differences were found in mean values for retinol-binding protein or for total carotenoids.

The mixed evidence from studies of serum vitamin A is not suprising, since homeostatic control maintains serum retinol within a narrow range and serum levels may not reflect what is in the tissues (74). The failure to find a relation- ship to blood levels in the more recent studies may reflect in part the narrow range of differences between individuals. Except in marked deficiency states, blood retinol levels do not indicate total body load. More important is that concentration differences at the target tissues may be far more relevant, and these have not been examined. In most studies to date, only total carotenoids, rather than the active (and less stable) beta-carotene, have been measured. Beta-carotene varies with blood lipids and, depending on diet, may account for only one-fifth of the total circulating carotenoids. Thus, the validity of these studies of blood levels of retinol and carotene to test the question of a protective effect of dietary retinol and beta-carotene against cancer is uncertain. Perhaps newer laboratory techniques will improve the results of prospective studies based on frozen sera, but it seems that clinical trials will be needed to obtain a definitive answer on the benefits of these compounds.

In one preliminary intervention trial, Gouveia et al (19) examined the effect of the synthetic retinoid Etretinate on 34 heavy smokers with bronchial metaplasia. The index of metaplasia scores dropped significantly in the 12 study subjects who completed 6 months of treatment. This preliminary study will need confirmation because the number of cases is small and the precision of the metaplasia score is uncertain.

Vitamins C and E

Vitamins C and E (also called alpha-tocopherol) appear to prevent the formation of nitrosamines, potential carcinogens resulting from metabolic reactions in the human digestive tract of nitrates, nitrites, and substances readily found in foods. Nitrates react with amines or amides in the digestive tract to form nitrosamines and nitrosamides, respectively. Nitrites include nitrite salts, such as sodium nitrite, added to meat for color, flavor development, and control of bacterial contamination; nitrate salts, used in food processing, that are readily reduced to nitrite in the body; and nitrogen oxides derived from "smoking" processes. Fermentation processes, such as pickling or brewing, permit conversion of a variety of nitrogen sources, including ammonia and amino acids, to nitrite.

Vitamins C and E compete with the amine or amide for the nitrosating agent. If the vitamin reacts first with the nitrosating agent, the formation of nitrosamines and nitrosamides is blocked.

Studies are needed to determine whether there is a maximum safe dose for long-term consumption of vitamin C. There are limited studies on the long-term side effects of alpha-tocopherol. Reports of adverse effects in humans receiving high doses of vitamin E for long periods of time (more than two years) are not numerous and have not generally been supported by solid epidemiologic evidence (61, 62). However, safety from a rare side effect is difficult to prove. Findings indicating that vitamin E may have unfavorable effects in pregnant women are preliminary and require further study.

Laboratory and animal research shows that vitamin C as well as alpha-tocopherol block the formation of nitrosamines. In some studies, large doses of vitamin C have completely protected rats against chemically induced liver tumors and have partially protected them from lung and kidney tumors. Other studies (59) have shown that oral vitamin C was capable of blocking the formation of bladder tumors induced by implanted tablets of a chemical with cancer-causing potential. It is believed that vitamin C prevented the oxidation of the chemical from a potential to an actual carcinogen. In tissue culture studies, vitamin C appears to prevent or reverse chemically induced cancer (5). Extending the findings from these animal and laboratory studies to the human situation requires carefully designed epidemiologic studies and clinical trials.

Epidemiologic studies suggest that fruits and vegetables containing vitamin C may offer specific protection for the upper digestive tract. For example, studies in northern Iran suggest that diets low in fruits and vegetables may be responsible for the high incidence there of cancer of the esophagus and, more specifically, that diets very low in fresh fruits and vegetables may contribute to cancer of the esophagus (1, 12, 33). In studies reported in 1980 and 1983, biochemical analyses and dietary surveys suggested that dietary constituents or deficiencies may contribute to the incidence of cancer of the esophagus in certain Chinese provinces, particularly rural Linxian (77). Similar factors have been implicated for the high incidence of stomach cancer in Colombia and Chile. Japanese who eat yellow and green vegetables daily appear to have a lower risk of lung cancer than Japanese who rarely eat these types of foods. This is true for both smokers and nonsmokers (31).

Changes in cancer incidence associated with diet modification have been reported in studies of Japanese from areas with high stomach cancer risk who migrated to Hawaii. Although the migrants continued to have a high risk in Hawaii, this stomach cancer risk was lower among their offspring born in Hawaii. Some investigators suggest that the Western-style diet, including foods rich in vitamin C, may have contributed to this lowered risk. Some studies show that food groups containing not only vitamin C, but also vitamin A, folic acid, or dietary fiber, as well as non-nutrient components of food such as phenol, seem to offer protection against various human cancers.

Some studies have tried to assess which of several available food components is responsible for the effect noted. These studies have calculated vitamin C intake from food intake data. Kolonel (36) reported that low vitamin C intake was associated with an increased risk of stomach cancer in groups of men in Hawaii; however, the difference between groups was small. However, Jain (32) found no difference between calculated vitamin C intake of colon cancer patients and normal people without colon cancer. One study that used a marker of vitamin C intake was done in China (1). The average excretion of vitamin C in the urine (a marker of vitamin C intake) of inhabitants of a region with high rates for cancer of the esophagus was only one eighth or one ninth that of residents of a low-risk area.

Although current data from human studies do not strongly support an association of vitamin C with several types of human cancer, there are some cases where pharmacological doses of the vitamin may prove useful in preventing some cancers. For example, oral vitamin C may block the formation of at least two types of carcinogens in the human bladder by causing high levels of vitamin C in the urine (65). This approach might be worth testing for people with recurrent bladder cancer. Clinical trials will be needed to test this approach.

Another example where pharmacologic doses of the vitamin may prove useful is in achlorhydria patients, who have low levels of stomach acids. This lowered acidity favors the formation of nitrosamines. Vitamin C may be useful in blocking nitrosamine formation in these patients who are at high risk for stomach cancer.

Some people produce feces that contain mutagens, or gene-altering agents

(9). Whether a mutagen might initiate changes in the large intestine leading to colon cancer cannot be determined yet because the ability of any particular mutagen to cause cancer in animals has not been adequately tested. However, the close relationship of mutagens and carcinogens suggests that this mutagen may possibly cause cancerous changes in the colon. Since supplemental vitamin C plus vitamin E have been shown to reduce mutagen production (15), these agents might help prevent colon cancer in persons at high risk.

Vitamin B_{12} and Folate

As early as 1944, scientists have investigated the potential of folic acid, a B vitamin, to inhibit cancer development (42). More recently, studies have shown that folic acid (or folate) plays a key role in the maturation and differentiation of normal cells (10). Cervical dysplasia in women taking oral contraceptives was improved by folic acid. Thus, folate may prevent the progression of precancerous lesions and, in some cases, promote a reversal to normalcy.

Selenium

Selenium is an essential element; however, as is true of many essential elements, toxicity may result at high levels through abuse of nutritional supplements. Seafood, organ meats, and grains grown in some geographic areas are rich in selenium. Intake varies in different populations because of soil content and the amount of meat eaten. Much of the selenium in the body and blood may not be physiologically active.

Numerous animal experiments have shown that selenium has a chemopreventive effect. The relevance of most of these studies to cancer risk in humans is not clear, since the levels of selenium used far exceeded recognized dietary requirements and often approached toxic levels. However, one experiment has shown that selenium deficiency and high levels of dietary polyunsaturated fats increased susceptibility to chemically induced tumor formation, whereas a dietary supplement of selenium close to the physiological requirement offered protection. The role of dosages in the broad range between the apparently nutritionally adequate level and the higher, effective level used in many antitumor studies has not yet been adequately investigated. The incidence of chemically induced colon cancer and liver tumors in rats can be reduced by adding certain forms of selenium to the drinking water. There is sufficient evidence to warrant further research on the anticancer effect of selenium.

The epidemiologic evidence on the relationship between selenium and cancer comes from a number of geographical correlation studies that associate cancer risk with estimates of individual (per capita) selenium intake, with selenium blood levels, or with selenium concentrations in the water supply or soil. In the northeastern United States, high rates of colon, rectal, and breast cancer have been correlated with industrialization, high intake of fat, and low soil selenium. In most areas studied, there is an inverse relationship between selenium level and cancer. However, whether this is a cause-effect relationship cannot be determined because of confounding effects such as industrialization. Moreover, it is not clear whether this relationship applies to all cancer sites or only to specific ones, such as the digestive tract. Rigorous epidemiologic studies of selenium and cancer have not been reported, and the effects of dietary selenium supplements on subsequent cancer development have not been studied.

Data related to selenium intake are being collected now in studies in China, Finland, and other countries where people are receiving selenium supplements or have low selenium intakes.

NCI Chemoprevention Human Trials

The findings from these laboratory, animal, and epidemiologic studies and early clinical trials suggest that certain dietary factors, vitamins, and trace elements may be potential cancer inhibitors in humans. To test this potential, the NCI has funded human intervention trials. These are listed in Table 2 by target site, risk group, chemopreventive agent, and principal investigator.

Table 2 Human intervention trials

Target site/ organ	Target/high risk group	Inhibitory agents	Principal investigator/ affiliation
All sites	Physicians (healthy volunteers)	Beta-carotene	Charles Hennekens, Harvard Med. School Brigham & Women's Hospitals, Boston
All sites	Dentists (healthy volunteers)	Retinyl palmitate, selenium vitamins E, B_6	Charles Hennekens, Brigham & Women's Hospitals, Boston
Cervix	Cervical dysplasia	Trans-retinoic acid	Earl A. Surwit, Univ. Ariz. Health Sci. Center, Tucson
Cervix	Cervical dysplasia	Retinyl acetate	Seymour Romney, Albert Einstein Coll. of Med., NYC
Cervix	Cervical dysplasia	Folic acid	Joseph Chu, Fred Hutchinson Cancer Res. Center, Seattle
Esophagus	General population from high risk area	Multiple vitamins and minerals	Philip Taylor, William Blot, NCI, Bethesda, MD; The Cancer Inst., Chinese Acad. Med. Sci., Beijing
Esophagus	Esophageal dysplasia	Multiple vitamins and minerals	Philip Taylor, William Blot, NCI, Bethesda, MD; The Cancer Inst., Chinese Acad. Med. Sci., Beijing

Table 2 *(continued)*

Target site/ organ	Target/high risk group	Inhibitory agents	Principal investigator/ affiliation
Colon	Familial polyposis	Vitamins C, E, wheat bran	Jerome DeCosse, Memorial Hospital for Cancer and Allied Diseases, NYC
Colon	Colon polyps	Beta-carotene	Phyllis Bowen, Univ. Ill., Chicago
Colon	Colon polyps	Beta-carotene, vitamins C, E	Robert Greenberg, Dartmouth Coll., New Hampshire
Lung	Persons with asbestosis	Beta-carotene (synthetic), retinol (vitamin A)	Gilbert S. Omenn, Fred Hutchinson Cancer Res. Center, Seattle
Lung	Asbestos	Beta-carotene (synthetic), Retinol	J. McLarty Tyler, Texas
Lung	Chronic cigarette smokers; discontinued cigarette smokers	Retinol; beta-carotene (synthetic)	Gary E. Goodman, Fred Hutchinson Cancer Res. Center, Seattle
Lung	Middle-aged smoking men	Beta-carotene (synthetic) vitamin E	Jussi Huttunen, Olli Heinonen, Natl. Public Health Inst. of Finland, Helsinki; Demetrius Albanes, NCI, Bethesda, MD
Lung	Chronic smokers	Vitamin B_{12}, folic acid	Carlos L. Krumdieck, Univ. Alabama, Birmingham;
Lung	Smoking men	Beta-carotene (synthetic)	Lewis Kuller, Univ. Pittsburgh
Skin	Basal cell carcinoma/ actinic keratoses	Retinol	Thomas Moon, Univ. Ariz., Tucson
Skin	Albinos	Beta-carotene (synthetic)	Gideon Luande, Muhimbili Med. Center, Tanzania
Skin	Basal cell carcinoma	Beta-carotene, vitamins C, E	Bijan Safai, Memorial Hospital for Cancer, NYC
Skin	Basal cell carcinoma, male military and VA hospital patients	13-*cis*-retinoic acid	Joe Tangrea, NCI, Bethesda, MD
Skin	Basal cell carcinoma	Beta-carotene (synthetic), retinol	Robert Greenberg, Dartmouth College, New Hampshire
Skin	Basal cell carcinoma, squamous cell carcinoma	Retinol 13-*cis* retinoic acid	Frank Meyskens, Univ. Ariz., Tucson

Literature Cited

1. Ackerman, L. V., Weinstein, I. B., Kaplan, H. S. 1978. Cancer of the esophagus. In *Cancer in China,* ed. H. S. Kaplan, P. J. Tsuchitaui, pp. 111–36. New York: Liss
2. Armstrong, B., Doll, R. 1975. Environmental factors and cancer incidence and mortality in different countries with special reference to dietary practices. *Int. J. Cancer* 15:617–31
3. Deleted in proof
4. Becci, P. J. 1978. Inhibitory effect of 13-cis retinoic acid in urinary bladder carcinogenesis induced in C57BL/6 mice by N-Butyl-N-(4-hydroxybutyl) nitrosamine. *Cancer Res.* 38(12):44–64
5. Benedict, W. F., Wheatley, W. L., Jones, P. A. 1982. Difference in anchorage-dependent growth and tumorigenicities between transformed C3H/10T1/2 cells with morphologies that are or are not reverted to a normal phenotype by ascorbic acid. *Cancer Res.* 42:1041–45
6. Bjelke, E. 1974. Epidemiologic studies of cancer of the stomach, colon, and rectum; with special emphasis on the role of diet. *Scand. J. Gastroenterol.* 9:1–53
7. Bjelke, E. 1975. Dietary vitamin A and human lung cancer. *Int. J. Cancer* 15: 561–65
8. Boutwell, R. K. 1982. Retinoids and inhibition of ornithine decarboxylase activity. *Am. Acad. Dermatol.* 6:796–98
9. Bruce, W. R., Varghese, A. J., Furrer, R., Land, P. C. 1977. A mutagen in the feces of normal humans. In H. H. Hiatt, J. E. Watson, J. D. Winsten, *Origins of Human Cancer, Book C: Human Risk Assessment,* ed. pp. 1641–46. Cold Spring Harbor: Cold Spring Harbor Lab.
10. Butterworth, C. E., Hatch, K. D., Gore, H., Mueller, H., Krumdieck, C. L. 1982. Improvement in cervical dysplasia associated with folic acid therapy in users of oral contraceptives. *Am. J. Clin. Nutr.* 35(1):73–82
11. Carroll, K. K. 1975. Experimental evidence of dietary factors and hormone dependent cancers. *Cancer Res.* 35:3374–83
12. Cook-Mozaffari, P. J., Azordegan, F., Day, W. E., Ressicaud, A., Sabai, C., Aramesh, B. 1979. Oesophageal cancer studies in the Caspian littoral of Iran: Results of a case-control study. *Br. J. Cancer* 39:293–309
13. Dales, L. G., Friedman, G. D., Ury, H. K., Grossman, S., Williams, S. R. 1978. A case-control study of relationships of diet and other traits to colorectal cancer in blacks. *Am. J. Epidemiol.* 109:132–44
14. DeWys, W. D., Greenwald, P. 1983. Clinical trials: a recent emphasis in the prevention program of the National Cancer Institute. *Semin. Oncol.* 10(3):360–64
15. Dion, P. W., Bright-See, E. B., Smith, C. C., Bruce, W. R. 1982. The effect of dietary ascorbic acid and alpha-tocopherol on fecal mutagenicity. *Mutat. Res.* 102:27–37
16. Doll, R., Peto, R. 1981. The causes of cancer: Quantitative estimates of avoidable risks of cancer in the United States today. *J. Natl. Cancer Inst.* 66:1193–1308
17. Elias, P. M., Williams, M. L. 1981. Retinoids, cancer and the skin. *Arch. Dermatol.* 17:160–82
18. Fujimaki, Y. 1926. Formation of cancer in albino rats on deficient diets. *J. Cancer Res.* 10:469–77
19. Gouveia, J., Mathe, G., Hercend, T., Gros, F., Lemaigre, G., Santelli, G. 1982. Degree of bronchial metaplasia in heavy smokers and its regression after treatment with a retinoid. *Lancet* 1 (8274):710–12
20. Graham, S., Dayal, H., Swanson, M., et al. 1978. Diet in the epidemiology of cancer of the colon and rectum. *J. Natl. Cancer Inst.* 61:709–14
21. Graham, S., Haughey, B., Marshall, J., et al. 1983. Diet in the epidemiology of carcinoma of the prostate gland. *J. Natl. Cancer Inst.* 70:687–92
22. Graham, S., Lilienfeld, A. M., Tidings, J. E. 1967. Dietary and purgation factors in the epidemiology of gastric cancer. *Cancer* 20:2224–34
23. Graham, S., Marshall, J., Mettlin, C., et al. 1982. Diet in the epidemiology of breast cancer. *Am. J. Epidemiol.* 116:68–75
24. Graham, S., Mettlin, C., Marshall, J., et al. 1982. Dietary factors of the epidemiology of the larynx. *Am. J. Epidemiol.* 116:68–75
25. Greenwald, P. 1985. Prevention of cancer. In *Cancer: Principles & Practice of Oncology,* ed. V. T. DeVita, Jr., S. Hellman, S. A. Rosenberg, 1:197–214. Philadelphia: Lippincott. 2nd ed.
26. Gregor, A., Lee, P. N., Roe, F. J. C., et al. 1980. Comparison of dietary histories in lung cancer cases and controls with special reference to vitamin A. *Nutr. Cancer* 2:93–97
27. *Health Consequences of Smoking: Can-*

cer. A Report of the Surgeon General. 1982. Washington DC: US DHHS, Off. on Smoking and Health, DHHS (PHS) 82–50179

28. Helms, P., Jorgensen, I. M., Paerregaard, A., Bjerum, L., Poulsen, L., Masbech, J. 1982. Dietary patterns in Them and Copenhagen, Denmark. *Nutr. Cancer* 4(1):34–40

29. Hill, D. L., Grubbs, C. J. 1982. Retinoids as chemopreventive and anticancer agents in intact animals (review). *Anticancer Res.* 2:111–24

30. Hirayama, T. 1979. Diet and cancer. *Nutr. Cancer* 1:67–81

31. Hirayama, T. 1977. Epidemiological evaluation of the role of naturally occurring carcinogens and modulators of carcinogenesis. In *Naturally Occurring Carcinogens, Mutagens and Modulators of Carcinogenesis,* ed. E. C. Miller, et al, pp. 359–80. Baltimore: University Press

32. Jain, M., et al. 1980. A case-control study of diet and colorectal cancer. *Int. J. Cancer* 26:757–68

33. Joint Iran-Int. Agency for Res. on Cancer Study Group. 1977. Esophageal cancer studies in the Caspian littoral of Iran: Results of population studies—a prodrome. *J. Natl. Cancer Inst.* 59:1127–38

34. Kark, J. D., Smith, A. H., Switzer, B. R., et al. 1981. Serum vitamin A (retinol) and cancer incidence in Evans County, Georgia. *J. Natl. Cancer Inst.* 66:7–16

35. Klein, A. J., Palmer, W. L. 1941. Experimental gastric carcinoma: A critical review with comments on the criteria of induced malignancy. *J. Natl. Cancer Inst.* 1:559–84

36. Kolonel, L. N., et al. 1981. Association of diet and place of birth with stomach cancer incidence in Hawaii Japanese and Caucasians. *Am. J. Clin. Nutr.* 34:2478–85

37. Kolonel, L. N., Hankin, J. H., Lee, J., et al. 1981. Nutrient intakes in relation to cancer incidence in Hawaii. *Br. J. Cancer* 44:332–39

38. Kolonel, L. N., Nomura, A. M., Hinds, M. W., et al. 1983. Role of diet in cancer incidence in Hawaii. *Cancer Res.* 43:2397s–2402s

39. Kummet, T., Meyskens, F. L. Jr. 1983. Vitamin A: A potential inhibitor of human cancer. *Sem. Oncol.* 10(3):281–89

40. Kvale, G., Bjelke, E., Gart, J. J. 1983. Dietary habits and lung cancer risk. *Int. J. Cancer* 31(4):397–405

41. Lasnitzki, I. 1955. The influence of a hyper-vitaminosis on the effect of 20-methylcholanthrene on mouse prostate glands grown in vitro. *Br. J. Cancer* 9:438–39

42. Leuchtenberger, C., et al. 1944. Folic acid: A tumor growth inhibitor. *Proc. Soc. Exp. Biol. Med.* 55:204

43. Liu, K., Stamler, J., Moss, D., Garside, D., Persky, V., Soltero, I. 1979. Dietary cholesterol, fat, and fibre, and colon cancer mortality. *Lancet* 2:782–85

44. Lower, G. M., Kanarek, M. S. 1981. Retinoids, urinary bladder carcinogenesis, and chemoprevention: A review and synthesis. *Nutr. Cancer* 3:109–15

45. Lubin, J. H., Burns, P. E., Blot, W. H., Ziegler, R. G., Lees, A. W., Fraumeni, J. F. Jr. 1981. Dietary factors and breast cancer risk. *Int. J. Cancer* 28:685–89

46. Lyon, J. L., Gardner, J. W., West, D. W. 1980. Cancer incidence in Mormons and non-Mormons in Utah during 1967–75. *J. Natl. Cancer Inst.* 65:1055–61

47. MacLennan, R., Da Costa, J., Day, N. E., et al. 1977. Risk factors for lung cancer in Singapore Chinese, a population with high female incidence rates. *Int. J. Cancer* 20:854–60

48. MacLennan, R., Jensen, O. M., Mosbech, J., Vuori, H. 1978. Diet transit time, stool weight and colon cancer in two Scandinavian populations. *Am. J. Clin. Nutr.* 31:S239–42

49. Marshall, J., Graham, S., Byers, et al. 1983. Diet and smoking in the epidemiology of cancer of the cervix. *J. Natl. Cancer Inst.* 70:847–51

50. Marshall, J., Graham, S., Mettlin, C., Shedd, D., Swanson, M. 1982. Diet in the epidemiology of oral cancer. *Nutr. Cancer* 3:145–49

51. Mettlin, C., Graham, S. 1979. Dietary risk factors in human bladder cancer. *Am. J. Epidemiol.* 110:255–63

52. Mettlin, C., Graham, S., Priore, R., et al. 1981. Diet and cancer of the esophagus. *Nutr. Cancer* 2:143–47

53. Mettlin, C., Graham, S., Swanson, M. 1979. Vitamin A and lung cancer. *J. Natl. Cancer Inst.* 62:1435–38

54. Miller, A., Kelly, A., Choi, N., Matthews, V., Morgan, R., Munan, L., et al. 1978. A study of diet and breast cancer. *Am. J. Epidemiol.* 107:499–509

55. Modan, B., Borel, V., Lubin, F., Modan, M. 1975. Low fiber intake as an etiologic factor in cancer of the colon. *J. Natl. Cancer Inst.* 55:15–18

56. National Cancer Inst. 1986. *Cancer control, objectives for the nation, 1985–2000. J. Natl. Cancer Inst.* In press

57. Nomura, A., Yamakawa, H., Ishidate, T., et al. 1982. Intestinal metaplasia in Japan. Association with diet. *J. Natl. Cancer Inst.* 68:401–5

58. Phillips, R. L., Snowdon, D. A., Burton, N. B. 1983. Cancer in vegetarians. In

Environmental Aspects of Cancer: The Role of Macro and Micro Components in Food, ed. E. L. Wynder, G. A. Leveille, U. H. Weisburger, Ch. 5, pp. 53–72. Westport, CT: Food and Nutrition Press

59. Pipkin, G. E., et al. 1969. Inhibitory effect of L-ascorbate on tumor formation in urinary bladders implanted with 3-hydroxyanthranilic acid. *Proc. Soc. Exp. Biol. Med.* 131:522–24

60. Reddy, B. S., Hedges, A., Laakso, K., Wynder, E. L. 1978. Fecal constituents of a high-risk North American and a low-risk Finnish population for the development of large bowel cancer. *Cancer Lett.* 4:217–22

61. Roberts, H. J. 1981. Perspectives on vitamin E as therapy. *J. Am. Med. Assoc.* 246:129–31

62. Salkeld, R. M. 1979. Safety and tolerance of high dose vitamin E administered in man: A review of the literature. OTC 150121. *Fed. Reg.* 44(53):16169–73

63. Deleted in proof

64. Shekelle, R. B., Liu, S., Raynor, W. J. Jr., et al. 1981. Dietary vitamin A and risk of cancer in the Western Electric Study. Lancet 2:1185–90

65. Schlegel, J. U. 1975. Proposed use of ascorbic acid in the prevention of bladder carcinoma. *Ann. NY Acad. Sci.* 258:432–37

66. Schuman, L. M., Maudell, J. S., Radke, A., et al. 1982. Some selected features of the epidemiology of prostatic cancer: Minneapolis-St. Paul, Minnesota, case control study, 1976–1979. In *Trends in Cancer Incidence: Causes and Practical Implications,* ed. K. Magnus, pp. 345–54. Washington/New York/London: Hemisphere Publ. Corp.

67. Smith, P. G., Jick, H. 1978. Cancers among users of preparations containing vitamin A. A case control investigation. *Cancer* 42:808–11

68. Sporn, M. B. 1980. Retinoids and cancer prevention. In *Carcinogenesis—A Comprehensive Survey. Modifiers of Chemical Carcinogenesis,* ed. T. J. Slag, pp. 99–109. New York: Raven

69. Sporn, M. B., Newton, D. L. 1981. Recent advances in the use of retinoids for cancer prevention. In *Cancer Achievements, Challenges and Prospects for the 1980s,* ed. J. H. Burchenal, H. G. Dettgen, pp. 541–48. New York: Grune & Stratton

70. Thompson, J. H., et al. 1980. Inhibition of 1 - Methyl - 1 - 1 - nitrosourea - induced mammary carcinogenesis in the rat by the retinoid axerphthene. *Arneim.-Forsch./Drug. Res.* 30–2(7):1128

71. Wald, N., Idle, M., Boreham, J. 1980. Low serum vitamin A and subsequent risk of cancer. Preliminary results of a prospective study. *Lancet* 2:813–15

72. Welsh, S. O., Marston, R. M. 1982. Review of trends in food use in the United States: 1909–1980. *J. Am. Dietet. Assoc.,* 81(2):120–28

73. Willett, W. C., Polk, F., Underwood, B. A., Stampfer, M. J., Pressel, S., et al. 1984. Relation of serum vitamins A and E and carotenoids to the risk of cancer. *N. Engl. J. Med.* 310(7):430–34

74. Willett, W. C., MacMahen, B. 1984. Diet and cancer—An overview, Parts 1 and 2. *N. Eng. J. Med.* 310:633–38, 697–703

75. Deleted in proof

76. Winn, D. M., Ziegler, R. G., Pickle, L. W., Gridley, G., Blot, W. J., Hoover, R. N. 1984. Diet in the etiology of oral and pharangeal cancer among women from the southern United States. *Cancer Res.* 44:1216–22

77. Yang, C. S., Sun, Y. H., Yang, Q. P., Miller, K. W., Li, K. Y., et al. 1984. Presented at Vitamin A and Cancer Prevent. Conf., NIH, Bethesda, Feb. 28–29, 1984

78. Ziegler, R. G., Morris, L. E., Blot, W. J., et al. 1981. Esophageal cancer among black men in Washington, D.C. II. Role of nutrition. *J. Natl. Cancer Inst.* 67:1199–1206

Ann. Rev. Public Health. 1986. 7:293–312

MEDIATING SOLUTIONS TO ENVIRONMENTAL RISKS

Sam Gusman

P.O. Box 2231, Taos, New Mexico 87571

Philip J. Harter

Suite 404, 2301 M Street NW, Washington DC 20037

INTRODUCTION

Regulatory and other legal processes have been used increasingly since the mid 1960s to make decisions concerning the management of public health risks. These processes tend to require specific findings of "fact" on the nature and degree of risk as a predicate to further action. Since a finding acts as a switch that will turn on or off future activity or liability, the stakes can be extraordinarily high in reaching the "right" result from the perspective of the respective parties. That in turn forces each one to take a more absolute position than the actual scientific base of information usually can bear.

Instead of supporting a unitary, unqualified conclusion, the science involved in risk assessment almost always contains significant uncertainties in terms of what is unknown because of a lack of data and in terms of the limitations of our current knowledge. The way we make many decisions involving assessment of environmental risks, in the face of inherently incomplete knowledge and a range of technical judgments, carries within what is represented as "fact" a substantial element of judgment and decision making. Whether intended to be or not, these judgments and decisions can have an immense bearing on subsequent decisions and events (17, 19).

Since the issues are so frequently cast in this kind of technocratic mode, it is often difficult under the common arrangement to reconcile the interested parties' varying perceptions of risk and their varying reactions to it. In short, it is difficult under the common arrangements to reconcile the differing and often competing values of our society.

293

0163-7525/86/0510-0293$02.00

Further, developing an appropriate course of action often requires a practical insight into the various options that are available for addressing and controlling risk. The context in which risk management decisions are usually made, however, can raise barriers to the full exploration of options.

The result, therefore, is frequently one of estrangement. Some will feel that decisions do not pay enough heed to science, or that legitimate concerns are not adequately heard, or that the means of making such decisions is not appropriate for making subtle but important political choices. Sometimes the major problem is that there is no suitable forum at all for making the decision so that it is made by default—the status quo is permitted to exist for lack of a means of changing it.

Direct negotiations among those who would be substantially affected by the outcome can sometimes be used to meet these concerns. Under appropriate circumstances, the affected parties may be in a better position than traditional decision makers—be it a court, an agency, or a legislative body—to establish the relevant information that can then form the basis of an enlightened political decision. In these cases, the parties will be able to determine what information is necessary for a reasonable decision; develop a "feel" for the range of uncertainty or of opinion on the technical issues; bring to bear a practical insight into the potential responses and their consequences, both positive and negative, from each vantage point; and actually develop a program for action under existing law that will be accepted politically and meet the needs of those who must live with it. In short, in such cases direct negotiation can provide a practical and effective means for coupling risk assessment with risk management.

All that sounds too good to be true. And, alas, it undoubtedly is, at least as a categorical matter applicable to all environmental risks. But we are gaining experience and insight into the use of direct negotiations to make complex decisions addressing environmental risks, and thus far it is quite promising. This paper reviews some of that experience and distills the criteria that will help predict whether the use of direct negotiations among those who will be affected by the outcome is likely to be an appropriate means for making the decision.

VARYING PURPOSES OF NEGOTIATION

Direct negotiations have been used successfully at virtually every stage of a controversy over environmental issues. They sometimes focus on only one aspect of environmental risk, such as the policy of what to do in response to a perceived risk or in determining the nature and extent of the risk. Sometimes they address the full range of issues. The nature of the discussions, the processes that are followed, who needs to be there, and the likelihood of success—indeed even the measure of success itself—may vary along with the purpose of the negotiations. Hence a clear notion is important at the outset of negotiations regarding what the goals of the undertaking are to be. Some different kinds of goals for negotiation are described below.

Even if negotiations do not lead to an agreement on a specific issue, they may still have substantial utility by making the parties more keenly aware of each others' needs and interests, thus enabling future controversies between them to be faced with broader understanding. Moreover, participants in negotiations can and do establish working relationships that can be used over time to resolve other issues.

Policy Recommendations

Policy dialogues generally involve discussions among a range of interests that could be expected to be antagonistic with respect to a major policy issue. The participants usually, but not invariably, take part in the discussions as individuals as opposed to official representatives of an interest, but they are invited to participate precisely because they are expected to articulate the position of the interest from whence they come. The discussions among them build on their collective expertise and practical insight as they identify the significant aspects that should be addressed and the actions that should be taken and by whom.

Often those with the power to make the decisions do not themselves participate in the discussions. Then, the purpose of the policy dialogue is to publicize the conclusions of the dialogue or to make recommendations to those who have decisional authority.

Establish Policy

Instead of making recommendations to those with the power to decide, the group itself may *de facto* have that power. In this case, the purpose and outcome of the negotiations will be to develop a general policy that will be followed in the future. The policy dialogue that resulted in the recommendation to create a private sector organization to facilitate the cleanup of toxic waste dumps was such an enterprise and resulted in the creation of Clean Sites, Inc. (6).

Another example is a dialogue among environmentalists, church representatives, and representatives of the major producers of pesticides in the United States. The dialogue was conducted with the understanding that agreements would be implemented voluntarily by statements of trade association policy and by individual member company actions. This group reached consensus on advertising practices to reduce misuse of pesticides in developing nations (7). The top ten US exporters of pesticides are among the association's member companies that have adopted the trade association policy statements as corporate policy. The group has continued its work and recently reached consensus on labeling practices for pesticides to be used in developing nations.

Develop Underlying Facts

Direct negotiations have also been used at the other end of the scale: deciding the "facts" about a particular issue. The quotation marks are to emphasize that in these matters the facts may be disputed and seen quite differently by the various parties. Thus, direct discussions concerning them can be of significant help in putting the matter into perspective. The Food and Drug Administration and the Environmental Protection Agency, for example, regularly convene advisory panels to review the factual basis of a pending issue. The value of these panels is both their technical expertise and also the variety of the viewpoints their members represent.

Lest anyone fear this would sell science short by submitting it to a plebiscite, it should be noted that scientists themselves have a potent voice in such matters. Indeed, a major purpose is to afford the interested parties the opportunity to raise the topics they believe are important and should be addressed. This approach, therefore, is not one to suppress good science but rather to provide a way of identifying, obtaining, and understanding the information that will be used in the course of making decisions on the management of risk.

The value of such an undertaking is to provide a forum to explore the issues by probing what is known, what is assumed, what the weaknesses are in the data, and what is unknown. It can also identify what remains to be done. For example, the Consensus Workshop on Formaldehyde, consisting of scientists from academia, government, industry, and public interest groups, "defined the consensus concerning a number of major points in formaldehyde toxicology and . . . identified a number of major deficits in understanding which are important guides to future research" (5).

Make the Decision

Direct negotiations among the parties have always played a major role in settling litigation. Indeed, the vast majority—more than 90%—of all lawsuits are either withdrawn or settled through negotiations among the parties (16). Some of these cases involve complex environmental issues. The lawsuit then provides the backdrop against which the parties negotiate a settlement, since each will need to bear in mind the potential outcome of that suit during the course of the negotiations.

But lawsuits frequently cram complex technical issues into strange molds to be determined under legal rules that are often only tangentially relevant to the real issues. One wonders, for example, whether it really was a concern for the endangered snail darter that led to the opposition to the Teleco Dam or whether the legal protection accorded it was a convenient weapon for those otherwise opposed (19). The power of direct negotiations is that they permit the parties to focus squarely on their actual concerns and attempt to work out a mutually satisfactory solution to the matter.

Direct negotiations among the interested parties have been used to resolve contentious environmental disputes involving particular sites. Some of these negotiations are to settle pending litigation, and some are conducted without suit having been filed but clearly looming in the background. In either event, the threat of litigation or some formal process is often an important part of the dynamics of the negotiations. As an illustration, the threat of delay that would result from litigation was an important reason for the corporate interests in at least one negotiation to sit down and meet with its opposition, even though it was confident that it would eventually win in court. Negotiations have resolved a wide variety of difficult environmental issues, including the environmental conditions that should be placed on a uranium mine, the placement of a hydroelectric generating station on a scenic part of the Hudson River, pollution resulting from a town dump, and the retrofitting of electric generating facilities to convert them from oil to coal (2, 3, 25).

In 1982 the Administrative Conference of the United States, a government agency charged with making recommendations to agencies on how to improve the process by which they make regulatory decisions, formally recommended procedures for negotiating proposed regulations (19). These recommendations contemplate that once some interested party—likely to be the agency itself, but sometimes a major party—believes a regulatory issue would be appropriately developed through direct negotiations, a neutral third party (called the convener) will conduct a review to determine whether the conditions for a successful negotiation, as described below, are met.

If it appears that these conditions are met, the agency would publish a notice that it is contemplating use of the regulatory negotiation process. The notice would invite comments on that decision as well as participation in the negotiations by those who would be substantially affected. The convener would likely serve as the mediator for the group as it identifies the issues, determines what facts are necessary for their resolution, develops those facts, negotiates an agreement on the regulatory issues, and prepares a document the agency can use as a foundation for a notice of proposed rulemaking. This course has been followed in the two EPA regulatory negotiations described below.

As to those issues not resolved during negotiation, the group may decide either to say it was unable to reach agreement or to announce the range of viewpoints. Both options are important and have materialized in actual negotiations. In the benzene negotiations described below, for instance, the parties chose to report only that they were unable to reach agreement, while at the Federal Aviation Administration, the group decided to submit a range of alternatives to the agency when it was unable to develop a single recommendation (9, 14).

In contrast with these examples, direct negotiations may be among government agencies with the authority to implement the agreement that emerges.

Historically, securing that kind of coordination among agencies has often been quite difficult, even rare. What the negotiation framework provides is a means to address environmental issues that cut across the jurisdictional lines of several agencies. A specific case is the negotiation among four local jurisdictions, four agencies of the State of Oregon, and four agencies of the federal government to develop plans, acceptable to all, for the development of port facilities—and the limitations on such development—in the estuary of the Columbia River (18). The complex agreement had no legal status in itself, but its language started to be used soon after the agreement was reached in the official plan submitted by the local jurisdictions to the state.

Direct negotiations, as indicated by this example, have the potential for actually creating politically viable agreements and decisions, and thus present a situation in which the parties may seek forums in which to embody agreements in law rather than forums in which to continue to attack each other.

WHEN TO NEGOTIATE

Parties will always seek to use whatever process for making decisions that they think will improve their own position. Thus, if a party believes it will be better off for using litigation or a traditional rulemaking proceeding or stonewalling, it is likely to attempt to direct the activity to that process. A frequently glossed over characteristic of direct negotiations is that they will only lead to an agreement when all the parties want this to happen. This is likely to be the case when:

COUNTERVAILING POWER   The outcome is genuinely in doubt because there is sufficient countervailing power among the parties so that each party is checked by another. This can, for example, be the case when the parties have been in conflict for a long time and have reached a *de facto* stalemate. In other instances, one of the parties may actually have the authority to make the ultimate decision, such as a government agency's authority to issue a regulation or a company's decision to build a plant. This putative ability may be illusory, however, when others have enough political clout or sufficient power of some other sort to make it clear that the decision cannot be made without incurring unacceptable costs. In general, when the outcome is in doubt for whatever reason, direct negotiation can be attractive since it provides the parties with the opportunity to avoid truly unacceptable outcomes. Uncertainty is a powerful motivation toward use of negotiation and avoidance of processes in which all may possibly be lost.

PARTIES   The parties that would be substantially affected by the outcome of the negotiations and who are necessary for its successful implementation are willing to participate or at least to not oppose the negotiations. Moreover, those parties need to be such that individuals can be selected to represent them, if not in a formal sense at least in such a way that their voice will be representative of the parties.

ISSUES ARE RIPE   The issues are ripe and ready for decision. Negotiating is hard work, and parties are not likely to undertake it unless they believe the issues are going to be resolved, if not by negotiation then by some other way. Moreover, issues need to be sufficiently crystallized that the group can address a specific problem. Groups are not particularly adept at grappling with a topic lacking in definition.

MULTIPLE ISSUES   A group of related issues has simultaneously surfaced, all affecting the same parties, and all in need of resolution. This can be helpful to a negotiation since the parties will frequently not all place equal weight or value on the same issues. Then a consideration of all the issues creates opportunities for each party to obtain in negotiations much of what it wants on the issues of highest importance from its viewpoint. It may be much more difficult to secure agreement when only one issue is presented.

DEADLINE   There is a realistic deadline. Any negotiation benefits from a deadline. That is certainly true in the abstract since no party will make its hard choices until it must. It is no coincidence that labor negotiations regularly settle a little past a midnight strike deadline. Moreover, in environmental issues, some party is likely to benefit from the status quo. Thus, having a deadline, in the form of some decision being made in the near future unless an agreement is reached, adds an important sense of urgency—"we *must* make a decision *now*"—and goes a long way to reducing potential for use of negotiations as a stalling tactic.

NO FUNDAMENTAL ISSUE   Parties are not called upon to negotiate any issue that they hold as a fundamental, basic value. By their very nature, such issues are not the stuff of compromise. Thus, negotiations need to be structured so as to avoid confronting such issues, or negotiations themselves may be inappropriate and some other means used to reach a decision. This is not to say that major, important issues cannot be negotiated, only that what is negotiated cannot go to the core of a party's very existence.

Negotiations are less likely to be appropriate if some authoritative determination is required that has legal significance in and of itself. Then, it may be necessary to use a traditional legal process for making the decision. For example, a party may believe that a particular case may set important legal precedent and, therefore, may be unwilling to enter into negotiations. Or, some party may want to make a point—"see, we told you we were right"—that can only come through the kind of hierarchical decision that is made by a court or an agency.

Sometimes, however, the fact that a legal process is required may wrongly suggest that negotiations are inappropriate. For example, if a permit is required before some action can be taken, it may clearly be appropriate to negotiate its terms and conditions with those interested and affected; though at least some form of a formal legal process may also be required, if all the parties are at the negotiating table and agree, the formal process should hold no surprises and the matter would be quickly resolved. This was the case after the Columbia River estuary negotiations when the state promptly approved locally recommended planning designations.

OTHER PROCEDURAL ISSUES

The desired outcome of negotiations is a "consensus" among the parties. Unfortunately, consensus is an elusive term. Its meaning can range from a simple majority to unanimity among all the participants (19). The parties to a negotiation can, of course, define it any way they choose. But its definition can have an important bearing on the negotiations themselves, and even on whether a party is willing to participate, since it determines the extent of a party's power. A party may fear that its position will not be given credence, that it lacks the resources to take on other participants, or that it will be on the losing side if "consensus" means anything other than "unanimity."

Unanimity is clearly a stringent definition, but it is the one usually used in environmental negotiations. This, of course, makes it difficult to achieve agreement, since any individual would have a veto. One way of dealing with this situation is to interpret consensus as meaning unanimity of interest groups rather than individuals. Then the parties can be consolidated into interest groups that can explore their own interests in caucuses before returning to the negotiating table. The caucuses can sometimes be a better forum to resolve the problems of dissenting individuals than would a meeting of the negotiating group as a whole.

Requiring unanimity can also have a powerful effect on coalescing a negotiating group since it provides an incentive for finding ways to deal with everyone's interests and needs. Each party must then decide whether, on the whole, it is better off with the agreement than without it. Without unanimity, parties can delude themselves into believing they can pick and choose among the issues that were discussed when, in fact, agreements are usually crafted so as to make the various parts of the agreement interdependent. If one party seeks to change or delete one part of an agreement, other parties will likely want to change other parts or repudiate the agreement as a whole.

A mediator (sometimes called a facilitator) can be significantly helpful in resolving complex, multiparty issues. A mediator is usually a rigorously neutral person who helps bring the parties together for the discussions and is dedicated to the process of the negotiations. The mediator's duties can include: building trust among the parties; helping the parties identify their own and the others' interests; helping frame the issues both within the respective parties and across the table; exploring alternative negotiating options by meeting with the parties and preparing outlines that serve to join the issues; and bringing the parties close enough together so that it is "safe" for them to talk directly and to express viewpoints openly.

A mediator has no independent power, however. It remains for the parties themselves to agree or disagree by means of their own negotiations. The purpose of the mediator is to help that process. The likelihood that a mediator will be helpful is directly proportional to the complexity of the negotiations themselves. That complexity can arise through the difficulty of the issues themselves, through the parties' unfamiliarity with direct negotiations (so the mediator serves an educational role), or through the parties' mutual antagonism.

If the parties to the negotiations are not in a position themselves to implement the resulting agreement, there must be some basis for them to expect that it will actually be implemented by those with the power to do so. Nonetheless, there are numerous examples of negotiations for which implementation did not occur. Perhaps this is a part of the infamous "not invented here" phenomenon, where an agency with the power to implement resists input from others. Perhaps it is part of the perennial optimism regarding the speed of implementation, which infects many areas of human endeavor. Especially with public policy issues, however, many forces are at work and implementation often should not be expected immediately.

It is therefore important at the outset of a negotiation to develop a "delivery system" to ensure that those in power will look favorably on the outcome if consensus is reached. That may mean, for example, having a commitment from the person with the authority to make the decision that he or she will adopt the consensus unless there is "good cause" not to do so; it may mean the agency's staff participates; it may mean the group as a whole has to be willing and able to wield sufficient pressure to make it happen; it may mean understanding at the outset that the consensus of the group will simply be one of the factors that influence long-term policy development (as in the case of the hazardous waste siting handbook described in the next section). But, without a before-the-fact understanding of the kind of implementation desired, the members of the group may ultimately be frustrated by what is perceived as an effort come to naught.

CASE EXAMPLES

Several detailed case examples will illustrate different kinds of anticipated outcomes of negotiation and different situations that may be encountered. Such illustration requires some description of the interest at stake and the nature of the substantive outcome.

Hazardous Waste Siting

The issues at stake in siting new hazardous waste management facilities touch central human desires of people in host communities for a healthy and pleasant environment and the concern that these will be threatened if a hazardous waste site is built nearby. The problems arise because of the inescapable generation of some residuals in industrial processes by which countless useful products are manufactured and the need to discard some of these residuals as wastes. Lacking a broad consensus on the policies that should govern siting, it is not surprising that serious controversies between host communities and would-be developers frequently arise.

It is easy to conclude that a national consensus is needed on ways to manage hazardous industrial residuals adequately and in a manner perceived as fair, but much harder to develop that consensus. From one point of view, each of the policy negotiations and dialogues on these issues can be viewed as a discrete activity, and one can examine each with respect to specific consequences. From another viewpoint, however, they all are a part of the ongoing, and as yet incomplete, process of developing a national consensus on the issues.

One underlying problem is that resolution of almost any aspect of the hazardous waste disposal controversy involves a balancing of a widely distributed benefit (the availability of products whose manufacture or use generates a hazardous waste) versus costs and risks that are concentrated on those few people who live near hazardous waste treatment or disposal facilities (2).

Mediation has not been used often to resolve specific hazardous waste siting controversies. Substantially more effort has been devoted to negotiation that seeks to set the policy framework within which specific siting controversies can be addressed (2).

Several of the earliest negotiations—policy dialogues—on hazardous waste siting policy among participants with highly diverse interests and positions on the issues were convened by The Conservation Foundation, the Keystone Center, and The New England Council during 1980 through 1983. These dialogues resulted in the preparation of a number of consensus statements in the form of a report or handbook (8, 20, 21, 23).

Taken together, these reports do not provide an unquestioning or unqualified consensus expression of need for new hazardous waste management facilities. To illustrate, immediately after acknowledging a need for "new and better" hazardous waste management facilities, The Conservation Foundation's hazardous waste dialogue group handbook went on to say, "As an initial step to reduce the risks posed by hazardous wastes, great effort should be directed toward insuring that the amount of hazardous wastes requiring special handling be reduced to the greatest extent possible through end-product and raw-material substitutions, treatment, recycling, and reuse. Disposal oriented options should be used as a last resort."

This kind of concern about the amount of hazardous waste that needs to be placed in the environment—raising the possibility of an expanded role for treatment, recycling, and reuse options—introduced an element of uncertainty into the debate about need for new hazardous waste disposal facilities.

There are other kinds of uncertainty also. For example, some confusion results from differing definitions of "hazardous waste" and, as a result, differing estimates of just how much hazardous waste is being generated (24). In these circumstances it can be hard to know how big the disposal problem is and how compelling the need is for new facilities. In assessing obstacles to siting of treatment facilities, the New England Council report mentioned both a lack of reliable information and the paralyzing effect of uncertainties.

The importance of efforts to reduce the generation of hazardous wastes has been brought into clearer focus by the work of a recent National Research Council Committee on Institutional Considerations in Reducing the Generation of Hazardous Industrial Wastes. Its final report, published in 1985, concluded that significant opportunities exist to reduce the generation of hazardous waste (4).

One of the Keystone dialogues addressed directly the question of whether new facilities are needed. Its report stated,

> Complete agreement among those who attended the Keystone workshop was not obtained on the issue of whether thorough consideration of the need for a proposed facility is a proper topic for a siting process. There was substantial agreement, however, that the question of need will be vigorously debated by a broad cross section of the community near a proposed site. Indeed, the group recognized that even if a new TSD (treatment, storage, disposal) facility were generally "needed" from a regional or state perspective, its "need" in the local area might still be contested by residents near the proposed site. The group generally felt, therefore, that a good siting process would accommodate serious discussion of the need for the proposed facility.

The New England Council report identified five major obstacles to siting new hazardous waste management facilities: obstacles to cooperation (for example, distrust of one another's motives), the paralyzing effect of uncertainties, insufficient public perception of the need for new treatment facilities, concern about lack of leadership by government officials, and, finally, a strong feeling that industry and government officials did not appreciate the feelings or perceptions that led to resistance to most siting attempts. The report also identified three broad strategies to help site new facilities: more reliable information and consistent policies, development of new "collaborative" entities to promote education, understanding, and cooperation, and clarification of the goals and strategies of government, especially state governments, in the siting process.

The Conservation Foundation Handbook includes a series of more than 100 detailed questions that the members of a dialogue group, comprised of private citizens, representatives of environmental and public interest groups, trade associations, industries and state government, agreed were important to ask as part of a continuing dialogue among all concerned parties to a siting process.

Recent policy dialogues have focused in greater detail on quite specific aspects of the overall problem. For example, Keystone Center decided to convene a dialogue group to address the issue of compensation for exposure to toxic substances (22). Another recent activity, also convened by the Keystone Center, took the handbook approach one step closer to the problems on decision making at individual sites. In 1984, as a result of the work of a Keystone Center dialogue group with special focus on the Galveston Bay area, a handbook was published by the Texas Department of Water Resources (26). It describes a siting process for new hazardous waste facilities in Texas that takes into account the particular problems and institutional arrangements in that area.

Other relevant, recent initiatives, all too recent to evaluate, have involved the development of institutional arrangements at the state level. Three states— Massachusetts, Rhode Island, and Wisconsin—have enacted legislation that specifically deals with negotiation between developers and local communities on hazardous waste siting issues (2). The Massachusetts statute is illustrative. It provides for mediation, but in the event the parties fail to reach agreement, a state-level council may declare an impasse and require binding arbitration of unsettled issues. The Rhode Island and Wisconsin statutes are similar in the sense that they also involve a referral to arbitration in the event that negotiations fail to reach across-the-board agreement between a host community and a would-be developer.

Overall, our review suggests that the time is not yet ripe for a national consensus on siting of specific new hazardous waste facilities to emerge with so broad a base of support as to allow substantial use of consensual mediation processes. It also suggests that the need at present is for additional dialogue on policy issues (such as public access to information, compensation for injury, reduction of waste generation, and the roles of state and local governments in siting controversies) to further define the framework within which specific siting decisions will be made in the future.

Site Cleanup

Quite a different history surrounds use of negotiations for decision making about the cleanup of abandoned hazardous waste disposal sites. A nearby dump site that is suddenly recognized as a hazard understandably engenders controversy about cleanup: how much money should be spent for cleanup, who should pay, what priority should be given to cleaning up that particular site now (as compared with cleaning up other sites), and what standards should be used for the cleanup. The local community may not trust the cleanup operation or its standards of final cleanup, but if the site is recognized as posing a threat, the community has incentives to want the job done soon and done well.

The Comprehensive Environmental Response, Compensation and Liability Act (CERCLA) is a 1980 federal statute that established a fund, widely known as Superfund, for cleanup. The initial implementation of this law was the subject of intense controversy. Allegations have been made of programmatic delays and negotiated private party cleanup agreements intended to keep Superfund expenditures low so that Congress would not need to reauthorize the fund in 1985 (1). The way CERCLA was implemented at the Environmental Protection Agency ultimately contributed to a change of leadership at EPA.

During the past few years, EPA has developed a more aggressive stance toward use of Superfund resources for site cleanup. It has invested in site-specific "remedial investigation" and "feasibility" studies to obtain a detailed assessment of physical conditions at sites and of alternative options for cleanup. Completion of these studies at a site is generally expected to occur prior to the start of cleanup, thus preventing what EPA has perceived as lengthy and inconclusive negotiations caused by inadequate knowledge of site conditions (1).

In an extensive review of CERCLA implementation and its relations to negotiation procedures, Dean Anderson points out that cleanup will be very slow, even under EPA's new policies intended to accomplish orderly, prompt cleanups. Anderson argues that negotiation could be used to improve the efficiency, lower the cost, and accelerate the cleanup rate of the CERCLA program. He proposes two reforms: first, that "EPA should modify its policies to encourage private party cleanups without recourse to the Fund (Superfund)" and, second, that "alternate dispute resolution techniques," of which environmental mediation and policy dialogue are prominent parts, "should be mobilized to provide this encouragement" (1).

Independently, another initiative has recently been taken by private parties, starting a process by which the first—and perhaps also the second—of Anderson's two proposed reforms may come to fruition. Sponsored by The Conservation Foundation, a policy dialogue among prominent members of the environmental community and the chemical industry led to publication of a consensus report (6) during 1984 entitled "Clean Sites and Private Action—A Plan to Accelerate Private Hazardous Waste Cleanup." This report acknowledges the necessity of governmental involvement and leadership while stating also that "Superfund legislation and the activity it creates cannot solve the hazardous waste problem alone in a satisfactory time frame." It proposes formation and funding of a new, independent nonprofit corporation, Clean Sites, Inc. (CSI), to be funded initially through a combination of foundation and industrial grants.

This policy dialogue, recommending the formation of a new institution, has had unusual impact. Clean Sites, Inc. is now a reality and has started its work. It would appear from its operating principles that it will foster negotiations, perhaps mediated negotiations, among potentially responsible parties to apportion liability.

CSI, in its operating principles, states that it would be "fully accountable to the public through a number of mechanisms, including the competence, integrity, and independence of its board and its careful attention to the interests of affected communities." These principles also state that its board "can be expected to use a variety of mechanisms to ensure that affected communities have confidence in the technical data that are used in cleanup plans and in the cleanups themselves." These commitments suggest that CSI will seek to bring all parties into direct negotiations on site cleanup issues.

Anderson, in discussing alternate processes for resolving disputes, offers additional insight into how this may develop. He reports on an interview with Lois Gibbs, President of Citizens Clearinghouse for Hazardous Wastes and a former Love Canal area representative (1).

> (She) stated that the key to citizen acceptance of a site remedy proposed by government or industry is review and approval of the clean-up plan by a technical consultant whom citizens trust, citing experience at the Bruin Lagoon at Kennerdell, Pennsylvania, the General Electric site at Fort Edwards, New York, and the Stringfellow site at Riverside, California. She added that complete removal does not remain the citizens' remedy of choice when this condition is satisfied.

Regulatory Negotiation

BENZENE   The Occupational Safety and Health Administration (OSHA) of the US Department of Labor issued a temporary emergency standard in 1977 to regulate the occupational exposure to benzene. Soon thereafter it issued a permanent standard. The first was overturned by the Court of Appeals and the second by the Supreme Court. Subsequently, several unions and public interest groups petitioned OSHA in 1983 to begin a rulemaking proceeding that would result in a new benzene standard. By that time, benzene had a long and particularly bitter history before OSHA.

OSHA denied the request for a new emergency temporary standard but announced that it would conduct a rulemaking proceeding on an expedited basis, promising to have a proposed standard in less than six months and a final standard in less than a year—an enormously compressed timetable for OSHA standards. It simultaneously announced that it was going to explore the use of mediation to develop the standard. OSHA then retained two mediators with complementary experience.

While it appeared in the abstract that the parties had a great deal to talk about and that the benzene standard met the criteria for direct negotiations, the mediators recommended against using the process to develop the draft standard because of the tight schedule OSHA had set for itself. No one wanted to take the responsibility for derailing that effort, and hence each felt it would be inappropriate to rely on an untested process, especially one that spawned substantial doubts in the face of such controversy. Given the history of the standard, it is not surprising that each side was highly skeptical that anything would come of direct discussions.

A meeting was held with a number of the parties and the head of OSHA to review the findings and to discuss the possibility of holding future discussions. Interestingly, that was the first time the various competing parties had met together to discuss their views on the benzene standard even after years of proceedings. The upshot was that OSHA's staff would proceed independently to develop its proposed standard, while the unions and the companies would meet again to explore whether they could develop their own recommendation to OSHA. OSHA agreed, however, that it would give any resulting consensus substantial weight when developing its notice of proposed rulemaking.

Representatives of the four major unions whose members would be affected by a benzene standard met several weeks later with representatives of the affected industries. OSHA's staff did not participate because of the schedule. The beginning of the meeting was unquestionably tense. The unions presented an outline of the provisions they would like to see in the new standard. That was followed by an exploration of the issues raised. The discussion focused on the practical aspects of various items. It afforded an exchange of ideas and concerns that is extremely rare in OSHA proceedings. The industry side presented its proposal at the next meeting, and it too was followed by clarifying discussions. The issues were joined in the third meeting.

Although the parties agreed that benzene could cause significant adverse health effects, they disagreed about the extent of the risk at low exposures. Given the dissention over the risk assessment, the parties focused on its management: They attempted to put it into overall perspective and then concentrate on what should be done in response to the risk, whatever its magnitude. They were able to rely on the technical work being done by OSHA that provided an analysis of the risk, the exposures, and the potential controls. The parties to the benzene discussions came up with creative proposals to meet the respective needs.

The negotiators were able to work out a tentative agreement across the board on a proposed standard and to submit it to their principals for ratification.

Unfortunately, for complex reasons generally outside the subject of the negotiations, the draft was not ratified and discussions were adjourned.

The parties had agreed at the outset that they viewed the standard as an interrelated whole and not a collection of free-standing parts, and hence they also agreed that they would either submit an entire proposed standard to OSHA or nothing. The group therefore was only able to report that it was unable to reach agreement. But so was OSHA. OSHA not only missed its deadline, but as of this writing, it is nearly two years behind schedule.

The experience offers us several lessons about the negotiation of complex, highly controversial technical issues. The first is that traditionally antagonistic parties can meet together and have productive discussions in good faith. Second, the negotiations should be viewed in the context in which they operate: That OSHA too failed to come out with a proposed rule removed an important deadline and also demonstrated the difficulty of the issues. Third, even if agreements are not reached at the end of negotiations, the parties may leave the table with useful insights into each other's needs that can aid the resolution of the issues at a later date and in another forum.

EPA REGULATORY NEGOTIATIONS   The Environmental Protection Agency announced in February 1983 that it was interested in using regulatory negotiation "to explore the extent to which face-to-face negotiations among interested parties could serve as a useful supplement to its current rulemaking process" (10). To that end, it solicited suggestions for potential topics to be the subjects of the negotiations. After receiving numerous suggestions, both from outside parties and from the staff, the agency settled on two topics: non-conformance penalties under the Clean Air Act and emergency exemptions under the Federal Insecticide, Fungicide, and Rodenticide Act (FIFRA).

EPA established a "Resource Pool" consisting of funds provided by the agency and some contributed by private entities. As described in the protocol that governed its use, its purpose was to provide the resources for "short term research and technical analysis for the group as a whole and by individual interests" and "to defray extraordinary expenses of participation for parties who would not otherwise be able to participate in the negotiations." For example, the first negotiating group decided that it would help its discussions to retain the services of a statistician to analyze the effects of various proposals. The second group decided to defray the travel expenses of some of the parties to attend the meetings.

The purpose of EPA's first regulatory negotiation was to develop a formula that would determine the penalties to be imposed on the manufacturers of heavy duty truck engines that fail to meet the emission control requirements of the Clean Air Act. The negotiating committee consisted of representatives of manufacturers, operators, importers, state agencies, environmentalists, and EPA itself.

The major issues to be considered in these negotiations centered on what cost factors should be included in calculating the penalties. The large companies wanted as many factors as possible to be included so they, who everyone assumed would be the technology leaders and hence not subject to the penalties, would not be at a competitive disadvantage for incurring the extra cost of meeting the requirements. The smaller manufacturers, who were more likely to be the laggards and hence subject to the penalty, wanted the penalties to be as low as possible. The environmental interests wanted to make sure that EPA would set stringent standards and not postpone their effective date to permit the slower companies to catch up before requiring compliance with a tight standard. Thus, they were interested in providing a safety valve that would enable EPA to set a low requirement while not putting out of business, the companies that were unable to meet it immediately. Moreover, they were interested in a formula that would fit with the overall strategy for implementing the Clean Air Act.

Together, the group determined which factors should be considered in calculating the penalty and how it would be applied. The Committee met several times in plenary sessions and much more frequently in working subgroups that addressed individual components of the rule. As with benzene, the parties explored alternative approaches and their potential effects. They reached a consensus on a proposed rule that EPA published in a *Notice of Proposed Rulemaking* (10).

Very few comments were received in response to the *Notice,* showing that the major issues had been raised and resolved satisfactorily during the negotiations. Less than six months later, EPA issued a final rule based on the negotiations (12). All in all the process went remarkably smoothly.

EPA's second regulatory negotiation concerned the procedures EPA would use in granting exemptions to state and federal agencies from certain requirements under the Federal Insecticide, Fungicide, and Rodenticide Act (FIFRA) to meet emergency conditions. The Committee consisted of representatives of 21 organizations including environmental groups, agricultural interests, pesticide manufacturers, and state and federal agencies, as well as the head of EPA's pesticide division. The parties agreed at the outset to ground rules, which provided in part (13):

> The Committee will make every effort to reach a total consensus on all issues. To the extent a consensus is reached on any issue, EPA is committed to using the agreement as the basis for a proposed rulemaking. The agreement reached will take the form of proposed regulatory language that will be signed by all parties. Specific offers and statements made during the negotiations will not be used by other parties as the basis for future litigation. The representatives attending any Committee meeting must be authorized to represent their organization.

The Committee identified 17 key issues that needed to be addressed and broke into three working groups to do so. The first focused on "Definition of Emergency and Crisis." The second was concerned with "Implementation."

And the third addressed "Health and Safety Considerations," including such items as how EPA should consider risk, how residues should be evaluated, and how to deal with chemicals for which the data are inadequate. The working groups met separately to develop tentative positions on their assigned topics and the results were then considered in plenary sessions of the whole Committee. The full Committee reached consensus not only on a proposed rule but also on its accompanying preamble. EPA then published the consensus as a notice of proposed rulemaking.

Thus, both of the EPA projects were able to reach consensus on proposed rules. Both did so in less than six months. In each, the parties were able to identify the significant issues raised by the regulation, develop the information necessary for their resolution (neither required the development of significant scientific material, however), and craft a politically acceptable result.

FLIGHT DUTY TIME   The Federal Aviation Administration is required to issue regulations governing the maximum periods of time that pilots may fly or otherwise be on duty and the minimum periods of rest that must come between their times on duty. The rule proved to be enormously controversial. The FAA had issued more than 1000 pages of interpretations of the regulation and had tried several times during the past 30 years to revise it, only to be frustrated in the attempt. It decided to use the regulatory negotiation approach in its latest effort, and it convened a committee of representatives of large and small airlines, pilots, public interest groups, and other aircraft operations, as well as several from the FAA itself (9, 14).

Several proposals were put forward during the negotiations by different interests and were discussed by the group as a whole. The participants were able to tell what the others "could live with" sometimes by what was not said more than by any affirmative agreement. The group was ultimately unable to reach a consensus on a single proposal, however. The various proposals together bounded the problem, and hence served to define a "region of acceptability." The negotiators left it up to the FAA to develop a single proposal within that range.

The FAA did so and submitted it to the committee for its review. The group concurred that it should be published as a *Notice of Proposed Rulemaking*. Given the controversial history of the rule, the comments on the notice were remarkably sparse—showing that most of the significant comments had been addressed in the actual negotiations. The FAA was then able to publish a final rule (15). While that alone is significant, it is even more significant that the agency has not been sued over the rule—something that is virtually assured for any rule of major consequence. Thus, the negotiations were able to reconcile the overall needs in an acceptable manner.

CONCLUDING REMARKS

We speak of mediation as if it were newly arrived on the scene. And, in a sense, it is. But negotiation of the issues dividing people is so prevalent in society as to be taken for granted and be a nearly invisible part of everyday discourse.

Then what is new about mediation? It is the context of its use that is new. In the United States, the formation of public policy has increasingly involved a jousting among experts (usually lawyers) representing clients' interests—and somehow the ethics of the courtroom have spilled over into this larger arena. It is almost as though all parties accept, without question, the necessity of a posture that involves arguing their cases to their client's strongest advantage. This posture is surely appropriate if there is an authority figure present that is willing and able to make wise decisions.

It is less appropriate if there is no such authority available—as is often the case for public health issues when different governmental agencies each hold a part of the jurisdictional pie. It is also less appropriate when procedural requirements indicate that the authority—perhaps a judge bound by legal precedents—may arrive at a legally correct decision, but perhaps not a wise one from the point of view of the substance of the issues on the table. Despite such defects, the adversarial system has mostly served its purposes well, and is certainly so well engrained as to be accepted, usually, as a matter of course. So, perhaps it is not so strange that the posture of the negotiator—involving a search not only for solutions that are acceptable from one's own point of view but which, by definition, must also be acceptable to other parties—has usually not come to mind naturally.

This is now changing. Increasingly, there is recognition that in some situations direct negotiation among the parties can offer advantages to each and, often, a net gain for society as a whole. We have presented some of the situations in which this may be the case. We have also described the ways in which negotiations can proceed, the role of a neutral third party as mediator, and some of the kinds of issues for which negotiation is a promising decision-making process. Finally, we have used several recent case examples to illustrate these points. In our view, mediated negotiation is increasingly accepted as a useful procedure, though still underutilized because many people still are not sure enough or sufficiently aware of the situations in which it can work to their advantage. We hope we have made it clear, by describing just where and when mediated negotiation may be useful, that there are situations in which it is the procedure of choice and others where it is not.

Our expectation is that the substantial recent interest in mediated negotiation will provide an ever broader number of people in decision-making roles with a better basis to make such distinctions. Then, mediated negotiation will simply be another procedural option—one among many—that is routinely considered when public policy controversies need resolution. There is a road yet to be traveled to reach that place.

Literature Cited

1. Anderson, F. R. 1985. Negotiation and informal agency action: The case of Superfund. Report to the Administrative Conference of the United States. *Duke Law J.* 85:261–380
2. Bingham, G., Miller, D. S. 1984. Prospects for resolving hazardous waste siting disputes through negotiation. *Natural Resources Lawyer* 17:473
3. Bingham, G. 1986. *Resolving Environmental Disputes.* Washington DC: The Conservation Found. In press
4. Committee on Institutional Considerations in Reducing the Generation of Hazardous Industrial Wastes. 1985. *Reducing Hazardous Waste Generation—An Evaluation and a Call for Action.* Washington DC: Natl. Acad. Press.
5. Consensus Workshop on Formaldehyde. 1984. *Environ. Health Perspect.* 58: 323–81
6. The Conservation Foundation. 1984. *Clean Sites and Private Action.* A consensus report by the Steering Committee on Hazardous Waste Clean-up. Washington DC: Convervation Found.
7. The Conservation Foundation. 1983. *Guidelines for advertising practices in the promotion of pesticide products in developing areas of the world.* Press release prepared by the Agr. Chem. Dialogue Group, accepted by Natl. Agr. Chem. Assoc.
8. The Conservation Foundation. 1983. *Siting Hazardous Waste Management Facilities, A Handbook.* Members of the Hazardous Waste Dialogue Group. Washington DC: Conservation Found.
9. Eisner, N. 1984. Regulatory negotiation: A real world experience. *Fed. Bar J.* 31:371–76
10. Environmental Protection Agency. 1985. Control of air pollution from new motor vehicles and new motor vehicle engines, nonconformance penalties for heavy-duty engines and heavy-duty vehicles, including light-duty trucks. Notice of proposed rulemaking. *Fed. Reg.* 50: 9204–30
11. Deleted in proof
12. Environmental Protection Agency. 1985. Nonconformance penalties for heavy duty engines. Final Rule. *Fed. Reg.* 50:35, 374–401
13. Environmental Protection Agency. 1985. Exemption of federal and state agencies of use of pesticides under emergency conditions. Notice of proposed rulemaking. *Fed. Reg.* 50:13, 944–59
14. Federal Aviation Admin. 1984. Flight time limitations and rest requirements for flight crew-members. Notice of proposed rulemaking. *Fed. Reg.* 49:12, 136–45
15. Federal Aviation Admin. 1985. Flight time limitations and rest requirements. Final rule. *Fed. Reg.* 50:29, 306–22
16. Galanter, M. 1983. Reading the landscapes of disputes: What we know and don't know (and think we know) about our allegedly contentious and litigious society. *UCLA Law Rev.* 31:4–71
17. Gusman, S. 1981. Mixing science and politics. *The Environ. Prof.* 3:195
18. Gusman, S., Huser, V. 1984. Mediation in the Estuary. *Coastal Zone Manage. J.* 11:273
19. Harter, P. J. 1982. Negotiating regulations: A cure for malaise. *Geo. Law J.* 71:1–118
20. Keystone Center. 1980. *Siting Non-Radioactive Hazardous Waste Management Facilities, An Overview.* Final report of the first Keystone Workshop on managing non-radioactive hazardous wastes. Keystone, Colo.: Keystone
21. Keystone Center. 1981. *Siting Non-Radioactive Hazardous Waste Management Facilities, A Second Look.* Final report of the second Keystone Workshop on siting non-radioactive hazardous waste management facilities. Keystone, Colo.: Keystone
22. Keystone Center. 1985. *Potential Approaches for Toxic Exposure Compensation: A Report on the Conclusions of a Keystone Center Policy Dialogue.* Keystone, Colo.: Keystone
23. The New England Council. 1983. *Toward A Solution.* The New England Hazardous Waste Siting Congress, Boston: New Engl. Council Inc.
24. Office of Technology Assessment. 1983. *Technologies and Management Strategies for Hazardous Waste Control.* Washington DC: US GPO
25. Talbot, A. R. 1983. *Settling Things.* Washington DC: Conservation Found.
26. Texas Department of Water Resources. 1984. *The Keystone Siting Process Handbook—A New Approach to Siting Hazardous Waste Management Facilities.* LP-194. Austin: Texas Dept. of Water Resources

Ann. Rev. Public Health. 1986. 7:313–35
Copyright © 1986 by Annual Reviews Inc. All rights reserved

GEOGRAPHIC ANALYSIS OF DISEASE AND CARE

Melinda S. Meade

Department of Geography, University of North Carolina at Chapel Hill, Chapel Hill, North Carolina 27514

The importance to health of customs of diet, dress, types of settlement and housing and of physical environmental factors such as climate, vegetation, altitude, and topography have been widely recognized since the time of Hippocrates' *Airs, Waters, and Places*. Geographical variation has been studied as geographic pathology, medical ecology, medical topography, geographical epidemiology, geomedicine, and other rubrics, but only in the past 30 years has the discipline of geography itself applied its perspective and methodology to the study of health, disease, and care. After presenting an introduction to the field, I address some of the major geographic questions as they apply to medical geography and offer an explanation and critique of the methodology and theory currently being used to answer them.

THE SUBDISCIPLINE OF MEDICAL GEOGRAPHY

Disease has long drawn some attention in geography's general role of providing information on the location of facts and events together with general knowledge of environmental conditions. The emergence of a systematic interest in medical geography can be dated from the first report of the Commission on Medical Geography (Ecology) of Health and Disease to the International Geographic Union in 1952, which has recently been published (25). It was another 15 years before the work of May in the United States (52, 53), Shoshin in the Soviet Union (83), Sakamoto-Momiyama in Japan (78), Jusatz in Germany (47, 75), Sorre in France (86), Learmonth in Great Britain and India (57), and others had resulted in the emergence of a subdisciplinary focus. It was five to ten years

313

0163-7525/86/0510-0313$02.00

more before comprehensive books of readings, research monographs, and the first texts defined its dimensions (6, 21, 51, 56, 65, 67, 70, 72, 80). The history and development of present trends in medical geography and its status in various countries today have also been reviewed elsewhere (7, 60, 64, 71), most notably in a recent festschrift to Andrew Learmonth (57).

Medical geography's strengths and weaknesses are those of its larger discipline. Geography is an integrative discipline whose practitioners conceptualize issues as readily at the global scale as at the microscale of a neighborhood or residential compound. Geographers are concerned with the character of places, with man-land relationships, spatial distributions, and differentiation of areas and formation of regions. Geography draws facts, concepts, and techniques freely from other social sciences. It views itself as a bridge to the natural sciences, having once been synonymous with meteorology, geology, and botanical discovery. Since true integration is so seldom achieved, one consequence for the discipline has been a tendency to fractionation. Geography has two major traditions, both sharing the special geographic methodologies of mapping and regionalizing.

The first tradition is concerned with man-land (or in today's terminology human-environmental) relations. It has evolved from "environmental determinism" (hot, wet climates cause lethargy and poor health) to "possibilism," in which the environment sets the ultimate constraints (one cannot get mosquito-transmitted diseases at 15000 feet elevation) but interacting cultural forms are varied, to a "cultural ecology" in which human existence is inextricably interwoven with the biosphere. The dimension of medical geography that developed from this tradition is concerned with such things as the malarial consequences of converting rain forest into agricultural land for population resettlement or the consequences of the shift in industrial structure in the US for siting of toxic waste contamination of air and water.

The second tradition is concerned with spatial analysis, or the explanation for variation over the earth's surface of almost anything. The trend over time has been from describing to explaining to, recently, optimizing locational decisions on the basis of the explanation. In medical geography this tradition has resulted in studies of phenomena as varied as the distribution of mortality, hospitals, and herbal remedies. The explanation has sometimes drawn upon the man-land tradition, but more often has rested on aggregate, ecological associations. The most theoretically advanced body of knowledge within geography lies in optimizing economic locational decisions, such as where to site a new industrial plant or construct a new interstate highway link. In American geography, the numerically largest group of medical geographers has found challenge and employment in locational analysis of the health care system.

The special and basic tool of geography has for centuries been the map. In recent times this has been most evident to the health profession in the form of various atlases of mortality (43, 75, 82). Statistical mapping for analytical purposes is much less known outside of the discipline. Dot distribution maps and choropleth maps (in which each areal data unit, such as a country, is shaded by its interval class) are widely used in public health studies, although they are sometimes poorly designed. Howe's (43, 44) sophisticated cartography, depicting population size, urban and rural location, and statistical significance of the differences in rates on incidence maps, contains enormous information that few nonspecialists have the ability to interpret—a matter that has greatly limited its utility. Maps of probability of occurrence using Poisson distributions for less common diseases (58, 96), trend surface mapping to generalize a pattern for analysis (2, 70), and the common two-factor maps using shading on two scales to depict such distributions as standardized death rates and median income levels simultaneously are seldom used outside the discipline. Forster (23) has pointed out the distortion of mapping population data on an areal base, but the use of population-based maps in which the size of the unit is proportional to the size of the population has been limited by the general lack of lay knowledge about how to make and interpret them.

A map is a powerful tool. It is a model of the world that through the use of line, point, and area symbols can integrate many dimensions of reality. Developments in computer technology are presently revolutionizing cartography. Many sources of social, economic, and health data are becoming available on a geocoded basis; that is, for areas which have been delimited with x and y coordinates. Patient addresses can now be sorted into census tracts. Satellite imagery of water pollution and changes in vegetation can be accessed and processed with microcomputers. A long-standing problem for medical geography has been the lack of location for data. It is common for health records on public files to have no addresses, for example, and data reported by economic class or by race are classified or even sampled in such a way as to remove the spatial dimension. Now computer cartography, remote sensing, and quantitative methodology are coming together into a specialization in *Geographic Information Systems.*

The focus of most research in geography is on accounting for spatial variation. Much of the remainder is concerned with integrating all the variation at a point or area to explain the character of places. Rather than proceed to review the literature in terms of the above traditions, I prefer to address them implicitly within a framework provided by five major geographic questions posed by Amedeo & Golledge (1, p. 13). A few of these questions have been better addressed within medical geography than the others, but the shorter review of research for the latter questions itself reflects the state of the subdiscipline.

WHY ARE PHENOMENA DISTRIBUTED IN CERTAIN AND SPECIFIC WAYS AS OPPOSED TO THE MANY OTHER WAYS THEY COULD BE DISTRIBUTED?

It is difficult to identify anything that occurs completely randomly or uniformly over the surface of the earth. Understanding spatial distribution forms the core of geography. The fact that the particular subject matter may be precipitation or cities, barn types or infant mortality often makes the field seem insubstantive and unfocused to nongeographers. A medical geographer does not specialize in the study of a type of cancer or schistosomiasis. Instead, the goal is explanation of the distribution of disease systems and health care, and ultimately integration of knowledge about the state of human health in places. Before one can explain a spatial distribution, however, it must be precisely described. Various forms of mapping have traditionally fulfilled this purpose, but more recently maps have also been abstracted into graphs and their x/y coordinate grid system has become the frame for classifying distribution of statistical frequency. Studies of patterns can be classified into those involving points, lines, areas, and surfaces.

A variety of techniques is used to describe dot distributions. Measures of standard distance, the two-dimensional equivalent of the standard deviation, can be used graphically to determine relative clustering or dispersion (91) or to establish zones of deviation from the centroid (minimal distance to all occurrences) location. The standard deviational ellipse also provides the direction of orientation and degree of circularity. Shannon (79) was able to compare for different ethnic and income groups in Washington DC the activity space (in which people went to work, shopped, went bowling, etc) with the care-seeking space in which clinics and physicians were located. In studies such as this, the shops, churches, hospitals, and interviewees are dots in two-dimensional space, and the ellipses contain two thirds of all the trip destination locations. Dot patterns can also be compared statistically to hypothetical distributions using various forms of nearest neighbor, quadrat analysis, and space-time clustering familiar to epidemiologists (49). The location and movement of lines (such as isolines, i.e. lines of equal values, connecting points with the same time of arrival for an epidemic) have been described mostly in diffusion studies within the framework of graph theory or network analysis. Areal patterns have been examined for space-time clustering. Surfaces can be constructed by adding to the x/y spatial locational dimensions height composed of standardized scores for variables. Thus Pyle & Lauer (74) described the market penetration areas of hospitals based on proportions of the population attending hospitals, and Gilg (28) described the initial, modal, and mean arrival time of fowl pest disease. These surfaces can then be subjected to correlation-regression techniques in trend surface analysis. For example, Angulo et al (2) used various quadratic surfaces to describe the spread of variola minor among preschoolers, adults, and others by the composition and size of households and vaccination levels.

Spatial Patterns

The nature of the areal units involved in analysis is of major concern to medical geography. However exact the description derived using the above methods, its use in statistical analysis is no better than its base. It is common for geographers as for other social scientists to use convenient administrative districts such as counties for their observations. Counties in the US, however, are not only of different sizes but are of different sizes in different areas, a spatial bias. The large number of small counties in an eastern state used in the same analysis with the small number of large counties in a western state involves different variances at the state level. This problem is compounded by the fact that most of the population lives in the east and that western densities are low, until one reaches the far west in California. Thiessen polygons and other techniques can be used to average observations over areas, removing political boundaries, but such techniques are in fact seldom used.

The arbitrary nature of the boundaries of the study units used, usually counties or states, is a more serious matter. The scale used for analysis is too often determined by what is conveniently collected rather than by what is appropriate. Encephalitis, for example, may be transmitted within a rural river lowland that runs through counties with large urban populations, but cases and populations are totaled for the counties. Maps of cardiovascular disease at the state level masked the high incidence of stroke among people on the coastal plain of the Southeast (61). The great internal variation of large old cities makes city-level reporting virtually useless for etiological analysis. Overcoming these serious problems of data quality often requires expensive fieldwork to collect microarea data that can be aggregated into appropriate units.

Different processes of disease causation result in different spatial patterns. The purpose of describing the spatial pattern so accurately is to fit a geographical model (14, 15, 24, 27, 42, 94) that explains its generation, and so to infer the process. For example, the concepts of distance decay and of spatial interaction as expressed in various models serve to order many spatial phenomena. *Distance decay* is the name given to the decline in intensity or frequency that commonly occurs with increasing distance. Distance is friction, whether measured as transportation costs or time, and it is an axiom that rational people are *distance-minimizers*. The gradient of the decline will decrease over time as an infection diffuses outward from its source. When distance decay is found, some contagious process, whether of ideas or of a disease agent, is usually inferred. An illness caused by the common water supply of a city, in contrast, would have a spatial pattern characterized by a large plateau and sudden fall off at the edge of the watershed. The effects of an occupational hazard would show no distance decay using data based on patient residence. Release of radiation, however, might result in a distance decay pattern from the site, one complicated by dosage or threshold considerations. Spatial interaction is often modeled in terms of *Central Place Hierarchy,* or the hierarchy of towns and cities that results from the necessity that various goods and services have different size populations to support them, and yet a location as near as possible to everyone. This results in a spatial pattern of small places with every-day goods and services scattered widely and rather uniformly, with regional cities having more specialized goods serving the area and interacting with larger, more specialized centers that also serve other areas. Central Place Hierarchy is easily visible in airplane connections or major sports franchise systems. It results in a spatial pattern of educational level, income, occupational structure, traffic, pollution, etc., ideally going from large urban to rural to small urban to rural and so on. These spatial patterns can be used to discover process. Central Place Hierarchy also figures, as explained below, in many efforts to optimize the location of health services.

Techniques emerging for analyzing spatial autocorrelation most powerfully distill the above spatial order. Autocorrelation is most familiar as the correlation of data pertaining to one year with that for the previous and following year, thus confounding the statistical requirement of each year being an independent observation. What happens in one period of time is influenced by what comes before and in turn influences what follows. Similarly, spatial autocorrelation involves the correlation of data for areal units because of propinquity. It has been a major statistical headache for geography (13) because of the usual assumptions of independence of observation. If one's units of observation are, say, census tracts or counties, it is not true that the observations are independent. The property values of one area, for example, certainly affect those of the adjacent area. In analyzing spatial autocorrelation, one correlates each spatial unit's value with those of contiguous units, then with those of units once removed, then twice removed, and so on. The resulting values are plotted as a correlogram with standardized scores on the y axis and lags, or units between, on the x axis. Glick (30–32) has pioneered the use of patterns of spatial autocorrelation for etiological explanation. He analyzed the spatial autocorrelation for cancer sites by counties, economic areas, states, and regions for the US. He also constructed transects of counties crossing the country north to south, east to west, and across major urban and rural areas. He found that in Pennsylvania, for example, the autocorrelation pattern for stomach cancer showed a sharp distance decay, indicating that the influence of one county seldom extended beyond the next. The autocorrelation pattern for bladder cancer showed a plateau of correlation over regions of four lags and then fell off sharply, indicating an areal environmental exposure. The autocorrelation pattern for lung cancer for males showed little relation between adjacent units, but small peaks of correlation at four lags and large peaks at nine lags to suggest that the central place hierarchy was important and so implicate pollution.

Glick deliberately studied the patterns of spatial autocorrelation at multiple scales so that he could systematically partition the spatial variation. Using nested analysis of the components of variance (42, 66), he focused attention on the relative importance of the different levels of the scale hierarchy as judged by the different proportion of total variation that can be ascribed to them. His analysis of lung cancer, for example, showed that male rates had significant proportions of variance at every scale, with the largest proportion at the county level, whereas the variation in female rates was due almost exclusively to county (local) level, with no influences at state or regional scale. He continued his investigation using spectral analysis, and suggested that a technique called *spatial transfer function modeling* (8) would be better for explaining the spatial variation than the usual multiple regression methods, which consider simultaneous effects and deal poorly with spatial spread effects over time (31).

Greenberg (37, 38) has refined such spatial variance-nesting methodology for analysis of the distributional changes of cancer. He has found a spatial convergence of cancer mortality in the US between 1950 and 1975 (52). Dividing counties into those that were strongly urban (10% of counties), moderately urban, and rural (69%), he found for 1950–1954 overall urban/rural ratios for cancers of the bladder, kidney, larynx, esophagus, lung, tongue, rectum, and large intestine of 1.9, and site ratios as high as 2.4. By the early 1970s, however, the ratio was only 1.2 overall and lower for white females. While cancer rates were converging and the white population especially was moving toward a homogeneous spatial pattern of cancer mortality for almost every type of cancer, cancer rates were diverging by sex and race subgroups of the population. In 1950–1955, white males had a cancer rate 7% higher than nonwhite males and 18% higher than white females. By 1970–1975, nonwhite male cancer rates were 22% higher than white male rates, and 65% higher than white female rates. White females had the greatest decrease in the decreasing rates (stomach, rectum, liver, cervix uteri, and corpus uteri) and the least increase in the increasing rates (lung, pancreas, multiple myeloma, melanoma, lymphoma, brain and central nervous system). Greenberg contends that the spatial convergence of cancer mortality in the US and other industrialized countries is caused by the diffusion of urban culture, with its risk factors of air and water pollution, cigarette smoking, alcohol consumption, diet, occupation, socioeconomic status, stress, and medical practices.

Covariation

Explaining spatial distribution often means analyzing spatial covariation, which is of course essentially what a map does visually. Statistically, a wide range of multivariate techniques are used, commonly including factor, canonical, and discriminant analysis, to determine what variables or sets of variables vary significantly with the study variable. Often the residuals or scores from the analysis can be mapped for the individual observation units to identify a spatial pattern that suggests additional variables that might be correlated. Researchers have learned to be wary of the ecological fallacy of using findings at one scale of analysis to explain relationships at another scale with different variance (10). As in the case of spatial autocorrelation, medical geographers need to focus on turning the scale-related changes in covariation into etiological tools (63).

Such a large literature exists on the associative occurrence of disease and socioeconomic and environmental factors that I shall limit my illustratory comments to one small focus on environmental patterns of cerebrovascular disease and certain cancers. There has been a great deal of international research on the associations of "The Water Factor," most often measured as water hardness but admitted to be unknown. In more than 16 countries, from Japan, Finland, and Britain to Canada and the US, studies have found elevated levels of stroke to be associated with soft water. As Comstock (17) has pointed out in his review of many studies, however, the more rigorous the analysis and the more micro the study area, the less association is found. One reason may be that the variance of cerebrovascular disease and soft water coincides at the scale of large areas but is overwhelmed by other variation at the microscale.

Takahashi (90) has analyzed the covariation of age-adjusted death rates for cerebrovascular disease over 46 prefectures in Japan with environmental and behavioral factors (N.B.: unlike epidemiological usage, in geographical terminology, "environment" does not include cultural, behavioral factors like smoking, diet, or exercise habits). These were followed up by microscale studies in two villages, one located in a high and the other in a low death rate area. He studied death rates, average annual temperature, annual sunshine duration, the occurrence of floor hearths or wood stoves, calcium/sulfate ratio for water quality, geochemical environment, rice production, the quantity of salt, dietary intake, blood pressure, and serum calcium, magnesium, and total base. People in the inland, higher stroke area had a stocky body index correlated with rice production, high rice consumption related to high salt consumption in miso soup and salted pickles, lower ambient temperatures, and lower serum calcium levels, but higher blood pressure. Thouez (92, 93) has studied water quality (copper, magnesium, lead, chlorine, nitrates, hardness, pH, potassium) in Quebec and its relationship to cerebrovascular disease and to certain cancers. Using regression and discriminant analysis, he found a negative association of water hardness and the incidence of malignant neoplasms of the stomach, rectum, prostate, and organs of the digestive system. He was stymied, however, by the inability to disaggregate municipal data on exposure for populations drawing drinking water from the St. Lawrence River or from underground aquifers.

There are numerous studies like the above: careful, comprehensive, statistically sound, flexible in scale and informed in their variable identification. Their findings usually are interesting. Their lack of a biologically plausible, theoretical model, however, limits their comparability between places and their general replicability. They do not purport, of course, to establish causal relationships, but only associative occurrences that should be followed up with individual-level, controlled studies. Most studies, either by confounding environmental factors and social/behavioral factors by indiscriminant mixing, or by focusing on a narrow and specific aspect, such as water hardness or salt consumption, do little credit to geography as an integrative discipline that speaks the language of both the physical and social sciences. Low levels of selenium in the soil and soft water have been implicated, for example, in the high stroke mortality of the Southeastern coastal plain. People living there, however, eat wheat from Nebraska and vegetables from Florida and California the same as other Americans, and they mainly draw their water from an underground aquifer shared with Mississippi and Florida. The particular soil and water conditions of the coast were associated with the development of particular cropping and landholding, and slave owning, systems of occupance. These in turn were followed by poverty, late industrialization, and recent urbanization that are in turn associated with certain occupational structures, migration and modernization stresses, diets, and life styles. The chain by which trace elements in the water or soil reach human beings is very complicated (62), and the mechanisms of how the population in its demographic, socioeconomic, and mobility complexity can be related to them needs to be specified before risk can be determined. One method being developed is to use areas of comparable socioeconomic/disease relationships as controls to study the environmental exposures of population in case areas where socioeconomic variables do not predict cerebrovascular disease (63).

Such a methodology would be a form of regionalizing. What is called *regionalization* in geography is simply classification to reduce variation.

Regionalization

Whether one defines uniform regions, delimited to be homogeneous for one or more variables, or functional regions based on the limits of interaction, one engages in classification to order the spatial variance in a distribution (1). By generalizing spatial complexity into regions, the regularities that underlie the variance may be discovered and regionalization may thus serve as the basis for inductive reasoning. This is important in geography because theory in many areas is not developed enough to support elaborate hypothesis generation through deduction. An efficient way to order variance is to group like things together and separate significantly unlike things. In a spatial sense, this means determining which subareas of a larger study area are homogeneous with respect to values of interest and thus constitute a region, whether or not they are contiguous.

Of all the multitudinous examples of regionalization in the literature, I shall focus on two very different ones that have been conceptually important for medical geography. The first is derived from urban ecological theory. Much is known about the ecological structure and evolution of American cities. The geographic model of a city shows types of residential, industrial, and commercial development and income and ethnic changes over time as expansion from the central business district in concentric circles. These rings are divided into sectors by major transportation arteries, which affect accessibility to the center and often separate types of land use. Girt (29) used these sectors within zones as quadrats within which he sampled his population to study the etiology of bronchitis in Leeds, England. His zones delimited the central business district, the transitional zone around that, a zone of small terraced housing and large housing (by sector), post-1918 residential areas, and ruralurbia. His sectors delimited middle, lower middle, and working class areas and industrial zones with lowest class residents. For his quadrats within these zones he carried out a sample interview survey and mapped the result, using probabilities of a Poisson distribution to determine that significant variation in bronchitis did exist between quadrats. He then proceded to study the effects of air pollution, construction type, dampness and fungi, crowding, past living conditions (derived by knowing the evolutionary history of these city regions), and industrial, commercial, and other land use. Girt's final model produced a simulated pattern of prevalence that closely resembled the real pattern.

Brownlea (9) studied the diffusion of hepatitis in Wollongong, Australia using diffusion models that are discussed below. Having defined what he called a "clinical front" moving outward from a center across his study area, he was able to identify areas in which the epidemic wave spread more slowly or quickly than predicted. He thus, in essence, defined three regions: where the infection spread as predicted by simple probability, where it spread faster than expected, and where it spread less quickly. His analysis of age structure, immigrant status, housing construction, lake and school location, sewerage systems, clay composition of the soil, and other variables related to these regions identified the importance of residential segregation by age for lowered resistance to spread (young families at risk) as well as the hazard of new construction with inadequate sewerage in low-lying areas with high clay content. Policy recommendations followed for urban planning.

The "landscape epidemiology" of Soviet and German medical geographers uses regionalization in a different way. Pavlovskii et al (68) defined a "natural nidus" to consist of the living community of plants and animals (biocenose) together with their necessary environmental conditions, among the members of which the zoonotic disease agent circulated continually. Defining the nidus of bubonic plague in Central Asia precisely meant determining the amount of detritus in the burrows, the pH of the soil, the depth of burrows relative to outside winter temperatures, the degree of predation by cockroaches and snakes and other creatures that ate larvae or eggs, the grass and other food necessary to maintain sufficiently rapid generations of susceptible baby rats, and even the exposure to the sun and slope of land (for drainage) on which burrows were found. When exact specifications for continual maintenance of the bacterium in circulation were ascertained, the landscape was analyzed to define regions in which these characteristics were found. One might, for example, specify south-facing slopes of a certain steepness that received enough rain to maintain a certain indicator grass. Burrows within this region could then be gassed. By proceding systematically, the ancient focus of plague in Central Asia has been greatly reduced. In a similar manner, when a project such as a new settlement or railroad construction in Siberia is proposed, the landscape is analyzed in detail to determine where various mosquitoes, ticks, reservoir fauna, and potential (anthropozoonotic) disease transmission occurs. Camps can then be located, and protective clothing or even hours of work can be adjusted to minimize health risk to the incoming population.

These ideas of landscape regions that define areas in which certain diseases may potentially be transmitted have allowed geographers to study health risks associated with population resettlement, road construction, or central place location in developing areas of the Third World. For example, Roundy (76) identified concentric zones of landscape habitat (home, residential compound, village, agricultural land, grazing land, far-ranging zone) that constituted nidi of hookworm, malaria, roundworm, contagion, and various vectored diseases. By studying the frequency and duration of exposure by purpose of the population to these zones, he was able to identify subgroups of the population most at risk of various infections and to propose some intervention strategies. I (59) used exposure to such landscape regions to analyze the health effects of land development programs in Malaysia, Kloos (48) for microscale analysis of schistosomiasis transmission in Africa, and Weil (95) to assess the health risks of agricultural development in Latin America. Armstrong (3, 4) developed this use of regionalization by defining regions around home, neighborhood, and workplace with characteristics relevant to nasopharyngeal cancer in Malaysia and using a case-control methodology to determine relative risk of exposure to them. A similar approach is now being used to analyze environmental exposures of the population in Savannah, Georgia relevant to cardiovascular disease (63).

WHY ARE THERE DIFFERENTIAL RATES AT WHICH GOODS AND IDEAS WILL SPREAD OVER AN AREA THROUGH TIME?

Tools such as plows and guns, ideas such as Christianity and relativity, and goods such as domesticated food crops and motor vehicles all spread, or diffuse, over space from a source area. Geography is concerned with how things spread across space. Geographers seek to comprehend the influence of such things as settlement systems, spatial structure, and human perception, so that speed and direction of diffusion can be predicted. Diffusion theory is one of the best developed bodies of thought in geography, but it has only recently been applied to disease. Previously the focus had been on the diffusion of innovations, such as new ideas or technologies (14). Several major types of diffusion may be identified relevant to disease spread. The first is *relocation diffusion*. This was initially intended to categorize such changes as the relocation of industry from inner cities to suburbs and the present shift of some industries abroad, or the resettlement of European ethnic groups in parts of the United States. It clearly characterizes the spread of many vectored disease systems, such as yellow fever, malaria, onchocerciasis, and schistosomiasis from the Old World to the New. Studies of relocation diffusion might be relevant to the shift of importance for Rocky Mountain Spotted Fever to the Southeastern piedmont, and might be useful for explaining why yellow fever has never spread to the dengue fever heartland of Southeast Asia. The necessary theory and methodology for modeling relocation diffusion of disease, however, lies largely within the subdiscipline of biogeography. Biogeographers have a long history of studying exotic introductions into island ecosystems and biological feedback in the formation and spatial shift of biotic communities. Biogeographers have not yet become involved with issues in medical geography. This unfortunate lack of connection also explains why landscape epidemiology has been so little used to investigate American zoonotic diseases.

Another type of diffusion, *expansion diffusion,* also sometimes deals with contagious processes, but since it is concerned with the role of newspapers, organizations, and other institutions more suited to the diffusion of ideas than of infectious agents, it is not considered further here. A few medical geographers have addressed topics such as the diffusion of medical technology (5) or the diffusion of the deinstitutionalization of the mentally ill at the state level (84), but most have been concerned with contagious disease. The two types of diffusion of major concern need to be discussed at greater length.

Contact Diffusion

Contact diffusion is alternatively known as contagious, or sometimes radial, diffusion. The brilliant work of Hagerstrand (39) introduced the subject to geography and was responsible for establishing the wave analog that has become widely accepted. As a wave spreads outward from its origin, distance decay results in not only a later time of arrival but also a lowering of frequency, or intensity. He suggested modeling the diffusion of an innovation using stochastic simulation. To do this, a "mean information field" is established by placing a grid over a surface of probabilities resulting from the adaptation of the normal bell curve to the two-dimensional surface. When the curve is centered over the introduced infection, the probabilities then reflect the distance decay evident in its more likely diffusion to someone nearby rather than on the other side of town. Cell probabilities can be adjusted to reflect population distribution, accessibility via transportation arteries, etc using empirical data until the real world is simulated well. The effects of projected changes in housing development, transportation, or even vaccination coverage can then be examined by simulation.

Brownlea (9) used this method to study the diffusion of infectious hepatitis in Wollongong, Australia. After ascertaining that the disease spread over time among a network of towns in the region, each town in turn serving as a radiating source before shifting to the inter-epidemic fill-in mode, he timed the movement of what he called the "clinical front" among the settlements. He then centered the probability surface on the origin of infection in Wollongong when it was a radiating node, and delimited where the diffusion wave should have moved outward to at successive time periods. By comparing the ideal "random walk" with the actual behavior of the epidemic, he was able to determine the effect of various demographic, environmental, and economic variables. Very young families, for example, accelerated the diffusion by 20% and a polluted lake did so by 10%, whereas older families slowed the wave by 10%, as did light sandy soil. His recommendations focused (*a*) upon the hazard of young, immigrant families crowding onto the low-lying river bottoms with their clay soil under conditions of inadequate sewerage infrastructure and (*b*) upon the public health importance of mixing age groups in residential areas.

At a more aggregated scale, the propensity for contact, or interaction, within a population can be summarized as *population potential,* which is derived from the gravity model. The *gravity model* is one of the most useful in geography, but it has been applied mostly to population migration and economic trade. It expresses the fact that distance retards or repells and places (through processes of spatial interaction) attract in a formula reminiscent of its namesake: the population of two places are multiplied together and divided by distance to some exponent (depending on the means of transportation involved). By interpolating isolines (lines of equal values), a surface of population potential is created. The measure reflects not only population distribution, as density does, but also direction, because people are measured relative to the location of all other people. The model is remarkably accurate in predicting such diverse interactions as the flow of telephone calls and the propensity for migration from place to place. At the local level, the multiplication of population (households, etc) and division by the distance between them gives the centroid, or center of population, for units such as counties.

Hunter & Young (46) used the gravity model to study the diffusion of influenza in England and Wales in 1957. After creating a population potential surface for the region, they located the centroid of influenza cases week by week. The infection was introduced into northwest England, and proceded up and along the ridge of population potential to London, spreading locally down the population potential gradient as it went. The study was one of the few in medical geography to use normative models to predict diffusion.

Haggett (40) adapted the Hamer-Soper diffusion model to geography and, alone and with Cliff (11, 12, 16, 41), has developed methods for analyzing the spread of multiple waves of infection and for timing the movement of the epidemic wave. To study the diffusion of measles in Cornwall, England, he transposed places onto a graph and used spatial autocorrelation to predict the movement of the infection according to various models: regional, urban-rural, local contagion, wave contagion, journey-to-work, population size, and population density. He developed a hybrid model upon findings that different kinds of spatial diffusion processes were most involved in different stages of the epidemic spread. Iceland next presented an opportunity to study the diffusion of measles over time in a system that could be closed. Hypothesizing, for example, that over the course of a century increased population density would lead to acceleration in disease diffusion, they found instead that the epidemic waves decreased in speed of movement. Epidemics became more frequent, more limited in extent, and in urban areas spread more slowly. There were, of course, important changes other than density involved, notably the increase in boarding schools and changes in the transportation infrastructure.

Hierarchical Diffusion

The final type of diffusion, *hierarchical diffusion*, refers to movement of innovations (or infections) through the spatial interactions characteristic of the urban hierarchy. The landmark study in medical geography was Pyle's (69) analysis of the diffusion of cholera in the US during the nineteenth century. In the 1820s, the disease spread as a function of distance. The farther a place was located from origin in three diffusion channels, the Atlantic coast, the Mississippi Valley, and the Great Lakes lowland (relative to Canadian sources), the later it received the epidemic. By the 1860s, rank in the urban hierarchy had become dominant: the larger the city, the sooner it received the epidemic irrespective of how far it was from New York City or other points of introduction. The residuals from this regression are themselves illuminating. There was still some early arrival of cholera along the Great Lakes, indicating the active cross-border contact that existed even at that time. Washington DC and San Francisco both received the epidemic much later than their urban rank indicated they should. Washington was such a pestilential place in summer that it was largely evacuated, and it did not receive the epidemic until Congress convened in fall and its population resumed its urban status. San Francisco, of course, was not yet integrated into the national urban system because the transcontinental railroad did not yet exist. Geographers especially like this study because it illuminates the developing spatial structure of this country in the nineteenth century quite aside from its disease focus.

Stock (89) also studied the diffusion of cholera. He recognized that the introduction of cholera to West Africa in the 1960s, historically for the first time, provided the opportunity to study the diffusion of disease in virgin territory. His comprehensive treatment analyzed the endangering and protective cultural behavior at microscale, including such customs as the bathing and mourning of the dead and the spatial distribution of kin, which provided the framework for diffusion as people fled infected villages. He found contact diffusion in the region around Lake Chad, and identified the role of coastal fishing in introducing the disease to internal river valley channel diffusion systems. He identified barriers, such as low population density, and corridor effects, such as transportation systems. More than all these things, however, the importance of urban hierarchical diffusion in countries such as Nigeria leaps out of his monograph. It was rank in the urban hierarchy, and not distance from Lagos, which determined when the epidemic arrived. Among other suggestions, Stock recommended to local public health officials who were trying with limited amounts of vaccine to carry out campaigns to control or retard the epidemic spread that they forget about neighbors, local shops, and contacts and head for the local bus station.

There is considerable interest in anthropology, epidemiology, and other disciplines in studying social networks to get at the process of disease diffusion. Social networks, of course, have territorial bases even in this age of what has been called neighborhood without propinquity, and several social geographers are well known for studying neighborhood and social networks. None have thus far expressed interest in disease diffusion. The closest study, in that it used household structure and socioeconomic and other neighborhood variables, was Angulo et al's (2) study of variola minor diffusion in Brazil.

Pyle (73) is presently completing years of work on a major study of diffusion of influenza in the US during the twentieth century. Given the importance of his work on other topics in medical geography, his monograph is eagerly anticipated.

WHY ARE THERE DIFFERENCES IN THE LOCATION CHOICES PEOPLE MAKE FOR THEIR INSTITUTIONS?

People, individually or collectively, choose where facilities and businesses are to be located. Industrialists have long recognized that choosing the correct site, relative to raw materials, market, and transportation, can determine success or failure. Zoning and planning are concerned with regulating location for the public, rather than individual, good. Locational analysis in geography has been concerned with such diverse phenomena as state capitols and McDonald's franchises, interstate highways, steel plants, new car manufacturing sites for General Motors and Honda, prisons, and toxic waste dumps. Only recently have the theoretical frameworks and methodologies been applied to health care.

Shannon & Dever (80) introduced a generation of graduate students to the spatial distribution of hospital beds, black and female physicians, specialists, and health technicians in this country. Students now read Pyle (72) to learn the relevance of urban hierarchy, or contemplate the difficulties of regionalizing Health Maintenance Organizations. A large literature has resulted in which analysis of covariation is used to describe the importance of amenities, population size and density, income, climate, neighborhood age, and office construction, among other variables, for the location of hospitals, clinics, physicians, and others. Gober & Gordon (33), for example, predict on the basis of distance decay that specialists who use hospitals frequently will be more spatially clustered around hospitals than general practitioners and others, and then proceed to analyze the distribution of physicians in Phoenix.

The first study for applying geographic approaches to locational analysis and optimalization for health facilities occurred in Sweden. The government of Sweden in the 1950s approached Godlund (34) and other geographers at the University of Lund to regionalize the new health care system then under development. In Sweden there is sparse population in the north, and dense settlement around Stockholm in the south. Some regional hospitals and medical schools already existed, along with a national transportation infrastructure. The problem was to optimize the location of a minimum number of additional teaching hospitals and other facilities in order to make health care most accessible to the population, recognizing that different levels of specialization demand larger thresholds of population size to support them economically. General practitioners, for example, need a relatively small population to occupy their time, whereas an eye surgeon may draw patients from a whole province. Similarly, every community hospital should be able to perform an appendectomy, but it takes a larger population to justify having a Catscan, and one excellent burn ward could serve all of Sweden. Yet, given the sparse distribution of the population in the northern half of the country and the difficulties of transportation, a facility located strictly by population service areas would be inaccessible to many people who needed it. National health service regions were delimited and facilities located according to the plan they developed.

In the 1960s, geographers involved in the Chicago Regional Studies (21, 67, 70) did the first, and in many ways still the best, comprehensive study of health facilities, physician and patient location, and behavior in an American city. Trend surface analysis was used to generalize morbidity and mortality experience, and socioeconomic, housing, and racial variables were factored into their major components for analysis of associative occurrence. Algorithms were developed to allocate patients to the nearest hospital with beds appropriate to the condition. The optimal pattern thus generated was then compared with empirical data to identify behavioral characteristics of the system. Changes in age structure and residential location were projected 15 years into the future and the location of future need for specific kinds of beds was forecast. These studies identified the importance of "social distance," as Jewish patients by-passed Catholic hospitals and welfare patients journeyed to the major facility that would receive them. They identified the importance of physician referral systems and the problems of neighborhood change. Such findings have been rediscovered by many geographers since those early studies.

Rushton (77) has contributed in many ways to the development of *location-allocation* modeling of health service. This family of models uses iterative algorithms to optimize spatial accessibility. One of his most important methodological contributions distributes the population of counties according to the health facility they use, to determine the "catchment area" of the hospital or family planning clinic, etc. The bed/population or physician/population ratios so commonly used can be quite misleading because people easily cross county lines to get care from physicians or hospitals. Only by market area type analyses can the spatial configuration of hospital accessibility be compared with population morbidity (74).

Location-allocation modeling has meant employment for a large proportion of medical geographers in urban and health planning offices as well as academic endeavor. Perhaps its purest expression has been the analysis of emergency medical service systems (54). Increasingly, however, researchers are focusing on the spatial behavior of users and providers (87), and have become more concerned with the framework for system constraints provided by the political economy and social attitudes (22). Smith's (85) analysis of locations for alcoholism treatment centers, and Dear's (18–20) body of work on the location of mental health treatment facilities and patients, have come to grips with externalities of fear, prejudice, and property values. This stream within medical geography is in confluence with a growing body of work on public policy, land use planning, and locational parameters of public (as opposed to private, profit-maximizing) facilities in general.

The locational parameters of health service continue to command the attention of many medical geographers, generate a vigorous literature, and provide useful methodologies for urban and regional planning (91). Enough studies have been carried out by now, however, that a more critical, second-generation perspective is developing. Although Pyle's early study related health care utilization to need, most studies have modeled only demand. Many studies based on utilization of facilities have in fact been tautological, because if distance affects utilization then those most affected by distance are not represented in demand based on utilization records. The importance of physical distance is not always obvious. Within cities, for example, the difference between two blocks and four blocks is not the same as the friction of five miles versus 30 in other areas. There is a threshold function. The importance of distance has been found to vary greatly with health complaint, as well as with income, education, and activity areas. Even where the relevance of distance seems most indubitable, in minimizing the time of emergency services, new findings about how utilizing higher, more specialized centers leads to deterioration of experience and performance in lower order centers—and hence higher mortality for those using them—have raised new doubts. The context of study of institutional location is broadening and becoming involved with political economy on one hand and more focused on individual behavior on the other.

WHY ARE THERE DIFFERENCES IN THE CHOICES OF DIRECTIONS AND LENGTHS OF MOVEMENTS PEOPLE MAKE?

The obverse side to optimal location of facilities is consumer behavior. This question asks not why things are located where they are, but why people choose to move as they do, or do not. Why do people retire to certain places and not others? Why do they live in certain residential neighborhoods? Why do they shop in one place and not another? How far will they travel for what purpose? Geographical methodologies for studying journey-to-work, multiple-purpose shopping trips, and the mental maps of spatial orientation were adapted to studying journey-to-physician, locational choice of physician as part of activity areas, and the nature of information about location, quality, and social barriers of care.

The focus of these studies, too, can be traced back to the Chicago research, with Earickson (21) studying the spatial behavior of hospital patients. Since then Stimson (87) has studied the spatial behavior of providers and users in Australia, and Shannon (81) has investigated the search for medical care within the social network of urban blacks. Shannon's (79) use of elliptical cells to analyze the spatial distribution of use of health services in comparison to overall activity space was an important conceptual contribution to this focus. This put health care consumer behavior into the context of other research on consumer behavior and locational preference. For example, the new primary care facilities diffusing across the US are efficiently located (as are bank branches and garages) in shopping centers or along major commuting routes where consumers can combine many purposes in a single trip.

This question is most often addressed by the subdiscipline of population geography. Many of the questions it asks about information flow and field, perception of distance, and the decisional locus of supportive social networks are relevant to selection of physician and facility, referral systems, and utilization. They are only beginning to be asked.

WHY ARE THERE DIFFERENCES IN IMAGES HELD BY INDIVIDUALS ABOUT THEIR COMMUNITIES AND SURROUNDING ENVIRONMENT?

Much of the literature that addresses this question is concerned with how individuals partition space, how they orient themselves in space, and how these cognition processes develop. Consideration of the social networks and individual identities involved has led to concern for neighborhood formation and sense of place. Geographers are also interested in people's perception of hazards such as earthquakes, tidal waves, floods, and hurricanes in the places where they live. One clearly could consider malaria as a hazard in such a context, but this has not notably been done. Knowledge of how people perceive space has of course been sought for the consumer-behavior research described above.

Some of the most interesting research that addresses this question in medical geography is concerned with utilization of traditional medical systems and their integration with biomedical systems in developing countries. Good (35, 36) has raised many geographical questions about how Africans perceive disease causation, prevention, and treatment and evaluate the use of the various health care systems concurrently available. Gessler (26) has reviewed the importance of African, Chinese, Ayurvedic, Unani, American Indian, and other non-biomedical health care sources, the nature and extent of Western biomedical health care availability in the Third World, and how consumers choose and shift among systems. Little is known of the effects of urbanization upon utilization of traditional medical systems, whether in Kenya, India, or Singapore, or upon recruitment and training of the next generation of practitioners, or about the source areas and trade of traditional pharmaceuticals. Several doctoral students are addressing this challenge through foreign area field work now.

INTEGRATION AND LIMITATIONS

Geography seeks to integrate all the variance at a point in space to understand the nature of place. This has in fact been seldom attempted by modern medical geography. Hunter (45) consulted for the World Health Organization on the project to control onchocerciasis in West Africa and criticized the region used for insecticide spraying. The region was ever expanding because the migration of black flies into the region on the monsoon wind shift prevented its separation from the larger area of which it was part. He recommended an integrated intervention program based on knowledge of population distribution and structure, the distribution of types of agricultural land and need for them, local clothing, house construction techniques, agricultural technology and seasonality, the regime of regional precipitation and fluvial dynamics, and the life cycle of the vector and its predators.

I (59) attempted to assess the overall consequences for health of population resettlement for land development in the forests of Malaysia. I considered the effects of such things as vegetational change on the vector and animal reservoirs of scrub typhus and malaria, women's support during child birth, population access to fresh vegetables and fruit, need for and use of health care, and consequences for intestinal parasites of introducing latrines. A major recommendation was that paving the road into the land projects before tree crops reach commercial production would enable the people to reach the services of market towns and would have favorable consequences for community nutrition, health care, and mental health.

There has been greater success in integrating material from many disciplines. The medical geography of health care has freely incorporated the concerns and findings from other disciplines about the social, economic, political, and cultural behavior of individuals and systems. It has in turn contributed its geographical perspective to the emergence of a social science of health care. Similarly, epidemiological design and methodology, parasitology, entomology, microbiology and other medical sciences, and the anthropology of medical belief, along with many other disciplinary insights, have been synthesized and used in explaining spatial distribution. Medical geographers are becoming better trained in the cognate fields relevant to their specialization, as economic and political and climatological geographers were before them.

Medical geography is reaching a stage of maturation in which it is becoming more introspective and critical. This is natural as a generation is now productive who specialized at both the master's and doctoral levels in the field. The limitations of methodology and the limits to medical contribution have been critiqued by Mayer (55), Stimson (88), and others. There is recognition in the field that changes in types of human behavior (transportation technology, electronic information processing, attitudes toward health promotion) change the structure of various spatial systems. There is philosophical concern for reasoning from (spatial) form to process, because it is known that more than one process can generate the same form.

Some limitations are endemic to the specialty. Medical geographers must usually take the medical data they are given. They are not competent to evaluate the differences between diagnosis of cancer of the rectum or colon, and are not usually even aware that there may be diagnostic variation across the study area. Geographers are generally ignorant of the physiology and chemistry that lie behind biological process, and this causes their hypotheses even about spatial form to be deficient.

Most medical geographers recognize these limitations and others, and are eager to collaborate with other health professionals and scientists. The subdiscipline is simply bursting with ideas on which to work. There is a growing concern, however, especially among students of the field, that there has been too much explaining and forecasting and too little effort to establish norms of action that may benefit society's health (22). Medical geography is entering a period of reassessment of its geographical goals before expansion of its field of research.

ACKNOWLEDGMENT

I wish to thank my colleague Wil Gesler for giving me pre-presentation access to the ideas and references of his paper. He and John Florin were kind enough to critique the manuscript for me, although the deficiencies in concept and coverage are of course my own.

Literature Cited

1. Amedeo, D., Golledge, R. G. 1975. *An Introduction to Scientific Reasoning in Geography*. New York: Wiley
2. Angulo, J. J., et al. 1979. *Soc. Sci. Med.* 13D:183–89
3. Armstrong, R. W. 1973. *Geogr. Anal.* 5:122–32
4. Armstrong, R. W. 1978. *Soc. Sci. Med.* 12D:149–56
5. Baker, S. R. 1979. *Soc. Sci. Med.* 13D:155–62
6. Barrett, F. A., ed. 1968. *Canadian Studies in Medical Geography*. Downsview, Ontario: York Univ. Geogr. Monogr.
7. Barrett, F. A. 1981. *Soc. Sci. Med.* 15D:21–26
8. Bennett, R. J. 1979. *Spatial Time Series*. London: Pion
9. Brownlea, A. A. 1972. See Ref. 56, pp. 279–300
10. Cleek, R. L. 1979. *Soc. Sci. Med.* 13D: 241–48
11. Cliff, A. D., Haggett, P. 1982. *Int. J. Epidem.* 11:82–89
12. Cliff, A. D., Haggett, P. 1983. See Ref. 57, pp. 335–48
13. Cliff, A. D., Ord, J. K. 1973. *Spatial Autocorrelation*. London: Pion
14. Cliff, A. D., Ord, J. K. 1981. *Spatial Processes: Models and Applications*. London: Pion
15. Cliff, A. D., Haggett, P., Ord, J. K., Bassett, K., Davies, R. B. 1975. *Elements of Spatial Structure: A Quantitative Approach*. Cambridge: Cambridge Univ. Press
16. Cliff, A. D., Haggett, P., Ord, J. K., Vessey, G. R. 1981. *Spatial Diffusion: An Historical Geography of Epidemics in an Island Community*. Cambridge: Cambridge Univ. Press
17. Comstock, G. W. 1979. *Geochemistry of Water in Relation to Cardiovascular Disease*, pp. 46–68. Washington DC: US Natl. Comm. for Geochem., Natl. Res. Council
18. Dear, M. 1976. *London Papers Reg. Sci.* 7:152–67
19. Dear, M. 1977. *Econ. Geogr.* 53:223–40
20. Dear, M. 1978. *Int. Reg. Sci. Rev.* 3:23–112
21. Earickson, R. J. 1970. *The Spatial Behavior of Hospital Patients*. Chicago: Univ. Chicago, Dept. Geography
22. Eyles, J., Wood, K. J. 1983. *The Social Geography of Medicine and Health*. New York: St. Martin's Press
23. Forster, F. 1966. *Br. J. Prev. Soc. Med* 20:156–71
24. Gattrell, A. C. 1983. *Distance and Space: A Geographical Perspective*. Oxford: Clarendon
25. Geddes, A. 1978. *Soc. Sci. Med.* 12(3/4D):227–37
26. Gesler, W. M. 1984. *Health Care in Developing Countries*. Washington DC: Assoc. Am. Geographers
27. Getis, A., Boots, B. 1978. *Models of Spatial Process: An Approach to the Study of Point, Line, and Area Patterns*. Cambridge: Cambridge Univ. Press
28. Gilg, A. W. 1973. *Trans. Inst. Br. Geogr.* 59:77–97
29. Girt, J. L. 1972. See Ref. 56, pp. 211–30
30. Glick, B. 1979. *Soc. Sci. Med.* 13D:123–30
31. Glick, B. 1980. See Ref. 62, pp. 170–93
32. Glick, B. 1982. *Ann. Assoc. Am. Geogr.* 72:471–81
33. Gober, P., Gordon, R. J. 1980. *Soc. Sci. Med.* 14D:407–18
34. Godlund, S. 1961. *Lund Studies Geogr.*, No. 21. Lund, Sweden: Univ. Lund
35. Good, C. M. 1977. *Soc. Sci. Med.* 11:705–13
36. Good, C. M., Hunter, J. M., Katz, S. H., Katz, S. S. 1979. *Soc. Sci. Med.* 13D:141–54

37. Greenberg, M. R. 1980. *Carcinogen* 1: 553–57
38. Greenberg, M. R. 1983. *Urbanization and Cancer Mortality: The United States Experience, 1950–1975*. New York: Oxford Univ. Press
39. Hagerstrand, T. 1952. *The Propagation of Innovation Waves*. Lund, Sweden: Gleerup
40. Haggett, P. 1975. *Processes in Physical and Human Geography*, pp. 373–91. London: Heinemann
41. Haggett, P. 1976. *Econ. Geogr.* 52:136–46
42. Haggett, P., Cliff, A. D., Frey, A. 1977. *Locational Analysis in Human Geography*. New York: Wiley
43. Howe, G. M. 1970. *National Atlas of Disease Mortality in the United Kingdom*. London: Nelson. 2nd ed.
44. Howe, G. M. 1981. *Soc. Sci. Med.* 15D:199–211
45. Hunter, J. M. 1981. *Soc. Sci. Med.* 15D:261–76
46. Hunter, J. M., Young, J. C. 1971. *Ann. Assoc. Am. Geogr.* 61:631–53
47. Jusatz, H. J. 1966. *Int. J. Biometeor.* 10:323–34
48. Kloos, H., et al. 1983. *Soc. Sci. Med.* 17:545–62
49. Knox, G. 1963. *Br. J. Prev. Soc. Med.* 17:121–27
50. Learmonth, A. T. A. 1975. *Prog. Geogr.* 7:201–26
51. Learmonth, A. T. A. 1978. *Patterns of Disease and Hunger*. Newton Abbot: David & Charles
52. May, J. M. 1950. *Geogr. Rev.* 51:9–41
53. May, J. M. 1958. *The Ecology of Human Disease*. New York: MD Publ.
54. Mayer, J. D. 1979. *Soc. Sci. Med.* 13D:45–57
55. Mayer, J. D. 1983. *Soc. Sci. Med.* 17:1213–21
56. McGlashan, N. D., ed. 1972. *Medical Geography: Techniques and Field Studies*. London: Methuen
57. McGlashan, N. D., Blunden, J. R., eds. 1983. *Geographical Aspects of Health*. London: Academic
58. McGlashan, N. D., Chick, N. K. 1974. *Austral. Geogr. Studies* 12:190–206
59. Meade, M. S. 1976. *Ann. Assoc. Am. Geogr.* 66:428–39
60. Meade, M. S. 1977. *Geogr. Rev.* 67: 379–93
61. Meade, M. S. 1979. *Soc. Sci. Med.* 13D: 257–66
62. Meade, M. S. 1980. *Conceptual and Methodological Issues in Medical Geography*, ed. M. S. Meade, pp. 194–221. Chapel Hill: Univ. North Carolina, Dept. Geogr.
63. Meade, M. S. 1983. See Ref. 57, pp. 175–96
64. Meade, M. S. 1984. *Adv. Med. Soc. Sci.* 2:341–59
65. Meade, M. S., Gesler, W. M., Florin, J. W. 1986. *Medical Geography*. New York: Guilford. In press
66. Moellering, H., Tobler, W. 1972. *Geogr. Anal.* 4:34–50
67. Morrill, R. L., Earickson, R. J., Rees, P. 1970. *Econ. Geogr.* 46:161–71
68. Pavlovskii, E. N., Petrischeva, P. A., Zasukhin, D. N., Oluf'ev, N. G. 1955. *Natural Nidi of Human Disease and Regional Epidemiology*. Leningrad: Medgiz
69. Pyle, G. F. 1969. *Geogr. Anal.* 1:59–75
70. Pyle, G. F. 1971. *Heart Disease, Cancer and Stroke in Chicago, A Geographical Analysis with Facility Plans for 1980*. Chicago: Univ. of Chicago, Dept. Geogr.
71. Pyle, G. F. 1976. *Econ. Geogr.* 52:95–102
72. Pyle, G. F. 1979. *Applied Medical Geography*. New York: Wiley
73. Pyle, G. F. 1980. See Ref. 62, pp. 222–49
74. Pyle, G. F., Lauer, B. F. 1975. *Econ. Geogr.* 51:50–68
75. Rodenwaldt, E., Jusatz, H. J. 1952–1961. *Welt-seuchen-atlas*. Hamburg: Falk. (3 vols.)
76. Roundy, R. W. 1978. *Soc. Sci. Med.* 12D:121–30
77. Rushton, G. 1975. *Planning Primary Health Services for Rural Iowa*. Iowa City: Univ. Iowa, Cent. for Locational Analysis, Inst. Urban & Regional Res.
78. Sakamoto-Momiyama, M. 1977. *Seasonality in Human Mortality: A Medico-Geographical Study*. Tokyo: Tokyo Univ. Press
79. Shannon, G. L. 1977. *Soc. Sci. Med.* 11D:683–89
80. Shannon, G. W., Dever, G. E. A. 1974. *Health Care Delivery: Spatial Perspectives*. New York: McGraw-Hill
81. Shannon, G. W., et al. 1978. *Int. J. Health. Serv.* 8:519–30
82. Shigematsu, I. 1981. *National Atlas of Major Disease Mortalities in Japan*. Tokyo: Japan Health Promotion Fdn.
83. Shoshin, A. A. 1962. *Principles and Methods of Medical Geography*. Moscow: Acad. Sci.
84. Smith, C. J., Hanham, R. Q. 1981. *Soc. Sci. Med.* 15D:361–78
85. Smith, C. J. 1983. *Econ. Geogr.* 59:368–85
86. Sorre, M. 1943. *Les Fondements Biologiques de la Geographie Humaine*. Paris: Colin

87. Stimson, R. J. 1981. *Soc. Sci. Med.* 15D:27–44
88. Stimson, R. J. 1983. See Ref. 57, pp. 322–34
89. Stock, R. 1976. *Cholera in Africa*. London: Int. African Inst.
90. Takahashi, E. 1981. *Soc. Sci. Med.* 15D:163–72
91. Tanaka, T., Ryu, S., Nishigaki, M., Hashimoto, M. 1981. *Soc. Sci. Med.* 15D:83–91
92. Thouez, J. P. 1978. *Canad. Geogr.* 18: 308–21
93. Thouez, J. P., Beauchmp, Y., Simard, A. 1981. *Soc. Sci. Med.* 15D:213–23
94. Unwin, D. 1981. *Introductory Spatial Analysis*. London: Methuen
95. Weil, C. 1981. *Soc. Sci. Med.* 15D:449–61
96. White, R. R. 1972. See Ref. 56, pp. 173–85

Ann. Rev. Public Health. 1986. 7:337–56
Copyright © 1986 by Annual Reviews Inc. All rights reserved

OCCUPATIONAL HEALTH: The Intersection Between Clinical Medicine and Public Health

Linda Rosenstock

Occupational Medicine Program, Department of Medicine, University of Washington, Seattle, Washington 98195

Philip J. Landrigan

Division of Environmental and Occupational Medicine, Department of Community Medicine, The Mt. Sinai Medical Center, New York, New York 10029

INTRODUCTION

Occupational health in the United States has historically been isolated from the mainstream of both clinical medicine and public health (16, 52). This has compounded the difficulties which result from the fact that occupational health is a hybrid specialty that exists at the sometimes uneasy intersection between these two realms. It is a specially that is involved not only with such classical issues of medicine as diagnosis and treatment of illness, but also with issues of engineering, law, and societal regulation. The challenge now confronting occupational health is to overcome its historical isolation and to develop and implement strategies that will strengthen its relationship with both clinical medicine and public health.

The forging of such relationships will be essential for the control of occupational diseases. Despite recent advances in the scientific basis of occupational health, successful reduction in the incidence of occupational disease will, in large part, rely on two factors:

1. the recognition and diagnosis of cases by physicians;
2. the development and implementation of surveillance, prevention, and control programs (57).

0163-7525/86/0510-0337$02.00

The first of these factors lies largely in the domain of clinical medicine; the second is in the domain of public health, involving expertise from such disciplines as epidemiology, biostatistics, toxicology, and industrial hygiene.

In this discussion, we trace the historical development of occupational health in the United States and describe the factors that led to its unfortunate isolation. We propose a strategy for the integration of occupational health into both clinical medicine and public health, a strategy that has as its goals the control of occupational disease.

HISTORICAL ISOLATION OF OCCUPATIONAL HEALTH

A major influence shaping the nature of occupational health and occupational health services has been the development of workers' compensation programs. Until the mid-1800s, employers had duties under common law to provide for the protection of their employees. There were few legal remedies then by which injured workers could recover monetary awards from employers, and industrial injury and death rates were on the rise. The pressures resulting from this situation produced a series of limited legislative acts called employers' liability acts; these acts to some degree facilitated employee recourse for work-related health problems (20). Some of these acts, such as the federal legislation covering interstate railroad employees, are still functioning today. But because of continued problems faced by the employees who had to bring legal actions to recover damages, and because of precedents established for increasingly large liability awards against the employer, both labor and management supported the introduction in the United States of workers' compensation programs (2). These programs flourished on a state-by-state basis in the early 1900s, following the model legislation developed first in Germany and later in most of Western Europe by the end of the nineteenth century.

Workers' compensation programs provide a no-fault insurance mechanism which almost entirely exempts employers from legal liability for work-related health problems. The programs are supposed to cover the costs of medical care, rehabilitation, and income support during periods of disability due to work-related injuries and illnesses (2, 54). Serious problems exist today in the operation of this system, particularly with the undercompensation of chronic occupational diseases; these issues, however, are beyond the scope of this discussion. With the advent of workers' compensation, a new field of specialized industrial medicine practice arose as physicians were hired by companies to represent employers within the bureaucracy of the compensation system. This development tended to increase further the isolation of occupational health practitioners.

Over the next several decades there were advances in engineering, toxicology, and industrial hygiene in the workplace, paralleling the small but growing specialization of occupational medicine. The isolation of occupational health services from general health services was recognized early by some observers of the rapidly emerging field of occupational medicine. B. J. Stern, author of a 1945 monograph, *Medicine in Industry,* expressed concern about the effects of this development on occupational medicine: "It has tended to sever industrial medicine from the mainstream of medicine and public health by dealing exclusively with hazards in the factory, shop, mine and mill, isolated from the worker's health in the community" (16, 68).

Decades later the post-World War II phenomenon of broad-based health insurance for large numbers of workers compounded this isolation of occupational medicine from mainstream medicine. These insurance benefits included, as part of negotiated wage agreements, broadened workers' access to the health care system, but almost always excluded coverage for work-related injuries or illnesses (16, 53). Health coverage for occupational conditions was left therefore to the province of the workers' compensation system and to industry-based occupational medicine programs.

Not only did these developments create a specialty of practice that was largely outside academic institutions and major sources of health care delivery (the office, the clinic, the hospital), but they also left the vast majority of American workers without access to occupational health services. Even today, of the approximately 100 million workers in the United States, most (70%) work in plants that do not have any medical care services, and fewer than 15% work in plants with physician services (39). Finally, the primary care practitioner ministered to most of the health problems of working people whether the problems were work-related or not, even though s/he was poorly prepared to accept this role (1, 9, 30, 52, 57).

DEVELOPMENT OF MODERN OCCUPATIONAL HEALTH SERVICES

Beginning in the 1970s, the practice of occupational health was significantly altered by the passage of several major pieces of legislation. In 1969, in response to a major mining disaster, Congress enacted the Coal Mine Health and Safety Act (renamed in 1977 the Coal Mine Safety and Health Act). In 1970 the Occupational Safety and Health Act (OSHA) was passed, creating NIOSH, the National Institute for Occupational Safety and Health, and OSHA, the Occupational Safety and Health Administration. As part of NIOSH's mission to provide research and training in occupational health, initially 12 (and now 15) Educational Resource Centers (ERCs) were established, providing education in occupational medicine, occupational nursing, and industrial hygiene. Most of the ERCs have been located in Schools of Public Health and have only minimally, if at all, been involved with the training of occupational health practitioners in primary care specialties (52). Aided by resources available as a result of the ERC initiative and by a growing awareness of the extent of the need, occupational health did achieve a greater prominence in the academic medical center in the last decade with the increasing number of hospital-based, academically affiliated, occupational medicine clinics (42, 48, 54). These clinics share a primary goal of providing diagnostic services to assess the work-relatedness of health problems; training and research activities are also integrated into the function of most of these clinics (54).

There is, however, a continuing shortage of trained occupational medicine specialists (2, 75): only about 1000 physicians have become board-certified in occupational medicine since the inception of that specialty's medical boards (subspecialty of American Board of Preventive Medicine) in 1955. A number of the primary care specialties have recognized the need to incorporate occupational medical training and practice into their disciplines; most recently, the American College of Physicians issued a position paper with the following two major summary positions (1):

1. Physicians, especially primary care internists, must address the occupational health care needs of their patients. Physician responsibilities in providing care to patients of working age include identification of occupational and other environmental health risks, treatment of disease and injury, and patient counseling about preventive behavior.
2. Physicians have a responsibility to improve the health of the population by working to prevent occupational and other environmental risks that cause injuries and disease.

The provision of occupational health services has recently expanded with the increase in the number of urgent-care centers and their older variant, the free-standing industrial medicine clinic. The latter is based outside of industry and usually contracts occupational services to small to medium-sized employers (17, 37). There is also evidence of growing interest in some sectors of the corporate community to incorporate the concept of a healthy workforce into planning for overall corporate growth and productivity (75). Partly in response to rising costs of workers' compensation (29, 45), Health Maintenance Organizations have been developed specifically designed to provide workers' compensation coverage (44). The most significant new trend arises from the changing economic pressures on the health care industry: occupational health services are likely to be used increasingly by large group practices and hospitals as a means to attract employee groups for personal health care (17, 32).

PREVENTION STRATEGIES IN OCCUPATIONAL HEALTH

Several special features of work-related conditions, particularly of chronic diseases of occupational origin, are of importance to the clinician, to the epidemiologist, and to those involved in designing and implementing prevention strategies. These principles are reviewed in more detail in a recent text of clinical occupational medicine (53).

1. The clinical and pathologic expressions of most occupational disease are indistinguishable from those of nonoccupational diseases. This is a crucial concept. Although a few hazards cause unusual patterns of illness, the common presumption that work-related symptoms are somehow unique is generally false.

2. For many occupational diseases, there is a latent interval between the onset of exposure and the first expression of disease. Most chronic diseases and all malignant sequelae follow this concept. This delay creates difficulties for the clinician who tries through history-taking to link these outcomes to often remote exposures, as well as for the epidemiologist and others investigating work-related diseases.

3. Many occupational factors act in concert with nonoccupational factors. Multifactorial causation has major importance for the clinician, the researcher, and the regulator. The often artificial distinction between work-relatedness and non–work-relatedness of disease, which stems from the necessary legal attribution of cause, often obscures important causal links and inhibits effective prevention strategies.

A now well-known example of multifactorial causation is the multiplicative effect of cigarette smoking and asbestos exposure on risk for lung cancer (60, 62, 63). Asbestos exposure multiples the risk for lung cancer (by about 2- to 5-fold) both for smokers and nonsmokers; this results in the dramatic increase in risk over background for the smoking asbestos worker. For example, if the relative risk in the smoker is 10, then combination of smoking with asbestos exposure may increase that risk to 20- to 50-fold, whereas the asbestos-exposed nonsmoker experiences an overall relative risk of 2–5 (12). The relative contribution of asbestos and smoking to risk has been the source of much controversy and millions of dollars in legal costs (26). Identification of this multifactorial effect has importance for the clinician, but its characterization was made possible by the epidemiologist, and those involved in prevention, including the regulator, need to consider its implications. In the setting of synergism, diminution of either of the causative agents can have a large impact on excess risk. Although most of the increased risk for lung cancer is seen among asbestos workers who smoke [92% of all their lung cancers would have been avoided had none been smokers (assuming a relative risk for smoking of 10, for asbestos exposure of 5, and for both, 50)], it is sobering to realize that 82% of all their lung cancers would have been avoided if none had been exposed to asbestos (59).

4. Occupational factors of importance may be difficult to ascertain by the clinician and may have as yet unestablished biological significance. Numerous problems of hazard identification still exist despite the increasing knowledge about a number of workplace toxins, for the following reasons: (a) about

50,000 chemicals are in wide use, of which about one half are toxic (72); (b) many toxins occur in mixtures, may be contaminants of other products, and are often not labeled; (c) hundreds of new substances are introduced annually into the workplace; (d) fear of litigation and privacy about proprietary formulations limit free flow of chemical information from employers and manufacturers; and (e) the toxicity of relatively few of these substances has been adequately evaluated (38).

5. The clinical effects of toxic exposure are related to exposure dose. Exposure-response relationships usually follow one of three patterns: (a) for direct acting toxins, both the incidence and severity of the resulting disease increase with progressively higher doses, and a safe threshold of exposure is often definable; (b) for substances producing hypersensitivity states, the severity of the response bears little relationship to exposure dose; however, for such substances, initially higher exposure doses will most likely cause a greater number of exposed persons to become sensitized; and (c) for substances that are carcinogens, there is no safe threshold, and dose will have a consistent and usually, although not necessarily, linear relationship to increased risk.

The Clinician's Tools

Not only is the physician critical to recognition of the effects of exposure to known occupational hazards in individuals, but in addition the alert clinician is in a unique position to identify new associations between workplace exposures and disease (34, 35). Perhaps in no other field does there remain so great an opportunity as in occupational health for the physician to identify new disease entities. Multiple instances exist of physicians who, sometimes after a problem has been brought to their attention by workers, have established a new link between an exposure and an adverse health outcome. Ramazzini, the father of occupational medicine, began this tradition at the beginning of the eighteenth century when he categorized the health problems of sewer workers, painters, and potters (46); and Pott in 1775 demonstrated that the frequency of occurrence of scrotal carcinoma was greatly elevated in young chimney sweeps (74).

More recent examples include the identification of the association between polyvinyl chloride manufacture and hepatic angiosarcoma (8); between neuropathy and exposure to dimethylaminopropionitrile (DMAPN) (28) and 2–5-butylazo-5-methylhexanae (BHMH) (21); and between aluminum smelting and progressive neurologic disease (31). In the next section we examine the tools available to the physician in aiding the recognition, treatment, and the prevention of occupational diseases.

THE OCCUPATIONAL HISTORY   Lack of awareness of occupational health hazards constitutes the most formidable obstacle to the clinician's successfully recognizing, preventing, and treating occupational disease. Without this awareness, the clinician is most unlikely to make a diagnosis of a work-related disease (49). The occupational history is the foundation on which most assessment of work-related conditions in individuals is based; the failure to obtain even the most rudimentary occupational history was first commented upon nearly 300 years ago by Ramazzini (46), and this continuing deficiency has been noted by many authors (7, 15, 41, 52).

The purposes of the occupational history include making accurate diagnoses of work-related diseases, preventing the development of such disease, preventing the aggravation by workplace factors of either work-related or other conditions, identifying and then preventing or alleviating the risk of exposure to workplace hazards, finding new associations between exposure and disease, and establishing the scientific basis for compensation of work-related disease (53).

Two main components of the occupational history are (*a*) the employment and exposure history and (*b*) the work-related health history. The work and exposure history obtains information about current and past jobs, including the nature of each job and industry in which a patient has worked, as well as information about the use of protective equipment and the presence of potentially hazardous exposures. Self-reported exposure histories have been demonstrated to have validity (55), but further investigation may be required to identify specific components of products and to document exposure levels. The work-related health history augments the traditional health history by asking the worker about the perceived relation, if any, between health problems and work exposures, the presence of similar symptoms or illnesses in co-workers, and the variation of symptoms with time at work or changes in work processes.

THE LABORATORY   Few findings in the physical examination are uniquely helpful or truly pathognomonic in diagnosing occupational diseases. Thus the often-portrayed blue gingival line (the "lead line") is rarely seen in modern adult lead intoxication (11), and typically-described basilar inspiratory pulmonary rales are neither sensitive nor specific to asbestosis (53). Rarely, a constellation of findings on physical examination may give evidence of multisystem involvement from an occupational exposure, such as the findings of peripheral neuropathy, dermatitis, and sinusitis in workers overexposed to certain solvents. More often, however, the occupational history, in conjunction with laboratory testing, is used to diagnose occupational disease, and the physical examination plays only an ancillary role.

A comprehensive review of available laboratory testing is beyond the scope of this discussion, but despite some overlap between categories, these can be broadly characterized as follows:

Functional tests   These tests are usually nonspecific to exposure or disease but provide valuable quantitative data on extent of injury. Spirometry, a test of pulmonary function, is a basic tool in assessing occupational lung disease (13).

Spirometry is useful in individual health assessment; it provides a reproducible portrayal of ventilatory function that can characterize the extent and nature of alterations from predicted function and can be used longitudinally to assess greater than expected decrements in function over time. Spirometry has also played a major role in both cross-sectional and prospective epidemiologic investigations in the detection of clinically obvious as well as subclinical lung dysfunction, with the result that detection of work-related lung disease has become feasible at an earlier stage than previously was possible. Such early detection may lead to improved prevention (13).

Early markers of dysfunction   These tests are usually nonspecific to exposure, but sometimes are specific to a particular disease. New technologies have been introduced over the past few decades that give evidence of early end-organ dysfunction and are promising as screening tools for preclinical occupational disease. Examples include tests of mutagenicity in urine following exposure to a wide range of carcinogens (66); of chromosomal aberrations in blood such as in benzene-exposed workers (66, 78); or urine assays of modified nucleosides (breakdown products of transfer RNA) such as in asbestos workers with mesothelioma and parenchymal or pleural fibrosis (65). Although these tests are only occasionally useful in individual health assessments and rarely in attributing disease etiology, they hold promise for epidemiologic studies as early markers of effects.

Biologic monitoring of exposure and effects   This last category of laboratory tests is usually specific to monitoring occupational diseases. Blood lead and urine arsenic determinations are examples of direct monitoring of toxins in human tissues, where levels have a reliable relationship to exposure dose. Detection of metabolities of toxins, such as hippuric acid in urine to detect extent of benzene exposure, may similarly allow a reliable assessment of exposure. A number of promising newer techniques allow for in vivo or in vitro assays of specific exposure effects, such as lymphoblast transformation test in beryllium-exposed workers with chronic beryllium disease (10), and bronchial inhalation challenge testing with a number of agents such as western red cedar (6). In addition to aiding attribution of cause in affected individuals, these tests are likely to play an increasing role by providing greater precision in epidemiologic investigations exploring exposure–effect relationships in occupational disease.

The Role of Epidemiology

By studying the occurrence of disease in populations, epidemiology provides a perspective in occupational health that is broader than that of clinical medicine, yet more specific to man than that of laboratory research. Through description of the patterns of occurrence of illness and through analysis of relationships between exposure and illness, epidemiology is a fundamental tool in the control of occupational diseases. This discipline provides a means to: (a) identify the etiologies of occupational disease; (b) identify the populations at greatest risk; (c) define precursor lesions that might serve as a basis for screening; and (d) provide a rational foundation for prevention interventions. Development of full knowledge of disease causation may not be possible through epidemiologic research. Determination of specific etiologies, however, is not always a necessary prerequisite to the prevention of disease. For example, John Snow's preemptive removal of the handle of the Broad Street pump in London in 1854 was effective in reducing the incidence of cholera, even though the causative organism *Vibrio cholerae* was not yet identified (64). Similarly, the observation of such associations as lung cancer and employment in coke ovens or chronic encephalopathy and solvent exposure may permit effective intervention long in advance of delineation of specific causative agent(s) or pathophysiologic mechanisms.

Given the economic implications that often result from determination of causality in occupational illness, rigorous criteria of causality have been developed for the assessment of putative cause-and-effect relationships in occupational epidemiology. The major criteria are presented below with comments about aspects specific to occupational disease (18, 19, 70).

EXPERIMENTAL DATA   Does evidence exist of a causal relation from true experiments in humans? This degree of proof is rarely available in chronic disease epidemiology in general and even less often in occupational epidemiology. When, however, these kind of data are available, such as from following prospectively the results of reductions in exposure in occupationally exposed cohorts, the resulting evidence provides powerful support for causality.

THE CONSISTENCY (REPRODUCIBILITY) OF THE ASSOCIATION   The evidence of a consistent finding of an association between an exposure and a disease observed in different places, circumstances, or times has been one of the key pieces of evidence showing causality in occupational epidemiology. The International Agency for Research on Cancer (IARC) has relied extensively on this criterion in assigning the strength of evidence about human carcinogenicity from occupational exposures, stating that "the most convincing evidence of causality comes when several independent studies done under different circumstances result in 'positive' findings" (25).

THE TEMPORAL DIRECTION OF THE ASSOCIATION   In addition to the prerequisite of exposure preceding illness, causality is best supported when appropriate latencies have occurred, usually on the order of several to as many as 50 years in the instances of occupational cancers (61).

THE STRENGTH OF THE ASSOCIATION   The greater the strength of the association, as measured by the relative risk (RR) or odds ratio, the more compelling is the suggestion of a causal link in occupational epidemiology. Monson has suggested a scheme of ranking the strength of the association as follows: No association demonstrated for relative risks of 1 to 1.2; weak association with a RR of 1.2 to 1.5; moderate association with a RR of 1.2 to 3; strong association with a RR of 3 to 10; and infinite association with RRs greater than 10 (36). Also important to consider is that fulfilling the criterion of reproducibility of findings may prove more compelling evidence of causality than the strength of the association, particularly if repeated but low-level excesses of increased risk are seen. Although statistical uncertainty of small numbers in any one study may raise doubts about the truth of an association, even small relative risks may have large public health impact when large numbers of workers are exposed to common exposures. Such may prove to be the case with fibrous glass and risk for lung carcinoma (58).

THE BIOLOGICAL GRADIENT OF THE ASSOCIATION (DOSE-RESPONSE RE-LATIONSHIP)   If an occupational exposure is related causally to a disease, the risk of developing the disease should be related positively to the extent and severity of the exposure (76, 77). Occupational diseases will sometimes defy this criterion; this has been observed when those employed for only brief durations have the highest levels of exposure. In these instances, duration of employment, often a good index for cumulative exposure dose, may appear to be protective for risk of disease. Selection out of the industry by those most affected, a component of the healthy worker effect, may also result in those with the shortest term of employment being most affected (14, 33, 67).

Sentinel Health Events (Occupational)

Sentinel health events (occupational) are a tool for the rapid identification of work-related disease. Recognizing that most physicians are currently ill-prepared to diagnose occupational diseases and that, in addition, health surveillance systems are inadequate for occupational disease surveillance, Rutstein and colleagues have expanded upon a previously described concept of the Sentinel Health Event (SHE) (56). An SHE was defined as a "preventable disease, disability or untimely death whose occurrence serves as a warning signal that the quality of preventive and/or therapeutic medical care may need improvement." An SHE (O) (occupational) is defined as a "disease, disability or untimely death which is occupationally-related and whose occurrence may: 1. provide impetus for epidemiologic or industrial hygiene studies; or 2. serve as a warning signal that materials substitution, engineering control, personal protection, or medical care may be required" (57).

The initially published SHE (O) list includes 50 work-related diseases, identifies the sequela(e) of concern (namely, unnecessary disease, unnecessary disability, unnecessary, untimely death), the industry and/or occupation where the disease is likely to be encountered, and the causative agent, if known. Only those conditions were included for which objective documentation of an associated agent or industry was available; this list was then reviewed by a working group on Preventable and Manageable Diseases. The SHE (O) list has a number of applications, including the following:

1. serving as a routine surveillance tool; the identification of an International Classification of Disease (ICD) code makes possible the linkage of events to most currently available data sets (e.g. vital registries);
2. serving as an episodic surveillance tool by follow-up of certain events, such as the monitoring of all mesotheliomas recorded on death certificates;
3. serving as a guide to the practicing physician by providing an overview of the industries and occupations and associated diseases that might be expected in a clinician's practice, and;
4. serving as a compendium of occupationally related diseases, with the potential to update the list periodically to reflect the changing state of knowledge about occupational diseases.

CASE STUDY: BENZENE AND LEUKEMIA

The history of the development of knowledge about benzene and its leukemogenic effects demonstrates the respective roles of clinical medicine and public health in the recognition and prevention of occupational diseases. Importantly, the epidemiologic research illustrates the increasing reliance on sophisticated techniques such as quantitative risk estimation. In addition, the regulatory response to the scientific evidence about benzene's toxicity demonstrates the influence of nonmedical factors, such as economics, in the prevention of occupational disease.

The association between benzene and leukemia was first described in case reports as early as 1928, and in the last 20 years reports of benzene-induced leukemia have outnumbered those of fatality from aplastic anemia, a long-recognized sequela of benzene exposure (50, 73). There was widespread reluctance among the occupational medical community to accept this leukemogenic effect, in part because benzene was one of the few suspected or known human carcinogens that did not initially prove carcinogenic in animal models. Recent test systems have, however, established benzene's animal carcinogenicity (51, 71).

Epidemiologic studies up until the late 1970s had demonstrated a variable excess risk of leukemia resulting from benzene exposure, with relative risks ranging from 2 to 24, depending on the study, type of leukemia identified as the outcome, and method of analysis (3, 23, 43, 73).

A retrospective cohort mortality study of about 1000 workers exposed to benzene in two Ohio rubber plants was undertaken by the National Institute for Occupational Safety and Health to evaluate this association more systematically (23, 47). In order to be eligible for inclusion, workers had to be employed for at least one day between 1940 and 1949, with vital status ascertained up until June 30, 1975. The preliminary results were published in 1977 (23). Final results were published in 1981 with vital status of 98% of the cohort ascertained; the report also provided a summary of the wealth of industrial hygiene information available concerning atmospheric benzene concentrations in the plants. Sources for exposure conditions included the Industrial Commission of Ohio, the Ohio Department of Health, the University of North Carolina and NIOSH (47). These data led to the conclusion that despite episodic excursions above allowable limits, for the most part exposures had been within the recommended standard in effect at the time of the exposure. Benzene standards in effect over the years covered by the study were changing, constantly being reduced (on the basis of benzene's irritant and nonmalignant hematopoeitic effects) as follows:

Year	Recommended standard
1941	100 ppm
1947	50 ppm, 8 hour time weighted average (TWA)
1948	35 ppm, 8 hour TWA
1957	25 ppm, 8 hour TWA
1963	25 ppm, ceiling
1969	10 ppm, 8 hour TWA

Evaluation of mortality experience of the cohort showed that there was a statistically significant increase in deaths from malignancies of the lymphatic and hematopoietic system (10 observed to 3.03 expected, $p<.01$); when leukemia deaths alone were analyzed, 7 cases were observed versus 1.25 expected [Standardized Mortality Ratio (SMR) = 560, $p<.001$]. A dose-response relationship was observed using duration of employment as an index of exposure dose, with the SMR of 200 for workers with less than five years of employment and 2100 for those employed five or more years (5 deaths observed vs .023 expected). These data were interpreted by the authors as demonstrating that risk for leukemia increased with higher levels of exposure to benzene. Although risk was demonstrated at levels generally allowable at the time of exposure, the data were insufficient to draw a dose-response curve that would allow a reliable quantitative risk assessment.

On the basis of the mounting epidemiologic evidence about benzene's carcinogenicity, NIOSH in 1977 recommended an emergency lowering of the then-allowable exposure level from 10 ppm to 1 ppm (40). OSHA responded and promulgated an emergency standard of 1 ppm airborne benzene. This standard was promptly challenged by the chemical industry. In a precedent-setting court decision, the Supreme Court in 1980 upheld an appeals court ruling that vacated OSHA's new benzene regulation (50, 51, 78). The court was split 5 to 4 in its decision; the plurality decided that OSHA had the burden of proving that benzene presented a "significant risk" to workers and of proving that the 1 ppm standard would reduce this risk. After examining the empirical studies and expert testimony, the majority of the court found that OSHA had not carried its burden of proof.

This decision was of particular interest because, although there was evidence available that the new standard would reduce the risk of benzene-induced leukemia, the actual risk reduction, namely, the number of lives that would be saved by imposing the lower exposure level, could not be precisely quantified. It is of considerable policy-making importance to consider whether regulatory standards can be impeded by the absence of available data to specify a quantitative risk assessment. The implications of the ruling were discussed by Justice Marshall in the dissenting opinion (22):

> The critical problem in cases like the ones at bar is scientific uncertainty. . . . The risk issue has hardly been shown to be insignificant, indeed future research may reveal the risk is in fact considerable. But the existing evidence may frequently be inadequate to enable the Secretary [of Labor] to make the threshold finding of 'significance' that the court requires today. . . . Such an approach would place the burden of medical uncertainty squarely on the shoulders of the American worker, the intended beneficiary of the Occupational Safety and Health Act.

Subsequent to the Supreme Court decision, however, quantitative risk assessment of benzene-induced leukemia was performed using new data as well as reanalyses of old data. The International Agency for Research on Cancer, IARC, projected that at a minimum, an excess of 140 to 170 leukemia deaths would occur per 1000 workers exposed during a working lifetime to 100 ppm; this determination extrapolates to 14 excess deaths as a low estimate and 170 deaths as a high estimate for lifetime exposures at 10 ppm (24, 49). In addition, NIOSH investigators subsequently have updated their initial mortality study with vital status ascertainment up until the end of 1981 (R. A. Rinsky, unpublished data). Through merging industrial hygiene data with personnel records, cumulative benzene exposure (ppm-years) have been calculated for each member of the workforce, allowing a more direct index of exposure rather than the problematic one of overall length of employment.

The overall SMR for leukemia in the updated analysis was 328 (9 observed vs 2.7 expected). When the workforce was stratified by cumulative benzene exposure (where an exposure of 1 ppm for one year equals one ppm-year), SMRs for leukemia followed a strong dose-response relationship: an SMR of

100 was found in workers with less than 40 ppm-years (equal to 40 years of exposure to 1 ppm), of 500 in those with 40 to 200 ppm-years, of over 800 in those with 200 to 400 ppm-years, and of over 2000 in those with 400 or more ppm-years exposure. Cumulative benzene exposure of 400 ppm-years is equivalent to a mean annual exposure over a 40-year working lifetime at 10 ppm, the currently enforceable US standard.

Justice Marshall may well have been right in his prediction about what future evidence about benzene-induced leukemia would show. Despite the newly available quantitative risk estimation, however, the standard remains at 10 ppm. The gap between available scientific evidence and implementation of prevention controls is striking in the case of benzene and leukemia.

BRIDGING THE GAP BETWEEN SCIENTIFIC EVIDENCE AND IMPLEMENTATION OF PREVENTION CONTROLS

Calkins and colleagues have suggested a framework for decision-making about potentially hazardous chemicals that involves three separate steps:

1. identification of the potentially hazardous substance, by using scientific research, including results of epidemiologic investigations, animal tests, and in vitro screening;
2. characterization of the risks from exposure, based on available descriptions of adverse effects, including quantitative risk estimation, the strength of the evidence about effects, and the sources and extent of exposure; and
3. policy decisions by governmental agencies, manufacturers, consumers, and other interested parties about what if any control measures should be instituted, such as regulating exposures, education, and material substitution (5).

Clinical medicine has its strongest role in Step 1 of the framework described above, namely, identification of the hazard. The astute clinician can find new associations between exposures and disease and bring these to the attention of the medical community and others involved in occupational health. Newly suspected hazards or diseases should generate further investigations, by case reports or epidemiologic studies to establish further evidence of a link beyond the index case. The practicing clinician can, using a system such as SHE (O), identify the presence of known associations in his/her practice. By so doing, a "follow-back" process can be initiated that, as with SHEs in general, may prove helpful in preventing occupational disease in other individuals.

Expertise from a number of public health disciplines is vital in Steps 1 and 2 of this framework, the characterization of risk. Increasingly, prospective epidemiologic investigations will need to employ sophisticated exposure indices. These will in turn provide more reliable data to perform quantitative risk estimation. Advances in biologic monitoring should also aid the development of biologic correlates of exposure for toxins amenable to measurement either directly or by measurement of their metabolites in tissues. In addition, the development of early biologic markers of disease that can identify subclinical toxic endpoints will aid in the identification and characterization of risk. More effective early detection and prevention of occupational diseases can occur when more refined tools have been developed to measure both outcome and exposure.

Finally, given the complexity of factors governing the institution of control measures, the clinician and public health practitioner must recognize their important role in developing and explaining the scientific evidence so that it can be correctly incorporated into policy that will further the occupational health of the population. The need for advocacy of furthering scientific understanding was recognized by the American College of Physicians (ACP). Its position paper on occupational medicine stated that "the ACP views as one of its responsibilities the provision of medical data necessary to help construct a sound scientific base for public policy development" (1).

SUMMARY AND RECOMMENDATIONS

The preceding discussion has focused on the historical isolation of occupational health and the potential contributions of clinical medicine and public health, especially epidemiology, to the recognition and prevention of occupational disease. As illustrated in the case of benzene and leukemia, factors much beyond these two realms of health have enormous influence on the actual implementation of prevention measures. Nonetheless, the scientific basis on which prevention should soundly rest can be significantly strengthened by implementing strategies that increase activities in occupational health in both clinical medicine and public health. A summary of recommended strategies to accomplish these goals is provided below.

Education of Clinicians

Given the central role of physicians, particularly those in primary care specialties, in recognizing and diagnosing known and suspected occupational diseases, it is imperative that physicians receive training in the basic concepts of occupational health. They also should be cognizant of the resources available for follow-up of known or suspected occupational diseases and hazards. The physician plays a critical role in most workers' compensation programs. One of the most important aspects of this role is to disclose findings of occupational diagnoses and health hazards to affected workers and to the public. In only a few states do physicians have a legal responsibility to report occupational illnesses and injuries. Until such time that there is a universal system of required reporting of occupational illnesses and injuries, the practitioner should be encouraged and educated to seek the most appropriate means of communicating known or suspected occupational health hazards. The avenues of reporting will vary with the situation but include publishing findings in scientific journals and relaying findings to workers and their representatives, to companies, to government agencies, and to the public. It is anticipated that the clinician will become increasingly involved in newly assigned roles of reporting should a partial or comprehensive system of occupational disease surveillance be established in the United States.

Integration of Occupational Health into Traditional Medical Services

Regardless of developments of occupational health services within industry or the extent of expansion of free-standing occupational medicine clinics, the patient with an occupational disease or injury is frequently treated only at traditional sources of medical care: in the primary care physicians' office, the clinic, or the hospital. Incorporating occupational health services into these areas involves more than simply the education of primary care practitioners. A wide range of medical personnel and others involved in administering health care can facilitate the appropriate recognition and evaluation of occupational conditions. An increasing number of workers receive all their health care from Health Maintenance Organizations or through Preferred Provider Organizations; if sophisticated diagnostic and treatment services within these organizations are not available, a mechanism needs to be established that does not make appropriate out-referrals impractical or unlikely. A feedback system of reporting known or suspected occupational conditions to appropriate agencies, employers, or unions needs also to be established. It is not always the treating physician who will best initiate these follow-up steps. Such is likely to be the case with visits to the Emergency Room, for example, which is often the first point of medical contact for the worker with acute but also chronic occupational health problems.

Further Development of Biologic Markers of Exposure and Effects

The development of early and more reliable markers of effects of toxic exposures can provide an early warning system in surveillance programs that test the adequacy of current control measures, and can allow more refined end points in epidemiologic investigations. Potential benefit to the individual is that detection of preclinical effects may favorably alter the natural history of work-related conditions by allowing changes in circumstance of work.

Elimination or reduction of exposure may be accomplished by technological improvements, work modification, or, if necessary, job transfer. Similarly, given the need for a better understanding of dose-effect relationships, improvement of existing technologies and support for development of new ones will facilitate better quantification of exposure dose.

Reporting Systems for Occupational Diseases

In addition to the need to expand existing programs within and outside industry for health surveillance and screening for defined populations of workers, there is an obvious need to develop broader reporting systems of occupational disease. There is also a need to address the lack of a standardized system for recording exposures, industries, and occupations, a deficiency already noted by the US National Committee on Vital and Health Statistics (69). One approach to improve reporting, possible without the development of new data systems, is to implement linkage of existing record systems. This linkage poses several methodologic difficulties and in and of itself would not be likely to provide direct evidence of disease etiology (4). Linkage of extant systems could, however, serve the following useful purposes: (*a*) identify high risk groups; (*b*) generate etiologic hypotheses; and (*c*) serve as a crude screening mechanism for significant effects. An example of linkage of existing records would be to use union or employment records to identify a cohort for the study; this cohort could then be followed for outcome effects through existing records, such as hospital discharge summaries or death certificates. Another example would be to link the occupational information derived from the decennial census with the National Death Index (NDI) (4).

Although only 12 of 50 states in the United States currently report occupation and/or industry on death certificates (27), a better use of information from such records could be derived by linking results from these states, which may demonstrate effects missed by smaller numbers in any single state. Even more desirable is the development of a national reporting system of mortality that is linked to occupational and industry identifiers.

The list of 50 SHE(O) can serve as a framework for a national system for occupational disease surveillance. Linking the SHE(O) list to the state mortality records that already encode occupational information can form an initial step in this process. A national system of physician reporting, partly derived from using this list as a source for potential reportable diseases, could be established for occupational illness. Public health agencies could use the list to monitor death certificates (even for states without occupational health information) as well as other events, such as claims filed through workers' compensation agencies. The follow-back of identified SHE(O)s can result in the initiation of steps to institute appropriate control measures.

Literature Cited

1. American College of Physicians. 1985. The role of the internist in occupational medicine: A position paper of the American College of Physicians. *Am. J. Ind. Med.* 8:95–99
2. Ashford N. A. 1976. *Crisis in the Workplace: Occupational Diseases and Injury: A Report to the Ford Foundation.* Cambridge: MIT Press
3. Aksoy M., Evelem, S., Dincol, G. 1974. Leukemia in shoe workers chronically exposed to benzene. *Blood* 44:837–41
4. Beebe, G. W. 1984. Record linkage: Methodologic and legal issues. *Arch. Environ. Health* 39:169–72
5. Calkins, D. R., Dixon, R. L., Gerber, R., Zarin, D., Omenn, G. 1980. Identification, characterization and control of potential human carcinogens: A framework for federal decision-making. *J. Natl. Cancer Inst.* 64:169–75
6. Chan-Yeung, M. 1973. Maximal expiratory flow and airway resistance during induced bronchoconstriction in patients with asthma due to western red cedar. *Am. Rev. Respir. Dis.* 108:1103–10
7. Coye, M. J., Rosenstock, L. 1983. The occupational health history in a family practice setting. *Am. Family Pract.* 28:229–34
8. Creech, J. L., Johnson, M. W. 1974. Angiosarcoma of liver in the manufacture of polyvinyl chloride. *J. Occup. Med.* 16:150–51
9. Cullen, M. R. 1985. Occupational medicine: A new focus for general internal medicine. *Arch. Int. Med.* 145:511–15
10. Cullen, M. R., Cherniack, M., Kaminsky, J. 1986. Chronic beryllium disease in the U.S. *Sem. Respir. Med.* 7:203–9
11. Cullen, M. R., Robins, J. M., Eskenazi, B. 1983. Adult inorganic lead intoxication: Presentation of 31 new cases and a review of recent advances in the literature. *Medicine* 62:221–47
12. Doll, R., Peto, J. 1985. *Effects on health of exposure to asbestos. Health and Safety Commission Report.* ISBN 011 8838032. London: Her Majesty's Stationery Off.
13. Ferris, B. G. 1978. Epidemiology Standardization Project. *Am. Rev. Respir. Dis.* 118:55–88
14. Fox, A. J., Collier, P. F. 1976. Low mortality rates in industrial cohort studies due to selection for work and survival in the industry. *Br. J. Prev. Soc. Med.* 30:225–30
15. Goldman, R. H., Peters, J. M. 1981. The occupational and environmental health history. *J. Am. Med. Assoc.* 246:2831–36
16. Goldsmith, F., Kerr, L. E. 1982. *Occupational Safety and Health. The Prevention and Control of Work-related Hazards,* pp. 27–76. New York: Human Sciences Press
17. Guidotti, T. L., Kuetzig, H. 1985. Competition and despecialization: An analytic study of occupational health services in San Diego, 1974–84. *Am. J. Indust. Med.* 8:155–65
18. Hill, A. B. 1965. The environment and disease: Association or causation? *Proc. R. Soc. Med.* 58:295–307
19. Hill, A. B. 1962. *Statistical Methods in Clinical and Preventive Medicine.* New York: Oxford Univ. Press
20. Hodd, J. B., Hardy, B. A. 1984. *Workers' Compensation and Employee Protection Laws,* pp. 1–22. St. Paul: West Publishing
21. Horan, J. M., Kurt, T. L., Landrigan, P. J., Melius, J. M., Singal, M. 1985. Neurologic dysfunction from exposure to 2-5-bytylazo-5-methylhexane (BHMH): A new occupational neuropathy. *Am. J. Public Health* 75:513–17
22. *Industrial Union Dept. v. American Petroleum Inst. (API).* 1980. 448 US 607:690
23. Infante, P. F., Rinsky, R. A., Wagoner, J. K., Young, R. J. 1977. Leukemia in benzene workers. *Lancet* 2:76–78
24. International Agency for Research on Cancer. 1982. *Monogr. on Eval. Carcinogenic Risk of Chemicals to Humans: Some Industrial Chemicals and Dyestuffs.* Lyon: IARC
25. International Agency for Research on Cancer. 1978. *IARC Monogr. on Eval. Carcinogenic Risk of Chemicals to Humans.* Lyon: IARC
26. Johnson, W. G., Heller, E. 1983. The costs of Asbestos-associated disease and death. *Milbank Mem. Fund Q.* 61:177–94
27. Kaminski, R., Brochert, J., Sesrito, J., Frazier, T. 1981. Occupational information on death certificates: A survey of state practice. *Am. J. Public Health* 71:525–26
28. Keogh, J. P., Pestronk, A., Wortheimer, D., Moreland, R. 1980. An epidemic of urinary retention caused by dimethylaminopropionitrile. *J. Am. Med. Assoc.* 243:746–49
29. Kurt, T. L. 1984. Workers' compensa-

tion: New worries for an old headache. *Occ. Health Safety,* March, pp. 68, 75

30. Levy, B. S. 1980. The teaching of occupational health in American medical schools. *J. Med. Educ.* 55:18–22

31. Longstreth, W. T., Rosenstock, L., Heyer, N. J. 1985. Potroom palsy? Neurologic disorders among three aluminum smelter workers. *Arch. Int. Med.* 145:1972–75

32. McCunney, R. J. 1984. A hospital-based occupational health service. J. Occup. Med. 26:375–80

33. McMichael, A. J. 1976. Standardized mortality ratios and the healthy worker effect: Scratching below the surface. *J. Occup. Med.* 18:165–68

34. Miller, R. W. 1981. Areawide chemical contamination: Lessons from case histories. *J. Am. Med. Assoc.* 245:1548–51

35. Miller, R. W. 1978. The discovery of human teratogens, carcinogens and mutagens: Lessons for the future. In *Chemical Mutagens,* ed. A. Hollgender, J. de-Serres, 5:101–26. New York: Plenum

36. Monson, R. R. 1980. *Occupational Epidemiology.* Boca Raton: CRC Press

37. Moxley, J. H., Roeder, P. C. 1984. New opportunities for out-of hospital health services. *N. Engl. J. Med.* 310:193–97

38. National Academy of Sciences. 1984. *Toxicity Testing: Strategies to Determine Needs and Priorities.* Washington DC: National Academy Press

39. NIOSH. 1977. *National Occupational Hazard Survey.* Vol. 3 DHEW (NIOSH) Publ. No 78-114

40. National Institute for Occupational Safety and Health. 1977. *NIOSH Revised Recommendations for an Occupational Exposure Standard for Benzene.* US Dept. of Health Education and Welfare. Public Health Serv. Center for Disease Control. (G 757-009/8)

41. The Occupational and Environmental Health Committee of the American Lung Association of San Diego and Imperial Counties. 1983. Taking the occupational history. *Ann. Intern. Med.* 99:641–45

42. Orris, P., Baron, S. 1983. Occupational medicine: A role for the primary care physician. *Hosp. Pract.* 18:195–202

43. Ott, M. G., Townsend, J. C., Fisbeck, W. A., Langner, R. A. 1978. Mortality among individuals occupationally exposed to benzene. *Arch. Environ. Health* 33:3–9

44. Powills, S. 1985. Minneapolis area HMO sponsors start new HMO for workers' compensation. *Hospitals,* June 1, 35–36

45. Price, D. N. 1983. Workers' compensation: Coverage, benefits and costs, 1983. *Social Security Bull.* 46:14–19

46. Ramazzini, B. 1974. *Diseases of Workers.* (Publ. in 1713, *Dr. Morbis Artifucum.*) Trans. W. C. Wright (Latin). New York: Hafner

47. Rinsky, R. A., Young, R. J., Smith, A. B. 1981. Leukemia in benzene workers. *Am. J. Ind. Med.* 2:217–45

48. Rosenstock, L. 1984. Hospital-based, academically-affiliated occupational medicine clinics. *Am. J. Ind. Med.* 6:155–58

49. Rosenstock, L. 1984. Occupational cancer: Clinical interpretation and application of scientific evidence. *J. Toxicol. Clin. Toxicol.* 22:261–82

50. Rosenstock, L. 1982. Leukemia and benzene. (Editorial.) *Ann. Intern. Med.* 97:275–76

51. Rosenstock, L. 1983. Leukemia and benzene. (Response to letter.) *Ann. Intern. Med.* 99:886

52. Rosenstock, L. 1981. Occupational medicine: Too long neglected. *Ann. Intern. Med.* 95:774–76

53. Rosenstock, L., Cullen, M. R. 1986. *Clinical Occupational Medicine.* Philadelphia: Saunders

54. Rosenstock, L., Heyer, N. J. 1982. Emergence of occupational medical services outside the workplace. *Am. J. Ind. Med.* 3:217–23

55. Rosenstock, L., Logerfo, J. P., Heyer, N. J., Carter, W. B. 1984. Development and validation of a self-administered occupational health history questionnaire. *J. Occup. Med.* 26:50–54

56. Rutstein, D. D., Berenberg, W., Chalmers, T. C., Child, C. G., Fishman, A. P., et al. 1976. Measuring the quality of medical care: A clinical method. *N. Engl. J. Med.* 294:582–88

57. Rutstein, D. D., Mullan, R. J., Frazier, T. M., Halperin, W. E., Meliuss, J. M., et al. 1983. Sentinel Health Events (Occupational): A basis for physician recognition and Public Health Surveillance. *Am. J. Public Health* 73:1054–62

58. Saracci, R. 1985. Man-made mineral fibers and health: Answered and unanswered questions. *Scand. J. Work Environ. Health* 11:215–22

59. Saracci, R. 1980. Interaction and synergism. *Am. J. Epidemiol.* 112:465–66

60. Saracci, R. 1977. Asbestos and lung cancer: An analysis of the epidemiologic evidence on the asbestos-smoking interaction. *Int. J. Cancer* 20:323–31

61. Schottenfeld, D. 1984. Chronic disease in the workplace and environment: Cancer. *Arch. Environ. H.* 39:150–57

62. Selikoff, I. J., Churg, J., Hammond, E. C. 1964. Asbestos exposure and neoplasia. *J. Am. Med. Assoc.* 188:142–46
63. Selikoff, I. J., Hammond, E. C. 1979. Asbestos and smoking. *J. Am. Med. Assoc.* 242:458–59
64. Snow, J. 1964. *Snow on Cholera.* New York: Hafner
65. Solomon, S. J., Fischbein, A., Shaema, O. K., Borek, E. 1985. Modified nucleosides in asbestos workers at high risk of malignant disease: Results of a preliminary study using discriminant analysis. *Br. J. Indust. Med.* 42:560–62
66. Sorsa, M., Hemminki, K., Vainio, H. 1982. Biologic monitoring of exposure to chemical mutagens in the occupational environment. *Teratogen. Carcin. Mutagen* 2:137–50
67. Sterling, T. D., Weinkam, J. 1985. The 'healthy worker effect' on morbidity rates. *J. Occup. Med.* 27:477–82
68. Stern, B. J. 1946. *Medicine in Industry.* New York: Commonwealth Fund.
69. US Dept. Health, Education and Welfare. 1977. Statistics needed for determining the effects of the environment on health. *Vital and Health Statistics* Ser. 4 No. 20. DHEW Publ. No. (HRA) 77-1457. Washington DC: US GPO
70. US Dept. Health, Education and Welfare. 1964. *Smoking and Health: Report of the Advisory Committee to the Surgeon General.* Washington DC: US GPO
71. US Dept. Health and Human Services (DHHS). 1981. *Second Annual Report on Carcinogens,* pp. 47–49. Washington DC: DSHS (NTP 81–43)
72. US Environmental Protection Agency. Office of Toxic Substances. 1976. *Core Activities of the Toxic Substances Draft Program Plan.* Washington DC: EPA Publ. 5604/4-76-005
73. Vigliani, E. C. 1976. Leukemia associated with benzene exposure. *Ann. NY Acad. Sci.* 271:143–51
74. Wagoner, J. K. 1976. Occupational carcinogens: Two hundred years since Percivall Pott. *Ann. NY Acad. Sci.* 271:1–4
75. Walsh, D. C. 1984. Is there a doctor in the house? *Harvard Bus. Rev.* 62:84–95
76. Waxweiler, R. J., Beaumont, J. J., Henry, J. A., Brown, D. P., Robinson, C. F., et al. 1983. A modified life-table analysis system for cohort studies. *J. Occup. Med.* 25:115–24
77. Weiss, N. S. 1981. Linking causal relationships: Elaboration of the criterion of dose-response. *Am. J. Epidemiol.* 113:487–90
78. White, M., Infante, P. F., Walker, B. 1980. Occupational exposures to benzene: A review of carcinogenic and related health effects following the US Supreme Court decision. *Am. J. Ind. Med.* 1:233–43

Ann. Rev. Public Health. 1986. 7:357–89

PRACTICE-BASED RECORDING AS AN EPIDEMIOLOGICAL TOOL

Maurice Wood, Fitzhugh Mayo, and David Marsland

Department of Family Practice, Medical College of Virginia, Richmond, Virginia 23298-0001

INTRODUCTION

An Historical Overview

Health care in the United States during the last 40 years has evolved in response to the burgeoning growth of new medical information. Prior to World War II, the majority of physicians were generalists and some, because of special interests, training or experience, developed expertise in some arena, but the needs of most communities were met by physicians who were prepared to be ubiquitous in their responsibilities.

After World War II, with the establishment of the National Institutes of Health (NIH) in the US and the concomitant increase in the availability of research funds from the federal government, research effort and, with it, educational activity in these areas increased. Subspecialty training programs in medical schools increased in number and size and by the early 1960s the majority of medical school graduates were entering subspecialty residency training programs. This movement had profound effects. Research was concentrated in hospital/laboratory settings. These were usually provided by the larger university hospitals, and studies therein generally assumed the capacity to extrapolate to the universe of medical care, including that outside the hospital.

If this assumption was appropriate in individual case studies, it was less so in inquiries that described the incidence and prevalence of morbidity in hospital practice. Discussions on the preferred management for specific conditions if extrapolated to the management of similar conditions in office practice resulted

357

0163-7525/86/0510-0357$02.00

in scenarios that were often difficult to undertake in such settings. The published medical literature reflected the lack of understanding by physicians of the difference between hospital and office practice. It induced a sense that two standards of care existed: a hospital standard and a more limited, and therefore inferior, standard in office practice. The academic "hubris" of excellence became self-fulfilling, as few opportunities existed for institutional physicians to experience community practice. Physicians seeking to practice in community settings found few effective training programs to prepare them for their role and frequently experienced cultural shock on beginning practice in the community. Many, therefore, gave up practice and, returning to the medical institutions, sought more specialized training.

As the number of physicians willing and able to practice away from large hospital settings decreased, their absence was first noted in the rural areas and smaller towns throughout the United States. As rural physicians died or retired, they were not replaced, but the growing metropolitan and suburban areas continued to have adequate numbers of physicians because the plethora of subspecialty-trained physicians were settling in the areas near large hospitals.

In the early 1960s, most state legislatures were providing limited fiscal support to affiliated medical schools. In the climate of social turmoil during that decade the need was increasingly expressed for more physicians in the rural areas and small towns of the United States. The criticism of the profession was such that in late 1963 the Council on Medical Education of the American Medical Association (AMA) constituted the Citizens Commission on Graduate Medical Education and appointed Dr. John S. Millis, PhD, from Case Western Reserve University, as the chair. Over the next two years this commission met 13 times. The final report was published by the AMA in August 1966 (1).

The report described the steadily increasing production of specialty-trained physicians since World War II, who practiced only in the immediate neighborhood of large hospitals, thus causing the paucity of physicians practicing in less well-populated areas lacking large hospitals. The commission recommended the production of a new type of physician—the "primary physician"—who would be the physician of first contact and would also have the responsibility for coordinating the provision of continuous, comprehensive care to individuals of all ages and both sexes, whether provided in the hospital or the office. Almost simultaneously, in November 1966, the AMA also published a report of the Ad Hoc Committee on Education for Family Practice, which had been chaired by Professor William Willard (2). This document, "Meeting the Challenge for Family Practice," identified the training necessary to produce family physicians capable of functioning as primary physicians and providing coordinated, comprehensive, and continuing care to individuals and families.

These seminal reports received positive reactions from consumer representatives. During the remaining years of the decade, helped by this support, the

American Academy of General Practitioners (AAGP) took steps to establish family practice as the twentieth specialty. This was done by instituting a certifying examining board for the specialty and seeking the formation of an accrediting committee under the jurisdiction of the Liaison Committee for Graduate Medical Education of the AMA to review and accredit training programs for postgraduate training in family practice. The review body was established in 1969 and the first board specialty examination for family physicians was held in 1970 (3).

New family practice training programs developed slowly in the early 1970s, but with the stimulus of federal and state government support, the number of programs created during the 1970s steadily increased. By 1982, there were 384 accredited family practice residency training programs in the US and approximately 2500 trained family physicians were being produced each year. The majority of medical schools had departments or divisions of family medicine with responsibilities for training both predoctoral and postdoctoral students in family practice. This growth occurred during a rapid increase in both the number of medical schools and the size of their classes. By the mid to late 1970s some academic departments of internal medicine and pediatrics were also training primary care physicians, mostly in tertiary care hospital settings, as distinct from the office practice "model unit" that was required for residency training in family medicine.

The Size and Nature of the Problem

The new family practice training programs were required to develop office practice settings in which resident physicians could experience the continuous comprehensive management of the health problems of a number of families over a period of three years. In the early 1970s the first attempts to develop curricula for this training highlighted the almost total absence of even the simplest information about the numbers and kinds of problems that individuals and families brought to a primary physician. However, in the health services literature as early as 1967 White (4) was drawing attention to the work of Crombie and the College of General Practitioners in England and reporting that "about 45% of the problems initially presented to primary care physicians cannot be given a diagnosis which fits the rubrics of the International Classification of Disease (ICD) except in the broadest categories. . . . Patients present to primary care physicians vague complaints, symptoms and problems, not labelled diseases" (4–6).

Last (7), in his seminal work, "The Iceberg—Completing the Clinical Picture in General Practice," used epidemiological methods to show the nature and size of some of the problems in England and Wales by adjusting the relevant data to a hypothetical "average general practice," which then consisted of about 2250 persons. He completed the clinical picture by estimating the number of people with undetected or potential disease who might be found on search, based on surveys of whole communities for a particular condition. This provided a detailed picture of the content of general practice in the UK at the level of practitioner-determined need and added an extra dimension of the community's unmet need.

Most of the early work was drawn from experience in practice in the United Kingdom. In the United States, prevailing opinion suggested that office practice in the US was different; therefore, such data could not be used for curriculum development in the new residency training programs. Assuming this to be true, there was in the US an obvious need for research into the content of primary care in terms of the morbidity, expressed in biological, psychological, and social terms.

The epidemiologic orientation reflected in such thinking was very different from the traditional definition of epidemiology. This, as stated by Last (8), is "the study of the distribution and determinants of health related states and events in populations and the application of this study to control of health problems." The difference lies in the definition of the term "population." As defined by Last, this is "all inhabitants of a given country or area considered together" (8). Such definitions prevented the application of traditional epidemiological concepts in describing the content of primary care and the development of rates for events in those settings. However, like the rest of medicine, epidemiology is dynamic, and all phenomena related to the health of populations are now addressed. Prior to World War II, infectious diseases were of seminal importance in the disease spectrum. Now the imperatives are the diseases due to aging and inappropriate lifestyle. This change has introduced epidemiological principle and data into the field of clinical decision-making and analysis, thereby influencing the probabilities of specific outcomes when alternative decisions are available. "Clinical epidemiology" is now fashionable. The term is used to describe the application of epidemiologic principle and the use of epidemiologic data, in the context of the personal health care of the individual members of groups or communities of patients. This has also been called "population medicine" and requires the development and use of person-defined data sets.

Such approaches encompass the work of the primary physician. Morris said of the modern world, "In a society that is changing as rapidly and as radically as our own . . . epidemiology has a special duty to observe contemporary social movements and their impact upon the people" (9).

In 1961, White et al (10) were more focused in stating, "Each practitioner or administrator sees a biased sample of medical care problems presented to him, rarely has any individual, specialty, or institution a broad appreciation of the ecology of medical care." A diagram of monthly disease prevalence estimates in the community and in hospital and university medical centers during the provision of medical care by physicians to adults 16 years old and over was used to illustrate the physician's limited view of disease (Figure 1).

Of 1000 adults in the community, 750 report one or more illnesses each month; 250 or 33% of those individuals contact a physician, nine or 1.2% are admitted to hospital, five or 0.7% are referred to another physician, and, finally, one is seen in a university medical center.

Two thirds of those reporting illness do not seek care; the vast majority of those who do are served outside the hospital or referral setting. Reports from the National Ambulatory Medical Care Survey (NAMCS) (11) in the United States have confirmed White et al's description. More recently, Regier et al (12) have shown that "at least 15% of the US population is being affected by mental disorders in any one year, but in 1975 only one fifth of those were served by the specialty mental health sector; whereas three fifths were identified in the general medical (primary care) sectors" (12). Goldberg & Huxley (13) concluded from an exhaustive review of the work in this field that "there is good reason to believe that there is an association between the psychiatric and physical morbidity in the primary care setting."

Henkin & Shapiro observed (14) that Mechanic (15) and Balint (16) have suggested that patients suffering from psychological symptoms feel uncomfortable presenting these complaints to a physician and instead present a variety of minor physical complaints, and that psychiatric symptoms may lower the

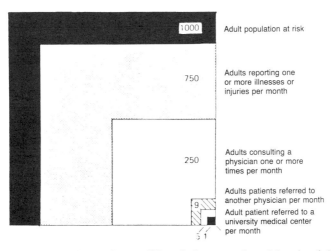

Figure 1   Monthly prevalence estimates of illness in the community and the roles of physicians, hospitals, and university medical centers in the provision of medical care (adults 16 years of age and over). Reproduced by permission from White, Williams & Greenberg (10).

patient's ability to cope with minor physical illnesses. Goldberg & Huxley (13) point out that Eastwood & Trevelyan in 1972 (17) observed that "the idea that individuals have a generalized psychophysical propensity to disease appears to be a valuable alternative model to that which seeks only a specific single cause and effect relationship." Many studies since then have supported this concept. Murphy & Brown (18) showed in a random sample of London women an increased likelihood of stressful life events preceding a new episode of physical illness. Aargaard and the Husfeldts (19) suggested that "poor health" in children is partly predicted by indices for long-term psychosocial stress. Kohn & White (20), in discussing determinants of health services use, observed, "Health and disease are multi-dimensional: there is considerable overlap between the bio-psychologic and social components and sometimes, though not necessarily, their severity or duration."

The constitution of WHO (1946) stipulated that "health is a state of complete physical, mental and social well being and not merely an absence of disease or infirmity" (21). The Alma Ata conference, "Health for All by the Year 2000" (22), re-emphasized the multifactorial determination of health and described new dimensions to health systems, stressing that people have the right and duty to participate individually and collectively in the planning and implementation of their health care.

White (23) in 1976 editorial, stated that future clinical research would be conducted with the cooperation of ambulatory patients in the doctor's office, the health center, the clinic, the outpatient department, and the home. He referred to the "new epidemiology," which Sir James McKenzie predicted would have to be the basis of clinical research in such settings (24), and then described the field of the new epidemiology. "It will involve patients and even non-patients at the earliest stages. . . . in the natural history of illness or disease (or the converse, sound health); it will start at the beginning. . . . Primary care research may be regarded as a long neglected frontier of research that is fundamental to a better understanding of the origins of ill health."

To achieve these objectives, White reflected on the need for new classifications of such elements as "symptoms," "reasons for visit," of human behavior and functional capacity. Further, he called for identification and definition of the terms and labels to be used and the means to calculate practice denominators that would encourage and enable more precise comparability within and among practices and institutions. This epidemiology constitutes the essential means to sound primary care research when linked with mechanisms for computer storage and retrieval of data (25–28).

In a more general sense, both Ryle in 1948 (29) and McWhinney in 1972 (30) had described the need for observational studies of the natural history of the presentation and evolution of the common, serious, and life-threatening illnesses seen in settings where the primary physician was the first contact for a person entering the health care system. An overwhelming need for such studies remains. The clinical practice of subspecialty medicine suffers as much from the resulting lack of information as that of primary care.

METHODS AND INSTRUMENTS

The National Scene

In the early 1970s, at the inception of family medicine as the twentieth specialty, a number of problems affected all of the primary care disciplines, including family medicine. There was scant scholarly activity, even in its broadest sense, in primary care settings. Primary physicians were, almost without exception, pragmatists who were task- and goal-oriented and service-committed. A superb exception was Hames in Evans County, Georgia, who had established a traditional epidemiological research model to undertake community-based research into cardiovascular problems among his practice population, which was synonomous with that of Evans County (31–33). However, his example only highlighted the uniqueness of the setting.

Further, there was an almost total absence of instruments capable of recording and retrieving data from the office setting without disrupting the normal process of care. Lack of these data—organized, classified, and analyzed to provide new information—made increased understanding of the content and process of primary care impossible.

The early research publications of the new discipline confirmed its epidemiologic orientation. They contained many descriptions of instruments usable in the office practice setting for recording (and retrieving) the demography and morbidity of the attending population. Much of this work came from the new departments and divisions of family practice in US medical schools, which were required to develop appropriate curricula for training predoctoral and postdoctoral students. The early academic primary physicians drew heavily on the experience in instrument development of the British College of General Practitioners, which made these instruments freely available to interested researchers in the United States and Canada (34–45).

These instruments included the age/sex register, i.e. a list of patients of a medical practice classified by birthdate and sex that was used in practice settings to provide denominator data for calculating age- and sex-specific rates (8, 34). A diagnostic index, usually in an E-book form, originally developed by Eimerl in the United Kingdom (46), provided a method for recording encounters in primary care by arranging them by problem or diagnostic category. This allowed tabulation of the number and frequency of persons seen, according to a problem or diagnostic category, over a given period. Methods of determining geographic site of residence using census tracts were also developed (38).

Shortly before this period, Lawrence Weed had developed his concept of the problem-oriented medical record (POMR) (47). In this record, the patient's history, physical findings, lab results, etc are formally organized to provide a cumulative record of "problems." The record includes Subjective and Objective (significant positive and negative) information, an Assessment of the definition of the problem, and Plans for diagnosis and treatment. This sequence of elements is known by the acronym SOAP. Once it was recognized that the POMR enables the recording and retrieval of clinical data, it was enthusiastically adopted by the new primary care training programs. The recording instruments had been previously developed in the United Kingdom and tested in numerous practice settings and through two national morbidity surveys in the United Kingdom by the early 1970s (48). All of these instruments were manual and could be completed by the physician or by the physician's staff.

The age and sex index used a minimum data set that included patient name, home address, telephone number, and marital status, in addition to date of birth and the sex. Other items like race, occupation, and years of education could be added if the need, opportunity, and commitment existed. The creation of a unique alpha-numeric number for each person allowed identification of the ambulatory care medical record of each person included in the index, and enabled the retrieval of that record from the medical record filing system for the purposes of clinical review or audit of the clinical care recorded in the chart.

The use of this unique identification number allowed the linking of the demographic information on the person with data on the diagnosis or definition of the problem determined by the primary physician using the Diagnostic Index. The restructuring of the medical record filing systems to allow charts to be grouped by census tract or other geographic unit, but linked with the unique patient numbers, enabled the analysis of the whole data set by distant computer after batch entry, without affecting data confidentiality.

Of equal importance were classifications appropriate for use in primary physician office settings. These also had evolved in the United Kingdom. They reflect the early work of the members of the College of General Practitioners, who noted that only about 50% of problems seen in the office setting could be classified by the then current *International Classification of Disease No. 7* (49). Repeated morbidity studies in office practice settings from other western countries had confirmed these findings (50–52).

All of these instruments were made available to members of the newly established specialty of family medicine in the United States. With appropriate modifications, necessary to reflect usual office practice in the United States and the steadily increasing commitment to problem orientation, they were published locally and then nationally in the newly established, peer reviewed *Journal of Family Practice,* which was first published in 1974 (53). *The Royal College of General Practitioners' Classification of Diseases* (1969) was modified for use with the POMR by the inclusion of a supplementary chapter categorizing psychosocial problems and adding "US" to its title (54, 55). Thus a literature base evolved that addressed the need for instruments and classifications usable in office settings without disrupting the office routine.

The Need for Data

The first and obvious need for the emerging primary care disciplines was data from which to develop an appropriate curriculum for the new residency training programs. Initially, most of the curriculum was borrowed from the long-established disciplines of internal medicine, pediatrics, obstetrics-gynecology, and the surgical specialties. However, the most difficult responsibilities for primary physicians lay in resolving problems presented in the office setting. Little or nothing was known of the sorts of problems people brought to the office-based physicians. No descriptions of the content of office practice in the US were then available.

Work began in 1973 at both the national and state levels to repair this deficiency. After many years of negotiation and preparation by staff and consultants at the National Center for Health Statistics, the National Ambulatory Medical Care Survey was begun in 1973 (11). The survey used a random sample of all physicians in all disciplines in the United States who provided ambulatory care. The careful, rigorous design required the recording of data on office visits by patients on certain days. Trained personnel visited each physician in the sample prior to the recording to explain the recording instrument and answer any questions. In addition, as one measure of evaluation, a post-study visit was made to the practice of each recording physician.

Data from the first survey (1974) appeared in 1975 (11). An average of three visits per person per year were provided by physicians in their private office practices during that year. The number of office visits increased with the patient's age and were higher for females than males and for whites than all others. Less than half of the office visits were to general and family practitioners, but the proportions varied between 65% of visits in nonmetropolitan areas to 35% of visits in metropolitan areas (where specialists could be expected to be highly concentrated). In 60% of visits, the physician had seen the patient before with the same problem; this proportion increased with the age of the patient, perhaps reflecting the increasing presence of chronic conditions. The most common reason for office visits, accounting for 80% of all visits, was for special examinations (prenatal care, follow-up after surgery, routine visit, etc); respiratory conditions accounted for 15% and circulatory conditions for 10% of all visits. These were the major disease categories. However, the important conditions were strongly age-related. Respiratory conditions accounted for 28% of all office visits for children, whereas circulatory conditions accounted for 29% of all visits for elderly people.

The seriousness of the principal problem was assessed by the physician: almost half were found to be "not serious" and another one third were found to be "slightly serious." Seriousness increased with age, but over two thirds of the visits by the elderly were still thought to be either "slightly serious" or "not serious."

At the end of 1975 and in the early part of 1976, similar data began to appear in the primary care literature. One example became known as the "Virginia Study." These data were recorded in multiple family practice settings in a single state over a prolonged period, (27). Geyman (56) in an editorial said of the Virginia Study that it reported on over half a million patient care problems collected over two years from urban, suburban, and rural practice settings in Virginia. In discussing the state of the art in primary care research he identified deficiencies in available coding systems, in agreed criteria for diagnosis, and in the reporting of behavioral problems.

This work showed that the fiftieth percentile of all 526,196 problems was contained in 23 descriptive diagnoses and the eightieth percentile in 102 diagnoses. Although most discussion of the Virginia Study concerned the educational resource it provided, McWhinney noted the importance of effective information systems in practice as an essential prerequisite for research (57). He postulated that every family practice setting would need an information system that provided at least an index of problems and diseases so that access to groups of patients for intensive observation over time would be available. He commented on the value of comparability of observations and noted that this required precise definitions of terms and agreement on classification systems. He identified a number of numerator problems, such as the extreme difficulty in identifying new problems so as to provide incidence rates and the difficulty of linking the presenting symptoms of patients with the final diagnosis across several visits.

Steward (58) and Hodgkin (59) discussed the limited recording of behavioral problems in the Virginia Study. McWhinney also discussed the difficulty of determining the co-morbidity of behavioral problems, which he attributed to a deficiency of the classification systems then available to primary physicians. Regarding the denominator of this study, he pointed out that because of the lack of a registered, and presumably committed, practice population in North America, practice rates derived from such data could only be presented in terms of the attending population, i.e. those persons who visited the practice over a period of time, and could not relate to the total population at risk, which was not defined.

McWhinney, in noting the dearth of information about the natural history of many common disorders and the cause and outcome of the many ill-defined illnesses seen by family physicians, called for more specific studies designed to test new hypotheses. Conceptual tools developed for other disciplines were inadequate in dealing with the multi-dimensional problems seen by family physicians in the office setting. McWhinney commented that progress in science occurs when information that is already available is perceived in new ways (57).

The Virginia Study was not presented as an epidemiological model but rather as the first attempt at a description of the provider-determined demand of patients attending the office of a primary physician. It reflected the steadily increasing interest of the new discipline in the morbidity content of office practice, as distinct from the hospital experience of generalists, which for many years had been the main focus of attention.

This study was followed by several smaller, similar studies from different regions of North America (60–63), which essentially confirmed that the distribution of morbidity in family practice settings across the United States held more similarities than differences.

The Denominator Problem

These studies highlighted the special problems of this first phase of primary care research in the US. Particularly, they focused attention on what became known as the "denominator problem." Work by Bass (64) Garson (65), and others in Canada involved the different methods available to determine the "at risk" population of a primary care practice. Kilpatrick (66) and Kretchmar (67) suggested that a practice denominator could be calculated when the frequency of "episodes of illness" (defined as a period of sickness for which there were one or more office visits) could be derived for persons using a particular source of ambulatory care, assuming that all or most of their care was obtained from that source.

Such a denominator would allow the determination of total crude rates of problems, encounters, procedures, tests, disposition, and other measures for individual practices and so enable comparison between practices. Although as Hill (68) has said, "crude rates should never be compared," the incorporation of age, sex specific data and the standardization of practice populations by age and sex and other demographic characteristics would allow more precise comparisons. The validation and replication of such a statistical method would represent a major step toward the development of an effective epidemiological model that would allow the determination of population statistics on demand.

In his work with data from the second national morbidity survey (1970–1971) in the United Kingdom, Kilpatrick (69) had shown that the frequency of "episodes of illness," brought to doctors' attention by 315,000 people in one year, followed a geometric distribution. It was hoped that fitting this mathematical model to the distribution of the number of visits or "episodes of illness" experienced by persons visiting a practice would, by backward extrapolation, provide an estimate of the number of persons with no visits in that year. The addition of this number to the number visiting in that year would then provide an estimate of the total practice denominator (69) (see Table 1 and Figure 2). [Underlying distribution: the percentage frequencies given in Table 1 yield a straight line relationship when plotted against the number of episodes on semi-logarithmic graph paper (Figure 2). This means that the ratio of successive episode frequencies is constant. The only discrete statistical distribution that has this property is the geometric distribution (151).]

Attempts in the United Kingdom and Canada to apply this model to episode rates of general practices showed some promise (70, 71). In these reports the calculated populations were within 5% of the registered population count in 50 individual practices. However, subsequent attempts to apply the same model to data derived from fee-for-service practices in the United States were unsuccessful. The difficulty was in clearly identifying "episodes of illness," as this was not a traditional concept in US practice. Likewise, attempts to apply the model to "office visits" for a new problem, on the basis that such visits would identify the beginning of an "episode of illness," were also unsuccessful, yielding wide-ranging estimates.

These attempts led Kilpatrick to comment in 1980, "A practice population is a nebulous concept, it is undefinable and cannot consistently be estimated. . . . Under the present health care system, we cannot use encounter records to do population based research" (72). He later tempered his statement: "The difficulties of epidemiological research in the US are not unique to primary care" (73).

Table 1   Distribution of episodes of illness (excluding prophylactic procedures and routine antenatal and postnatal care)[a,b]

Number of episodes	Frequency	Frequency (%)	Percentage predicted
0	127,569	40.4	40.0
1	71,261	22.6	24.0
2	46,656	14.8	14.4
3	28,716	9.1	8.7
4	16,997	5.4	5.2
5	10,336	3.3	3.1
6	5,950	1.9	1.9
7–9	6,427	2.0	2.2
10–14	1,467	0.5	0.6
15+	110	0.0	0.0

(a)	Total number of episodes	=	473,426
(b)	Total number consulting	=	187,920
(c)	Total number of people at risk	=	315,489
(a)/(b)	Episode rate per patient consulting	=	2.5193
(a)/(c)	Episode rate	=	1.5006

[a]Source: Second National Morbidity Survey, Table 9, males and females; Office of Population Studies and Censuses and the Royal College of General Practitioners, 1974.
[b]Reprinted with permission from *Journal of Royal College of General Practitioners*, 1975, 25:686–90.

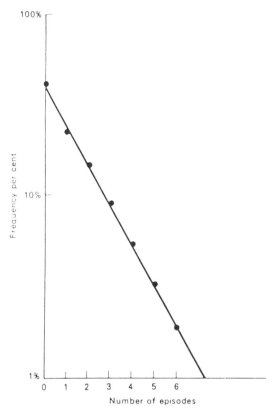

Figure 2   Reproduced by permission from the *Journal of the Royal College of General Practitioners*, 1975, 25:686–90.

In support he quoted such authorities as Doll & Peto (74): "Even in the US as a whole available population estimates seem surprisingly unreliable." With regard to cancer registration, "It is difficult to arrange a system . . . which ensures that each patient gets counted exactly once."

A high level of interest in the denominator problem continues among primary care researchers and their biostatistical colleagues. More recently, Krogh-Jensen (75) suggested a double negative binominal distribution of visit frequencies that allowed the determination of non-attender rates in 250 practices in Denmark. Schach (76) suggested that a Poisson log normal distribution, applied to the same data set, may be an adequate model to estimate the proportion of non-attenders in the 250 general practices in Denmark. As yet, these approaches have not been tested in other settings.

J. E. Anderson presented another interesting approach (personal communication, 1985). He evaluated the quadratic odds estimator (QDE) as described by Smith (76a), by using data from two prepaid Ontario primary care practices with patient populations of confirmed size, and developed a mathematical model. This model "functioned well in fulfilling the evaluation criteria with the . . . practice whether applied to illness episodes or patient visits. It provided accurate estimates both in the aggregate and in subsets and it was consistent over time." Anderson argues that the reason for the failure of most mathematical models so far is that "attending patients have been lumped together to generate an estimate of non-attenders that includes both full and part time patients." As "the proportion and behavior of part-timers in the attending group is variable, it is no wonder that the models have failed." He suggests that if it is possible for practices to reliably identify their full time (regular) attending patients, it may be feasible to estimate the number of regular non-attenders, as was done in his study. A separate model could then used to estimate the part-time patients and those attending and not attending during the study period. For study purposes the part-time attending patients could be reduced to full-time equivalents. He further suggests that the basic methodology exists and that the solution to the denominator problem will come from work in practices with populations of known size.

In the same vein, Kilpatrick recently pleaded for comparative studies among practices in different settings over several years—particularly among those with different systems of registering patients, i.e. state-required and practice-required registration and those using indirect methods of estimating practice size (73). In his view, such studies would allow the evaluation of observational methods drawn from other disciplines, such as the capture-recapture methods used in estimating wildlife populations. More traditional methods are presently being tested, including the utilization correction factor method comparing the sociodemographic and utilization statistics of small-setting patient populations with those of state or national samples by using health interview survey methods (77). Such comparisons allow the determination of weighting factors, which, when applied to specific demographically determined strata, may permit generalization of the data product from such populations to the larger population.

Numerators and Episodes

The considerable attention paid to the "denominator problem" in primary care research has somewhat overshadowed an issue of equal or greater importance. There is also a "numerator problem": considerable difficulties are encountered in clearly and accurately identifying the numerators required for the development of various crude rates for comparison purposes. Patients do not always present with clear cut diagnoses in primary care, but mostly with a mix of ill-defined problems, complaints, feelings, and concerns. Even traditional labels (diagnoses) may be applied differently, as physicians use various criteria for defining them (78). Thus, in retrospective studies using medical records it is often impossible to know which criteria have been used to determine the use of a specific rubric. Similarly, for prospective cohort studies to be considered valid and reliable, it is necessary to include only cases that meet previously agreed criteria of definition of the diagnosis to be used. Further, Bentsen has shown that physicians asked to specify the major diagnosis during primary care office recording disagreed in 15% of cases (79). Primary care researchers have addressed the first difficulty by agreeing and setting diagnostic criteria for commonly used disease labels in primary care. These take the form of inclusion and exclusion criteria for over two thirds of the rubrics listed in the *International Classification of Health Problems in Primary Care No. 2 (ICHPPC-2)* (80). This classification is the authorized version of the *International Classification of Diseases,* nineth version, for use in primary care settings. It is also known by the World Health Organization as *ICD-9 General Medicine* (ICD-9-GM). The version of *ICHPPC-2* that lists inclusion criteria is known as *ICHPPC-2 Defined* (81), and was developed by international consensus by the Classification Committee of the World Organization of National Colleges, Academies, and Academic Associations of General Practitioners/ Family Physicians (WONCA). Increasingly, these criteria are being accepted by primary care researchers and evaluators throughout the world as a baseline against which to measure their own locally determined criteria.

Diagnostic accuracy is further confounded by the difficulty of defining an episode of illness. Anderson (82) has pointed out that this epidemiological construct is based on the concept of there being a single identifiable cause for an illness or disease. "There appears to be a distinct tendency to associate episodes with a diagnosis." The paradigm of a "single identifiable cause" was established with death certification, where it has created some problems, but the difficulties of this approach in the clinical situation are much greater. The model of portion of a death certificate, below, is drawn from Anderson [(82) reprinted with permission of Praeger Publishers] and illustrates the point effectively.

Medical certificate of death:

		Duration
Immediate cause of death	A. Acute myocardial infarction	7 days
Antecedent causes (Underlying cause last)	B. Arteriosclerotic heart disease	4 years

Whereas in epidemiologic terms the cause of death may be considered a single episode of disease, in clinical terms it actually represents two distinct problems.

The effect of this oversimplification is to underestimate the frequency of important clinical problems in family practice settings, and it "compounds the difficulty of attempting to base denominator estimates on the episode count" (82). Anderson suggests that an "episode is a clinical problem rather than a diagnosis" and claims that because clinical problems are the focus of primary care practice and teaching they should also be the focus of research. This seems most apt as the need for research in primary care increasingly involves studies of the patient's reason for visiting a primary care provider, which is only rarely a disease.

If we accept that the data from primary care records are deficient in terms of 1. the definition of a true denominator because of the difficulty of defining the true population at risk; 2. the definition of numerators because of (a) problems of diagnostic accuracy, (b) different behavioral responses to the same illness or problem by both patients and physicians, and (c) difficulty of defining an episode of illness, we have to answer the question: What is the purpose of such recording? Anderson (82) states that the only justification is to identify possible changes in morbidity distribution over time, but he agrees with Kilpatrick (73) that the rate problems are not unique to primary care but also affect the application of epidemiological principles to research in other fields (83, 84). To reject the use of practice recording because of difficulties which to some degree are universal is inappropriate. Without question the data product from recording in primary care practice is effective in "identifying patterns of physician intervention in illness and health" (84). Lillienfeld, on primary care, noted that "the data . . . have their greatest utility in studying the effects of 'time,' 'place,' and 'person,' of specific health problems" (85).

In addressing the larger picture of data recording in practice, Cherkin commented (86): "In spite of this high level of interest [in the denominator problem] . . . there is now a body of opinion which suggests that clinical trials, case control studies, cohort studies, studies of the natural history of disease, and family studies, among others, do not require known practice populations or numerators and can be performed in primary care practice."

With these complications, uncertainties, and difficulties of data recording and analysis compounding the already incredibly varied nature of morbidity in primary care settings, it is evident that research in these environments must be both difficult and expensive, not only in terms of instrumentation but also in people and in time. However, it is an imperative that the work be done in these settings. From NAMCS (11) the evidence is overwhelming that the major proportion of all care is provided in such settings; studies are essential to confirm the impression that there is considerable cost benefit in continuing to expand the availability of cost-effective ambulatory primary care services (87–89).

Additionally, the paucity of such data, particularly from person-oriented data sets rigorously followed over time, embarrasses health planners and public health administrators and managers in fulfilling their responsibilities to organize the provision of health services for the public good. Fries has commented on these problems under the aphorism, "The world outside the laboratory is more complex than that within" (90).

In reflecting on chronic disease, Fries states, "Meaningful analysis of chronic disease outcome requires a more complex biological, psychological and social model of disease and the development of new techniques to deal with this complexity. . . . The many inferences upon chronic disease outcome include social and economic considerations, patient compliance with therapy, and complicated inter-relationships among multiple risk factors and out-comes." He claims that the traditional form of reductionist univariate experi-ment cannot adequately account for such complex relationships and recom-mends the development of chronic disease computer data banks to follow large numbers of patients from many settings over time. He stresses the need for rigor in standards of data collection, quality control, and evaluation and for reliable and valid outcome measures. Fries further predicts that a chronic disease data bank can help resolve some of the many questions still extant concerning the natural history of some illnesses, the risk factors for certain outcomes, and the costs and benefits of different treatments. He provides powerful arguments in favor of the use of structured rigorously audited clinical records as an effective epidemiological instrument.

Clinical Studies

Over the past few years the primary care literature has begun to support Cherkin's observation that certain studies in primary care do not require known practice populations or numerators (86). An exhaustive list of clinical studies that incorporated practice-based recording or chart review would be unreward-ing. However, the following studies are offered as an illustration of the diversity of the published material available from practice-based recording. Most of the studies involve the use of data drawn from medical records in primary care centers. They reflect the capacity of this method to study disease, its diagnosis, management, and outcome in environments differing in size from a single practice to a collaborating group of 38 practices. The range of clinical subjects varies from the definition of disablement drawn from 7000 records in 38 practices (91) to the diminishing incidence and prevalence of duodenal ulcer and its association with psychiatric disorder and chronic pulmonary disease derived from a practice population of 13,131 registered patients in Scotland (92). Hypertension, its diagnosis, management and control also figure promi-nently (93, 94). The epidemiology of urinary tract infection is discussed in a one-year morbidity study of 741 cases (95) and its seasonal variation and prevalence is described in a three-year retrospective study of 654 cases (96). Psychiatric diagnosis and consultation are discussed in two studies reflecting the importance of psychopharmacology and time-limited psychotherapy in the diagnosis and treatment of depression (97, 98). Other studies include clinical trials reflecting an interest in antibiotic prescribing (99), smoking cessation (100), the use of survey techniques to investigate urban lead toxicity in the population served by a family practice center (101), and, more recently, an evaluation of 249 cases of lymphadenopathy in a family practice (102). The method of data abstraction from the medical record figures prominently in studies of children. Clinical issues are addressed, such as failure to thrive, a study of 312 children drawn from three primary care centers (103); middle ear disease, a prospective follow-up of 2570 children from birth to the first five years of life in five primary care centers (104); compliance with treatment of otitis media, a study of 295 patients at four primary care offices (105); telephone management of febrile young children, a retrospective chart review of 311 febrile children in one center (106); social factors and life events as predictors for children's health; a one-year prospective study of the children in one general practice (107); and a comparison of physician home and office visits to families with newborns within the first two weeks of life (108).

All of these studies involved the use of data drawn from medical records in primary care centers and provide illustrations of the usefulness of such data even when the numbers of patients included are small and the period of the study is short.

Patients' Reasons for Visiting a Provider

The dynamic nature of primary care research has recently led to the development of instruments to record the patient's reason for entering a health care system (109–111). The resulting capacity to record effectively this long-neglected element of information may represent one of the major potential strengths of practice recording. Kerr White has commented (112) "that symptoms are the input of the health care system while diagnoses are an output." This "output" ignores the preceding health care process and renders impossible the study of the presentation and evolution of the problems, and the investigations and the treatment undertaken. These elements, which represent many of the patients' reasons for encounter, are virtually unresearched in primary care. There is no detailed knowledge of how patients' reasons for encounter, be they symptoms or other elements, evolve into diagnoses and subsequent interventions, treatment, and disposition. In no other settings can this process can be researched; whatever method of research design is used will incorporate practice-based recording.

Review of the clinical studies available in the primary care literature of research abstracts for 1980–1982 reveals that the majority deal with provider-determined diagnoses (113–115). Only three abstracts were concerned with patients' reasons for visit or the presentation of symptoms, and only one published paper could be identified (116). All physicians, including primary care physicians, have paid lip service to the value of this information for many years, but it has not been routinely collected and incorporated into the problem-solving process. One reason may be that no acceptable classification system existed to facilitate the collection of such data. The first attempt to develop such a classification was the Reason for Visit classification of the National Ambulatory Medical Care Survey (RFV/NAMCS) (117, 118).

Under the stimulus of the World Health Organization Alma Ata Conference held in the USSR in 1978 (21), the Unit of Development of Epidemiological and Health Statistical Services of WHO initiated the development of a reason-for-encounter classification to enable the accumulation of data on patient-perceived needs in primary care. These data were seen as essential to the reassessment of priorities in the planning and administration of health care services that would be necessary to achieve the goals of the Alma Ata Conference, condensed in the aphorism, "Health for All by the Year 2000."

The group responsible for this work produced a Reason For Encounter Classification (RFEC), which was field tested in eight countries and five languages in 1984 (119, 120). This is a relatively simple classification based on two axes, chapters and components, and uses a three-character alpha-numeric code for each rubric. Chapters, which are named by body systems or more general terms, are the reasons health care is sought and are designated by an alpha symbol. Five of the seven components, which are subdivisions of each chapter, contain rubrics identified by the same two-digit numeric code and relate to elements of the process of investigation or treatment in primary care settings. These component titles are Diagnostic, Screening and Preventive Procedures, Treatment Procedures and Medication, Test Results, Administrative Reasons, and Referrals or Other Reasons. Component 1 relates to the symptoms and complaints that patients bring to physicians; the final component, 7, Diagnoses and Diseases, incorporates all diagnoses contained in the *International Classification of Health Problems in Primary Care No. 2 (ICHPPC-2)* (121, 122). This classification by a technique of optional hierarchial expansion (123) can be directly related to all codes contained in the *International Classification of Diseases No. 9 (ICD-9)* (124).

The analyses of the field trial data showed that most reasons for encounter take the form of a symptom or a complaint. It provided a list of 60 most common reasons for encounter; these represented, jointly, 58% of all the data collected. Cough, fever, and sore throat ranked first in all countries, followed by blood pressure problems and various aspects of hypertension. Clustering analyses revealed significant clusters in each of three problem areas: hypertension, acute respiratory infection and acute gastrointestinal infection play a prominent role in all countries involved in the field trial. Cough and fever are often associated with sore throat and rhinorrhea. Diarrhea and vomiting correlate and are often accompanied by fever and sometimes coughing. As would be expected, hypertension, taking the blood pressure, and giving a prescription are associated (120). The field trial data analyses were used to modify the classification. A final version of the tabular list, which is expected to continue in its present form during the life of *ICD-9,* has been completed, along with a manual for use and an alphabetic index.

The classification can be used to classify three of the four elements of problem-oriented medical recording; namely the subjective information or reason for encounter, the assessment leading to the diagnosis, and the plan for intervention and disposition. This diagnosis, which will be expressed in the rubrics of the *ICHPPC-2*, can be linked by optional hierarchial expansion to *ICD-9*. In view of this, in April 1984 the reason-for-encounter classification was provisionally designated the International Classification of Primary Care (ICPC) (125). Arrangements are currently underway to ensure that the full tabular list, its manual for use, its alphabetical index, and a list of abbreviated titles will be published, with the endorsement of WHO, during 1986. This will allow the testing of the classification in all cultures and settings.

It is significant that broadly the same generic reasons for visiting a primary care provider were manifest in all countries taking part in the field trial. Because developing countries rarely have even marginally trained providers available at the level of first contact with their health care system, reason-for-encounter classifications need to be linked semantically with age and culture-specific lists of lay terms. Additionally, classifications of patient functional status, also age-, gender-, and culture-specific, need to be developed to complete the spectrum of primary care recording instruments necessary to describe, define, and explore the dimensions of the primary care process in all cultures. Work is already under way by WHO in these areas.

In parallel with this effort, which is directed to the needs of the developing world, research in primary care settings in the industrial countries of Europe and North America is exploring the progression from patient's expressed reasons for encounter through the process of provider-determined diagnosis to intervention and/or disposition. Better understanding of the issues involved in this progression could lead to improved communications between patients and physicians and the assumption by patients of a greater share of the responsibilities for the management of their problems (H. Lamberts, personal communication, 1985).

Minimum Data Sets (MDS)

The effective use in primary care settings of such instruments as described above requires a commitment by the primary care providers to collect, routinely, demographic information on the attending population. A basic requirement for this purpose is agreement by the recorders on a minimum data set of items to be collected with standard definitions and under specific circumstances. Wood has commented that patient care requires at least a minimum amount of demographic and clinical information about the patient; this can serve as a baseline for the measurement of both the process and the outcome of the care provided (127).

The concept of a minimal data set is usually decried by clinicians as being incompatable with good clinical care because they assume it limits the amount of information to be collected. However, "the essential element is the acceptance of the minimum data set by all users and providers of care and the agreement to record *at least* these items of information on all clinical records. Other items of information may be recorded and used in addition to the minimum data set, but the minimum data set items would invariably be present in the clinical record" (127). The MDS may be limited to age and sex, but can also incorporate race and ethnicity, marital status, and socioeconomic status determined by various parameters. A standard MDS is available for general use in the Uniform Ambulatory Medical Care Data Set (UAMCDS), developed and reported by the United States National Committee of Vital and Health Statistics (USNCVHS) (128, 129).

Examples of the use of this approach are seen in the MDS used by the recording physicians in the NAMCS, discussed above. NAMCS uses a denominator of all physicians in the United States providing ambulatory care and selects a small but precise sample as a means of accessing the US attending-patient population. A simple encounter form is used to record the MDS at the time of contact with the patient (130–132).

Collaborative Research

More recently this approach has been used in the Ambulatory Sentinel Practice Network (ASPN), which is a network of primary care practices throughout the US and Canada committed to collaboration for research purposes (133). In all data recording in primary care settings, researchers are faced with the difficulty of a small attending population of patients at any one individual practice. Some important and life-threatening problems and diseases occur infrequently in the average primary care practice, hence rendering the study of such conditions difficult in a single setting where the attending population is small. The solution to this problem is to enable collaboration between the providers in those settings.

Collaboration between providers for the purposes of service, education, and research is an imperative in primary care. For research purposes it probably began in the 1950s in the United Kingdom, as a result of the association between the Office of Population and Census Statistics (OPCS) and a number of volunteer recording practices of the then College of General Practitioners (CGP). The purpose was to describe the demography and morbidity of general practice populations in the United Kingdom (134, 135). This collaboration was remarkably successful, and it stimulated other examples of collaborative endeavor. In 1960, Scott collected reports on the prevalence of megalocylic anemia from 4700 practices, covering a total population of just over 16 million persons, which represented one third of the current population of the United Kingdom. These reports showed a gradient from high prevalence in the north and west to lower rates in the south and east, which has not yet been explained (136). The British College of General Practitioners also collected clinical reports from 1373 physicians on 10,000 children born with congenital abnormalities between 1954 and 1960. These reports showed a previously unreported summer excess among children born with partial absence or other defects of their upper and lower limbs (137).

Other collaborative systems have become well established, such as the Sentinel Stations in The Netherlands begun in 1970 (138). About 50 general practitioners are involved. Their practices are located so that their populations reflect the demographic and geographic distribution of the Dutch population as a whole. The physicians are asked to keep a weekly account of the number of patients they see with certain diseases and conditions by using a standard reporting format. Similar networks have developed for descriptive research purposes in New Zealand (139) and the US (140–142), but only recently have these became sophisticated enough to allow research on specific morbid conditions. This type of research requires the careful formulation of the question, its expression in the simplest of hypotheses, and the need for standardization of definitions, terms, procedures, and recording methods. Inevitably this requires the development of precise protocols that include glossaries of terms and appropriate classifications. The creation of person-specific data sets within these practice settings allows follow-up studies and even prospective studies over the considerable periods necessary to produce results.

A "network" is the association of large numbers of similar primary care practices for the purpose of sharing an agreed minimum data set of demographic and morbid information on a practice-attending population, recorded prospectively in a valid and reliable manner. Two US examples have been mentioned, the Cooperative Project in New England (141) and the Virginia Data System (27). In 1980, the North American Primary Care Research Group (NAPCRG) sponsored the development of a North American Sentinel Practice Network, which subsequently received support from the Rockefeller and Kellogg Foundations and is now known as the Ambulatory Sentinel Practice Network (ASPN) (133). ASPN is based on the recording methods pioneered by The Netherlands Sentinel Stations (138). Over the past four years, ASPN has completed studies on spontaneous abortion, headache, and pelvic inflammatory disease. Headache was defined as proposed by the Ad Hoc Committee on Classification of Headache (1962). During a 14-month period, 3847 persons made 4940 visits for headache to ASPN practices. Eighty-two percent (82%) of these patients visited only once, and 90 patients (2%) made more than three visits. Investigation procedures were used in a minority of headache episodes; 3% of patients seen over the 14-month period had a computerized tomography (CT) scan; 5% were referred to other physicians; and 2% hospitalized at some time during the study (143). ASPN is currently analyzing these data from the standpoint of the cost of managing headache in primary care and the use of CT scans. In addition, new and follow-up studies on chest pain, spontaneous abortion, diabetes mellitus, and herpes are in progress. Many other studies are in the planning and development stages.

The network consists presently of 50 practices in the United States and Canada and is projected to reach 80 practices by the end of 1985, involving more than 200 physicians and their staffs and an attending patient population of over 600,000. Early data from ASPN shows the expected similarities and differences between the age and sex distribution of ASPN attending patients and the US population identified at the 1980 census (133) (see Figure 3).

The problems and diseases that can be monitored by such systems are many. The range can best be illustrated by the following list of subjects of the weekly returns from the Sentinel Stations of The Netherlands between 1970 and 1983 (144) (see Table 2).

In the United States, Fries has recently addressed collaborative research in discussion of the Chronic Disease Data Bank (90). He presents eight principles that enable the development of such systems. "These principles mandate the development of chronic disease computer data banks. . . . there must be large numbers of patients included, preferably from diverse settings" (90).

All of this requires person-oriented data systems that use a form of problem-oriented medical record. Fries described a "time oriented medical record" that displays clinical information in the form of flow sheets, with time represented

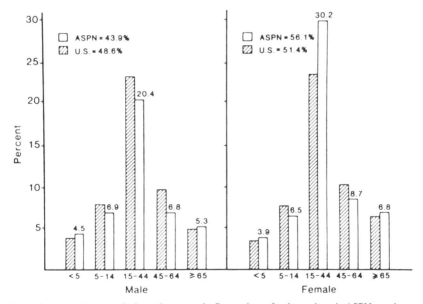

Figure 3   Ambulatory sentinel practice network. Comparison of active patients in ASPN practices and US populations, 1980 census. Reproduced by permission from the *Journal of Family Practice* 18(2):275.

Table 2 Subjects on the weekly returns 1970–1983

Subject	1970	1971	1972	1973	1974	1975	1976	1977	1978	1979	1980	1981	1982	1983
Influenza (-like illness)	x	x	x	x	x	x	x	x	x	x	x	x	x	x
Exanthema e causa ignota	x													
Acute diarree e causa ignota	x													
Consultations for family planning	x	x	x	x	x	x	x							
Request for abortion	x	x	x	x	x	x								
(Attempted) suicide	x	x												
Rubella (-like illness)		x								x	x	x	x	x
Otitis media acuta		x												
Abortus provocatus		x	x	x	x	x	x	x	x	x	x			
Accidents		x												
Tonsillectomy or adenotomy		x												
Prescription of morning-after pill			x	x	x	x	x	x	x	x	x	x	x	x
Sterilization of the man performed			x	x	x	x	x	x	x	x	x	x	x	x
Prescription of tranquillizers			x	x	x									
Consultation for drug-use			x	x	x					x	x	x		
(Suspicion of) battered child syndrome				x	x									
Sterilization of the woman performed						x	x	x	x	x	x	x	x	x
Consultation with regard to addiction to smoking					x									
Measles						x	x	x	x	x				

	1	2	3	4	5	6	7	8	9
Alcoholism	x								
Ulcus ventriculi/duodeni	x								
Skull traumas in traffic	x	x					x		
Certificate for another dwelling issued	x								
Psoriasis		x					x		
Prescription of antihypertensive or diuretic		x					x		
Cervical smear		x		x	x	x	x	x	x
Mononucleosis infectiosa		x			x	x	x	x	x
Prescription of medicine for infection of the urinary tract							x		
Hay fever				x	x	x		x	x
(Suspicion of) myocardial infarction					x	x		x	x
Traumas in sport				x			x	x	x
Diabetes mellitus				x			x	x	x
Parkinson's disease				x			x	x	x
Accidents in the private sector				x				x	x
Spontaneous abortion or *partus immaturus*									
Partus at gravidity ≥ 28 weeks				x				x	x
Penicillin (prescriptions and side effects)				x				x	x
Depression								x	x

on the horizontal axis. This type of record is in use and is taught in most primary care training programs, particularly those of family practice. Graduates of such programs are well qualified to be members of sentinel practice networks and recording members for chronic disease data banks.

Community-Oriented Primary Care

Another application of epidemiologic principles to medical records in primary care has recently been discussed in a report of a study of community-oriented primary care (COPC) by the Institute of Medicine of the National Academy of Sciences (145). COPC was defined as "the provision of primary care services to a defined community, coupled with systematic efforts to identify and address the major health problems of that community, through effective modifications in both primary care services and other appropriate community health programs." Seven widely different study sites in the US were selected from a total of 147 possible sites. These seven sites were presented as case studies. In its conclusions, the IOM Committee urged that extreme caution be used in generalizing the observations beyond the case studies themselves, because the findings were derived from a nonrandom sample of the identified possible sites. The Committee noted, "In all the health problems identified by the study sites, there were only a few that first came to light as a result of an epidemiologic study. Most problems had been previously recognized, although an epidemiologic study often served to identify the correlates of the problem and to provide information that enabled the practice to target its efforts on the individuals or the subset of the community at higher risk." Although COPC "is not the prevailing mode of practice in the US nor was the study able to find an example of the COPC model that is fully developed," the recent rapid growth in numbers of health maintenance organizations (HMOs) and other prepaid systems in the United States can lead to increasing interest among primary care practitioners "in the individuals or the subsets of the community at highest risk." In these circumstances, the recording of demographic and morbidity information on members of the community served by COPC practices will become an essential epidemiological tool to enable secondary and tertiary preventive care. This will be similar to the experiences in other countries with prepaid systems (146).

THE ROLE OF PUBLIC HEALTH PROFESSIONALS

Schools of public health came into being to train professionals to provide services to safeguard the health of populations, communities, and groups, rather than individuals. The separation from the clinical training schools seemed to be an appropriate step in the beginning to allow concentration on the development of epidemiological and biostatistical skills. That this approach was effective is no longer in question. A cadre of highly trained professionals has developed with the purpose of providing the greatest good for the largest number of people in the community. The functional paradigm that has evolved is based on the model used in the control of infectious disease. Case finding has been concentrated in institutional settings, hospitals, laboratories, public health clinics, and the community at large.

This model has been so effective that until recently there has been little need to develop and use different paradigms. However, recent concern with the problems of an aging population and the need to develop population descriptors of the prevalence of chronic disease, disabilities, handicaps, occupational diseases, and of the functional status of individual members of the community have highlighted the limitations of the infectious disease model.

Traditional sample surveys will continue to be necessary, but these are expensive and time consuming to develop and undertake, and in addition they are episodic. Other methods, such as surveillance systems based on collaboration between physician recorders have recently begun to be used. A prime example, established by the Centers for Disease Control (CDC), is the use of a cadre of 125 practicing physicians drawn from the membership of the American Academy of Family Physicians (AAFP). These physicians reported, on a weekly basis, the occurrence of influenza-like illnesses[1] among their practice populations. The system has now been underway since the 1982–1983 season. The *Morbidity and Mortality Weekly Report* from the CDC commented (147), "When influenza type A (H1N1) virus predominates . . . and outbreaks occur predominantly in healthy young populations, influenza epidemics may not be reflected by increases in national mortality attributable to pneumonia and influenza because the elderly are spared." The report states further that it is especially useful to have a rapidly repeated quantitative assessment of influenza morbidity available. Following a pilot study in the 1982–1983 season, weekly reports from family practitioners in all regions of the country have generally corresponded with other indicators of influenza virus activity.

This cautious statement has since been consistently reaffirmed (148, 149). Surveillance by family physicians has been able to provide more sensitive indicators for national influenza epidemicity than was previously available, and the indicators have shown consistency over time (see Figure 4). Recently, similar surveillance systems in Canada have confirmed that the time of first isolation of an influenza virus precedes the onset of an epidemic by three to five weeks (150).

Increasing familiarity with such a system will improve the data product qualitatively and quantitively. The model can probably also be applied to the

[1]Defined as having a fever of 37.8°C (100°F) or greater and having at least a cough or sore throat.

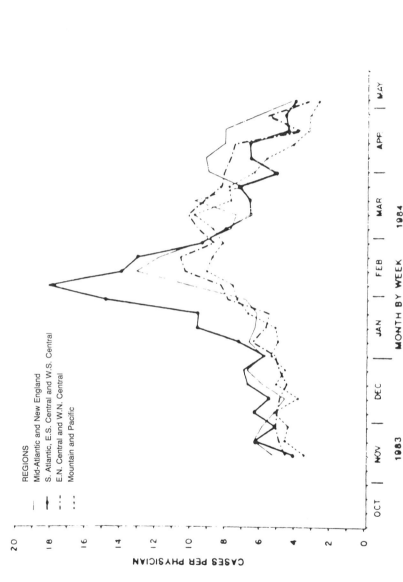

Figure 4 Cases of influenza-like illness reported from physicians by geographic area—United States, 1983–1984 season. Cases reported to CDC by approximately 125 physician-members of the American Academy of Family Physicians research panel. A case was defined as a patient with a fever of 37.8°C (100°F) or greater and having at least a cough or sore throat. Reproduced by permission from *Morbidity and Mortality Weekly Report* 33(29):421, DHHS, Centers for Disease Control, Atlanta (1984).

monitoring of other conditions or problems that lend themselves to similar levels of definition.

It is remarkable that neither the public health establishment nor the organizations representing family physicians and other primary care specialties have recognized the usefulness and availability of such a resource until now. Manifold opportunities exist at regional and local levels for cooperation among public health officers and representatives of state and local chapters of organizations, such as the AAFP, for surveillance of a spectrum of problems important to the community, including both acute and chronic problems.

Literature Cited

1. *The graduate education of the physician.* 1966. Rep. Citizens Commission on Grad. Med. Educ. J. S. Millis, Chm. Chicago: Am. Med. Assoc.
2. *Meeting the challenge of family practice.* 1966. Report of Ad Hoc Comm. on Educ. for Family Pract. of Counc. on Med. Educ. W. R. Willard, Chm. Chicago: Am. Med. Assoc.
3. *The Core Content of Family Medicine.* 1966. Rep. Comm. on Requirements for Certification. (Joint Comm. of Am. Acad. Gen. Pract. and AMA Sect. Gen. Pract.) In *Trans. 1966 Congr. of Delegates of the AAGP,* Kansas City
4. White, K. L. 1967. Improved medical care statistics and health service systems. *Public Health Rep.* 82:847–57
5. Crombie, D. L. 1963. Diagnostic Process. *J. Coll. Gen. Pract.* 6:579–89
6. *J. Coll. Gen. Pract.* 1963. Records and statistical unit. 6:195–232
7. Last, J. M. 1963. The iceberg—Completing the clinical picture in general practice. *Lancet* 2:28–31
8. Last, J. M. 1983. *Dictionary of Epidemiology.* New York: Oxford Univ. Press
9. Morris, J. N. 1967. *Uses of Epidemiology.* Edinburgh/London: Livingstone
10. White, K. L., Williams, T. F., Greenberg, B. G. 1961. The ecology of medical care. *N. Engl. J. Med.* 265:885–92
11. National Center for Health Statistics. 1975. *National Ambulatory Medical Care Survey: 1973 Summary.* Rockville, Md: DHEW Publ. No. (HRA), 1976–1771
12. Regier, D., Goldberg, I. D., Taube, C. 1978. The de facto U.S. mental health service system: A public health perspective. *Arch. Psychiatr.* (35):685–93
13. Goldberg, D., Huxley, P. 1980 *Mental Illness in the Community.* London: Tavistock

14. Henkin, J., Shapiro, S. 1979. The demand for medical services by persons under psychiatric care. In *Social Consequences of Mental Disorders,* ed. J. K. Wing, L. N. Robbins. New York: Springer
15. Mechanic, D. 1977. Illness behavior, social adaptation, and the management of illness. A comparison of educational or medical models. *J. Nerv. Mental Disorders* 165(2):1979–87
16. Balint, M. 1964. *The Doctor, His Patient and The Illness.* New York: Pitman
17. Eastwood, M. R., Trevelyan, M. H. 1972. Relationship between physical and psychiatric disorder. *Psychol. Med.* 2: 363–72
18. Murphy, E., Brown, G. W. 1980. Life events, psychiatric disturbance and physical illness. *Br. J. Psychiatr.* 136: 326–38
19. Aagaard, J., Husfeldt, P., Husfeldt, V. 1983. Social factors and life events as predictors for children's health. A one year prospective study within a general practice. *Acta Paediatr. Scand.* 72:275–81
20. Kohn, R., White, K. L. 1976. *Health Care: An International Study.* London: Oxford Univ. Press
21. World Health Organization. 1978. *Alma Ata 1978: Primary health care.* Rep. Int. Conf. Primary Health Care, Alma-Ata, USSR, Sept. 1978. Geneva: WHO. Reprinted 1982. *Health for All* Ser. 1
22. World Health Organization. 1982. *Basic Documents,* p. 1. Geneva: WHO. 32nd Ed.
23. White, K. L. 1976. Primary care research and the new epidemiology. *J. Family Pract.* 3(6):579–80
24. Mair, A. 1973. *Sir James McKenzie, M.D., 1853–1925. General Practitioner.* Edinburgh/London: Churchill-Livingstone

25. Mayo, F. 1973. Educational directions: Quality primary care from quality records. *J. Clin. Comput.* 1(6):28
26. Wood, M., Mayo, F., Marsland, D. W. 1975. A systems approach to patient care, curriculum and research in family practice. *J. Med. Educ.* 50(12):1106–12
27. Marsland, D. W., Wood, M., Mayo, F. 1976. A data bank for patient care, curriculum and research in family practice: 526,196 patient problems. *J. Family Pract.* 3(1)
28. Wood, M. 1973. The way ahead in primary care. *J. Clin. Comput.* 2(6):20–28
29. Ryle, J. 1948. *The Natural History of Disease.* London: Oxford Univ. Press. 2nd ed.
30. McWhinney, I. R. 1972. Beyond diagnosis. An approach to integration of behavioral sciences and clinical medicine. *N. Engl. J. Med.* 287(8):384–87
31. Hames, C. G., Sauer, H. I. 1979. Cardiovascular disease death rates for counties in Georgia. *J. Med. Assoc. Georgia* 68
32. Kark, J. D., Smith, A. H., Hames, C. G. 1980. The relationship of serum cholesterol to the incidence of cancer in Evans County, Ga. *J. Chronic Dis.* 33
33. Hames, C. G., Heyden, S. 1981. Risk factors and hypertension. *J. Med. Assoc. Georgia* 70:337–38
34. Farley, E. S., Froom, J. 1974. An integrated system for recording and retrieval of medical data in a primary care setting. Part I: The age-sex register. *J. Family Pract.* 1(1):44–46
35. Froom, J. 1974. An integrated system for the recording and retrieval of medical data in a primary care setting. Part 2: Classification of diseases. *J. Family Pract.* 1(1):47–48
36. Froom, J. 1974. An integrated system for the recording and retrieval of medical data in a primary care setting. Part 3: The diagnostic index -E book. *J. Family Pract.* 1(2):45–48
37. Froom, J. 1974. An integrated system for the recording and retrieval of medical data in a primary care setting. Part 4: Family folders. *J. Family Pract.* 1(2):49–51
38. Farley, E. S. 1974. An integrated system for the recording and retrieval of medical data in a primary care setting. Part 5: Implications of filing charts by area of residence. *J. Family Pract.* 1(3–4):43–47
39. Froom, J. 1974. An integrated system for the recording and retrieval of medical data in a primary care setting. Part 6: The problem-oriented medical record. *J. Family Pract.* 1(3–4):48–51
40. Froom, J. 1975. An integrated system for recording and retrieval of medical data in a primary care setting. Part 7: The encounter form and the minimum basic data set. *J. Family Pract.* 2(1):37–41
41. Treat, Donald F. 1975. An integrated system for the recording and retrieval of medical data in a primary care setting. Part 8: Individual patient's medical record. *J. Family Pract.* 2(1):43–53
42. Newell, J. P., Bass, M. J., Dickie, G. L. 1976. An information system for family practice. Part 1: Defining the practice population. *J. Family Pract.* 3(5):517–20
43. Bass, M. J., Newell, J. P., Dickie, G. L. 1976. An information system for family practice, Part 2: The value of defining a practice population. *J. Family Pract.* 3(5):525–28
44. Newell, J. P., Dickie, G. L., Bass, M. J. 1976. An information system for family practice. Part 3: Gathering encounter data. *J. Family Pract.* 3(6):633–36
45. Dickie, G. L., Newell, J. P., Bass, M. J. 1976. An information system for family practice. Part 4: Encounter data and their uses. *J. Family Pract.* 3(6):639–44
46. Eimerl, T. S. 1960. Organized curiosity. *J. Coll. Gen. Pract.* 3:246–52
47. Weed, L. L. 1968. Medical records guide and teaching. *N. Engl. J. Med.* 278:593–600, 652–57
48. Eimerl, T. S., Laidlow, A. J. eds. 1969. *A Handbook for Research in General Practice.* Edinburgh/London: Livingstone. 2nd ed.
49. Crombie, D. L. 1963. Diagnostic process. *J. Coll. Gen. Pract.* 6:574–89
50. Lough, J. D. 1967. Content of general practice: A survey of 42 practices. *N. Zealand Med. J.* 66:23–27 (Suppl.)
51. Murco, C. 1984. Content and process of general practice. Preliminary Report. *Austr. Family Physician.* 13(2):126–28
52. Curry, L., MacIntyre, K. 1982. The content of family practice. Do we need more studies? *Can. Family Physicians,* 28:124–26
53. 1974. *J. Family Pract.* Vol. 1, No. 1
54. *Coded Classification of Disease.* 1972. (A problem-oriented adapt. of R. Coll. Gen. Pract.'s *Classification of Diseases.* 1969.) Richmond: Med. Coll. Virginia, Dept. Family Practice
55. *Coded Classification of Disease.* 1971. (Adapt. of R. Coll. Gen. Pract.'s *Classification of Diseases.* 1969.) Rochester, NY: Family Med. Program, Highland Hosp.
56. Geyman, J. P. 1976. Towards the definition of family practice: A quantum jump. *J. Family Pract.* 3(1):1
57. McWhinney, I. R. 1976. Research im-

plications of the Virginia study. *J. Family Pract.* 3(1):35–36

58. Steward, W. L. 1976. Clinical implications of the Virginia study. *J. Family Pract.* 3(1):7–10

59. Hodgkin, K. 1976. Educational implications of the Virginia study. *J. Family Pract.* 3(1):11–12

60. Haight, R. O., McKee, C. A., Barkmeier, J. R. 1979. Morbidity in the first year of a family practice and its comparison to the Virginia Study. *J. Family Pract.* 9(2):295–99

61. Shank, J. C. 1977. The content of family practice: A family medicine resident's 2½ years' experience with an E-book. *J. Family Pract.* 5(3):385

62. Robertson, D. L. 1981. Symptoms encounters during a 3-year family practice residency. *J. Family Pract.* 13(2):239

63. Hollison, R. V., Vazquez, A. M., Warner, D. H. 1978. A medical information system of ambulatory care research and curriculum in an army family practice residency: 51,113 patient problems. *J. Family Pract.* 7(4):787–95

64. Bass, M. 1976. Approaches to the denominator problems in primary care research. *J. Family Pract.* 3(2):193–95

65. Garson, J. Z. 1976. The problem of the population at risk in primary care. *Can. Family Physician* 22:71

66. Kilpatrick, S. J. 1976. An empirical study of the distribution of episodes of illness reported in the 1970–71 National Morbidity Survey. *Soc. Sci. Med.* 9:139

67. Kretchmar, A. L., Shacklett, G. E. 1977. *The use of a probabilistic model to estimate the population base for practice statistics.* Presented at the 8th Ann. Meet. Int. Epidemiol. Assoc., Puerto Rico, Sept. 1977

68. Hill, A. B. 1977. *A Short Textbook of Medical Statistics.* London: Hodder & Stoughton

69. Kilpatrick, S. J. 1975. The distribution of episodes of illness—A research tool in general practice. *J. R. Coll. Gen. Practitioners* 25:686–90

70. Crombie, D. L. 1974. Changes in patterns of recorded morbidity. In *Benefits and Risks in Medical Care,* ed. D. Taylor. London: Off. Health Econ.

71. Bass, M. 1976. Approaches to the denominator problem in primary care research. *J. Family Pract.* 3(2):193–95

72. Kilpatrick, S. J. 1980. Success and failures in the analysis of family medicine data bases. In *New Challenges for Vital & Health Records.* Proc. 18th Natl. Meet.

Public Health Conf. on Records Stat., Natl. Cent. Health Stat., Hyattsville, Md. DHHS Publ. No. (PHS) 81–1213. Washington DC: GPO

73. Kilpatrick, S. J. 1984. A solution to the denominator problem? In *Primary Care Research,* ed. S. J. Kilpatrick Jr., R. M. Boyle, p. 153. New York: Praeger

74. Doll, R., Peto, R. 1981. The causes of cancer: Quantitative estimates of avoidable risks of cancer in the U.S. today. *J. Cancer Inst.* 66:1192–1308

75. Krogh-Jensen, P. 1983. Estimation of the practice population. *Gen. Pract. International* 3:129–34

76. Schach, E. 1983. Comparison between practices: Estimating the size of the practice population. The *Eur. J. Gen. Pract. Family Med.* 3:141–44

76a. Smith, B. W. H. 1984. *The denominator problem in primary care: Four solutions.* Proc. NAPCRG 12th Ann. Meet. Orlando, Fla. (Abstr.)

77. Mayo, F., Marsland, D., Wood, M. 1986. Denominator definition by the utilization correction factor method. *Family Pract. Int. J.* In press

78. Anderson, J. E. 1980. Reliability of morbidity data in family practice. *J. Family Pract.* 10:667–83

79. Bentsen, B. G. 1976. The accuracy of recording patient problems in family practice. *J. Med. Care* 51:311

80. *ICHPPC-2.* 1979. *International Classification of Health Problems in Primary Care.* New York: Oxford Univ. Press. 2nd ed.

81. *ICHPPC-2 Defined.* 1983. *International Classification of Health Problems in Primary Care.* New York: Oxford Univ. Press 3rd ed.

82. Anderson, J. E. 1984. The utility of routine encounter reporting in primary care research. In *Primary Care Research,* ed. S. J. Kilpatrick Jr., R. M. Boyle, pp. 3–20, New York: Praeger

83. *Acute respiratory infection.* 1981. Summary report of a symp. of the surveillance of viral respiratory infection in Europe (Madrid, June 1980), *WHO Chron.* 35:20–27

84. Bebbington, P., Hurry, J., Tennant, C. 1980. Recent advances in the epidemiological study of minor psychiatric disorders. *J. R. Soc. Med.* 73:315–18

85. Lillienfeld, A. M. 1976. *Foundation of Epidemiology.* New York: Oxford Univ. Press

86. Cherkin, D. C. 1984. Learning to live without practice denominators. Guest editorial. *J. Family Pract.* 19(4):437–39

87. Eddy, D. M. 1984. The economics of cancer prevention and detection: Getting

more for less. *Cancer* 5 (Suppl. 1):1200–9
88. Weinstein, M. C. 1983. Cost-effective priorities for cancer prevention. *Science* 224:17–22
89. Schottenfeld, D. 1980. Fundamental issues in cancer screening. *Colo-Rectal Cancer: Prevention, Epidemiology & Screening*, ed. S. Winawer, pp. 167–74. New York: Raven
90. Fries, J. F. 1984. The chronic disease data bank: First principles to future directions. *J. Med. Physiol.*, pp. 161–80
91. Fleming, D. M., Elliott-Binns, C. P. 1985. Disability as identified from family practice records. *Br. Med. J.* 290:287–90
92. Sklaroff, S. A. 1963. The use of national health service general practice records in epidemiological inquiries. *Br. J. Prev. Soc. Med.* 17:177–84
93. Forsyth, R. A. 1980. Hypertension in a primary care Practice. *J. Family Pract.* 10(5):803–7
94. Zismer, D. K., et al. 1982. Improving hypertension control in a private medical practice. *Arch. Int. Med.* 142:297–99
95. Steensberg, J., et al. 1969. Epidemiology of urinary tract diseases in general practice. *Br. Med. J.* 4:390–94
96. Anderson, J. E. 1983. Seasonality of symptomatic bacterial urinary infections in women. *J. Epidemiol. Community Health* 37(4):286–90
97. Katon, W., Williamson, P., Ries, R. 1981. A prospective study of 60 consecutive psychiatric consultations in the family medicine clinic. *J. Family Pract.* 13(1):47–55
98. Richards, H. H., Midha, R. N., Miller, S. 1982. A double blind study of trazodone and mianserin in the treatment of depression in general practice. *J. Int. Med. Res.* 10:147–56
99. Robinson, J. D., et al. 1982. Antibiotic prescribing in a family medicine residency program. *J. Family Pract.* 15(1):111–17
100. Wilson, D., et al. 1982. Randomized clinical trial of supportive follow-up for cigarette smokers in a family practice. *Can. Med. Assoc. J.* 126:127–29
101. Galazka, S. S., Rodriguez, G. A. 1982. Integrating community medicine in a family practice center: An approach to urban lead toxicity. *J. Family Pract.* 14(2):333–38
102. Williamson, H. A. 1985. Lymph adenopathy in a family practice: A descriptive study of 249 cases. *J. Family Pract.* 5:449–52
103. Mitchell, W. G., Gowrell, R. W., Greenberg, R. A. 1980. Failure to thrive: A study in a primary care setting.
Epidemiology and follow-up. *Pediatrics* 65:(5):971
104. Teele, D. W., et al. 1983. Middle ear disease and the practice of pediatrics. *J. Am. Med. Assoc.* 29(8):1026–29
105. Reed, B. D., et al. 1984. Compliance with acute otitis media treatment. *J. Family Pract.* 19(5):627–32
106. Soman, M. 1984. Telephone management of febrile young children in a family practice setting. *J. Family Pract.* 19(3):329
107. Aagaard, J., Husfeldt, P., Husfeldt, V. 1983. Social factors and like events as predictors for children's health. A one year prospective study within a general practice. *Acta Paediatr. Scand.* 72:275–81
108. Currie, A. L., et al. 1983. Newborn home visits. *J. Family Pract.* 17(4):635–38
109. *To develop a classification of the reasons for contact with primary health care services.* 1980. Working party rep. to Int. Classification of Diseases Unit, WHO, Geneva
110. Lamberts, H., Meads, S., Wood, M. 1984. Classification of reasons why persons seek primary care: Pilot study of a new system. *Public Health Rep.* 99(6):597–605
111. Meads, S. 1983. The WHO reason for encounter classification. *WHO Chron.* 37:159
112. White, K. L. 1967. Improved medical care statistics and health service systems. *Public Health Rep.* 82:847–57
113. Lipkin, M. Jr., White, K. L., eds. 1981. *Primary Care Research in 1980: Collected Abstracts of Four Societies.* New York: Rockefeller Found.
114. Lipkin, M., Boufford, J., Froom, J., White, K. L., eds. 1982. *Primary Care Research in 1981: Collected Abstracts of Five Medical Societies.* New York: Rockefeller Found.
115. Lipkin, M., Boufford, J., Froom, J., Schonberg, S. K., White, K. L., eds. 1982. *Primary Care Research in 1982: Collected Abstracts of Five Medical Societies.* New York: New York Univ. Med. Cent.
116. Robertson, D. L. 1981. Symptoms encountered during a three year family practice residency. *J. Family Pract.* 13(2):239–44
117. Meads, S., McLemore, T. 1974. *The national ambulatory medical care survey: Symptom classification.* DHEW Pub. No. (HRA) 74–1337. Rockville, Md.: HRA
118. Schroeder, D., Appleton, L., McLemore, T. 1978. *A reason for visit classification for ambulatory care. Vital*

Health Stat. Ser. 2, No. 78, DHEW Pub. No. (PHS) 78–1352. Hyattsville, Md.: Natl. Cent. Health Stat.

119. Deleted in proof

120. Lamberts, H., Meads, S., Wood, M. 1984. Why go to a doctor? An international study with the reason for encounter classification. Huisarts, En Wetenschap 27:234–44

121. Deleted in proof

122. Deleted in proof

123. Anderson, J. E., Lees, R. M. 1978. Optional hierarchial expansion as a means of increasing the flexibility of a morbidity classification system. J. Family Pract. 6(6):1271–75

124. World Health Organization. 1977. Manual for the International Classification of Diseases, Injuries and Causes of Death. Geneva: WHO

125. Minutes of the WHO working party for the development of an international classification for primary care, Richmond, Va., April 4–8, 1984

126. Deleted in proof

127. Wood, M. 1978. Collection of data. J. Family Pract. 7(1):91–100

128. National Committee on Vital and Health Statistics. 1981. Uniform Ambulatory Care Minimum Data Set. DHHL Publ. No. (PHS) 81–161. Hyattsville, Md.: US Dept. Health Human Serv., Public Health Serv., Off. Health Res., Stat., Technol., NCHS

129. Wood, M., DeLozier, J. 1981. The uniform ambulatory care minimum data set. Top. Health Record Manage. 1(3):45–54

130. Tenney, J. B., White, K. L., Williamson, J. W. 1974. National Ambulatory Medical Care Survey: Background in methodology. United States, 1967–72. Vital Health Stat. Ser. 2, No. 61, DHEW Pub. No. (HRA) 74–1335. Washington DC: GPO

131. Natl. Cent. Health Stat. 1975. National Ambulatory Medical Care Survey, 1973 Summary: United States, May 1973–April 1974. Vital Health Stat. Ser. 13, No. 21, DHEW Pub. No. (HRA) 76–1772. Washington DC: GPO

132. Natl. Cent. Health Stat. 1977. National Ambulatory Medical Care Survey of visits to general and family practitioners: January through December 1975. Adv. Data from Vital and Health Stat. No. 15, DHEW Pub. No. (PHS), 78–1250. Washington DC: GPO

133. Green, L., et al. 1984. Ambulatory sentinel practice network: Purpose, methods and policies. J. Family Pract. 18(2):275–80

134. Research Committee. 1958. Morbidity, Continuing Observation and Recording Off. J. R. Coll. Gen. Pract. 1:107–28

135. Morbidity Statistics from General Practice. 1958–1962. (3 vols.) London: Gen. Register. Off., Her Majesty's Station. Off.

136. Scott, E. 1960. J. Coll. Gen. Pract. 3:44

137. Eimerl, T. S., Laidlaw, A. J., eds. 1969. A Handbook of Research in General Practice, pp. 22–25. Edinburgh/London: Livingstone

138. Continuous Morbidity Registration Sentinel Stations Annual Report. 1970. Utrecht: Netherlands Inst. for General Practice

139. Deleted in proof

140. Nelson, E. C., et al. 1981. The cooperative information project: Part 2: Some initial clinical, quality assurance and practice management studies. J. Family Pract. 13(6):867–76

141. Nelson, E. C., et al. 1981. The cooperative information project: Part 1: A sentinel practice network for service and research in primary care. J. Family Pract. 13(5):641–49

142. Deleted in proof

143. Becker, L. 1985. Headache in primary care: A report from ASPN. Presented at the North Am. Primary Care Res. Group (NAPCRG) Ann. Meet., Seattle, Wash.

144. Foundations of The Netherlands Inst. for General Practice. 1982. Continuous Morbidity Registration Sentinel Stations. Utrecht: Ministry of Welfare, Public Health, and Culture, Chief Med. Officer of Health.

145. Div. Health Care Serv. Inst. of Med. 1984. COPC: A Practical Assessment, Vol. 1 and 2. Washington DC: Natl. Acad. Press

146. Watt, G. 1983. The application of COPC practices in a Welsh Mining Village. In COPC: New Directions for Health Services Delivery, pp. 243–49. Washington DC: Natl. Acad. Press

147. Morbid. Mortal. Weekly Rep. 1984. 33(10): 134

148. Morbid. Mortal. Weekly Rep. 1985. 34(4): 62–63

149. Morbid. Mortal. Weekly Rep. 1984. 33(29): 421

150. Tarrant, M. 1985. Viral Watch Project. Alberta: Can. Coll. Family Physicians, Newsletter No. 5

151. Ord, J. K. 1967. J. R. Stat. Soc. Ser. A 130:232–38

Ann. Rev. Public Health. 1986. 7:391–409

REIMBURSEMENT INCENTIVES FOR HOSPITAL CARE

John P. Bunker

Division of Health Services Research, Stanford University School of Medicine, Stanford, California 94305

Ralph W. Schaffarzick

Blue Shield of California, San Francisco, California 94120

The open-ended reimbursement of hospitals, physicians, and other providers by the government and by private third party payors has played a major role in the increasing costs of health care as well as the types and amounts of health care received by the American public. In the pages to follow we review the effects of cost reimbursement and other methods of financing on the use of hospital care, on the outcome of medical care practices, and on medical innovation and its diffusion. We examine the likelihood that changes in method of reimbursement will achieve their intended effects of eliminating or reducing unnecessary care and improving the efficiency with which medical care is delivered, and we also consider secondary effects of reimbursement on the quality of medical care and on its distribution.

Reimbursement Incentives for Cost-effective Hospital Care

How a hospital is paid, whether by cost reimbursement, as part of a prepaid premium, or by Medicare's new Prospective Payment System, markedly affects the incentives for hospital care. Fully insured cost reimbursement for hospital care and fee-for-service reimbursement for physicians and other health professionals in the past have encouraged the provision of all medical care and diagnostic tests that might be of value and have provided no incentives for cost-effective care, which we define as care that maximizes net benefits. Ignoring, for the moment, the difficulty in equating marginal costs in dollars with marginal benefits measured in improvement in the quality or length of

391

0163-7525/86/0510-0391$02.00

life—and ignoring the great uncertainty with which the benefits of care can be measured—it is widely recognized that if neither the patient, nor the physician, nor the hospital need consider cost, then care in which marginal benefits are less than marginal costs, but more than zero, will be provided (37, 25). The monitary advantages to the physician of providing services in hospital, rather than in the office, provide additional strong incentives to hospitalize (5a).

In contrast to the economic incentives of cost reimbursement and fee-for-service to err in the direction of overtreatment and overhospitalization, the prepayment of a lump sum to provide all necessary and appropriate medical care provides incentives to limit care to those procedures and diagnostic tests that can be clearly shown to be effective, to minimize the use of hospitalization or other costly interventions for diagnosis and treatment, and possibly to undertreat. Prepayment, or capitation, is the standard method of reimbursement of Health Maintenance Organizations (HMOs). The success of this approach in limiting cost is reflected in a hospital admission rate for patients cared for by physicians in prepaid group practice which has, in the past, been 25% lower than for the patients of physicians who are reimbursed on the basis of fee-for-service (30).

THE PROSPECTIVE PAYMENT SYSTEM   In the Social Security Amendments of 1983, the Congress introduced for beneficiaries of the federally funded Medicare Program a new method of reimbursement, the Prospective Payment System (PPS), that incorporates some of the good features of prepayment, but retains some of the perverse economic incentives of cost reimbursement/fee-for-service. Prospective reimbursement, in which a set fee for each of 468 diagnostic categories ("diagnosis-related groups," or DRGs) is paid for hospital services, introduces, as does prepayment to an HMO, strong incentives to provide cost-effective and efficient care. It also provides strong incentives to improve the quality of the information on which cost-effective judgments are made; it strongly encourages the rigorous application of technology assessments to new, as well as existing, medical technologies; and it strongly discourages the in-hospital application of untested technologies (38).

A major objective of the Prospective Payment System, and its anticipated impact, is to decrease the intensity of services provided to hospitalized patients, but with a single, important loophole: surgery. The hospital component of surgical procedures, excluding only those that are experimental, is individually identified and allowed to inflate reimbursement for a given DRG to levels that differ little from those of the immediate past. "Thus, DRGs may more appropriately be termed 'diagnosis-and-treatment-related groups' " (39). This feature of the Medicare Prospective Payment System perpetuates existing incentives for the hospital to encourage surgical intervention and is one of the features that distinguishes it from the prepayment HMO, in which a single annual, or monthly, charge is made which covers all medical care, including surgical services, that may be provided.

In contrast to surgical procedures, there is no itemized incremental fee for medical or diagnostic procedures, with a single exception. Thus, gastroscopy carried out by the gastroenterologist, or a GI series by the radiologist, for which substantial hospital service charges have routinely been made in the past, bring no additional income to the hospital under prospective reimbursement. The exception is cardiac catheterization in patients admitted with a cardiac diagnosis, for which a separate DRG acknowledges the procedure and reimburses at a higher rate.

Fee-for-service physicians continue to have a strong incentive to admit patients for medical and diagnostic procedures (5a), whether or not in conflict with the fiscal interests of the hospital. Current "customary, prevailing, and reasonable" fees paid by the government's Medicare Program, as well as by private insurers, reward physicians more per unit of time for procedural than for "cognitive" services, and this imbalance in reimbursement is widely acknowledged to be a major cause of the emphasis on procedure-oriented medicine and the relative neglect of the equally or more important physician function of decision making and counseling (3). A call for fee schedules that will be "technology-neutral" has been made (34, 46), and the American College of Physicians and the American Society of Internal Medicine have proposed more equitable reimbursement for cognitive services (3). The possible extension by the government of prospective payment to the reimbursement of physicians would help to reverse at least the incentive for intensity of services for hospitalized patients, but only significant moves in the direction of capitation or major changes in existing fee schedules (5a, 34, 46) can be expected to lessen the incentives for surgical over medical care, for invasive medical or surgical procedures over "cognitive" medical services, and for hospital over ambulatory care.

REIMBURSEMENT INCENTIVES TO HOSPITALIZE   While introducing incentives for reducing the intensity of at least medical and diagnostic services to hospitalized patients, the Prospective Payment System does nothing to discourage hospitalization itself, thus retaining a second major perverse incentive of fee-for-service reimbursement. Indeed, since a fixed fee is provided for each hospitalization and this fee is based on average cost, the economic incentives of prospective payment encourage more admissions of less than average complexity as a way of attempting to offset financial losses that may be incurred by patients whose care demands greater than average use of resources. It has been predicted for this reason that admissions will rise (19, 28b, 56).

Contrary to prediction, hospital admissions for patients over 65 in age have fallen continuously since early 1983, and for those under 65 since 1981, and the annual rate of increase in total hospital expenditures, while still rising, has fallen from 16.2% to 5.4%. That the "medical marketplace" is not responding to prospective payment in the way expected may be due to other activities occurring at the state and regional levels, such as the federally mandated Peer Review Organizations (PROs), to a much heightened awareness within the private sector of the need to use our medical resources more economically, and possibly to the "announcement effect" of a program with such far-reaching potential impact. In California, for example, pro-competitive strategies have been encouraged in an attempt to control health care costs, and state law now allows the use of selective hospital contracts to negotiate with "preferred providers" to provide care at discounted fixed prices (52). Other states (e.g. Massachusetts, New York, and Maine) have attempted to control costs by establishing a revenue cap on payments to hospitals. In Massachusetts, for example, there are accompanying penalties for cost increases, and rewards for savings that may be achieved (10).

REIMBURSEMENT INCENTIVES FOR AMBULATORY CARE   The continuing fall of hospital admission rates, especially if this represents a shift in site of care from the in-hospital to an ambulatory setting, would represent a major accomplishment. There is clear evidence that this is already happening in surgery, where a rapid growth of ambulatory surgery in the so-called "surgi-centers" has occurred at the expense of hospital admission. While this should be a highly desirable trend, ambulatory surgery is still largely unregulated, data on the volume and costs of ambulatory surgery are not yet available, and standards of performance are only just beginning to be developed at the state level. If the bias toward surgical intervention in the closely monitored hospital environment is of concern, the possible overuse of surgery in the unregulated ambulatory setting should be of greater concern (15), and it will be important to monitor its growth and costs carefully.

Reimbursement and the Distribution of Hospital Services

In the cost-unconscious environment of the immediate past there has been widespread uneven distribution of hospital services. In a series of path-breaking studies, Wennberg and his associates have demonstrated large variations in the volume of hospital care received by populations, depending on where they live (54) and in per capita health care expenditures, (53). Wennberg made surveys of the frequency of surgery and hospitalization in such states as Vermont, Iowa, Maine, and California. He divided individual communities of a county or state into what he called "hospital markets" or "hospital service areas" in which most of the population used one local hospital or group of hospitals. He then gathered information about the rates of use of medical treatments, diagnostic tests, and surgical procedures in various hospital markets by examining comprehensive, population-based health insurance records (such as Medicare and Medicaid) and hospital discharge records. He found that many "hospital markets" had "highly variable rates of use for most specific medical treatments, diagnostic tests, and surgical procedures, and by widely different resource use rates" (54). For example, he observed (54),

> In Maine, by the time women reach seventy years of age in one hospital market the likelihood they have undergone a hysterectomy is 20 percent while in another market it is 70 percent. In Iowa, the chances that male residents who reach age eighty-five have undergone pros-tatectomy range from a low of 15 percent to a high of more than 60 percent in different hospital markets. In Vermont the probability that resident children will undergo a tonsillec-tomy has ranged from a low of 8 percent in one hospital market to a high of nearly 70 percent in another.

Similarly, Wennberg has shown that Americans living in some cities or towns in New England and in Iowa are twice as likely to undergo surgery or to be hospitalized for nonsurgical conditions as those living in other cities or towns of those states. Moreover, contrary to what one might expect would result from such wide variations in treatment, there is no evidence that the health of populations in areas with low hospitalization and operation rates suffers as a result.

That method of reimbursement is not solely responsible for the large variations in services is strongly suggested by the fact that similar variations are observed in Great Britain and in Norway (35) and among HMOs (30, 55), where all or almost all medical services are provided on a basis of capitation or prepayment. Method of reimbursement must be considered at least partly responsible, however, for there are no incentives under-cost reimbursement/ fee-for-service in the United States, or under the National Health Services of Great Britain and Norway, for physicians to balance marginal costs with marginal benefits of the care they provide. Hence, Wennberg attributes most of the variation to differences in physician practice style. The US Government's new Prospective Payment System introduces no incentives to correct variations, and might well encourage their perpetuation. Prepayment, by itself, seems unlikely to be much better, in view of the large variations observed in Great Britain under their National Health Service and among prepaid HMOs in this country.

Reimbursement and the Regionalization of Hospital Care

A growing body of evidence indicates that complex medical procedures, such as total hip replacement, open heart surgery, and prostatectomy, are performed more safely and at lower cost in institutions carrying out relatively high volumes of these procedures (21, 22, 23, 32). Method of reimbursement and, in particular, current and proposed changes in reimbursement can be expected to have a profound impact on the distribution of medical technology—that is, on

regionalization of services, on specialization of individual technological procedures, and on the diffusion of new medical technologies into general practice.
In the past health professionals have made relatively little effort to regionalize
medical technology, except for a few highly specialized services such as burn
care, neonatal intensive care, and organ transplantation. The government,
itself, has been reluctant to limit coverage for its beneficiaries to specific
institutions (37).

THE HIGHER COSTS OF INFREQUENT SURGERY   The higher cost per case in
institutions carrying out complex procedures (particularly those involving
substantial capital outlay) on an occasional basis (20, 23) could be offset by
higher charges, which have, in the past, been automatically reimbursed by the
government and by private third party payors. Higher costs of such procedures
in low-volume hospitals can also be hidden in charges for other services by
cross-subsidization. (Indeed, cost-accounting methods in most institutions
have not been sufficiently precise to allow accurate estimation of the costs of
many procedures. This shortcoming is in the process of fairly rapid improvement in response to prospective reimbursement.)

Prospective reimbursement provides a very strong incentive to determine
which procedures are profitable and to limit or discontinue those that lose
money. Thus, it offers a strong incentive for institutions to collaborate in
concentrating many such specialized procedures, with not all institutions providing every procedure.

Individual states have acted to encourage regionalization. For example, the
Massachusetts State Legislature, responding to the State Rate Setting Commission, has enacted a revenue cap (called the maximum allowable cost) that
"encourages regional planning by allowing hospitals to distribute among themselves the revenue allowance for services that are terminated as a result of
mergers or cooperative agreements" (10).

A PRIVATE EFFORT TO REGIONALIZE   In the private sector action has also
been initiated to promote regionalization of complex, expensive procedures. In
1982, for example, Blue Shield of California's Medical Policy Committee
determined that it would pay for percutaneous transluminal coronary angioplasty (PTCA) only those physicians who could satisfy the criteria defined
by the PTCA Registry of the National Heart, Lung, and Blood Institute
(NHLBI). In 1984 the Blue Shield of California's Medical Policy Committee
applied this principle of selective coverage to human heart and liver transplanta-
tions. In the cases of heart and liver transplants, not only must an institution and
transplantation team document their skills, resources, and commitment, but
also they must demonstrate a level of successful outcomes comparable to that of
established entities. At this writing the National Center for Health Services

Research and Health Care Technology Assessment is considering a recommendation to the Health Care Financing Administration (HCFA) that selective coverage be employed in the case of heart transplantation for Medicare beneficiaries. A next logical step could be negotiations by the private carriers and HCFA with qualified centers for reasonable payment rates.

UNDESIRED EFFECTS OF REGIONALIZATION?   The trend toward regionalization/specialization is not guaranteed to be beneficial, despite its obvious advantages in theory. Stern & Epstein (50), in their review of anticipated institutional responses to prospective payment, suggest that the resulting "specialization is likely to have desirable effects on quality and efficiency," but warn that institutions that provide a particular service more cheaply may do so by, providing care of a lower quality, and/or by admitting patients who need less care, that is, by skimming off more profitable patients. Davis and her associates (13) express concern that "hospitals might be induced to stop performing technologically complicated procedures, or from investing in innovations that would increase the safety with which they are performed."

Efficiency in Resource Allocation and Hospital Care

"The rationale for uniform payments [under the Prospective Payment System] is the assumption that differences in efficiency rather than differences in characteristics of the patient population or in the quality of care are responsible for interinstitutional differences in the cost of providing care" (50). The same might be said for prepayment or capitation.

EFFICIENCY OF HOSPITAL CARE   Within a narrow definition of efficiency at the institutional level, we see that regionalization, discussed in the preceding section, may improve efficiency. Institutions that provide highly technical services such as total hip replacement and coronary artery bypass graft on an occasional basis report poorer results on average. This is reflected in higher postoperative mortality and higher average prices, and thus these services are inefficient. In the case of total hip replacement, readmissions for correction of complications are also greater in low-volume institutions, further adding to the costs and decreased efficiency (23). To the extent that prospective reimbursement provides strong incentives for regionalization, as discussed above, efficiency of health care delivery should be enhanced.

EFFICIENCY OF POPULATION-BASED CARE   A broader definition of efficiency would be one based on the health outcomes and costs of care provided to a population. A prototype application of such a population-based definition of efficiency would be to compare efficiency in the prepaid HMO with that of fee-for-service practice. Luft lists reasons why the HMO can be expected to be more efficient in the delivery of care (31). Manning, Newhouse, and their associates at the Rand Corporation (33), in their randomized comparison of several methods of reimbursement, found that total resources used were 28% lower for those patients assigned to care in a prepaid group practice than for those assigned to care by physicians reimbursed by fee for service, and that outcomes of care for the majority of patients were comparable (J. E. Ware, Jr., personal communication, 1985).

INEFFICIENCY OF CARE IN SMALL AREAS   The large inequality in the distribution of medical care among the small geographic areas discussed in a preceding section provides a different perspective on the question of efficiency. Wennberg and his associates report that the health of populations living in Vermont hospital service areas where hospitalization and surgery rates are low is similar to that in high-use areas (54). When efficiency is measured in terms of age- and sex-adjusted per capita costs among populations living in neighboring areas, a major factor contributing to these differences is the difference in admission rates, not in cost per admission.

   The decision to hospitalize a patient, particularly for medical conditions, is strongly affected by the number of beds per capita. For historical reasons that seem to have little to do with patient needs, the number of hospital beds per 1000 population in the United States shows great variation, as does the closely related number of hospital employees and the consequent per capita expenditures for hospitalization. When a community possesses more beds, those beds are used for a variety of medical conditions that in less bedded areas are more often treated in an ambulatory setting, as predicted by "Roemer's Law" (J. E. Wennberg, personal communication, 1985). Wennberg has observed several communities, such as Iowa City, Iowa, and New Haven, Connecticut, with low overall hospitalization costs where most services are delivered in university hospitals. The low per capita costs are achieved by an efficient, low admission rate, not because of low costs per case. He concludes that the implicit standards of care associated with the low rates of hospitalization are compatible with state-of-the-art medicine as practiced in academic medical centers. If the admission criteria used in such markets could be made explicit, their adoption into more general use would pave the way for a reduction in the demand for hospital care and the freeing of resources that could be allocated to build new systems of ambulatory care. The potential savings may be very large. The 1982 costs to the Medicare program for medical care (Part A and Part B reimbursement) for residents of Polk County, Iowa, which includes Des Moines, was $1753 per capita, while for Johnson County, which includes Iowa City, where most services are provided in the University of Iowa Medical Center Hospital, costs were 40% less, $1002 per capita (J. E. Wennberg, personal communication, 1985).

PREVENTION MAY BE MORE EFFICIENT THAN CARE   Another large source of health care inefficiency, of yet a different sort, should be considered if "efficiency in use of medical resources means that the last dollar spent on any particular type of care purchases medical benefit worth no less than the last dollar spent for any other type of care" (1). A large and growing body of evidence points to investment in prevention as a much more efficient way to improve the public health than many forms of curative therapy. Although society invests large sums in the artificial heart, with the prospect of prolonging a small number of lives, much smaller expenditures in heart disease prevention can be shown to save a much greater number of lives (14, 29). Similarly, many more lives can be saved by programs to assist smokers to stop smoking than by surgical procedures that attempt to cure smoking-related disease, and these programs are much less expensive.

Will Cost Constraints Decrease Quality?

Proponents of fee-for-service reimbursement for medical services claim that medical care in the United States is the best in the world, and that the method by which we finance medical care is essential in maintaining our supremacy. As a corollary, it is also claimed that any departure from the current system of payment will lead inevitably to a lowering of the quality of care in this country. Milt Freudenheim reports, in the *New York Times* of July 30, 1985, that "more than 60 percent of the 7,800 physicians responding to a preliminary survey by the American Medical Association said that quality of care had already deteriorated or that they feared such a decline" as a result of federal cost controls. Under the headline, "Medicare Payment Plan Is Blamed for Hasty Release of Aged Patients," *The Wall Street Journal,* on June 25, 1985, gives anecdotal reports of elderly patients prematurely discharged. While few in number, the prominence of such reports in the press gives credence to the belief that quality of care has fallen.

Robert J. Blendon and David E. Rogers, vice president and president, respectively, of the Robert Wood Johnson Foundation, writing in the *Journal of the American Medical Association* in October 1983, warn of the risk of damage to the public health in the process of "cutting medical care costs" (5). The Congressional Office of Technology Assessment in a July 1984 report entitled "Medical Technology and Costs of the Medicare Program," expresses concern that "in some cases, the substitution of low cost technologies for high cost technologies may result in a decline in quality of care" (37). And Henry Aaron and William Schwartz predict that cutting costs and reimbursement will lead to withholding of services, such as hemodialysis and kidney transplant in the elderly, that are demonstrably effective in supporting life and improving its quality (1).

CUTTING COST WITHOUT CUTTING QUALITY   Only a few (16, 24) seem to
have entertained the possibility that cost constraints can be accompanied by
improvements in the quality of care. But if prospective payment or other forms
of reimbursement reform provide incentives for more cost-effective care, and
for improving methods by which to measure cost effectiveness and the wider
application of these methods, there should be the real possibility of improving
the quality of care by eliminating care that is ineffective, and care that is even
harmful (7). At the very least, quality of care can be expected to increase as the
result of greater regionalization of complex medical technologies and withdrawal of such care from most low-volume hospitals, where the outcomes of
complex procedures such as total hip replacement and coronary artery bypass
surgery have been shown to be poor (21, 22, 23, 32).

It can also be anticipated that correction of the current marked imbalance in
services provided to different geographic segments of the population will lead
to an improved public health. Bunker argues that much of the care provided in
areas of high procedure and hospitalization rates is of poor quality in that risks
may exceed benefits (leading to iatrogenic illness) and that selective lowering
of rates can improve the quality of care (7).

The examples of low-cost/low-utilization hospital service areas where most
services are provided by members of medical school faculty also argue that it is
safe and in the public interest to lower the use of hospitals. But the economic
incentives built into the Medicare Prospective Payment System, which pays a
flat amount for a given diagnostic group, is not geared to reward hospitals in
hospital service areas with low per capita admission rates. Indeed, Wennberg
and his associates warn that low-use markets face a danger of DRG-induced
rationing, particularly for medical admissions (56). In low-utilization areas,
physicians must be assumed to screen more carefully, admitting only the very
sick to the hospital. Since the amount of money reimbursed per DRG is
determined by average costs across low- and high-utilization areas, it is
weighted by the less ill and less costly patients who are admitted more often in
high-utilization areas. In the long run, as the "fat" is taken out of the system,
patients with particularly severe examples of a given illness may well face the
danger of under service. The irony is that the penalties of rationing will be felt
most severely by patients admitted to those hospitals which, from the perspective of the government (the amount of Trust Fund dollars spent per capita),
should be considered most efficient.

THE QUALITY OF CARE IN HMOS   It is assumed by many that prospective
payment by inpatient case is a temporary measure and will be followed in the
near future by some form of prepayment or capitation, at least for beneficiaries
of the federally funded Medicare and Medicaid programs. The impact of
prepayment on the quality of care is, therefore, of paramount interest. Whether

prepaid HMOs, for which the Kaiser plans offer the prototype, offer care of a quality equal to that provided by the fee-for-service sector has long been debated. Cunningham & Williamson, in a 1980 summary of published studies of the quality of care in HMOs compared to that in other settings, concluded, "There is little question that facility-based HMO care is at least comparable to care in other health facilities, if not superior" (11). Their conclusion was based on 27 studies, in 19 of which the general quality of health care was considered superior in the HMOs studied, and in eight the quality of care was found to be similar or the results inconclusive.

Luft, in his 1981 review book entitled *Health Maintenance Organizations,* like Cunningham & Williamson, reports care provided by HMOs to be comparable to that found in other settings and that the "specific financial incentives of HMOs seem to have little direct effect on quality" (31). He goes on to suggest that those who expect "HMOs to provide substantially better care would be disappointed"—but those who expect "HMOs to skimp on quality to cut costs would find little evidence to support that contention." The recently completed Rand randomized comparison of different methods of reimbursement, cited above (33), supports the view that the outcomes of treatment of adult patients cared for by physicians in prepaid group practice is as good for the majority of patients as those for patients cared for by physicians reimbursed by fee for service.

PHYSICIANS MUST CHANGE THEIR PRACTICE STYLE   In a subsequent section we discuss the need for better and more comprehensive data on health care outcomes as indices of the quality of medical care. Even with better data, it is quite possible that we will not be able to compare, conclusively, the quality of care provided by different systems of reimbursement or organization of medical services. Nevertheless, we believe that it is reasonable to conclude from the foregoing that much saving can be achieved without loss of quality. In order to do so, Lester Thurow, in his 1985 *Shattuck Lecture* before the Massachusetts Medical Society, suggests that physicians' practice styles "would have to shift from one based on the motto 'Do no harm' to one based on the precept 'Employ a treatment only when you are sure that it will make a noticeable improvement.' Instead of optimistically using new procedures that 'just might' work when old procedures don't, doctors would not employ new procedures until they could be proved to work well. Experimental procedures would not become commonplace overnight. Heroic measures would not be employed unless there was a high probability that they would work" (51).

Hospital Access to Medical Care for the Poor and Uninsured

Prospective payment by the government and cost-conscious negotiated pricing in the private sector have begun to attack hospitals' ability to provide uncompensated care to the poor and uninsured. With the sharp decline of cost reimbursement, providers—mainly hospitals—are no longer able to crosssubsidize care for the uninsured by increasing charges to the insured. Indeed, in the case of government-supported patients receiving medical care under the Medicare or Medicaid programs, payments are already made with marked discounts below charges, with little or no surplus left in the system to cover the costs of care for patients without insurance coverage, private or government provided.

That the poor and uninsured use fewer medical services (2, 59) and are in poorer health (2, 36) is established beyond any reasonable doubt. Access to medical care for the poor was markedly improved by Title XIX of the Social Security Act of 1965, which established the Medicaid program, but is now decreasing as a result of a continuing annual decrement in federal funding for health care for the poor and uninsured (27, 36). The congress is not unmindful of the problem. John Iglehart, in his Health Policy Report column that appears in the *New England Journal of Medicine,* reports, "Many advocates of the market approach have pointed out to the administration that unless policies are designed to protect the uninsured, support for making price the overriding consideration in the care transaction will erode" (27); and Mr. Iglehart quotes the remarks of Senator Durenberger at a September 24, 1984, hearing on medical care for the economically disadvantaged, to the effect that "as we create a price-sensitive health care marketplace, accommodations must also be made. These accommodations are necessary on moral as well as on economic grounds to assure access to quality services for all who need health care. We never want to return to a two-tiered system, with one standard of care for those who can pay and a second, substandard, for those who cannot" (27). Congressional action to date includes an extension of Medicaid coverage to low-income pregnant women and to children not previously meeting narrow eligibility requirements in some states. Senators Kennedy and Durenberger and Congressman Stark have introduced legislation that will require employers to offer the opportunity to buy insurance to those laid off from work and to widows of deceased employees, but the goal of comprehensive coverage for the health needs of the poor remains a distant one.

EQUALIZING ACCESS FOR THE POOR THROUGH TAX SUBSIDIES   The most comprehensive approach to correcting or lessening inequities in access is embodied in a series of legislative proposals to modify the existing tax treatment of employer contributions to health benefits of the employed. Alain Enthoven, in testimony before the Senate Finance Committee on July 19, 1985 (18), stated,

The present tax treatment of health insurance has been the main cause of the paradoxical situation that millions of people are overinsured and causing inflation in health care, while millions of other people are underinsured or have no coverage at all. . . . [In so doing] the government is subsidizing the efforts of upper income people to bid up the prices and standards of care that the uninsured must then pay for directly and that the government must then pay for through Medicare and Medicaid. . . . [If] the social policy goal of tax subsidies to health insurance should be to motivate and help everyone, whether employed or not, [to] purchase a good quality comprehensive cost-effective health plan, and to discourage people from purchasing an inefficient overly costly health plan, . . . the way to do this is to subsidize everyone's purchase of a health plan up to a limit judged to correspond to the price of a good quality cost-effective plan, and not to subsidize choices above that limit.

From 1979 to 1983, a number of bills have been proposed in the Congress to limit tax-free employer contributions toward their employees' health insurance premiums. "These tax cap proposals would have saved the budget billions of dollars and would have greatly improved the economic rationality of the financial incentives in the health care system. But, by themselves they would have done nothing for the self-employed and others without tax-free employer contributions. [In 1985] Senator Durenberger introduced S.1211, the Health Equity and Fairness Act of 1985, which contained . . . substantial improvements over previous tax cap proposals."

Enthoven (17, 18) has recommended "that the Congress go beyond the approach of these bills and create a refundable tax credit or direct subsidy to qualified health plans equal, for example, to 40 percent of premium payments up to a limit on subsidized premiums of $60 per month for an individual, $120 for a couple, and $180 for a family in 1986, indexed to GNP per capita. Such a credit would be equally valuable to a person with a low income as to a person with a high income. It would give everyone an incentive to buy a health plan up to the subsidized limit, but would make them fully cost conscious above that limit."

THE STATES ACT TO EQUALIZE ACCESS   In the absence of federal action, some states have moved to provide coverage for the unemployed and uninsured. "Maryland, New Jersey, and Massachusetts reimburse providers through an all-payer rate-setting system that includes an allowance for charity and bad debt in each payment made to hospitals" (27, 59), and Florida taxes hospitals to create a pool to pay for care of the uninsured. Iglehart, in his health policy report (27), summarizes actions taken by some other states.

Reimbursement Incentives for Innovation and Diffusion of Medical Technology

The dominant method of payment for medical care in the past by fee-for-service to physicians and cost reimbursement to hospitals provided a strong economic incentive for innovations and unrestrained diffusion of medical technology. "The result," in the words of a spokesman for the Health Industry Manufacturers Association, "was an inflationary but extremely dynamic medical marketplace that produced and adopted a vast array of new diagnostic and therapeutic tools with substantial benefits for patients and providers" (42). Unfortunately, not all medical innovations are successful. In a review of published clinical trials of surgical and anesthetic innovations, Gilbert, McPeek & Mosteller found that only one out of every seven represented a substantial advance, and less than half were judged to be even modest improvements over existing procedures (26). It can be assumed that the success rate in unpublished trials is even less.

The path to improved medical care through new and improved medical technology should lie through encouragement and well-funded support of biomedical innovation coupled with careful and well-funded clinical trials and technology assessment. The funding of biomedical innovation, from the government and from industry, has been generous (57), but the funding for clinical trials has been poor and that for technology assessment almost non-existent (8, 9). The importance of technology assessment has been recognized for some years, and the creation by the Congress in 1978 of the National Center for Health Care Technology (NCHCT) was in recognition of this need. While created in response to an important need, NCHCT was perceived by the medical profession as a threat to professional autonomy, and by industry as a threat to biomedical innovation. Opposition of the American Medical Association (6) and of the Health Industry Manufacturers Association (45) at appropriation hearings before the House Subcommittee on Health and Environment on March 20, 1981, were instrumental in the subsequent demise of NCHCT.

EVALUATION OF NEW MEDICAL TECHNOLOGY   While the Congress is only now beginning to show renewed interest in the importance of evaluation of new medical technology, the private sector has responded to increasing cost constraints by mounting cost effective initiatives such as the Medical Policy Committee of Blue Shield of California (44) and the Clinical Efficacy Assessment Program (47, 58) of the American College of Physicians. A major goal is to advise private insurers whether a given technology can be shown to be effective and therefore appropriate for reimbursement, or whether, if experimental, innovative, and unproven, it should not be covered in standard medical insurance policies.

When computed tomography (CT) was introduced in the early 1970s, this significant, expensive imaging technique was initially retarded in its diffusion by the Food and Drug Administration and the Certificate of Need (CON) process (49). After evaluation of its safety and efficacy by technology assessment entities such as the Blue Shield Medical Policy Committee, however, there was rapid diffusion into most major hospitals. Hospital administrations were motivated by demands from medical staffs and by the need for prestige to acquire CT instruments in large numbers, the CON process notwithstanding.

By way of contrast, we are now observing the process of diffusion of magnetic resonance imaging (MRI), a technique that is nonionizing but even more costly than CT (49). The efficacy of MRI is now clearly established for imaging the brain (especially in the posterior fossa) and cervical spinal cord. Additionally, MRI can distinguish between white and gray matter, and thus reveal demyelinating processes such as found in multiple sclerosis. In the current health care economic environment, however, hospitals are more circumspect about making capital investments in MRI. Instead, radiologists from several different hospitals, with assistance from capital investors, are forming consortia for establishing free-standing MRI facilities to serve several "markets."

The government itself, as the major medical insurer of the elderly through Medicare, must make similar judgments. The Health Care Financing Administration relied for reimbursement advice on the National Center for Health Care Technology during the Center's brief existence and currently turns to the Office of Health Technology Assessment (OHTA) of the National Center for Health Services Research and Health Care Technology Assessment.

PAYING FOR MEDICAL INNOVATION   As the effort to exclude from routine reimbursement those medical and surgical procedures judged to be experimental or investigational becomes more sophisticated and more widely applied, the freedom to introduce and diffuse such innovations and to receive reimbursement has become increasingly limited (43). The implementation of prospective payment by the government (4, 13, 39), and, in the private sector, the growing movement toward selective contracting with "preferred provider organizations," and the continuing growth of prepaid group practice add further severe fiscal constraints on the introduction of new technologies.

To counter the imminent loss of reimbursement for clinical investigation, investigators have urged that additional DRGs or procedure codes for research procedures be established (48, 60). In response to the call for a research DRG, Carolyn Davis, then chief of the Health Care Financing Administration (HCFA), pointed out that the Social Security Amendments of 1965, in establishing the Medicare program, expressly excluded payment for research costs (12). While excluding research costs, HCFA will, however, reimburse for the routine costs of institutionalization of patients on research protocol, as it has in the past. What has changed is that whereas under cost reimbursement the costs of the considerable additional laboratory tests and diagnostic procedures of the usual research protocol were automatically paid, under prospective reimbursement, payment will be limited to the flat fee established for the particular DRG under which the patient is admitted. Opportunities for the "bootlegging" of research costs for patients covered by private insurance will similarly be sharply reduced in the process of selective contracting for hospital and physician services and as investigational costs are identified by more sophisticated cost accounting and excluded from reimbursement.

As it becomes increasingly difficult to divert funds for research from the routine patient care budget, it also becomes increasingly urgent that new funds be identified to support clinical investigation. Medicare Trust Funds may be used for clinical trials at the discretion of the Prospective Payment Assessment Commission and the Secretary of Health and Human Services. Similarly, private insurers, such as Blue Shield, can and do authorize reimbursement for the costs of clinical investigation on a selective basis. What is needed is a markedly enhanced comprehensive federal and private mechanism for funding and administering technology assessment, including clinical trials (9, 28).

Conclusions and Summary

Medicine has entered a new era of cost-consciousness fueled by strong monetary incentives for cost-effectiveness and efficiency in the care of hospitalized patients. Hospital admission rates for privately insured as well as Medicare-entitled patients have fallen, despite perverse incentives to increase admissions. Additional perverse incentives that persist favor surgical over medical care and procedure-oriented over "cognitive" services. Large variations in the amounts of hospital care provided to populations in different geographic areas persist and appear to be unrelated to methods of reimbursement. Access to hospital care for the poor and uninsured remains a large and unresolved problem.

While it is clear that large changes in hospital care are taking place, it is not clear how much of the change is forced by cost constraints and how much represents a response by health professionals to new data from studies of hospital utilization (32, 54) and to increasing peer pressure for adherence to professional standards and concensus. If change is to be rational, it will be necessary to mount a markedly enhanced national effort to evaluate the outcomes of medical and surgical care by clinical trials and technology assessment. Practicing physicians themselves must be actively involved in the effort to develop and apply standards of care based on better outcome data, their performance must be monitored, and they must be provided with appropriate feedback of their performance as the basis for peer review and self-regulation.

The ultimate success of efforts to improve medical care in general and hospital care in particular, in an era of limited resources and cost constraints, will depend in large measure on our ability to develop new medical technologies that are cost-saving rather than cost-increasing, a few modest examples of which have appeared within the past few years (40, 41). The basic research from which most medical innovations emerge is well funded by the National

Institutes of Health. What is needed, in addition, is an equally well-funded program of support for the development and evaluation of new medical technologies.

ACKNOWLEDGMENTS

Research for this review was carried out while Dr. Bunker was a Henry J. Kaiser Senior Fellow at the Center for Advanced Study in the Behavioral Sciences. The authors are indebted to Alain C. Enthoven, Jinnet Fowles, Harold S. Luft, and John E. Wennberg for their review of an earlier draft and for their many helpful suggestions. We are grateful to Dawn Ward for her meticulous preparation of the manuscript, and to Margaret Marnell and Judith Engerman for editorial assistance.

Literature Cited

1. Aaron, H. J., Schwartz, W. B. 1984. *The Painful Prescription: Rationing Hospital Care*. Washington, DC: Brookings Inst. 161 pp.
2. Aday, L. A., Fleming, G. V., Andersen, R. 1984. *Access to Medical Care in the U.S.: Who Has It, Who Doesn't*. Chicago: Pluribus Press. 229 pp.
3. American Society of Internal Medicine. 1981. *Reimbursement for physicians' cognitive and procedural services: A white paper*. Unpublished. 4 pp.
4. Anderson, G., Steinberg, E. 1984. To buy or not to buy: Technology acquisition under prospective payment. *The New Engl. J. Med.* 311:182–85
5. Blendon, R. J., Rogers, D. E. 1983. Cutting medical care costs: Primum non nocere. *J. Am. Med. Assoc.* 250:1880–85
5a. Blumberg, M. S. 1980. Health status and health care use by type of private health coverage. *Milbank Mem. Fund Q.* 58:633–55
6. Boyle, J. 1981. Testimony presented before the Subcommittee on Health and Environment, House Committee on Energy and Commerce, U.S. House of Representatives, March 20, 1981
7. Bunker, J. P. 1985. When doctors disagree. *NY Rev. Books*, April 25
8. Bunker, J. P. 1980. Hard times for the national centers. *N. Engl. J. Med.* 303:580–82
9. Bunker, J. P., Fowles, J., Schaffarzick, R. 1982. Evaluation of medical-technology strategies. *N. Engl. J. Med.* 306:620–24, 687–92
10. Caper, P., Blumenthal, D. 1983. What price cost control? *N. Engl. J. Med.* 308:542–44
11. Cunningham, F. C., Williamson, J. W. 1980. How does the quality of health care in HMOs compare to that in other settings? *Group Health J.* 1:4–13
12. Davis, C. K. 1985. The impact of prospective payment on clinical research. *J. Am. Med. Assoc.* 253:686–87
13. Davis, K., Anderson, G., Steinberg, E. 1984. Diagnosis related group prospective payment: Implications for health care and medical technology. *Health Policy* 4:139–47
14. Eddy, D. M. 1985. More on cost-effectiveness. Appendix 6, *Artificial Heart and Assist Devices: Directions, Needs, Costs, Societal and Ethical Issues*, pp. 56–57. The Working Group on Mechanical Circulatory Support of The Natl. Heart, Lung, and Blood Inst. Washington DC: NHLBI
15. Egdahl, R. H. 1983. Ways for surgeons to increase the efficiency of their use of hospitals. *N. Engl. J. Med.* 309:1184–87
16. Enthoven, A. C. 1978. Cutting cost without cutting the quality of care. *N. Engl. J. Med.* 298:1229–38
17. Enthoven, A. C. 1984. A new proposal to reform the tax treatment of health insurance. *Health Affairs* 3(1):21–39
18. Enthoven, A. C. 1985. Statement on the tax treatment of fringe benefits. Testimony presented before the Senate Finance Committee, July 19, 1985
19. Enthoven, A. C., Noll, R. G. 1984. Prospective payment: Will it solve Medicare's financial problem? *Issues Science Technol.* 1:101–16
20. Finkler, S. A. 1979. Cost-effectiveness of regionalization: The heart surgery example. *Inquiry* 16:264–70
21. Flood, A. B., Scott, W. R., Ewy, W. 1984. Does practice make perfect? Part I:

The relation between hospital volume and outcomes for selected diagnostic categories. *Med. Care* 22:98–114

22. Flood, A. B., Scott, W. R., Ewy, W. 1984. Does practice make perfect? Part II: The relation between volume and outcomes and other hospital characteristics. *Med. Care* 22:115–24

23. Fowles, J., Bunker, J. P., Oda, M., Schurman, D. J., Osborn, P. N., Loftus, M. 1985. *Outcomes of total hip replacement using Northern California Medicare claims data: A pilot study.* Final report to the Natl. Center for Health Serv. Res., Rockville, Md. 27 pp.

24. Fuchs, V. R. 1976. A more effective, efficient and equitable system. *West. J. Med.* 125:3–5

25. Fuchs, V. R. 1986. Paying the piper, calling the tune: Implications of changes in reimbursement. *Front. Health Serv. Manage.* 2: In press

26. Gilbert, J. P., McPeek, B., Mosteller, F. 1977. Statistics and ethics in surgery and anesthesia. *Science* 198:684–89

27. Iglehart, J. K. 1985. Medical care of the poor—a growing problem. *N. Engl. J. Med.* 313:59–63

28. Institute of Medicine. 1983. *Planning Study Report: A Consortium for Assessing Medical Technology.* Washington DC: Natl. Acad. Press. 34 pp.

28b. Lave, J. R. 1984. Hospital reimbursement under Medicare. *Milbank Mem. Fund. Q.* 62:251–68

29. Lubeck, D. P. 1981. *A cost-benefit analysis of disease treatment and prevention.* Doctoral dissertation, Univ. Calif., Berkeley. Springfield, Va.: Natl. Techn. Information Serv. (P.B. 882 194556)

30. Luft, H. S. 1978. How do health-maintenance organizations achieve their "savings"? Rhetoric and evidence. *N. Engl. J. Med.* 298:1336–43

31. Luft, H. S. 1981. *Health Maintenance Organizations: Dimensions of Performance.* New York: Wiley. 468 pp.

32. Luft, H. S., Bunker, J. P., Enthoven, A. C. 1979. Should operations be regionalized? *N. Engl. J. Med.* 301:1364–69

33. Manning, W. G., Leibowitz, A., Goldberg, G. A., Rogers, W. H., Newhouse, J. P. 1984. A controlled trial of the effect of a prepaid group practice on use of services. *N. Engl. J. Med.* 310:1505–10

34. Moloney, T. W., Rogers, D. E. 1979. Medical technology—A different view of the contentious debate over costs. *N. Engl. J. Med.* 301:1413–19

35. McPherson, K., Wennberg, J. E., Hovind, O. B., Clifford, P. 1982. Small-area variations in the use of common surgical procedures: An international comparison of New England, England, and Norway. *N. Engl. J. Med.* 307:1310–14

36. Mundinger, M. O. 1985. Health service funding cuts and the declining health of the poor. *N. Engl. J. Med.* 313:44–47

37. Office of Technology Assessment, US Congr. 1984. *Medical Technology and Costs of the Medicare Program.* July. Washington DC: Natl. Tech. Information Serv. OTA-H-227

38. Office of Technology Assessment, US Congr. 1983. *Diagnosis Related Groups (DRGs) and the Medicare Program: Implications for Medical Technology—A Technical Memorandum.* July. Washington DC: Natl. Tech. Information Serv. OTA-TM-H-17

39. Omenn, G. S., Conrad, D. A. 1984. Implications of DRGs for clinicians. *N. Engl. J. Med.* 311:1314–17

39a. Prospective Payment Assessment Commission. 1985. *Report and recommendations to the Secretary, US Dept. Health Human Serv.,* April 1, 1985. Washington DC: US GPO

40. Reeder, G. S., Krishan, I., Nobrega, F. T., Naessens, J., Kelly, M., Christianson, J. B., McAfee, M. K. 1984. Is percutaneous coronary angioplasty less expensive than bypass surgery? *N. Engl. J. Med.* 311:1157–62

41. Ricardo-Campbell, R., Eisman, M. M., Wardell, W. M., Crossley, R. 1980. Preliminary methodology for controlled cost-benefit study of drug impact: The effective of cimetidine on days of work lost in a short-term trial in duodenal ulcer. *J. Clin. Gastroenterol.* 2:37–41

42. Roe, W. I. 1985. Medical technology under PPS: An uncertain future. *Hospitals* 59:88–92

43. Romeo, A. A., Wagner, J. L., Lee, R. H. 1984. Prospective reimbursement and the diffusion of new technologies in hospitals. *J. Health Econ.* 3:1–24

44. Schaffarzick, R. W. 1985. Cost containment: Technology assessment and health benefits determination. *Quality Rev. Bull.* 11:222–25

45. Schoellhorn, R. A. 1981. Federal technology assessment programs should be limited. *Med. Instrum.* 15:291–92

46. Schroeder, S. A. 1984. Curbing the high costs of medical advances. *Business Health,* July/August, pp. 7–11

47. Schwartz, J. S., Ball, J. R., Moser, R. H. 1982. Safety, efficacy, and effectiveness of clinical practices: A new initiative. *Ann. Int. Med.* 96:246–47

48. Smits, H. L., Watson, R. E. 1984. DRGs

and the future of surgical practice. *N. Engl. J. Med.* 311:1612–15

49. Steinberg, E. P., Sisk, J. E., Locke, K. E. 1985. X-ray CT and magnetic resonance imagers. *N. Engl. J. Med.* 313: 859–64

50. Stern, R. S., Epstein, A. M. 1985. Institutional responses to prospective payment based on diagnosis-related groups. *N. Engl. J. Med.* 312:621–27

51. Thurow, L. C. 1985. Medicine versus economics. *N. Engl. J. Med.* 313:611–14

52. Trauner, J. B. 1985. The California health care market—Where is it headed next? *Front. Health Serv. Manag.* 1:4–30

53. Wennberg, J. E. 1982. Should the cost of insurance reflect the cost of use in local hospital markets? *N. Engl. J. Med.* 307:1374–81

54. Wennberg, J. E. 1984. Dealing with medical practice variations: A proposal for action. *Health Affairs* 3(2):6–32

55. Wennberg, J. E., Barnes, B. A., Zubkoff, M. 1982. Professional uncertainty and the problem of supplier-induced demand. *Soc. Sci. Med.* 16:811–24

56. Wennberg, J. E., McPherson, K., Caper, P. 1984. Will payment based on diagnosis-related groups control hospital costs? *N. Engl. J. Med.* 311:295–300

57. White, J. K. 1985. Health care innovation in an era of cost containment. *Health Affairs* 4(2):105–18

58. White, L. J., Ball, J. R. 1985. The Clinical Efficacy Assessment Project of the American College of Physicians. *Int. J. Technol. Assess. Health Care* 1:169–74

59. Wilensky, G. R., Berk, M. L. 1982. Health care, the poor, and the role of Medicaid. *Health Affairs* 1(4):93–101

60. Yarbro, J. W., Mortenson, L. E. 1985. The need for diagnosis-related group 471. *J. Am. Med. Assoc.* 253:684–85

Ann. Rev. Public Health. 1986. 7:411–39

PUBLIC HEALTH ASPECTS OF NUCLEAR WAR

Jennifer Leaning

Harvard Community Health Plan, One Fenway Plaza, Boston, Massachusetts 02215

Alexander Leaf

Department of Preventive Medicine and Clinical Epidemiology, Harvard Medical School, Massachusetts General Hospital, Boston, Massachusetts 02114

PHYSICAL EFFECTS OF NUCLEAR EXPLOSIONS

Although the destructive power of conventional weapons has greatly increased, the advent of the first atomic bombs heralded the introduction of a huge increase in destructive capability, a jump from tons to kilotons, expressed as equivalent weight of TNT (dynamite). The advent of the hydrogen bomb increased the energy yield by another three orders of magnitude, to megatons of TNT. The total of all explosives used in the Vietnam War is estimated at some four megatons. A single hydrogen bomb can exceed this many-fold, and many of the hydrogen bombs existing in today's arsenals individually exceed the total of all explosives used in wars since the discovery of gun powder.

The total nuclear weapons in today's arsenals include more than 12,000 megatons (Mt) of explosives. This amounts to three tons of dynamite for every man, woman, and child on earth!

The compactness of nuclear bombs is another important feature. The weight, for example, of the materials needed for a 20-megaton bomb is some ten tons (52). If the same explosive yield was produced by dynamite, the weight of the dynamite would exceed that of any man-made structure, even the great Pyramid of Cheops (70). This feature allows the enormous explosive power of a hydrogen bomb, or bombs, to be carried distances of 10,000 kilometers or more by intercontinental missiles, which can now be targeted with great accuracy.

Nuclear weapons are qualitatively similar to conventional weapons' blast and thermal effects, although orders of magnitude larger. They differ quali-

411

0163-7525/86/0510-0411$02.00

tatively, however, by introducing a new dimension in destruction, namely radiation effects that may amplify enormously the lethal effects of nuclear weapons.

The unprecedented destructive nature of a thermonuclear explosion results from the enormous energy released in a small space during a very brief period (80). This results in temperatures higher than those in the interior of the sun, and enormous pressures. This enormous energy is dissipated as blast (50%), heat (35%), and radiation (15%). Radiation includes 5% that is released immediately as gamma rays and neutrons and 10% as radioactive fallout. The damaging effects of each of these forms of energy on humans and the environment are considered here; the interested reader is referred elsewhere to accounts more detailed (3, 44, 46, 48, 61) than can be included in this chapter.

The destructive capacity of a nuclear bomb depends foremost on its size, which is expressed by its explosive yield in an equivalent weight of TNT (kiloton equals 1000 tons; megatons equals one million tons of TNT). Each MX missile carries ten warheads of 370 kilotons each. [The bomb that decimated Hiroshima, killing 90,000 to 110,000 persons out of a population of approximately 340,000 (48), was a mere 12.5 kiloton explosive.] With the capacity for more accurate targeting there has been a tendency to reduce the size of individual warheads. The destructive area of an explosion increases only as the two thirds power of the energy of the explosion. It is therefore possible to do more damage with several smaller bombs than with fewer larger-megaton bombs possessing the same total energy.

The altitude above a target at which a bomb bursts affects its destructive action. Ground bursts will most effectively destroy targets such as hardened underground weapon silos because they can maximize the overpressure from the blast at the site of the target. The full impact of the explosion will be felt on the targeted object and the intense heat will vaporize all matter in the immediate neighborhood of the explosion. The vaporized material is lifted by the hot air into the atmosphere, and subsequently its radioactive burden of debris from the bomb itself and radioactivity induced in the vaporized earth and material by neutron bombardment is deposited on the earth as radioactive fallout. With ground bursts from bombs of one megaton or larger, some of the radioactive debris may be carried into the stratosphere, from which it is deposited globally but only slowly over a period of months to a year or so. Radioactive decay occurs during its long sojourn in the stratosphere so that by the time the fine particulate matter descends to earth it no longer represent an external radiation hazard. The major remaining radioactive elements of biological importance are iodine-125, cesium-137, and strontium-90, which when ingested create an internal radiation hazard. With smaller bombs of today's arsenals the radioactive debris will only rise into the trophosphere, from which it returns to earth much sooner, with less of its radioactivity decayed.

When the explosion is too high for the fireball to reach the ground there will be no local fallout except for material that may be washed out by rain—the black rain of Hiroshima—and the radioactivity from fission products remains in the atmosphere. The latter is known as an airburst. The altitude below which a 100-kiloton bomb will produce local fallout is 350 meters and for a one-megaton bomb, 860 meters.

The radiation consequences of an attack on nuclear power installations—reactors, reprocessing plants, spent fuel and radioactive waste storage sites—has recently received attention (30). Any nuclear war that includes attacks on industrial targets is likely to destroy nuclear reactors. A nuclear ground burst would vaporize such facilities, sucking their radioactive contents up with the fireball into the mushroom cloud along with the fission products from the bomb. From an attack that included a nuclear industry of 500 GWe (500 billion watts), the accumulated average per capita dose of radiation to the world's population, starting one week following the explosions, would be three times larger than if nuclear installations were not attacked. This translates into an expected tens of millions more people dying of cancer (56).

ACUTE MEDICAL EFFECTS

Radiation

Radiation injury may result from the direct effect of the neutrons and gamma rays created at the moment of the explosion, the external radiation in the environment from radioactive fallout, and the internal exposure from the global fallout of cesium-137 and strontium-90, which enter the food chain and are ingested. Although alpha and beta particles are produced in thermonuclear explosions, their pathway even in air is too short to create a hazard. Only if the local fallout contaminates the bare skin is it likely to cause radioactive burns.

The effects of exposure to ionizing radiation depend not only upon the total dose absorbed but on the duration of exposure. The longer the period over which a given radiation dose is absorbed the less biological damage it will cause. For our purposes, we consider whole-body exposure for periods up to seven days as an acute radiation dose. Table 1 shows the exposure doses in rads to humans, along with the generally accepted morbid consequences. It should be realized that the LD_{50} dose of 450 rads has been estimated from accidental radiation exposures following which the victims have generally received optimal care under peacetime civilian circumstances. It is being cogently argued that under wartime and post-attack circumstances such treatment facilities will not exist and that the LD_{50} dose would be considerably smaller, perhaps around 250 rads (71). These doses may be compared with those used in the radiation treatment of cancers in man. Such treatments may involve as much as 4000 rads, but the radiation is delivered over a longer period of time generally and,

Table 1 Effects of radiation on man

Acute dose (6–7 days) rem	Lethal[a] (probability) %
600	90
450	50
300	10
200	severe illness
less than 50	no acute symptoms but 0.4–2.5% cancer

[a]Death in a few weeks.

most importantly, to a very limited portion of the body. The figures in Table 1 refer to total body exposure to radiation. A chest X ray delivers 0.02 rads and a bowel series approximately 1.0 rad, by comparison.

A major deleterious effect of low-dose, nonfatal radiation exposure, in addition to increasing the incidence of later cancers, is its ability to compromise the body's immune responses. Thus even small doses, not lethal alone, acting synergistically with the many other nonlethal burns, blast wounds, and the inevitable infections, may be expected to result often in death in the aftermath of a nuclear war (11).

The three recognized clinical syndromes of acute radiation injury are the cerebral, the gastrointestinal, and the hematopoietic syndromes (37). Their features are briefly summarized in Table 2. These clinical pictures have been delineated largely from accidents occurring in the peacetime applications of radioactivity and from animal experiments in the past.

The cerebral syndrome results from large doses of 2000 to 4000 or more rads. It results within a few hours in lethargy, headache, vomiting, tremors, incoordination, obtundation, seizures, coma, and in death in 8 to 48 hours. There is no treatment and no survivors from this syndrome. This is the kind of result for which enhanced emission or neutron bombs were designed—no damage to tanks or physical surroundings but sufficiently high neutron fluxes to incapacitate and kill.

The gastrointestinal syndrome occurs with radiation doses of 500 to 2000 rads. In the immediate aftermath of a nuclear attack nausea and vomiting among survivors is likely to be very common. There is no simple way to distinguish in which cases it is simply the result of psychic reaction to the experience and in which it portends serious radiation injury. Other GI symptoms will not appear for several days, but the development of diarrhea that is bloody is a most ominous sign. Under the unsanitary conditions that will prevail, bacterial or viral enteritis is the expectation not the exception; but blood in the stool portends a more serious diagnosis of acute radiation illness.

Table 2   The acute radiation syndrome (37)

	Cerebral form	Gastrointestinal form	Hematopoietic form
Threshold dose	2000 rads	500 rads	100 rads
Characteristic signs and symptoms	convulsions; tremor; ataxia; lethargy	diarrhea; fever; disturbance of electrolyte balance	leukopenia; purpura; hemorrhage; infection
Time of death	within 2 days	within 2 weeks	within 2 months

The major effect of radiation on the biologic system is to prevent cells from dividing. Thus manifestations of its effects are most evident on organs in which cell turnover is most rapid. The lining of the gastrointestinal cells and the circulating white cells in the blood and bone marrow are the two most vulnerable systems. If radiation injury blocks cell mitosis, the last functional mucosal cell will slough off in three to four days, leaving a denuded, atrophic intestinal mucosa vulnerable to infection and bleeding. Death results in a week or so after onset from blood and body fluid loss, and infections with endogenous flora quickly becoming invasive. With radiation-induced suppression of the body's immune response this is soon followed by septicemia and death. It is possible under peacetime conditions with maximal use of modern medical resources that some of these cases could be salvaged. Under wartime conditions, without the antibiotics, plasma, intravenous fluids, transfusion services, and bacterial-free environments, the GI syndrome will invariably be fatal.

Lesser radiation exposure of 100 to 500 rads is likely to produce the hematopoietic syndrome. Within 24 to 48 hours of exposure nonspecific nausea and vomiting may occur, associated with a transient increase in body temperature. This is likely to be followed by a seven to ten day asymptomatic period. After this period the victim may begin to note lassitude with progressive, persistent fevers and sweats. In another few days petechiae will appear together with nose bleeds and bleeding gums. Routine examination of the blood will reveal a progressive decline, or virtual disappearance, of white blood cells, especially of neutrophils, with platelet counts of about 50,000 or less. The thrombocytopenia and leucopenia may worsen and then gradually improve over a period of two to five weeks. If the individual does not die from infection or generalized internal bleeding, recovery should occur. With antibiotics to control infection, platelets and whole blood transfusions to combat blood loss and thrombocytopenia, recovery is possible. But the weeks to months duration of the illness and the requirement for sophisticated medical care mean that many of the individuals with this acute radiation syndrome will die under post-attack conditions.

In Hiroshima and Nagasaki, people near the hypocenter of the blast received lethal radiation doses from the immediate gamma and neutron radiations of the bombs. With the much larger bombs that now exist in strategic arsenals it will be fallout radioactivity that will be the source of radiation injury rather than the emanations of the bomb itself. With large bombs the lethal area for blast extends beyond the range of the immediate gamma rays and neutrons so that people will be killed by blast rather than radiation. With small tactical weapons acute radiation from the thermnonuclear explosion could again become significant—with neutron bombs, such is the intention.

Lindop, Rotblat & Webber (56) have recently examined the effect of the different LD_{50} values for radiation on the number of casualties and deaths that would be expected following assumed attacks on London. For a single one-megaton bomb (half-fission, half-fusion) exploded at 580 meters above the center of London the fireball would touch the ground, giving rise to local fallout. Using a procedure employed by the US Office of Technology Assessment (61), they calculated that the total number of fatalities from heat and blast would amount to 560,000 out of a London population of 7 million. They further calculated the effect of receiving local fallout radiation by exposure in one day and over seven days—the latter is the period during which the accumulated dose is nearly equal to the dose at infinity. Calculations were made assuming four values for the LD_{50} of 3, 4, 6, and 8 Gray (800 rads) and protection factors (PF) of 1, 5, 10, and 20. A protection factor of 1.0 indicates no shielding from radiation exposure. A protection factor of 5.0 is often used as an average value for urban populations. The deaths ranged from 1.87 million with no shielding and LD_{50} = 3 Gray (300 rads) to a low of 140,000 with LD_{50} = 8 Gray (Gy) and a protection factor of 20. At the conditions most often assumed in the literature, LD_{50} = 4 Gy and PF of 5, the radiation deaths come out to be the same as the total from blast and heat. With another perhaps more likely scenario London is attacked by four weapons totaling 8 Mt, three of which are ground bursts, all within the Greater London Council but on its periphery. From blast 1.08 million deaths and from heat 0.27 million deaths would occur. Using the same method of calculating radiation fallout deaths for LD_{50} = 4 Gy and PF = 4 gives deaths due to radiation to be twice the deaths from blast. These examples illustrate some of the assumptions made in dealing with estimates of a very complex system in which crude average values must be assumed as the best guess of what would happen if such thermonuclear explosions should occur. The examples also put into perspective the terribly lethal consequences that may result from radiation, which in these calculations involve only the gamma rays from the fission after deposition on the ground.

Burns and Blast Injuries

The burn and blast casualties of nuclear war are similar in essential respects to what has been seen in past wars and disasters, with the significant exceptions that these injuries are created in enormous number and are potentially complicated by the additional factor of radiation. The blast wave created by nuclear explosions inflicts injuries on people through a number of phenomena (39):

1. The massive shift in environmental pressure as the air front hits the human body (primary effect);
2. The projection of missiles into the human body (causing either penetrating or nonpenetrating injury);
3. The sudden displacement of the human body against a standing rigid surface;
4. The collapse of structures on people either within or adjacent to them.

The extent and nature of human injury in this context depend on the biomechanical parameters of the explosion, whether caused by nuclear weapons or other means. Experimental literature has defined in detail the physical characteristics of the blast wave, but injury correlates are confined to animal models (39, pp. 548–59). The medical literature describes the injuries seen in settings ranging from conventional war to terrorist bombings, but cannot retrospectively establish precisely the physical characteristics of the explosions (20). A few general conclusions emerge from experience of these settings, and apply to a taxonomy of injuries to be expected.

Skull fractures, intra or extracerebral hemorrhage, and cervical spine injuries occur at high overpressures (5–6 psi) that create peak wind velocities that drive people into a rigid surface or drive a blunt object against the skull. At much lower overpressures (1–2 psi), buildings may still collapse and cause severe head injury to those trapped within or nearby (39, pp. 175–89, 553–57).

A particular entity called blast lung has been identified among soldiers killed by explosions during the First and Second World Wars and among experimental animals. The lesion appears to be caused by the primary effect of the overpressure as it produces a shock front that initially compresses the chest wall against the spinal column and then, in its displacement phase, releases it. Human body displacement and blunt projectiles can also create this injury. Physical structures within the thoracic cage most prone to damage in this context are those at tissue interfaces and hollow viscera. Acute deaths can also arise from the sudden propagation of air emboli into the cerebral and cardiac circulation, and from pulmonary hemorrhage and pulmonary edema (21).

The eardrum is very susceptible to rupture from the primary effect of blast wave; such injury has been found in approximately 36% of hospitalized casualties in a series from the bombing in Northern Ireland and among 45% of those who died, indicating its association with severe injury (20, p. 961). Data on threshold incidence range from 2 to 5 psi (39, p. 552).

Long bone fractures arise from displacement phenomena or from the trauma inflicted by external structures. Lacerations, abrasions, and contusions form the majority of wounds encountered among survivors of blast injury and are due primarily to the effect of penetrating missiles accelerated to high velocities by the blast wave (50). In the winds created by the blast, almost any object can be transformed into a penetrating missile; in conventional war and terrorist bombing the examples range from shards of glass to table legs (20). Lacerations causing extensive soft tissue destruction or wounds penetrating deeply create ideal conditions for serious infections such as gas gangrene; damage to major vessels or organs can also prove life-threatening. Many victims of blast injury suffer numerous minor cuts and abrasions, thus facing long-term risk of infection from retained fragments of glass, wood, and other contaminated material.

Abdominal injuries are relatively uncommon among survivors of blast injury occurring on land, prompting speculation that most serious abdominal injuries do not survive to reach the hospital (50).

The current approach to the treatment of blast victims relies on skilled assessment of casualties, immediate resuscitation of most severe cases, sorting by priority for operating room time, assignment of appropriate specialty teams, and decisive treatment of individual wounds and internal injury. With extensive organization, a new facility, and years of practice, the surgical teams at the Royal Victoria Hospital were prepared to handle, on a one-time basis only, the sudden arrival within one hour of 50 to 100 casualties (68).

The thermal energy released from nuclear weapons explosions can cause human burns by direct radiation, or by igniting clothing or other materials that secondarily engulf people in flames. Over 90% of burns seen among survivors of Hiroshima and Nagasaki were from direct radiation, termed "flash" burns (39, p. 566). Flame burns, resulting from exposure to secondary fires or contact with ignited clothing, are identical to the burns seen in conventional war or peacetime disasters.

First degree burns, affecting only the epidermis, can cause transient dehydration and pain but require no emergency treatment. Second degree burns (or partial thickness burns) result in blistering of the skin. In severe cases, full thickness or third degree burns occur. This last category, if extensive at all, will heal only with skin grafts; partial thickness burns heal by slow regrowth of skin from the wound base.

At the thermal energy levels delivered by the explosion of a 1 Mt bomb, measured in cal/cm^2, the range for flash burns is extensive. At nine to ten miles from ground zero, assuming a fraction of the population is exposed, approximately 82% of that population might be expected to receive first degree flash burns on exposed surfaces and 18% would suffer second degree burns. The thermal flux in that area would be approximately 5 cal/cm^2 (39, pp. 563–65).

Serious burns requiring emergency intervention and three to six weeks of intensive care are second or third degree burns extending beyond 20% of the body surface area (BSA); or those in critical locations (from the viewpoint of infection and function), such as the face, neck, perineum, and hands. Pulmonary and airway burns (either thermal or toxic) are also in this category (19). Failure to recognize that people with these injuries will require early and significant intravenous fluid and electrolyte replacement, scrupulous treatment of infection, and possibly aggressive airway support has led in the past to significant mortality among initial survivors of major burn disasters (7, 14). Other factors contributing to increased mortality from burns include extremes of age and combined traumatic and burn injury. The interaction of either burn or blast with radiation injury has also enhanced mortality in all settings, clinical and experimental (39, pp. 588–90). Marked delay in wound healing, extending to immunological collapse and overwhelming sepsis, have been observed in both blast and burn subjects suffering acute radiation exposures in the hematopoietic range (16, pp. 120–21; 39, pp. 588–90).

To manage successfully the care of one seriously burned patient may require the services of an intensive care unit, several physicians and nurses, hundreds of units of blood products, and scores of operations. Still, with the utmost skill, perserverance, and capacity, we can promise only marginal chances of survival to those over middle age with a greater than 50% BSA burn (24, 26).

THE MEDICAL RESPONSE

The availability of prompt and effective medical care during combat has been regarded as important to the morale of combat troops as well as for their potential salvage in event of injury. The large number of casualties, civilian as well as military, that are probable with virtually any use of nuclear weapons during hostilities between the major powers make any meaningful medical response unlikely. In this section we attempt to analyze first the potential needs versus available resources for a single megaton air burst over an urban center, as may occur as part of a counter-value attack on civilian populations, or as an initial or counter force strike at military and key industrial sites. The medical needs versus available resources will then be examined for a major nuclear attack on the United States.

Our example for the consequence of a single air burst of a one megaton nuclear weapon over an urban center will be Boston. A report of the Arms Control and Disarmament Agency of our State Department (4) indicates that the population of Boston (1979) was 2,844,000 and that a single one-megaton air burst over central Boston would produce 695,000 prompt fatalities and 735,000 surviving injured. Thus one-half of Boston's population would be killed or seriously injured. Boston has 5186 registered physicians. If one assumes the same proportion of physician casualties as for the general population, 50% of physicians would survive uninjured. (In fact, the Massachusetts Commissioner of Health estimated 80% of physicians and 70% of nurses to be prompt casualties.) But with 2593 uninjured surviving physicians and 735,000 seriously injured, each physician on the average would have 284 injured to treat. The futility of providing care for such numbers is indicated by the calculation that if each injured were seen for 15 minutes and each physician worked a 16 hour day, it would take 4.4 days for all injured to receive an initial medical contact. But the injuries would be serious burns, trauma, and radiation exposures, and these are among the most demanding of medical care and resources.

Examination of available hospital facilities indicates further disparity between needs and resources. Boston has 12,816 hospital beds, but the hospitals are concentrated in the urban target area so that of 48 acute care hospitals 38 would be destroyed or badly damaged. Thus 83% of the beds would be destroyed, leaving approximately 2135 beds for the care of 735,000 seriously injured survivors or 344 per hospital bed!

These stark figures fail to take into consideration the damage that would occur to the entire physical structure, the social organization upon which the medical care system is based, and the psychology of survivors. Medical facilities today exemplify almost the epitome of dependence on an intact and sophisticated socioeconomic organization. With electric power gone, transportation nonexistent, shortage of medical supplies, inadequate health workers of all skills, any semblance of the kind of modern sophisticated intensive medical care required by the seriously injured would be lacking. Were such an attack a single catastrophe and the remainder of the country intact, help could certainly be mobilized to come in from the outside. But even resources in the US as a whole are not scaled to approach the needs that would follow a single thermonuclear explosion over an urban center such as Boston. It is estimated that the intensive care beds that could be mobilized in the country to care for severe burns number between one and three thousand. But the burns created by a single bomb burst, as depicted, would number tens of thousands so that make-shift, less than optimal, care is all that could be provided for those injured even with ideal triage making best use of US medical resources. The same would apply were radiation and blast injuries considered, though with a single urban center affected, damage to the ecosystem, starvation, cold, and other long-term effects would be avoided.

One can sense that in any large nuclear attack the medical deficiencies to cope with casualties even for a single bomb burst over a single city would be multiplied many-fold. Abrams (1) has made quantitative assessments of the medical resources that would survive a nuclear war versus the medical needs. His scenario, designed by FEMA (Federal Emergency Management Agency), was that of a massive nuclear war (CRP-2B) in which the United States is exposed to 6559 megatons of nuclear explosives; the targets of attack, in order of priority, are military bases and equipment, industrial centers, and population concentrations of 50,000 or more. The following is a summary of Abrams' analysis.

In 1981, 73% of the population of the United States lived in or near cities with more than 50,000 inhabitants. Approximately 80% of the country's medical resources (hospital beds and personnel, blood, drugs, and medical supplies) were also located in these vulnerable areas. Estimates of casualties published by federal agencies, together with data from the Hiroshima-Nagasaki experience, suggest that with no shelters or evacuation there will be 93 million survivors of whom approximately 32 million will have been injured. Twenty-three million Americans will have radiation sickness of varying severity, while 14 million will have suffered trauma and/or burns, allowing for combined injuries as observed in Japan. Thus a total of 9.1 million burns and 9.8 million blast injuries would occur, with 4.9 million having combined trauma and burn. Among the 9.8 million blast victims, probably 6 million would have open wounds; head, thoracic, abdomen, and extremity injuries would number in the hundreds of thousands.

Approximately 80% of medical personnel and resources would be destroyed. The surviving 48,000 physicians would have 32 million casualties, or there would be one physician for every 663 patients. Of the trauma and burn victims approximately 55% will require hospitalization. This will mean 64 patients for each available hospital bed, and the patients and beds may be in widely separated localities. Estimates of the needs for blood products, replacement fluids, and other resources show gross disparities from available supplies. Adding the problems with transportation of wounded and supplies, lack of power, and total socio-psycho-economic chaos, it is very clear that no meaningful medical response is possible for the injured survivors in the aftermath of a nuclear war.

CIVIL DEFENSE AND PREPAREDNESS

Since the Federal Civil Defense Act of 1950 established national responsibility for civil defense policy and program, the key controversies have centered on the strategy and feasibility of protecting the population from nuclear war (9, 51). Participating in assessments of Soviet threat and the effects of nuclear weapons, Federal civil defense agencies have oscillated between a focus on in-place fallout shelters and population evacuation. Fallout shelters, initially endorsed, began to seem less acceptable as the massive blast and thermal power of nuclear weapons became more widely understood. Reports of the explosive force of the Bikini hydrogen bomb then suggested that population evacuation from target areas might be the only reasonable response; and then, as the potentially lethal effects began to be discussed publicly, the pendulum swung back to fallout shelters. Although the Cuban missile crisis marked a near-approach to war, its longer-term effect (the signing of the Limited Test Ban Treaty in 1963 and the easing of cold war tensions) dampened public interest in civil defense issues. From the mid-1960s until the late 1970s, the Federal civil defense agencies engaged primarily in research on shelter efficacy and strategic evacuation, linking their analysis to military and political evaluation of warning and escalation scenarios (8, 29). In the mid-1970s, interest in civil defense revived, as developments in weapons technologies and in nuclear strategic doctrine converged in policies that undermined deterrence, emphasized flexible response, and stressed Soviet first-strike capability (38, 40). Responding to studies by the Defense Department and the National Security Council, Carter in 1978 issued Presidential Directive 41, which mandated a civil defense policy designed to ensure population survival in the event of nuclear war. Based on a model of population evacuation developed by civil defense agencies in preceding years, the plan, called crisis relocation, projected a $2 billion expenditure over five years (3, 51, pp. 155–67).

In 1980, the newly organized Federal Emergency Management Agency (FEMA), which incorporated all previous disaster and civil defense agencies under one roof, adopted crisis relocation as its main strategy. Reagan recommended a $4.2 billion expenditure over seven years in support of this strategy, so that FEMA could set up a system for responding to a period of "heightened international tension" by evacuating 150 million citizens from the 250 largest urban areas. Within a three- to five-day period, this population was expected to travel by all available means over a several hundred mile radius to designated host areas, where shelters would have been prepared or "expedient" shelters built at the time to afford protection from fallout during the first two weeks after the postulated nuclear attack (12, 20).

Vigorous public debate about the viability of crisis relocation rested on three main points (53, 73):

1. The actual evacuation and shelter plans were not feasible and could not produce what was projected within the time and budget proposed;
2. The plan was strategically destabilizing in that its existence would heighten Soviet anxiety and its implementation in the midst of crisis might provoke a Soviet first strike;
3. The effects of nuclear war on the continental United States were sufficiently dire and pervasive to obliterate long-term survival prospects and to dwarf any short-term mitigation crisis relocation might arguably introduce.

Hit by public criticism and Congressional skepticism FEMA, in 1983, revised its policy, proposing a merger of disaster and war response in the program called the Integrated Emergency Management System (IEMS) and arguing that evacuation and shelter were key strategies in responding to a range of disasters, including nuclear war (38). Despite this shift, public misgiving about FEMA's overall direction has continued to constrain annual funding allocations for the agency's programs (18).

In March 1983, Reagan introduced the Strategic Defense Initiative (SDI), a ballistic missile defense system designed to destroy in space the incoming enemy missiles before they reached the US land mass and capable, according to its advocates, of providing a degree of population protection and security against attack previously unobtainable. Controversy regarding the ultimate nature of the defense this system might confer has been intensified by recent new data on the effects of nuclear war. As in the past, tension between what the program can promise and what nuclear weapons can deliver continues to define the polarity of the debate.

INTERMEDIATE AND LONG-TERM MEDICAL EFFECTS

Fallout and Radiation Effects

The amount of local fallout released in a given attack is usually expressed in the form of a fallout map, derived from summing up the radiation released from individual warhead explosions and distributing it according to composite meteorological conditions. These maps abstract from local fallout patterns, which depend on specific terrain and wind characteristics that may vary tremendously from the standard. Concentrated local areas of fallout, called "hot spots," pose unpredictable hazards, and the concept of a composite wind velocity obscures the fallout risk posed by departures from the average.

These maps describe the distribution of radioactive fallout across a given geographic area as though the radiation were received at all points simultaneously. In actuality, the fallout is delivered over time, so that the leading edge of the eliptical radioactive plume, traveling from the point of detonation, reaches points downwind at times determined by meteorological conditions. The radiation contained in local fallout decays in intensity over time by a factor of ten for every seven-fold increase in elapsed hours, measured by convention from a unit-time reference of one hour (or H + 1) after detonation. Exposure to radioactive fallout can be expressed either in terms of dose rate, specifying some point in time after the explosion, or in terms of cumulative dose, which usually incorporates a factor of biological repair. Cumulative dose sums all radiation received to infinite time, constituting 9.3 times the initial unit-time reference dose (69).

The main sources for data on human response to high dose radiation are the populations of Hiroshima and Nagasaki exposed in 1945 to airbursts of fission weapons. Two other populations undergoing investigation are the residents of the Marshall Islands, accidentally exposed to fallout from the Bikini Atoll thermonuclear test in 1954, and a Utah population exposed at school age to fallout from tests conducted in the years 1951–1958. Other data sources include occupational experience, clinical trials, and accidents at research and industrial sites.

The chief factors affecting human response are radiation dose, dose-rate, and the age of the exposed population. The US government after World War II suggested a range of 360 to 450 rads as the LD_{50}, depending on midline (organ target) or body surface dose. This dose range has been reexamined from the perspective that synergistic stress in wartime populations might reduce the LD_{50} to a range as low as 150 to 250 rads (bone marrow dose) (57, 71, pp. 1–9).

Repeated observations, leading to the theory of biological repair rates, indicate that a given dose of radiation will inflict more severe consequences in humans if delivered all at once, in a single dose, than if fractionated and given in multiple, smaller doses over time. The dose-fractionation effect pertains only to acute exposures, however; for long-term sequelae, like cancer induction, the dose effect appears to be cumulative, whether fractionated or not. It has been assumed that fractionation of moderate doses (such as those that may on average apply in the first few months after the attack) would eliminate or markedly reduce health risks; but the literature suggests instead that moderate doses be evaluated on a cumulative basis (57, pp. 500–9; 60).

Developing humans, whether *in utero,* infants, or young children, are particularly sensitive to radiation, in terms of both acute response and long-term susceptibilities. Older people have also been found to be less resistant than middle-aged adults to the effects of acute doses of radiation. The available data are too limited, however, to assign a dose-response value to either the very young or the elderly (60, p. 42; 69, p. 53).

The health consequences of acute radiation exposure (within the first seven days after attack) have been described above. Here the focus is on the effects of exposure to moderate doses over the first several months to several years following a war, an exposure range and duration that would apply to a population initially seeking shelter and then emerging to forage for food and water. For these weeks and months, radiation exposures to much of the surviving population in the Northern Hemisphere might range from 0.1 to 10 rads per day. The doses would accumulate on the burden already received during the early shelter period.

The NCRP suggests a minimum threshold dose for acute symptoms of 0.14 rads per day, or 1 rad per week (60, p. 19). So far as is known at present, fractionated or protracted exposures at the overall rate of 1 rad/week for six years (about 300 rads total) have little chance of causing any acute symptoms, although it is possible that some signs of significant radiation effect can be demonstrated by means of laboratory methods. It remains an unsettled question whether protracted doses slightly above this range would produce clinically significant morbidity or mortality.

The mortality effects of doses in this range are suggested in data from medical and accidental exposures to intermediate levels of radiation. Over one year, exposures to a daily dose of 1.5 rads produces a 10% probability of death, climbing to a 90% probability for exposures of 6 rads per day. These data were obtained from people suffering from other diseases, and it is recommended in the report that, to extrapolate these findings to healthy populations, the threshold daily exposures should be raised by a factor of three (57, pp. 501–2). However, as Rotblat and Greer have both recently argued, a large proportion of survivors may well suffer from malnutrition, infectious disease, and other untreated illnesses and might succumb to mortality curves similar to the ones in this study (42).

Conception and production of healthy children may be adversely affected by doses in this range. Permanent sterility requires exposures to high acute doses, estimated at over 600 rads for men, 300 to 400 rads for women (17). Temporary azospermia, however, lasting one to three years, can result from acute exposures to 20 to 50 rads; and persistent azospermia can be produced by doses as low as 0.2 rads if sustained on a daily basis over two to five years (5, 16). Human sensitivity to radiation during intrauterine and early postnatal life has been well documented. Defects in fetal central nervous systems are detectable at maternal exposures to acute doses of 10 rads (17, pp. 481–85); the incidence of microcephaly among infants exposed at 6 to 11 weeks of age to radiation released at Hiroshima and Nagasaki was markedly increased above nonexposed populations (16, pp. 152–56). Fetal wastage in Hiroshima has been difficult to estimate, since most pregnant women had been evacuated from the city, but was prominent among the pregnancies investigated in Nagasaki (16, pp. 152–56).

As the radioactivity in local fallout decays in intensity over the first several months, the surviving population becomes subject to what has been called the long-term consequences of radiation exposure. Contributing to these consequences are the effects of global, or delayed, fallout that ultimately result in contamination of the human food chain. These long-term radiation effects are expressed in terms of increased cancer incidence and genetic mutation rates.

Radiation exposure appears to increase the incidence of certain cancers but not change the time at which these cancers currently arise in human life cycles. Among the cancers increased in survivors of Hiroshima and Nagaski were leukemia, cancer of the breast, lung, stomach, thyroid, colon, and urinary tract and multiple myeloma (49). A dose-response curve could be drawn only for the case of leukemia, which in years of peak incidence occurred at a rate of ten times that in the nonexposed population (31). The leukemia data are now the subject of review, prompted by new estimates of dosimetry for neutron and gamma radiation released at Hiroshima (59). The International Commission on Radiation Protection (ICRP) estimates cancer risks for populations exposed to varying levels of radiation. Employing a linear dose-response curve, which has been criticized as understating incidence at lower doses, the ICRP calculates the excess risk of death from all cancers for both sexes as 12.5×10^{-3} per 100 rems. In the setting of nuclear war, those with nonlethal cancers (estimated as double the number of lethal cancers) might, in absence of adequate medical care, experience an accelerated mortality (47).

The main genetic effect of ionizing radiation appears to be an increase over the present incidence of spontaneous mutations in human populations, which occur at an annual rate of 10% of all live births. The doubling dose in humans (that required to double the current background incidence) has been widely estimated to range from 15–250 rads (62). Contrary to evidence from other human and from animal data, and without a generally accepted explanation for this finding, there is no sign of significant genetic damage in the F_1 generation from Hiroshima and Nagasaki (75). Incorporating these conflicting lines of evidence, the Committee on the Biological Effects of Ionizing Radiation (BEIR III) suggests that exposing a population to one rem will induce 5 to 65 significant genetic mutations per million live births in the first generation (17, p. 85).

In discussing the effects of fallout on human populations in a given nuclear war scenario, it has become customary to define the shelter strategy the population may adopt. The radiation protection afforded by shelters is based on the fact that the intensity of radioactivity decays with time and is reduced by shielding. The term "protection factor" (PF) is used to identify the protection conferred by a given shelter construction. For the United States, in the post-attack setting, FEMA has defined a shelter as adequate if it affords a PF of 40 or above, thus reducing the interior dose rate to one fortieth of the prevailing external level (43). As a ratio, the safety this factor affords is relative to the intensity of the external dose. Since it assumes a uniform radiation field, the concept also requires that the shelter be circumferentially sound. A PF of 40 offers little margin for error: If winds were to shift and levels greater than expected delivered to shelter residents, a PF of 40 could not protect Northeast residents from levels of 10,000 rads per hour; and in the Midwest, areas normally upwind from SAC and ICBM bases could, in variable wind conditions, be exposed to levels of 30,000 rads per hour (74).

In addition to the protection factor, the other main variable affecting shelter efficacy is consistency of shelter use. After nuclear war, it is suggested that the population remain sheltered for a period of two to four weeks, until ambient radiation has decayed to permissible levels. In areas where initial levels would be high, the extent to which people abide by the injunction would be critical. Aside from the difficulty of reliably determining the external doses, pressures to exit during the early time frame might be irresistible: lack of food or water, accumulated wastes or dead bodies, poor air, deprivation of light, claustrophobia, inability to live with ongoing uncertainty. Every foray would increase one's cumulative dose, and reduce the protection afforded by the shelter. In a critique of official civil defense assessments of shelter use, the Arms Control and Disarmament Agency describes a realistic pattern of shelter stay for a US population after nuclear war. In this analysis, the pattern resulted in degrading the PF of 40 to a range between 12 and 20 (64). Similar adjustments have been made in other accounts employing sheltering strategies (25).

Radiation casualties from acute and intermediate effects of fallout from nuclear war have been estimated for a variety of scenarios. In a major nuclear war on North America, described by the US Defense Civil Preparedness Agency in 1976, 6559 megatons would release sufficient fallout to kill from 19 million to 67 million, the range dependent on assessments of sheltering strategies and use (78). In a revision of the scenario developed by *Ambio,* the Journal of the Royal Swedish Academy of Sciences, Harwell developed a scenario for nuclear attack on US military and industrial targets in which the explosion of approximately 2500 megatons resulted in approximately 62 million deaths from fallout alone (44, pp. 1–83). World scenarios, with estimates of fallout effects, are contained in the *Ambio* study and in a report of the World Health Organization (48, pp. 1–42). Relying on different attack parameters, both studies find radiation deaths from a major nuclear war to number in hundreds of millions. Increased cancer incidence and genetic defects would affect tens of millions of those surviving the acute consequences of war extending to both hemispheres.

Infectious Diseases

Among the initial injured survivors with burns, blast wounds, and acute radiation syndromes, infections will take a heavy toll. In the absence of antibiotics and medical care generally, infections will be the terminating factor among the surviving injured who die in the first few weeks.

The intermediate period following the attack we will take to include the shelter period, when survivors attempt to sustain themselves in fallout shelters amid intensive radiation and fires about them and deprivation from food, water, and sanitation within the shelters. This intermediate period will blend into the late period characterized by efforts to survive in a chaotic primitive economy and to rebuild some semblance of social and economic order. During both the intermediate and subsequent intervals, infection is likely to be a major cause of morbidity and mortality, together with starvation and freezing, as discussed below.

A very important factor in the prevalence of infections among survivors will be the generalized suppression of the immune system caused by ionizing radiation, which will make survivors much more susceptible to both the occurrence and devastation of infections. Federal estimates indicate that 23 million survivors of a large scale nuclear attack will suffer from radiation sickness (28). This indicates a mean dose of some 200 rads or more. But the number of persons receiving less than 200 rads but a dose still sufficient to depress the immune response will be at least double the number suffering from acute radiation sickness. Furthermore, it is now appreciated that ultraviolet radiation can also compromise the immune response (22, 41, 63). With depletion of the ozone layer by nitrous oxides, exposure to UV-B will increase. It is expected that all survivors will have some degree of compromise to their immune systems. Protein malnutrition and starvation, which will be rampant, will further interfere with the ability of survivors to fend off infections.

With these factors decreasing the ability of survivors to cope with infections, there will be an additional number of factors acting to increase the spread of disease. Abrams (2) has considered the problem of infections in the intermediate postattack period. The brief discussion below follows his analysis.

Individuals in both large public shelters and those confined to basements and other underground occupancy will be vulnerable to the spread of infection. In crowded public shelters lacking adequate forced ventilation, the heat and humidity will favor the spread of respiratory infections. The absence of adequate waste disposal and toilet facilities, together with vomitus, open wounds, corpses, flies, and diarrheal stools, will quickly result in spread of gastroenteritis and hepatitis.

Once radioactive decay has made it safe for people to leave shelters even for a few hours daily, conditions favoring spread of communicable diseases will continue. Sanitary water supplies, properly prepared and refrigerated food, sewage and waste disposal and treatment will be seriously compromised or totally lacking. Enteric diseases to which Americans are likely to be highly vulnerable will spread: infectious hepatitis, *E. coli* infections, salmonellosis, shigellosis, amoebic dysentery, typhoid, and even cholera may be expected. These are the diseases that have marched in the wake of wars in the past, but conditions after a nuclear war would be more conducive to their occurrence than any prior known situation.

There will be millions of human corpses left in the wake of a nuclear war; these will pose a further threat to sanitation. With all the other survival problems to cope with, it is not likely that burial or cremation will quickly remove this source of infection and contamination. Rats and other scavenging animals are likely to be the major undertaker force.

Insects generally are much more resistant to radiation than are humans, animals, and birds. Thus few of their natural enemies will remain, but the lack of sanitation and undisposed corpses will feast them. An explosion of flies is anticipated as well as of other insects, and these will serve as transmitters of diseases, the enteric diseases, but also such diseases as typhus, malaria, dengue fever, and encephalitis will appear and increase.

Other infectious diseases that exist among us but are held in check by good sanitation, nutrition, housing, and medical treatment will increase under post-attack conditions: tuberculosis, hepatitis and all enteric diseases, penumonias, influenza, meningitis, whooping cough, diphtheria, streptococcal infections, poliomyelitis, and many others that we currently associate with the over-crowded, underdeveloped world and that are fostered by poor sanitation, malnutrition, crowding, and lack of immunization and medical care. Other epidemic diseases that have been essentially suppressed in our country will return, such as cholera, malaria, plague, yellow fever, and typhus. Thus infections will take a heavy toll on survivors, even as they had from antiquity until the present century, and in the presence of widespread immune suppression their lethal effects should be anticipated as devastating.

Food and Nutrition in the Aftermath of a Nuclear War

Terrible as the acute effects of a thermonuclear war might be, the long-term effects will be even more disastrous. Careful analyses predict the failure of agriculture and a consequent lack of food in the aftermath of a nuclear war (48, 76). Hunger and starvation would be widespread not only among the survivors in the combatant countries but throughout the world in both the northern and southern hemispheres. Hundreds of millions would starve to death in the first few years following an all-out nuclear war. The report of the World Health Organization (48) indicated this potential disaster, and the SCOPE study (45) arrives at the same conclusion through a careful analysis of the probabilities. The occurrence of widespread starvation throughout the world is based upon the following considerations:

The granaries of the world contain at any given time relatively small stores of grains and cereals. In recent years about two months' supply of cereals have been available at the present consumption rate (34). The United States could survive approximately a year on its grain stores, but portions of the stores would undoubtedly be damaged directly by the thermonuclear explosions. Blast, fire, and radioactive contamination would render other stores unavailable for consumption. Furthermore, crops in the field would be damaged to an unpredictable extent.

Transportation from the sites of production to the sites of need is likely to be destroyed. Roads, bridges, rail, and port facilities are likely targets for an aggressor intent on destroying an opponent's industrial competence to sustain a war. Little of the food that appears in the large markets today is grown locally. In Massachusetts more than three quarters of the food arrives from out of state by truck or rail, and supplies on hand would last only a few days. In a nuclear attack most of these supplies in urban areas will be destroyed. Most of the developed world depends upon transportation for food supplies. In the north-eastern United States some 80% of the food consumed is imported. Eighty-five percent of the United States' corn is grown in eleven midwestern states; one sixth of the wheat is grown in Kansas alone; two thirds of the soybeans are grown in the Great Lakes states and the corn belt; rice is grown mainly in Arkansas, Louisiana, Texas, Mississippi, and California; fruit and vegetable production is nearly as regionally concentrated (76). In the absence of transportation, surviving crops could not be moved to places of need.

In the United States and other developed countries food is supplied by a complex network of businesses that involve not only farming, animal husbandry, and fishing, but also the production of farm machinery, pesticides, fertilizers, petroleum products, and commercial seeds. Mass food production also requires slaughterhouses, grain elevators, cold storage plants, flour mills, canning factories, and other packaging plants. Transportation, storage, and the marketing and distribution of foods through both wholesale and retail outlets are also involved. In the event of a breakdown in this vast agribusiness, an inevitable consequence of nuclear war, there would no longer be means to harvest, process, and distribute what crops survived. There would be much spoilage.

The social and economic structure of society would be a major casualty of a nuclear war. Money would have little or no value and food and other necessities would be obtained, if possible, by barter. As people became desperately hungry, survival instincts would become dominant and armed individuals or marauding bands would raid and pilfer what supplies and stores existed. Warehouses would be ransacked; law enforcement would not exist.

Supplies of fuel, fertilizers, agriculture chemicals, and seed would soon be exhausted. Beasts of burden as well as tractors would not be available. Food production would become very labor intensive, a reversion to the primitive farming methods in the Middle Ages or earlier (35). Insects, resistant to radiation, would proliferate, and pesticides would not be available for their control. The insects would further reduce the yield of what crops might survive. Radioactivity would render some fields unusable for weeks or months.

The destruction of sanitation, refrigeration, food processing methods, especially in remaining urban areas, will result in contamination of food with bacteria, particularly with enteric pathogens. Spoiled meat and carrion of domestic animals, and even of human corpses, are likely to be eaten by starving persons, as has happened in major famines in the past. Civilized man has lost resistance to many such pathogens acquired from foods and waters contaminated by excreta, by flies, other insects, and rodents, which are likely to proliferate in the aftermath of a nuclear war.

Water supplies may be seriously reduced and frequently contaminated with radioactivity. Dams and large irrigation projects may well be targeted, certainly in a counter-value attack. Reduced rainfall would interfere with agricultural productivity, and radioactive fallout would contaminate reservoirs and surface waters with long-lived radioactive isotopes.

The many surface fires will cause much soot and dust to enter the atmosphere, thus absorbing solar infrared energy (15, 23, 81). and reducing the average temperature at the earth's surface in the northern hemisphere. This will interfere with the maturation and the ripening of grain—the staple of our diets. "Nuclear winter" seems a likely consequence of the large amounts of soot in the atmosphere. If temperatures are decreased by tens of degrees for periods of weeks during the spring and summer growing season, as most climatic models predict, the effects upon agriculture will be devastating. During most of the growing season a sharp decline in temperature for only a few days may be sufficient to destroy crops. Since most of the wheat and coarse grains are grown in the temperate regions of the northern hemisphere, which would be the zones most affected by a "nuclear winter," a nuclear war, especially during the spring or summer, would have a devastating effect on crop production and food supplies for at least that year. The United States and Canada are literally the bread baskets for the world. Rice is even more sensitive to temperature reduction than are the grains grown in the northern hemisphere, so this staple for much of the developing world would also be eliminated.

Man's adaptation to cold is calorically expensive. A "nuclear winter" would increase metabolic needs just when dietary calories would be least available.

The effects on agriculture may be long term due to deterioration of the quality of the soil following a nuclear war. Death of plant and forest coverage due to fire, radiation, and lack of fertilizers will leave the soil vulnerable to erosion by wind and rain. Desertification will occur. Coarse grasses and shrubs will provide ground cover, making agriculture and animal husbandry less productive.

Hunger and starvation, as we note, will not be limited to the combatant countries alone or even to just the northern hemisphere. It will be truly a global occurrence. Even without the possible climatic effects of a "nuclear winter" spreading to the southern hemisphere, millions will die of starvation in noncombatant countries. Today a large portion of food exports goes to parts of the world where millions of people are suffering undernutrition and hunger (76). The World Bank estimated, on the basis of 1980 data, that some 800 million persons in developing countries, amounting to 61–70% of their populations, have deficient diets (67). Using a slightly more stringent criteria, the Food and Agriculture Organization of the United Nations estimates that some 16 to 23% of the global population, or 436 million persons, have food intake levels that are inadequate and barely permit survival [amounting to $1.2 \times BMR$, a level of caloric intake below which survival is not possible (33)]. The World Health Organization in addition identifies at least 450 million children presently suffering from varying degrees of protein malnutrition (65). A large number of these persons are dependent directly or indirectly on the food supply and price structure made possible by the food exports of North America. A disruption of these supplies would thus have grave consequences for most of the populations of developing countries.

It is these considerations that make it almost certain that hunger and starvation will decimate survivors of a major nuclear war. The developing countries in fact may be the main victims of this famine, as their populations may not be as immediately reduced by the direct effects of nuclear war as would the populations of the combatant countries.

SOCIOECONOMIC EFFECTS

The diversion of funds from all social programs, including health and medical care, by the huge military expenditures is today a central issue in the congressional debates over the federal budget. The diversion of a large part of the world's resources—estimated at some 660 billion dollars in 1982 (77)—to preparations for war leaves far fewer resources available for health services and for other programs that would improve the quality of life. The developing countries have also been deflecting their resources to military items during the period 1960–1978—4.3% of their gross national product, compared to 5.6% for the NATO countries (77)—despite the enormous medical and social needs of these developing countries. Two billion people live on incomes below $500 per year; 600 million persons have no jobs or are less than fully employed; 11 million babies die before their first birthday; two billion people lack a dependable supply of safe water to drink; 450 million suffer from hunger and malnutrition; 120 million children of school age have no school (77). Money can be spent to strengthen industrial production and improve health and social conditions, or for military purposes, but the huge expenditures on the latter preclude the former.

After a major nuclear war, devastation to the advanced economies of the world will be practically complete (35). Transportation centers, heavy industries, energy sources and supplies are prime targets. Skilled personnel clustered about such facilities would almost all be included in the tens or hundreds of millions of immediate casualties. The destruction of the capability of an opponent to wage and sustain hostilities is a goal of modern warfare; in a nuclear war the sources of economic strength on both sides will be eliminated.

Money, banking, investments, and all the trappings of advanced economies, as well as central government authority, would disappear in the combatant countries. The destruction of sources of electricity, oil, and gas, as well as means of transportation, would render useless what industry survived direct damage. A reversion to a medieval economy would occur, and survivors would lead a labor-intensive marginal existence. The Dark Ages would return, with a disease-ridden, shortened life-span for survivors (35).

If such will be the fate of combatant countries, what will happen to the bystanders? A recent report from the Royal Society of New Zealand depicts a very similar outcome in a noncombatant country in the southern hemisphere (72) because of dependence on foreign trade, which would be disrupted.

Under primitive economic conditions following a nuclear war, Galbraith (35) indicates that neither capitalism nor communism would have significance. Both concepts are creations of advanced levels of industrialization, which would no longer exist. Thus adherents to either political/economic philosophy would find that the very principles for which the nuclear war was ostensibly waged would be the certain victims of that war.

CLIMATE AND ENVIRONMENTAL EFFECTS

Recent data suggest that the injection into the atmosphere of massive quantities of smoke, dust, and toxic vapors from the mix of air and ground bursts that would characterize a nuclear war might cause shifts in light flux and temperature of sufficient magnitude to threaten many biological systems, including human. Damage estimates depend on a series of assumptions and on choice of parameters among atmospheric models. Repeated iterations now confirm the probability that a "nuclear winter" will follow a major nuclear war, and discussion now focuses on the spread, intensity, and duration of the effects.

The initial consequences of airbursts over cities and forests would be to generate millions of tons of optically dense smoke spreading into the troposphere. High yield surface bursts would inject millions of tons of dust into the stratosphere. Over a period of several weeks, the mixture of smoke and dust would extend throughout the atmosphere of the northern hemisphere and would begin to create a pall over the southern half of the globe.

In the more severe scenarios for the northern hemisphere, this shroud of particles would block and absorb the transmission of sunlight and cause some reduction of light and a potentially marked decrease in temperature at the land surface. For the 5000 megaton case, it is estimated that within three weeks of these detonations, land temperatures would drop to $-18°C$ (0°F) and the intensity of light in midday might be significantly diminished. More mild projections suggest ambient temperature reductions of 5 to 10°C with slight changes in light flux. These effects, depending upon the scenario, would persist for one to three months and might extend for up to one year (27).

During this first year, as the soot and dust began to clear, scattered by winds in the upper atmosphere and washed out by rainfall, the effects of ozone depletion in the upper atmosphere would become apparent. Nitrous oxides, produced by the massive combustions, would reduce stratospheric ozone by approximately 30% resulting in a two-fold increase in UV-B light flux at the land surface of the northern hemisphere. Over several years, this increased intensity would abate, as ozone levels in the atmosphere began to regenerate and again block transmission of sunlight in these wave lengths (44, pp. 136–40).

These shifts in light and temperature, descending within the first few weeks postwar, would impose serious hardship on the initial survivors. Among the interacting stresses would be the morbid effects of exposure. Humans require shelter and clothing to survive in the temperatures "nuclear winter" would produce. Damp or windy conditions would accelerate the onset of hypothermia and possible death. Those at the extremes of age or already weakened by injury, hunger, or disease would be less able to compensate for the cold by increasing their activity or metabolic rates (66).

The issue of "nuclear winter" also raises new uncertainty about access to water supplies during the first several months after a nuclear war. Because pumping and storage systems would have been extensively destroyed, people would have to depend on rainfall and fresh water in lakes and streams. During the first several months of the "nuclear winter", however, precipitation over the land masses of North America (the coastal areas might experience severe storms arising from clashing temperature fronts) is predicted to be well below pre-war levels. Most of the surface water in North America is found in lakes: Under conditions defined by the more severe scenarios, the majority of water bodies accessible to the remaining US population would be frozen to a depth of 0.5 to 1 meter for two to six months postattack (44, pp. 101–11). Breaking through to water beneath the ice and then transporting it would require sustained energy expenditure, a requirement which, in settings of markedly constricted food resources, might become highly significant.

PSYCHOLOGICAL FACTORS

The psychological factors relating to nuclear war have come under increasing study. For purposes of discussion these psychologic factors may be subdivided into two categories:

1. effects of living under the continuous threat of nuclear annihilation;
2. psychologic responses to a nuclear attack.

Effects of Living Under the Continuous Threat of Nuclear Annihilation

There have been several surveys of both children and adults to assess reactions to the continuous threat of nuclear annihilation (6, 13, 58). Standard opinion surveys of adolescent populations indicate that adolescents have concerns about nuclear annihilation occurring during their lifetimes. In 1984, Gallup (36) surveyed 514 teenagers aged 13–18 as a representative national cross-section. Fifty-one percent indicated it was "somewhat likely" that a nuclear war will be started during their lifetime; 15% of the group thought it is "very likely" to happen during their lifetimes. About half of the group surveyed say the possibility of nuclear war has influenced their plans for the future and 25% describe the influence as serious. Other surveys by direct interview or question-naire have been performed in the United States, the Soviet Union, and other countries (6, 13, 58). The results of such studies indicate that many youngsters, particularly from white collar families, are perplexed and bewildered by the threat of nuclear war. Some are frankly troubled or frightened. Helplessness and a sense of powerlessness may accompany the realization as well as fear about the future. The current generation of adolescents is thought to view their futures less hopefully and more pessimistically than previous generations. Russian children seem to share the same fears and anxieties as do American children.

Despite the widespread concerns among children and adolescents about nuclear war and their futures, there is no evidence yet that such beliefs lead to psychopathology in later years. Probably the effects will be much more subtle than to create overt psychopathic behavior. What will be the price to society of a generation growing up pessimistic about their futures? Perhaps lack of respect for authority, eroded self-confidence, and feelings of powerlessness and frustration? Will it lead to seeking quick gratifications, political extremes, increased crime, or even psychotic behavior? We don't know yet. It is deplor-able to frighten children in this manner. The evidence is that these fears are not discussed with parents or peers but borne alone. Nevertheless, adults have always frightened children. Tales of dragons, monsters, the Grimm's fairy tales, and even Little Red Ridinghood are all aimed at frightening the little rascals. In fact, one might argue, the prevalence of fear that the nuclear threat engenders among our children is a good sign because it at least indicates the children are aware that a serious problem exists.

Adults appear to take a much more complacent view about the threat of a nuclear war. Understanding that a nuclear war would be an unprecedented disaster seems insufficient to mobilize most adults to actions that would stop the nuclear arms race with its increasing potential for destruction. Much has been written and said regarding the seemingly apathy of most adults to the course that the super powers are accelerating and which activists regard as likely to result in mutual self-destruction. Psychic numbing, denial, and other psychologic dodges have been proposed to account for the apathy (55). Fiske (32) concludes that remaining relatively unworried and inactive, despite the horrific possibili-ties of a nuclear war, is not irrational if people are correct in judging that their activities have no consequences. The tendency of activists to view this general apathy as irrational or even as evidence of mass mental illness may not be warranted, she thinks.

By contrast, other psychologists and sociologist have concluded that psychic numbing and denial dominate most people's reaction to the horrible consequences of a nuclear holocaust (10, 55). Breznitz points out that it is often difficult to distinguish between lack of concern and active denial. Since children worry and adults generally don't, the presence of active denial is suggested. Denial as a psychologic defense in the event of seemingly overwhelming disaster may be life saving. However, denial does have its dangers: it delays treatment and promotes procrastination; it may even lead to fainting, which is the ultimate form of denial. Breznitz (10) postulates several levels of denial:

1. denial of personal relevance;
2. denial of the urgency of the issue;
3. denial of vulnerability;
4. denial of personal responsibility—"nothing I can do about it!"

Further levels of denial include denial of information. Most people are at the fourth level of denial, he believes. Furthermore, nuclear war is easy to deny. It is an abstract, not a concrete, issue; we have no experience of it; there are many urgent, immediate competing things on our minds. People are not motivated by abstract fears but rather by immediate benefits; life insurance is sold not on the fear of the future disaster but that it makes one feel better today. Preventive actions for the future are not motivational.

Psychological Response to a Nuclear Attack

Experience on which to delineate the psychological response to nuclear attack is fortunately limited. The situation in 1945 in Hiroshima and Nagasaki, when the population didn't know what struck them, didn't know that unseen and unfelt radiation was a potential cause of injury or death, may have created a different psychological response than would occur in the aftermath of a major nuclear exchange today inflicted on a public knowledgable about the likely consequences. Nevertheless students have looked at the Hiroshima-Nagasaki experience, and also to reactions to other major sudden disasters—floods, earthquakes, fires, large industrial accidents, and selected portions of previous wars—to understand what human psychological responses may be anticipated.

The single small bombs of 12.5 and 20 kilotons that exploded over Hiroshima and Nagasaki, respectively, would now be regarded as small tactical weapons for battlefield use compared to the megaton-sized bombs now aimed at potentially 18,500 strategic targets. Nevertheless, insights have been gained from the responses of survivors (54). John Hersey has recounted the horror that survivors in Hiroshima witnessed (46). After encountering so much horror, survivors found that they were incapable of emotion. They behaved mechanically and felt emotionally numb. Most survivors focused on one ultimate horror that had left them with profound pity, guilt, or shame: a baby still half-alive on its dead mother's breast, loved ones abandoned in the fire, pathetic requests for help that had to be ignored, piles of dead bodies heaped up in streams, a mother and her fetus still connected by the umbilical cord, both dead.

Those who have had a brush with death are left in a heightened state of emotional turmoil. This effect is short-lived, and soon gives way to the "disaster syndrome." Survivors appear dazed, stunned, and bewildered (82). Their reactions are not the ones associated with panic. By contrast, after a disaster victims are apathetic, docile, indecisive, unemotional, and they behave mechanically. They are still in a state of high autonomic arousal, but appear to be paying for their period of terror by emotional and behavioral exhaustion. The survivors are left in a diminished condition, feeling helpless in the face of massive damage and the impossibility of repairing their shattered world. Following the stage of numbing, psychotic disorders are uncommon. Depression, anxiety about cancer, fears of death, and generalized complaints of fatigue, dizziness, irritability, and difficulty coping are common among survivors and may persist for many throughout the life of the exposed generation (79).

Literature Cited

1. Abrams, H. L. 1984. Medical resources after nuclear war: Availability vs. need. *J. Am. Med. Assoc.* 252:653–58
2. Abrams, H. L., VonKaenel, W. E. 1981. Medical survivors of nuclear war: Infection and the spread of communicable disease. *N. Engl. J. Med.* 305:1226–32
3. Adams, R., Cullen, S., eds. 1981. *The Final Epidemic*. Chicago: Univ. Chicago Press. 254 pp.
4. Arms Control and Disarmament Agency, US Dept. State. 1979. *U.S. Urban Population Vulnerability*, pp. 66–124. Washington DC:US GPO
5. Ash, P. 1980. The influence of radiation on fertility in man. *Br. Med. J.* 53:271–73
6. Beardslee, W. R., Mack, J. E. 1983. Adolescents and the threat of nuclear war: The evolution of the perspective. *Yale J. Biol. Med.* 56:79–91
7. Beecher, H. K. 1943. Resuscitation and sedation of patients with burns which include the airway. *Ann. Surg.* 117:825–33
8. Berger, H. M. 1978. *A Critical Review of Survival and Recovery after a Large-Scale Nuclear Attack*. Marina del Ray, Calif.: R & D Assoc.
9. Blanchard, B. W. 1980. *American Civil Defense 1945–1975: The Evolution of Programs and Policies*, pp. 26–190. Ann Arbor: Univ. Microfilms Int.
10. Breznitz, S. 1986. Hope and denial of stress in the nuclear age. *Proc. Inst. Med., US Nat. Acad. Sci., Symp. on Med. Implications of Nuclear War*. Washington DC: National Acad. Press
11. Brooks, J. W., Evans, E. T., Ham, W. T., Reid, J. D. 1952. The influence of external body radiation on mortality from thermal burns. *Ann. Surgery* 136:535
12. Cent. Defense Information. 1982. President Reagan's civil defense program. *The Defense Monitor* 11(5):1–8
13. Chivian, E., Mack, J. P., Waletsky, J. P. 1986. Soviet children and the threat of nuclear war: A preliminary study. *Am. J. Orthopsychiatry*. In press
14. Churchill, E. D. 1972. *Surgeon to Soldiers: Diary and Records of the Surgical Consultant, Allied Forces Headquarters, WWII*, pp. 12–25. Philadelphia: Lippincott
15. Committee on the Atmospheric Effects of Nuclear Explosions. 1985. *The Effects on the Atmosphere of a Major Nuclear Exchange*. Washington DC: Nat. Acad. Press. 193 pp.
16. Committee for the Compilation of Materials. 1981. *Hiroshima and Nagasaki: The Physical, Medical, and Social Effects of Atomic Bombings*, pp. 73, 152–53. New York: Basic
17. Committee on the Biological Effects of Ionizing Radiation (BEIR III). 1980. *The Effects on Populations of Exposure to*

Low Levels of Ionizing Radiation. pp. 497–98. Washington DC: Nat. Acad. Press

18. Comptroller General. 1983. *Management of the Federal Emergency Management Agency—A System Being Developed.* Washington DC: US Gen. Account. Off. 105 pp.
19. Constable, J. D. 1982. Burn injuries among survivors. In *Last Aid,* ed. E. Chivian et al, pp. 202–10. San Francisco: Freeman
20. Cooper, G. J. 1983. Casualties from terrorist bombings. *J. Trauma* 23:955–67
21. Coppel, D. L. 1976. Blast injuries of the lungs. *Br. J. Surg.* 63:735–37
22. Cripps, D., Horowitz, S., Hong, R. 1974. Selective T cell killing of human lymphocytes by ultraviolet radiation. *Cell. Immunol.* 14:80–86
23. Crutzen, P. J., Birks, J. W. 1982. The atmosphere after a nuclear war: Twilight at noon. *Ambio* 11:115–25
24. Curtis, P. A., Yarbrough, D. R. 1972. Burns. Sabiston D. C., Jr., ed. In *Textbook of Surgery,* ed. D. C. Sabiston, pp. 272–93. Philadelphia: Saunders
25. Daugherty, W., Levi, B., vonHippel, F. 1986. Casualties due to the blast, heat, and radioactive fallout for various hypothetical nuclear attacks on the U.S. See Ref. 10, pp. 7–8
26. Dimick, A. R. 1981. Triage of burn patients. In *Thermal Injuries. Topics in Emergency Medicine,* pp. 17–20. Aspen, Colo.: Aspen Systems Corp.
27. Ehrlich, P. R., Harte, J., Harwell, M. A., Raven, P. H., Sagan, C., Woodwell, G. M., et al. 1983. Long-term biological consequences of nuclear war. *Science* 222:1293–1300
28. Federal Emergency Management Agency (FEMA). 1980. *Short- and Long-term Health Effects of the Surviving Population of a Nuclear War.* US Senate Comm. on Labor and Human Resources, Subcomm. on Health and Sci. Res. Hearings of the 96th Congr. 2nd session. Washington DC: GPO
29. Feinberg, A. 1979. *Civil Preparedness and Post-Attack U.S. Economic Recovery: A State of the Art Assessment and Selected Annotated Bibliography.* Marina del Ray, Calif.: Analytical Assessments Corp.
30. Fetter, S. A., Tsipis, K. 1981. Catastrophic releases of radioactivity. *Sci. Am.* 244:41–47
31. Finch, S. C. 1979. The study of atomic bomb survivors in Japan. *Am. J. Med.* 66:900
32. Fiske, S. T. 1986. Adults' images, feelings, and actions regarding nuclear war: Evidence from surveys and experiments. See Ref. 10
33. Food and Agriculture Organization of the United Nations. 1981. *Agriculture Toward 2000.* Rome: Food and Agriculture Organ.
34. Food and Agriculture Organization of the United Nations. July, 1985. *Food Outlook No. 6.* Rome: FAO
35. Galbraith, J. K. 1981. Economics of the arms race—and after. In *The Final Epidemic,* ed. R. Adams, S. Cullen, pp. 48–57. Chicago: Univ. Chicago Press. 253 pp.
36. Gallup, G. 1984. *The Gallup youth survey,* released October 17, 1984. New York: Associated Press
37. Gerstner, H. B. 1958. Acute radiation syndrome in man. *US Armed Forces Med. J.* 9:313–54
38. Giuffrida, L. 1982. Testimony before the House Committee on Armed Services, Military Installations and Facilities Subcommittee, 97th Congr. 2nd session, March 12, 1982, pp. 927–43
39. Glasstone, S., Dolan, P. J. 1977. *The Effects of Nuclear Weapons,* pp. 80–86, 132–53. Washington, DC: US GPO
40. Gray, C., Payne, R. 1980. Victory is possible. *Foreign Policy* 39:14–19
41. Greene, M., et al. 1979. Impairment of antigen-presenting cell function by ultraviolet radiation. *Proc. Natl. Acad. Sci. USA* 76:6591–95
42. Greer, D. S., Rifkin, L. S. 1986. The immunological impact of nuclear warfare. See Ref. 10, pp. 1–17
43. Haaland, C. M., Horwedel, B. M. 1979. *Instrumentation Requirements for Radiological Defense for Crisis Relocation Planning,* pp. 11–12, 20, 38–39, 60. Oak Ridge, Tenn.: Oak Ridge Nat. Lab.
44. Harwell, M. A. 1984. *Nuclear Winter: The Human and Environmental Consequences of Nuclear War.* New York: Springer-Verlag. 179 pp.
45. Harwell, M. A., Hutchinson, T. C. 1985. *The Environmental Consequences of Nuclear War, Vol. 2: Ecological, Agricultural, and Human Effects.* Chichester, U.K.: Wiley
46. Hersey, J. 1946. *Hiroshima.* New York: Knopf. 116 pp.
47. International Commission on Radiological Protection Recommendations. *ICRP No. 26.* Cited in Ref. 90, p. 47
48. International Committee of Experts in Medical Sciences and Public Health. 1984. *Effects of Nuclear War on Health and Health Services.* Geneva: WHO. 176 pp.
49. Kato, H., Schull, W. J. 1982. Studies of

the mortality of A-bomb survivors. *Rad. Res.* 90:395–432

50. Kennedy, T. L., Johnston, G. W. 1975. Civilian bomb injuries. *Br. Med. J.*, Feb. 15, p. 383

51. Kerr, T. J. 1983. *Civil Defense in the U.S.: Bandaid for a Holocaust?* pp. 1–132. Boulder, Colo.: Westview Press

52. Lapp, R. E. 1962. *Kill and Overkill.* London: Weidenfeld & Nicholson

53. Leaning, J., Keyes, L., eds. 1984. *The Counterfeit Ark: Crisis Relocation for Nuclear War.* Cambridge, Mass.: Ballinger. 337 pp.

54. Lifton, R. J. 1968. *Death in Life: Survivors of Hiroshima.* New York: Random House

55. Lifton, R. J. 1982. Beyond psychic numbing: A call to awareness. *Am. J. Orthopsychiatry* 52:619–29

56. Lindop, P., Rotblat, J., Webber, P. 1985. Radiation casualties in a nuclear war. *Nature* 313:345–46

57. Lushbaugh, C. C. 1974. Human radiation tolerance. In *Space Radiation Biology and Related Topics*, ed. C. A. Tobias, P. Todd, pp. 494–501. New York: Academic

58. Mack, J. E. 1984. Resistance to knowing in the nuclear age. *Harvard Educ. Rev.* 54(3):260–70

59. Marshall, E. 1981. New A-bomb studies alter radiation estimates. *Science* 212:900–3

60. National Council on Radiation Protection and Measurements. 1974. *Radiological Factors Affecting Decision-Making in a Nuclear Attack. NCRP Report* 42:18. Washington DC: NCRP

61. Office of Technology Assessment, Congr. of the US. 1979. *The Effects of Nuclear War.* Washington DC: US GPO. 151 pp.

62. Oftedal, P. 1984. Genetic damage following nuclear war. World Health Organization. *Effects of Nuclear War on Health and Health Services,* pp. 1–32. Geneva: WHO

63. Parrish, J. A. ed. 1983. *The Effect of Ultraviolet Radiation on the Immune System.* Johnson & Johnson Baby Products Co., USA. 213 pp.

64. Pugh, G. E. 1980. *Estimating the Behavioral Degradation of Fallout Protection Factors for Use in Damage Assessment Calculations,* pp. 1–15, A22–A33. Arlington, Va.: Decision-Science Applications, Inc.

65. Report by the Director General to the World Health Assembly. March 15, 1983. *Infant and Young Child Nutrition.* Geneva: Document WHA 36/1983/7

66. Reuler, J. B. 1978. Hypothermia: Pathophysiology, clinical settings, and management. *Ann. Int. Med.* 89:519–27

67. Reutlinger, S., Alderman, H. 1980. Prevalence of calorie deficiency diets in developing countries. *World Bank Staff Working Paper No. 374.*

68. Rodgers, H. W., Robb, J. D. A. 1973. Surgery of civil violence. *Recent Adv. Surg.* 22:321–31

69. Rotblat, J. 1981. *Nuclear Radiation in Warfare,* pp. 73–92. Cambridge, Mass.: Oelgeschlager, Gunn & Hain.

70. Rotblat, J. 1984. Physical effects of nuclear weapons. In *Effects of Nuclear War on Health and Health Services,* pp. 41–64. Geneva: WHO. 176 pp.

71. Rotblat, J. 1986. Acute radiation mortality in a nuclear war. See Ref. 10

72. Royal Society of New Zealand. 1985. *The Threat of Nuclear War: A New Zealand Perspective,* pp. 26–31. Wellington, New Zealand: Royal Soc. New Zealand.

73. Scheer, R. 1982. *With Enough Shovels: Reagan, Bush and Nuclear War.* New York: Random House. 283 pp.

74. Schmidt, L. A. 1981. *A Study of Twenty-four Nationwide Fallout Patterns for Twelve Winds,* pp. 123, 135, 205–6, 213. Arlington, Va.: Inst. for Defense Analyses

75. Schull, W. J., Masanori, O., Neel, J. V. 1981. Genetic effects of the atomic bombs: A reappraisal. *Science* 213:1220–27

76. Scrimshaw, N. S. 1984. Food, nutrition, and nuclear war. *N. Engl. J. Med.* 311:272–76

77. Sivard, R. L. 1983. *World Military and Social Expenditures.* Washington DC: World Priorities, Box 25140. 46 pp.

78. Sullivan, R. J., Heller, W. M., Aldridge, E. C. Jr. 1978. *Candidate U.S. Civil Defense Programs.* Arlington, Va.: System Planning Corp.

79. Thompson, J. 1986. Pathological consequences of disaster: Analogies for nuclear war. See Ref. 10

80. Tsipis, K. 1983. *Arsenal: Understanding Weapons in the Nuclear Age,* pp. 29–44. New York: Simon & Schuster. 342 pp.

81. Turco, R. P., Toon, O. B., Ackerman, T. P., Pollack, J. B., Sagan, C. 1983. Nuclear winter: Global consequences of multiple nuclear explosions. *Science* 222:1283–92

82. Wallace, A. F. 1956. *Tornado in Worcester.* Nat. Acad. Sci. Disaster Study No. 3. Washington DC: Natl. Acad. Press

Ann. Rev. Public Health 1986. 7:441–71

DELAYED HEALTH HAZARDS OF PESTICIDE EXPOSURE

Dan S. Sharp and Brenda Eskenazi

School of Public Health, University of California, Berkeley, California 94720

Robert Harrison

Division of Occupational Medicine, University of California, San Francisco, California 94143

Peter Callas and Allan H. Smith

School of Public Health, University of California, Berkeley, California 94720

INTRODUCTION

Pesticides have profoundly improved the human condition. Their dramatic effects in preventing crop loss and controlling vectors of disease have led to their acceptance and expanded use throughout the world (21). However, the powerful chemicals for killing pests have raised concern that they are agents of environmental pollution and human disease.

The greatest concern involves potential delayed health effects of pesticide exposure, rather than the relatively well understood acute effects. This concern is especially great in developed nations, where the delicate balance between starvation and food production and between mass epidemics and vector control has ceased to be an issue. Indeed, particularly in developed countries, pesticides help to increase life expectancy and thus to manifest the adverse effects of long-term exposure (113).

In this review we focus on the delayed health hazards of pesticide use and present the evidence for pesticides causing various cancers, deleterious reproductive outcomes, and subtle neurologic sequelae.

Epidemiologic evidence provides the focus of the review. In some cases, however, pertinent animal and clinical research is presented to support or

441

0163-7525/86/0510-0441$02.00

contrast with significant epidemiologic conclusions about specific pesticides' hazards. In the concluding section, we suggest future directions and priorities for research for each of the three types of delayed health outcomes: cancer, reproductive, and neurotoxic. In each case further advances in knowledge will be enhanced by changing epidemiologic research methods and focus. Replicating the study designs and focus of the past may merely add to the confusion, rather than generating information for prompt and effective public health action.

CANCER HAZARDS

Many methods and study populations have been used to investigate the relationship between pesticide exposure and cancer. In some studies it is not clear whether pesticides or other agents are related to increased rates of cancer. Studies of farming occupations constitute an indirect, albeit consistent, line of inquiry into the carcinogenicity of pesticides.

A second line of inquiry has been the study of pest control operators and cohorts of workers with known exposure to pesticides. Rarely have these studies been able to address effects of specific pesticides, but appear to implicate some type of pesticide exposure in association with a cancer outcome.

Specific agents of primary concern for cancer are phenoxy herbicides and related compounds, dioxin impurities, arsenicals, and organochlorines such as DDT. These agents have engendered considerable attention in the scientific literature, and have given rise to a large number of studies attempting to assess risk of cancer to specific pesticides.

We first examine implied exposures to pesticides (the farmer studies), then present the studies involving definite but nonspecific pesticide exposure, and, last, review studies of specific agents.

The Farmer Studies

The farmer studies have generally shown an increased level of certain cancers in agricultural occupations. Table 1 briefly summarizes a number of these studies (3, 7, 14, 22, 24–28, 37, 46, 107, 124, 133). Many of these attempted to assess possible modes of exposure by examining relative cancer mortality rates in smaller geographical units, such as counties with higher production of poultry and greater pesticide use. All the listed studies showed elevated relative risks of the listed cancers for farmers or listed agricultural occupation. Greater or newly significant associations were noted upon stratification by production or usage of the products listed in the last column. The relative risks for these studies are generally less than three.

The outcomes for these studies were determined on individuals. However, the measures of exposure and stratification are either indirect indexes of

Table 1 Summary of farmer studies

Ref.	Region	Outcome	Type of Activity
(46)	California	leukemia Hodgkin's lymphoma multiple myeloma	farming farming farming
(107)	Washington	leukemia multiple myeloma	poultry farming
(133)	SE USA	multiple myeloma uterine cervix ovarian cancer	poultry farming farming
(14)	Nebraska	leukemia	corn, insecticide, poultry, cattle, hogs
(3)	Texas	leukemia	farming
(24)	Iowa	leukemia lymphoma multiple myeloma prostatic cancer stomach cancer	farming farming farming farming farming
(26)	Iowa	leukemia	poultry, herbicides
(27)	Wisconsin	lymphosarcoma reticulum cell sarcoma	none noted cattle/dairy, small grains/insecticides, wheat
(25)	Iowa	multiple myeloma non-Hodgkin's lymphoma prostatic cancer stomach cancer	poultry, hogs, insecticides, herbicides poultry, hogs, herbicides, milk production none noted corn, cattle, milk production
(7)	Britain	soft tissue sarcoma	farming
(22)	Illinois	non-Hodgkin's lymphoma prostatic cancer	farming farming
(28)	Wisconsin	multiple myeloma	poultry, insecticides, fertilizers
(37)	N Carolina	melanoma prostatic cancer brain cancer non-Hodgkin's lymphoma leukemia	whites: poultry, cattle, dairying whites: poultry, cattle nonwhites: peanuts, chemical use nonwhites: corn, tobacco, peanuts, chemicals nonwhites: none noted
(124)	New Zealand	lymphoma multiple myeloma both	farming farming orchard (poultry)

exposure (e.g. occupation) or group summaries (e.g. county usage or production of product). Thus, the exposure and stratification measures have characteristics of ecologic measures, and are fraught with problems of validity and precision. Any inferences drawn about causality from these significant associations are tenuous. However, features common among studies lend credibility to inferences that may be pursued with more direct epidemiologic and experimental approaches.

Studies that stratified on age at death (14, 26–28, 46) demonstrated, with only one exception (28), significantly higher rates of leukemia, multiple myeloma, and lymphomas in younger people (usually less than 65 years) and/or in later birth cohorts (usually born after 1900).

Seven studies (14, 25, 26, 28, 107, 124, 133) found significant associations between high levels of exposure to poultry, and leukemias, multiple myeloma, and lymphomas. Five of these seven also demonstrate associations with pesticide use. This consistency across some studies suggests the possibility of interaction between agents. Indirect evidence for relationships between animal and human leukemias and lymphomas mediated by viruses have been studied in cattle, cats, and poultry (124). The evidence is not unequivocally suggestive of a relationship. However, the issue of exposure to multiple agents, such as viruses and chemicals and their interaction, has not yet been adequately studied.

Pesticide User Studies

Pesticide user studies involve cohorts of workers with known exposure to pesticides, but to multiple agents under a variety of conditions. Thus, it is not always clear which agent, or combination, may be responsible for observed associations.

Barthel (10, 11) found that a cohort of 1658 male agricultural workers using pesticides and employed between 1948–1972 in the German Democratic Republic manifested significantly higher rates of lung cancer (SMR=2.0), independently of smoking status. A positive trend was noted between cancer rate and duration of employment, thereby suggesting a dose-effect relationship. It was not possible to disentangle specific pesticides as possible causal agents due to the multitude of agents (e.g. arsenic, asbestos, chlorinated dibenzodioxins, DDT). The likelihood of the cause being arsenicals was assessed by examining lung cancer rates of those workers employed before 1960 and those employed after 1960, when arsenicals were banned. No differences were found.

Riihimaki et al (137, 138) examined a cohort of 1926 Finnish male workers involved with brush control who were exposed to 2,4-D, 2,4,5-T, and other agents between 1951–1971. The follow-up period was from 1972–1980; 16,694 person-years were represented. Only 26 cancer deaths were noted with 36.5 expected. No lymphomas or soft tissue sarcomas were observed.

The authors point out, however, that the small size of the cohort and brief follow-up period limited the utility of this study.

Blair et al (13) demonstrated significantly increased lung cancer mortality rates (SMR = 1.35) in a cohort of 3827 licensed pesticide applicators in Florida. A positive trend was noted between duration of licensure and cancer rate. It was not possible to assess smoking habits among the cohort, and the possibility of confounding accounting for the association cannot be excluded.

Wang & MacMahon (167) demonstrated elevated Standardized Mortality Ratios (SMR) for skin (1.73) and bladder cancer (2.77) in an historical cohort study of 16,126 males employed at least three months between 1967–1976 in one of three nationwide pest control companies. Only the bladder cancer SMR was statistically significant. The lung cancer SMR was 1.15.

One of the few studies focusing on women examined the association between ovarian mesothelial tumors and nonspecific herbicides use (39). Sixty incident cases of this tumor diagnosed between 1974 and 1980 by the National Cancer Institute in Milano, Italy, were matched with 135 other cancer controls on year of diagnosis, age, and residence district. Herbicide exposure potential was assessed by interview. A significant odds ratio of 4.4 suggested an association. Stratification by age demonstrated a marked increase in the odds ratio to 9.1 for women under 55 years.

Phenoxy Herbicides, Chlorophenols, Dioxins, and Amitrole

Phenoxy herbicides were introduced commercially in the 1940s. They later catapulted into public view when linked to various adverse reproductive and cancer sequelae, although whether phenoxy herbicides or their dioxin contaminants are responsible for the apparent association with various human cancers is still controversial.

Hardell (61) in 1977 noted that five patients in a series of seven cases of mesenchymal tumors had extensive exposure to phenoxy herbicides. This paper heralded publication in *The Lancet* of a large number of letters-to-the-editor, an editorial, and a review article over the next five years (12, 29, 31, 34, 41, 57, 62, 64, 66, 72, 77, 84, 108, 112, 119, 141). These reflected the ongoing epidemiologic research and contentions of that period. After 1982 one further letter suggested disproportionate rates of Hodgkin's disease among sawmill and pulp workers exposed to chlorophenols in British Columbia, Canada (52).

These letters and articles delineated three lines of epidemiologic evidence in studying the association among various mesenchymally derived tumors and phenoxy herbicides, chlorophenols, and dioxins. These were the Swedish studies, the industrial cohort studies, and the New Zealand studies.

THE SWEDISH STUDIES   In 1974, Axelson & Sundell (5) examined a cohort of railway workers engaged in brush control. Between 1957–1972 six cases of cancer were detected in 207 workers exposed at least 45 days to herbicides and representing 1747 person-years of observation. While statistically significant increases in rates were noted for those workers exposed to the possible human carcinogenic herbicide, amitrole (81), none was noted for those exposed to any of the phenoxy herbicides. In 1980 Axelson et al (6) updated their study of this cohort. With 348 workers followed up to 1978 for 5541 person-years, a total of 17 tumors were observed, with only 11.8 expected. The excess was noted particularly in workers exposed to both amitrole and phenoxy herbicides. Examination of workers exposed just to phenoxy herbicides, and accounting for a ten-year latency period, revealed a statistically significant increased rate of stomach cancer (2 observed, 0.33 expected).

In 1979 Hardell & Sandstrom (69) published results of a case-control study of 52 cases of soft tissue sarcoma registered from the three northern-most counties in Sweden. A detailed assessment of exposure to specific phenoxy herbicides such as 2,4,5-T, 2,4-D, and MCPA was undertaken by mailed questionnaire and telephone follow-up. Population-based controls were chosen for living cases. Controls from the National Registry for Causes of Death were chosen for dead cases. The odds for exposure in cases was 5.7 times that of controls. In most circumstances exposure was to multiple agents. Exposure to phenoxy herbicides and chlorophenols was 5.3 and 6.6 times more likely to be reported in cases than in controls, respectively. An odds ratio of 9.9 was noted when the analysis was limited to the 21 living cases and their controls. The odds ratio was 3.8 for the 31 dead cases. This study was followed by a series of four additional ones (45, 63, 67, 68).

Exposure to phenoxy herbicides and chlorophenols in 110 cases of soft tissue sarcoma and in 220 controls from five southern Swedish counties (45) was assessed in order to confirm the findings in northern Sweden. The overall odds ratio for exposure to phenoxy herbicides was 6.8. When stratified on exposure just to 2,4-D and MCPA, the odds ratio remained significant at 4.2. It was claimed that these agents were not contaminated by 2,3,7,8-TCDD, a potent carcinogen in animals, as was 2,4,5-T, thus suggesting evidence for the carcinogenicity of phenoxy herbicides in their own right. However, Hay (72) claimed that such an inference could not be unequivocally justified, since 2,4-D was often contaminated with dichloro and trichloro dioxins. When occupation was used as an index of exposure the relative odds of exposure dropped to an insignificant 1.4. This observation seemed to underscore the importance of better methods of assessing personal exposure to agents of concern; although it also raised the issue of recall bias in falsely elevating odds ratios when exposure is assessed from interview data.

Hardell et al (67) extended their studies to include malignant lymphomas, demonstrating in 169 cases with 338 controls an overall relative odds of exposure of 5.3. When exposure just to phenoxy herbicides was examined, the odds ratio remained significant at 4.8, and a dose-effect relationship was suggested for exposure to chlorophenols by using duration of exposure as the surrogate measure for dose. The issue of 2,3,7,8-TCDD contamination could not be assessed. Hardell & Bengtsson (65) reanalyzed these data in order to assess possible confounding effects by SES and concurrent disease/health conditions but were unable to demonstrate any such confounding.

Hardell (63) next examined the relationship between colon cancer and herbicide exposure. The study was motivated by criticisms that use of general population controls would result in recall bias. Cancer cases would be expected to recall differentially past chemical agent exposure in such a way as to falsely elevate the odds ratio. Hardell (63) expected to find no significant measure of association using colon cancer cases and population controls. Odds ratios of 1.3 and 1.8 for exposure to phenoxy herbicides and chlorophenols, respectively, were not statistically significant, confirming his expectation. Hoar et al (76) have demonstrated similar findings in failing to find a significant association between herbicide use and colon cancer in Kansas farmers between 1976–1982. Using colon cancer as a control, Hardell (63) reanalyzed the previous studies of soft tissue sarcoma in northern Sweden (69) and malignant lymphoma (67), and reported significant overall relative odds of exposure of 5.5 and 4.5, respectively.

Finally, Hardell et al (68) examined the role of herbicide exposure in nasal-pharyngeal cancer. Seventy-one cases, and 541 controls derived from previous studies (67, 69), demonstrated a statistically insignificant odds ratio of 2.1 for phenoxy herbicide exposure, but a significant 6.5 for chlorophenol exposure. There was some suggestion of an interaction between chlorophenol exposure and woodworking occupations, but poor statistical power limited such inferences.

THE INDUSTRIAL COHORT STUDIES   Three US studies (32, 122, 178) of workers exposed to a variety of dioxins and phenoxy herbicides in manufacturing facilities were published in 1980. Two of the studies (32, 178) examined cohorts of workers involved in acute accidental exposures.

Cook et al (32) examined 61 males between 1964–1978 who were accidentally exposed to 2,3,7,8-TCDD in 1964. Forty-nine of these men developed chloracne as a result of this accident, thus indicating significant exposure. Three cancers developed during this period (one a fibrosarcoma), with 1.6 expected ($p=0.13$). Orris (120) raised several criticisms of this study, the most cogent being that an insufficient latency period had transpired to detect any real carcinogenic effect from this accidental exposure.

Zack & Suskind (178) reported cancer outcomes of a cohort of 121 males accidentally exposed to 2,3,7,8-TCDD in 1949. Development of chloracne was a criterion for inclusion into the study. Between 1949–1978 100% follow-up revealed 9 cancer deaths, with 9.04 expected. However, three of these were lymphatic or hematopoietic in origin (0.88 expected, $p=0.047$), and one was a primary dermal fibrous histiocytoma (0.15 expected). Although the cohort size was small, the degree of exposure was significant, as indicated by development of chloracne.

Ott et al (122) examined a cohort of 204 workers involved in manufacture of 2,4,5-T for at least one month between 1950–1971. Only one lung cancer death was noted, in a worker who happened to be a smoker.

In 1983 Zack & Gaffey (177) reported the mortality status of 884 white male employees of the Nitro, West Virginia, Monsanto plant who had been employed at least one year between 1955–1977. The nine cases of bladder cancer were significantly in excess of expected (0.91). However, the plant had used a bladder carcinogen, para-aminobiphenyl, between 1941–1952 in rubber processing. One case of generalized liposarcoma was reported.

Honchar & Halperin (77) suggested that although each of these US manufacturer studies failed to report an excess risk for soft tissue sarcoma, in combination the three reported soft tissue sarcoma cases might be significant. Four additional cases were subsequently identified (31, 84, 112).

In 1984 Fingerhut et al (49) reviewed the seven cases, examining the pathologic evidence directly for the correct diagnosis of soft tissue sarcoma by using two reviewers. Two of the seven cases were independently reported by both reviewers as carcinomas.

Although Fingerhut's reassessment (49) moderates the degree of association suggested by the four cohort studies (32, 122, 177, 178) and their addendums (31, 84, 112), the five confirmed cases still represent an excess number. However, three of these five cases did not directly work in manufacturing, and the extent of their exposure to 2,3,7,8-TCDD is in doubt.

Thiess et al (157) examined mortality outcomes in a cohort of 74 workers in the Federal Republic of Germany who were accidentally exposed to dioxins in 1953, 66 of whom developed chloracne. Mortality status was determined for 100% of the cohort up to 1979, representing 1698 person-years of observation. Several internal and external control populations were used. The most significant finding was an excess of stomach cancer in the exposed cohort (3 observed, 0.7 expected). No lymphatic, hematopoietic, or soft tissue sarcomas were noted.

The recent Danish study by Lynge (98), however, demonstrated 5 soft tissue sarcoma cases (1.84 expected) in a cohort of 3390 males (49,879 person-years of observation) involved in the manufacture of phenoxy herbicides prior to 1982. The primary herbicides manufactured were 2,4-D and MCPA, and the likelihood of dioxin contamination was thought to be minimal. No excess of malignant lymphoma was noted. The study differs significantly from the other industrial cohort studies reported so far by virtue of the large cohort size.

A number of studies attempted to assess various clinical and laboratory indices of workers exposed primarily to dioxins (16, 100, 123, 154). These studies were often plagued by poor participation rates (16, 154). The nonspecific nature of various measures of liver function, lipid metabolism, and peripheral nerve function limit the inferences one can draw about risk of disease, especially of cancer.

THE NEW ZEALAND STUDIES   To test the association between herbicide exposure and soft tissue sarcoma Smith et al (148) initiated a case-control study comprising 102 male soft tissue sarcoma cases registered nationally between 1976–1980. They randomly selected 306 controls from cases of other cancers, matched on age and registration year. Using occupation as the indicator of exposure, an odds ratio of 1.03 was noted for those designated as general agricultural and forestry workers. Examination of only farmers raised the odds ratio to 1.45, but this was not statistically significant. A more thorough assessment of exposure by telephone interview of 80 of these cases and 92 controls failed to reveal any odds ratio greater than 1.6 for various categories of exposure to phenoxy herbicides (146, 150). None of these were statistically significant.

A second case-control study of non–Hodgkin's lymphoma also failed to reveal an association with phenoxy herbicides (odds ratio = 1.4) or with chlorophenols (odds ratio = 1.3) (125). Cases were more likely to have done fencing work or been employed in meat processing, but no conclusions could be reached about possible causative agents.

The design of the New Zealand studies is comparable to that of Swedish case-control studies. Tumor registry data identified incident cases. Both occupational and personal exposure data were determined by questionnaire and/or telephone interview. The New Zealand soft tissue sarcoma study's use of other cancer patients as controls contrasts with the Swedish use of general population controls. However, the New Zealand non–Hodgkins lymphoma study utilized both cancer and general population controls, and the two control groups gave comparable results. The lack of concordance between the Swedish and New Zealand studies therefore requires some explanation.

One possible explanation is that the 2,4,5-T herbicides used in New Zealand might have been less contaminated with dioxins. Unfortunately, the exact levels of contamination in New Zealand phenoxy herbicides during early use are not available. However, evidence from the southern counties Swedish study (45) detracts from this explanation, since significant relative risks of exposure were noted from use of phenoxy herbicides free from 2,3,7,8-TCDD contamination.

VIETNAM VETERAN STUDIES   Studies of Vietnam veterans exposed to Agent Orange have been limited in their assessment of cancer outcomes. A study of mortality patterns involving 4558 Vietnam era veterans in New York State suggested no excess of deaths from death certificate diagnoses of soft tissue sarcoma and lymphomas (92). However, a study of veterans in The Commonwealth of Massachusetts did demonstrate significantly greater numbers of veterans with death certificate diagnoses of soft tissue sarcoma and kidney cancer (2). A longer period of follow-up for this cohort and other Vietnam Veteran studies are needed to encompass a reasonable latency period.

CONCLUSIONS   Neither phenoxy herbicides nor dioxins can be unequivocally stated to cause cancer in humans. However, animal data refute claims that they are harmless. For example, an extensive investigation of over 20,000 ewes at slaughter demonstrated significant increases in the prevalence of small intestinal adenocarcinoma in sheep exposed to phenoxy and picolinic herbicides (116). Tumor rates appeared to be independent of exposure to 2,3,7,8-TCDD-contaminated phenoxy herbicides. More importantly, the experimental animal data are consistent enough that the International Agency for Research on Cancer has concluded that 2,3,7,8-TCDD is a potent rodent carcinogen (81).

The Swedish case-control studies provide the strongest evidence for causality in humans. However, the industrial cohort studies are inconsistent in suggesting such associations, and the New Zealand study demonstrates no association. Inconsistent findings such as these are unlikely in the presence of true causal associations. The possibility of different levels of dioxin contamination of phenoxy herbicides in these populations has already been raised. Similarly, the possibility of interaction of more than one exposure or characteristic should not be overlooked. Swedish populations might be exposed to two necessary agents (one being phenoxy herbicides or dioxin contaminants) that cause cancer; industrial cohorts and New Zealand populations might not be exposed to the second factor.

Arsenical Pesticides

The carcinogenic potential of arsenic, having been suspected for almost a century (127), is well established (80). Arsenical pesticides are rarely used for this reason. A number of the nonspecific exposure studies (10, 11, 13) have suggested a role for arsenicals in demonstrating increased rates of lung cancer in occupations using pesticides. A possible role of arsenic in association with human lymphatic and hematopoietic cancers has also been suggested (4, 121, 125).

Ott et al (121) demonstrated a significant increase in respiratory cancers in 173 decedents with occupational exposure to arsenical insecticides. Using proportional mortality analysis, they demonstrated that 16.2% of deaths in the arsenical-exposed group were due to respiratory system cancer, as compared to 5.7% in controls. The study also demonstrated a dose-effect relationship where dose was assessed by a determination of time-weighted average concentration-months.

Mabuchi et al (99) attempted to assess the role of arsenical pesticide exposure in a manufacturing plant cohort of 1393 workers employed between 1946–1977. They were able to determine the status of 82% of the cohort. When limited to just the 1050 males (87% follow-up, 19,248 person-years of observation), 23 deaths from lung cancer were noted (13.7 expected regionally, 8.7 nationally). A dose-effect relationship was noted in workers exposed to high levels of arsenicals, using duration of exposure as the measure of dose. Accounting for 15+ years latency increased the SMR to 16.7. Unfortunately, the investigators were unable to account for possible confounding effects from smoking. Nevertheless, they felt the evidence was strong enough to infer causality.

In contrast to the strong epidemiologic evidence for arsenic's role as a respiratory carcinogen, animal data demonstrate no causal role for arsenic in the genesis of cancer, and in some cases even an antagonistic effect (51, 117). Nordberg & Andersen (117) have suggested that environmental exposure to arsenic is always coupled with exposure to other metals, sulfur dioxide, or organic carcinogens. Some epidemiologic studies have also suggested that arsenic acts more as a promoter of lung cancer than as an initiator (19, 43). An interactive effect with smoking was noted in a study by Pershagen et al (129), thus supporting arsenic's role as a promoter (128).

Organochlorine Pesticides

The organochlorine pesticides include products such as DDT, chlordane, heptachlor, aldrin, and dieldrin. The IARC (81) has listed some of these agents (e.g. DDT) as "probably carcinogenic to humans," although it also categorizes them as being inadequately assessed for human carcinogenic potential. Their carcinogenicity has been demonstrated in animal studies, but insufficient data has accrued from human studies. In particular, DDT has demonstrated significant liver, lymphatic, and lung neoplastic activity in rodents, while dieldrin is more equivocal in suggesting such activity (81).

A number of studies assessed the level of agents such as DDT and dieldrin in adipose tissue and blood in cancer patients. These studies extend back into the 1960s, and are reviewed in the *IARC Monograph* literature (79, 81, 82). The results of such studies have not been conclusive in assessing causality.

A report by Infante et al (78) is representative of a number of case reports implicating organochlorines as possible causal agents for a variety of blood dyscrasias. They presented six cases with various disorders and history of chlordane exposure, as well as summarized 25 similar cases reported in the literature since 1955. One cannot assess the reliability of these associations in case reports without comparative population data.

In response to these reports, Wang & Grufferman (166) conducted a case-control study of aplastic anemia mortality in North Carolina males for the period 1968–1977. Using stated occupation on the death certificate, they were unable to show an association between the disease and any occupation involved with pesticide use. Failure to detect an association does not necessarily eliminate the likelihood of one because of inaccuracies introduced in using occupation recorded at time of death as an exposure index.

The Swedish case-control studies of soft tissue sarcoma, lymphomas, and colon cancer assessed DDT exposure and failed to demonstrate any association (45, 63, 67, 69). Some studies have shown associations between organochlorine pesticide exposure and development of hypertension, cerebrovascular disease, and arteriosclerotic cardiovascular disease, but not for any cancer (109, 168, 174). Ditraglia et al (38) reexamined two cohorts previously studied by Wang & MacMahon (168), adding two more industrial plants involved in organochlorine pesticide production. With 2141 workers (171 lost to follow-up, 46,566 person-years of observation) there was no suggestion of increased death rates from 12 categories of cancer.

Human evidence for organochlorine carcinogenic potential is not strong. However, limitations in these studies as well as consistent animal data suggest that these agents could be human carcinogens. Their persistence in the environment, and continued use in third world countries in the case of DDT, mandate further study.

REPRODUCTIVE HAZARDS

Dibromochloropropane (DBCP), 2,4,5-T, and DDT were all used for many years before they were suspected of having reproductive toxicity. However, only in the case of DBCP, which had profound effects on male fertility, were these suspicions confirmed. Why then, was it so difficult to confirm or refute our suspicions about DDT and the phenoxy herbicides?

1. Their effects might not be as profound as those for DBCP.
2. Many of the studies lacked adequate statistical power to examine outcomes such as individual congenital malformations. For some populations, such as in Seveso, Italy, and Vietnam, baseline information on reproductive outcomes was unknown.
3. Accurate exposure data were lacking, particularly for the studies on Agent Orange and the ecologic studies in which not only the levels of exposure, but also who was exposed, were unknown.

We are left with unconfirmed suspicions based on inconsistent data that exposure to phenoxy herbicides, particularly Agent Orange, may be associated with congenital malformations such as neural tube defects and facial clefts, with molar pregnancies, and with spontaneous abortions. Similarly, an association between exposure to organochlorine pesticides (particularly DDT) and spontaneous abortion and premature delivery are only suspect at this time.

Dibromochloropropane (DBCP)

The human reproductive toxicity of DBCP is more apparent than for DDT or the phenoxy herbicides. Interest in the reproductive effects of DBCP was sparked when wives of DBCP production workers in a northern California chemical plant complained about an inability to become pregnant. Studies by Whorton and co-workers (106, 170, 171) showed that almost half of the workers had lower than normal sperm counts compared to less than 10% in nonexposed workers. Testicular biopsy studies revealed hyalized seminiferous tubules with no spermatogenic activity in the workers with azoospermia (90, 132, 171).

Although changes in sperm count were noted, changes in sperm morphology were not related to DBCP exposure (54, 86). The degree and length of exposure was directly related to sperm count. Pesticide applicators or farm workers exposed to DBCP had some reduction in semen quality but to a lesser extent than production workers and formulators (54, 140). Production workers with abnormal counts had worked longer than three years. One year after exposure ended, six of nine oligospermic men became normospermic, two of nine showed improvement but remained oligospermic, and none of the 12 azoospermic men showed any improvement (106). In other studies approximately a third of azoospermic men improved after four years without exposure (56, 130).

Some studies have not found dose-related reductions in sperm counts following DBCP exposure. However, workers were examined one year after exposure (97), or were exposed for less than three years (90).

Serum levels of follicle-stimulating hormone tended to be increased in exposed workers (42, 97, 131, 132). Elevated levels of luteinizing hormones have been found in some studies (42, 170), but not in others (131, 132). In most studies (131, 132, 140) testosterone levels are unaltered by DBCP exposure, although one study found depressed levels in exposed workers (90).

Two studies have observed a preponderance of female offspring in DBCP-exposed workers (56)—a finding suggestive of increased rates of Y-chromosome non-dysjunction. Kharrazi et al (87) found an increase in the rate of spontaneous abortions in the wives of pesticide applicators after their husbands' exposure (20%) compared to before (7%). However, their baseline rate was rather low, suggesting under reporting.

No studies have examined the offspring of women who have been exposed.

Phenoxy Herbicides and Their Contaminants

Studies investigating human reproductive effects focus on five major populations:

1. Vietnam veterans exposed to Agent Orange (a mixture of 2,4-D and 2,4,5-T contaminated with TCDD);
2. Vietnamese civilians exposed to Agent Orange;
3. men exposed to phenoxy herbicides in production or in application;
4. residents in Seveso, Italy, accidentally exposed to TCDD;
5. residents living near areas sprayed with phenoxy herbicides.

VIETNAM VETERANS   There has been enormous public concern about the exposure of Vietnam Veterans to Agent Orange and its possible effects on their offspring. Nevertheless, studies of veterans done in the United States, Australia, and Vietnam have been largely inconclusive. In a case-control study of infants born between 1968–1980, the Centers for Disease Control found no difference in the proportion of fathers who served in Vietnam and those who did not (9% in both groups) (44). However, rates of spina bifida, facial cleft, and neuroblastoma increased with the father's estimated dose of Agent Orange. The Australian study (165) of infants born between 1966–1979 found that only 1.5% of the fathers in each group served in Vietnam, and that Australian soldiers were exposed to much smaller quantities of Agent Orange than American soldiers (30).

The United States Air Force is following a cohort of over 1000 men (Ranch Hands) who flew aircraft that sprayed Agent Orange. The initial studies showed no differences between the Ranch Hands and other unexposed veterans in semen quality and number of children fathered (91). Based on the veteran's report the study found a significant increase in miscarriage rate in one exposed group (officers), a higher overall rate of birth defects compared to unexposed controls (in part due to a cluster of skin anomalies), and a larger number of neonatal deaths in postexposure years compared to pre-exposure years.

Hatch (71) reviewed a few of the unpublished studies examining the offspring of Vietnamese veterans. Two studies found a slightly increased risk for birth defects, particularly of the neural tube and facial clefts, in offspring of fathers who served in South Vietnam, where most of the exposure to Agent Orange had occurred. Another study found that wives of veterans who served in South Vietnam had twice the number of miscarriages (16% versus 8.5%).

VIETNAMESE CIVILIANS   Investigations of civilian populations in Vietnam suffer from both poor exposure estimates and inaccurate birth records (71). Two studies of Vietnamese civilians found congenital malformations of the neural tube and the palate with potential herbicide exposure. Meselson and co-workers (103) examined the records of children who received surgery at Saigon Children's Hospital, the major hospital for surgical correction of congenital malformations in South Vietnam, and noted a major change in the relative frequency of spina bifida and pure cleft palate in the two years of heavy spraying (1967 and 1968). Kunstadter, at the National Academy of Sciences (89), observed similar peaks in rates of cleft lip in 1963, 1966, 1969 (the highest), with a subsequent decline. However, Kunstadter (89), with access to dates, times, and location of spraying, found no link between maternal residence (within five miles of spraying) and overall risk for birth defects or risk for a specific birth defect.

A number of studies investigated the association between molar pregnancy and herbicide exposure. The initial studies (35) found no increase in molar pregnancy and stillbirths in the years of heavy spraying (1966–1969) compared to the years of light spraying. However, most of the pregnancies occurred in Saigon and were relatively unexposed. When these pregnancies were eliminated from the analysis (103), almost twice the rate of molar pregnancies was noted in the heavy spraying years, and the highest rate of stillbirths was in the province of Tay Ninh (68 per 1000)—an area heavily exposed.

Hatch (71) cites an investigation in Vietnam—matched for maternal age, parity, and social conditions—that observed a ten-fold excess in herbicide exposure in women hospitalized for molar pregnancy compared to women with normal deliveries. Because the incidence of molar pregnancies increased about 10 years after heavy spraying in South, but not in North Vietnam, Hatch (71) suggested that the effect might be maternally mediated.

OCCUPATIONAL EXPOSURE   In general, women whose husbands have worked with chlorophenols have not had a higher rate of infants with congenital malformations, spontaneous abortions, stillbirths, or infant deaths (161). Even men with relatively high levels of TCDD exposure, as evidenced by chloracne, demonstrated no increase in fathering infants with congenital malformations or in their wives' having pregnancies that ended in spontaneous abortion (100, 111, 154). However, these studies are limited by small numbers and by recall of pregnancies up to 30 years previously.

Smith et al (149) compared reported reproductive histories of pesticide applicators (mostly 2,4,5-T) in New Zealand to those of agricultural contractors. Since wives often help their husbands in the field, they may have also been exposed. Smith et al found no significant differences in congenital malformations, stillbirths, miscarriages, and overall fertility rates. In addition, analysis specifically for 2,4,5-T use did not identify any reproductive hazard (147).

Only one study yielded a positive association between men exposed to pesticides, but not specifically to phenoxy herbicides (8). The study compared the rates of spina bifida, anencephaly, and facial clefts for offspring of fathers whose job title suggested exposure to agricultural chemicals (e.g. farmers, gardeners) with rates in offspring of fathers with all other occupations. Defect rates were consistently higher (no significance levels given) for a variety of agricultural occupations, including gardeners and agricultural workers. However, a case-control study by Golding & Sladden (55) of infants born with anencephaly, spina bifida, and facial clefts was unable to confirm these findings.

THE SEVESO ACCIDENT   The release of TCDD from a plant producing trichlorophenol occurred in July 1976 in Seveso, Italy. More than two weeks elapsed before the health authorities responded by relocating children and pregnant women. A number of Italian investigators claimed that the rates of spontaneous abortion increased following the accident (20, 160), and that these rates did not completely drop until after 1978. However, no differences were observed when rates were compared across high, moderate, and low contamination areas (136). There were also claims that rates of congenital malformation had increased in the contaminated areas. Bruzzi et al (20) reported an excess between 1977–1980 in the overall rates of multiple malformations in the contaminated areas compared to the less contaminated areas, and an excess in hypospadias, hemangiomas, and neural tube defects (mostly spina bifida) compared to other Italian registries.

The true effects of the Seveso accident could not be determined for a number of reasons:

1. No baseline rates existed.
2. Numbers were too small.
3. Exact numbers of induced abortions were unknown.
4. Cases of chloracne ($n=53$) existed outside the "exposure zones," and thus the exposed population could not be readily defined.
5. Political turmoil surrounding the management of health services prevented the immediate collection of data.

ECOLOGIC STUDIES   Ecologic studies pose many problems for the epidemiologist. Although this type of study is relatively inexpensive and simple to implement, interpretation may be difficult, since little is known about individual exposure. Field & Kerr (48) compared the annual combined rate of anencephaly and meningomyelocele in New South Wales with the previous year's use of 2,4,5-T in all of Australia. A linear correlation was found. Highest rates were for conceptions in the summer, supposedly the season of maximal spraying. A study of a different area of Australia (18) demonstrated an increase in facial clefts for infants conceived in spring and summer months; the authors suggested that these were related to pesticide use. No levels of statistical significance were provided in the above studies.

In contrast, an investigation by Hanify et al (59) in New Zealand evaluated the relationship between malformations (confirmed by hospital records) and aerial spraying (monthly density). Rates of heart malformations, hypospadias, and talipes were elevated in the years of spraying (1972–1976) compared to years prior to use of 2,4,5-T. When more precise estimates of exposure (reflecting year, area of exposure, and fractional removal rate) were used, only talipes remained significantly correlated with exposure.

Other studies have reported equivocal or negative relationships between estimates of 2,4,5-T exposure and birth defects. No relationship was observed between previous year's usage of 2,4,5-T in Hungary and cystic kidney, facial clefts, anencephaly, spina bifida, and still births (158). Nelson et al (115) subdivided 75 Arkansas counties into high ($n=15$), medium ($n=9$), and low ($n=51$) exposure groups based on their rice acreage. Higher rates of facial clefts were found in the low- and high-exposure counties than in the medium.

Perhaps the ecologic study that stirred the most controversy was the "Alsea" study (162). Women from Oregon coastal areas had complained about miscarriages, which they thought might be due to the spraying of 2,4,5-T in nearby forests. The EPA responded with an ecologic study examining the spontaneous abortion rate of women of that area who were hospitalized between 1972–1977. An increased rate in the study population compared to two control areas, one rural the other urban, was noted. The study area rates peaked during June. The EPA noted that poundage of 2,4,5-T used correlated with rates of spontaneous abortion when a lag time of two to three months was imposed. This study has been criticized for a number of reasons:

1. Only a small part of the study area was sprayed.
2. The rates of spontaneous abortion were within the expected rates.
3. No potential confounders were assessed.
4. Differences in medical care between rural and urban areas confused comparisons.
5. The area of study was a vacation area with an influx of people during the summer, thus affecting estimates of both the case population and the target population.

Organochlorine Pesticides

Organochlorine pesticides such as DDT pass through the placenta, with an average level in the newborn blood reaching around a third of that in maternal blood (1, 135). These pesticides are stored in human fat, and levels are higher in breast milk than in maternal blood (144, 173). Although DDT is no longer in use in most parts of the world, its residues are persistent (1). However, information is scarce on human reproductive effects of DDT and organochlorine pesticides in general.

Limited evidence suggests that DDT body burden is related to premature delivery or spontaneous abortion. Procianoy & Schvartsman (134) reported

DDT levels significantly higher in the cord blood of preterm infants ($M=33$ wk) than of term infants in Brazil. In an Indian study (142) comparing cases of premature abortion or delivery (10–32 wk) and term deliveries, DDT levels were five times higher in placental tissue of cases. The highest DDT levels were seen in the most premature deliveries.

Although DDT levels have been shown to be elevated in the cord blood of infants delivered prematurely or in fetuses spontaneously aborted, the DDT levels in their mothers are not consistently elevated. DDT levels were not found to be higher in blood of women who had spontaneous abortions than in those who had normal pregnancies (118). Procianoy & Schvartsman (134) found that mothers of preterm ($M=33$ wk) and term infants had comparable DDT levels. However, Saxena et al (142) found that women having spontaneous abortions and mothers of premature infants had 10 times the DDT levels of mothers with term infants.

A number of theories attempt to explain the elevated DDT levels seen in the preterm infants or aborted fetuses. Saxena et al (143) proposed that organo-chlorine pesticides are known to have weak estrogenic effects, and may precipitate labor. Procianoy & Schvartsman (134) suggested that preterm infants may have an increased placental permeability to DDT; or, more DDT is found in the blood because preterm infants have less adipose tissue. They suggested that the latter hypothesis is supported by the significant negative correlation of birth weight and DDT levels. However, in a larger study (36) of women and their newborns ($n=350$), where only 3% of the infants were preterm [compared to 44% in Procianoy & Schvartsman's study (134)], birth weight did not correlate significantly with DDT levels.

Conclusions

Apart from male infertility due to DBCP, the most impressive result of the findings for human reproductive effects from exposure to pesticides is their inconsistency. This inconsistency is particularly apparent in the wide range and large numbers of studies of phenoxy herbicides. The inconsistency stems from one of two causes: either the effects are weak at exposure levels experienced by humans, and therefore difficult to detect epidemiologically; or there are no effects, and the apparent findings result from multiple comparisons—each study looking at a variety of outcomes, some of which are by chance statistically significant.

NEUROTOXIC HAZARDS

The nervous system has been recognized as a target organ for pesticide toxicity for several decades. Indeed, the desired pesticidal action of the organophosphates (OPs) is caused by the inhibition of acetylcholine esterase and the subsequent accumulation of the neurotransmitter, acetylcholine. The initial use of organophosphates in chemical warfare led to a large literature describing the biochemical mechanisms of action and the clinical observations of excess cholinergic activity in humans (114). The suggestion that chronic neurobehavioral sequelae may result from acute organophosphate intoxication or chronic lower level exposure is important in light of the continued risk of OP poisoning to the estimated 2.5 million seasonal and migrant farm workers and 340,000 pesticide production workers in the United States.

The emphasis in this review is on organophosphates. However, organophosphates are not the only pesticides with neurotoxic effects. Organochlorines were widely used until organophosphates were substituted for them in the 1960s and 1970s.

The chlorinated hydrocarbon insecticide, chlordecone, was responsible for over 75 cases of neurologic disease among workers at the Life Sciences Products Company in Hopewell, Virginia in 1975 (156). Tremor and opsoclonus were the most frequent abnormalities, with signs and symptoms gradually diminishing over 18 months. However, several workers continued to manifest a mildly incapacitating tremor after four years. Chlordecone appears to be unique in that chronic sequelae have not been reported following acute intoxication with other chlorinated hydrocarbon insecticides.

Peripheral neuropathy has been reported following occupational exposure to the phenoxy herbicides, 2,4,5-T and 2,4-D (111, 123, 145). Neurologic toxicity has also been noted from acute exposure to pesticides containing arsenic, the fumigant methyl bromide, and rodenticides containing thallium (9, 74, 75, 93). Scattered reports of prolonged sensory or motor neuropathy have been recorded (156). However, the main concern about neurotoxic effects of pesticides involves organophosphates.

Organophosphates

Acute OP poisoning can generally be measured with in vitro measurement of red blood cell or plasma cholinesterase, although central nervous system symptoms may be absent with mild depression of cholinesterase values (73). Continued case reports of acute poisoning among farm workers exposed to residual crop levels have emphasized the need for baseline cholinesterase measurement, continuing surveillance, and further coordination of emergency treatment by local health care professionals (105). In California alone, over 1200 cases of suspected pesticide poisoning are reported yearly, the majority due to organophosphates.

In addition to the neurologic signs and symptoms of acute intoxication, organophosphate pesticides may cause two delayed or chronic effects from acute high dose or chronic low dose exposure: (*a*) delayed polyneuropathy, consisting of a symmetrical distal axonal degeneration, and (*b*) neurobehavioral effects.

ORGANOPHOSPHATE POLYNEUROPATHY   Most reported cases of organophosphate neuropathy have been caused by tri-ortho-cresyl-phosphate (TOCP), which has been responsible for thousands of paralytic cases due to contaminated alcohol [Ginger Jake paralysis (110)] and cooking oil. The pesticides mipafox, trichlorphon, tamaron, trichlornate, and leptophos have also been reported to cause such a neuropathy. Acute exposure is followed within 8 to 18 days by progressive lower extremity weakness and subsequent hand weakness associated with varying degrees of sensory loss. Recovery is generally poor.

The mechanism of this toxic effect is due to the inhibition of neurotoxic esterase (NTE), although recently Seifert & Casida (143a,b) have clearly demonstrated a second target of action. These agents act to enhance brain cytoplasmic microtubule protease activity and thus alter levels of high molecular weight proteins associated with cytoplasmic microtubule stability and assembly. It is unclear, however, whether these actions are an effect rather than a cause of neurotoxicity (143a).

Elegant assays have been developed for neurotoxic esterase activity utilizing the hen, where inhibition of approximately 75% or greater of whole hen brain NTE one day after dosing is used as an indicator of neurotoxic potential. Good correlation has been found between inhibition of brain NTE and functional ataxia 10 to 14 days later. Johnson has reviewed this subject extensively (85).

ORGANOPHOSPHATE NEUROBEHAVIORAL EFFECTS   The acute effects of organophosphate intoxication result from the nicotinic, muscarinic, and central nervous system manifestations of cholinergic excess. Individuals may have difficulty concentrating, and may be confused and drowsy. Symptoms begin within 24 hours after exposure, and, if severe anoxia has not occurred, complete symptomatic recovery usually occurs within ten days. However, follow-up of survivors of acute pesticide poisoning suggests that a few individuals may continue to experience persistent neurobehavioral symptoms.

The effect of a single dose of an organophosphate anticholinesterase was assessed by Bowers et al (17) in normal volunteers by using serial administrations of a behavioral checklist. Impaired concentration and increased distraction were noted at whole blood cholinesterase levels of less than 40%. Tabershaw & Cooper (155) examined 117 individuals three years after systemic poisoning by organophosphates. Continued visual disturbances, gastrointestinal symptoms, headaches, and nervousness were the most common complaints. No control group was examined, however. Harmon et al (70) assessed six patients 9 to 48 months after organophosphate poisoning but did not administer a standard questionnaire to elicit symptoms. The neurologic examination was normal.

Chronic exposure to organophosphates has been anecdotally reported to cause impairment in concentration in agricultural and scientific workers as well as agricultural pilots (53, 102, 126, 151). Metcalf & Holmes (104) interviewed 56 men with organophosphate exposure and reported disturbed memory and difficulty in maintaining alertness and appropriate focusing of attention. Work history, cholinesterase levels, and severity and duration of exposure were unknown. Whorton & Obrinsky (172) noted persistent complaints of blurred vision in 12 of 19 farm field workers examined four months after organophosphate poisoning.

Rodnitzky & Levin (139) were the first to assess a variety of neurobehavioral functions in subjects occupationally exposed to organophosphates. Twenty-three farmers and pesticide applicators exposed to organophosphates, matched for age and education with a control group of farmers, were given a battery of neuropsychiatric tests. Plasma cholinesterase was slightly depressed among the pesticide applicators. All workers were asymptomatic. No visuomotor or memory abnormalities were found, although pesticide control applicators scored significantly higher on the Taylor Manifest Anxiety Scale (94).

As it was known that organophosphates in large doses induce prominent electroencephalographic (EEG) changes and convulsions in humans and other higher mammals, Burchfiel et al (23) investigated the persistent effects of a single dose of sarin on the primate EEG. Seizures were induced by a single injection of sarin while the animals were paralyzed and artificially respired. Spectral analysis of serial EEGs over a one-year period revealed a persistent increase in the relative amount of beta voltage in two out of three treated monkeys, compared with none of the controls. Duffy et al (40) followed up this finding with EEG studies of 77 industrial workers with histories of accidental exposure to sarin at least one year previously: 41 of the 77 had at least three exposures within the six years preceding the study; 38 industrial workers from the same plant served as controls. Spectral analysis revealed increased beta activity in both the total of exposed and the highly exposed subgroup compared with controls. Visual inspection of the tracing was inconsistent and showed decreased alpha activity with nonspecific abnormalities. Despite real statistical differences, expert visual inspection did not permit diagnosis of individual subjects.

Methodologic Issues

Research on the neurobehavioral effects of pesticides is fraught with inconsistencies and methodologic problems not unique to the study of pesticides (15, 47, 50, 60, 101, 159, 163, 164). Study results are limited by the neuropsychologic and neurophysiologic tests used to evaluate workers, the sensitivity of these tests, their validity, and their reliability. It is often unclear what significant findings mean to the workers' performance and functioning. Test administrators often are not blind to exposure status. Appropriate worker control groups matched on age, education, and habits are usually not employed. The lack of a comparative population leads to problems in interpretation, since exposed groups may function within normal limits but show deficits relative to controls. Another possible comparison is with baseline or pre-exposure performance. However, baseline performance, although assumed from the subsequent pattern of performance, is rarely known.

The recent use of computers to administer versions of the standard paper and pencil tests to large groups of worker populations has minimized tester variability, cost and time of administration, and problems in data storage. However, use of computers has also raised other problems in the field of neurobehavioral toxicology. For example, the computer versions of these tests have not been well validated on large control populations. Even when validated, normative data should not preclude the use of control populations on a study-by-study basis.

In summary, the discipline of neurobehavioral toxicology is in its infancy. Our knowledge of delayed neurobehavioral effects of pesticide exposure is limited by our techniques to assess these effects and our understanding of what performance on these tests mean to human function.

FUTURE DIRECTIONS

Improvement of future research in delayed health hazards of exposure to pesticides will necessitate changes in the direction and emphasis of epidemiologic research. These changes are specific to the three types of outcomes discussed in this review.

Cancer Hazards

The present epidemiologic approach to detecting human cancer hazards faces two major concerns:

1. The effect of cancer latency is that cancer hazards cannot be detected by traditional means for 20 years or more after sufficient numbers of the population have been exposed. This problem has fueled the move to increasing reliance on animal studies. However, use of genetically pure strains of animals in constant environmental conditions and on controlled diets may not detect human risks, particularly if interaction of several agents and conditions is involved.

2. The magnitude of exposure to particular chemicals, at least in the industrialized world, is declining with improved industrial practices and increasing environmental awareness. While this trend is highly desirable, it reduces the likelihood of epidemiologic studies detecting an effect. Therefore, it is imperative that cancer epidemiology turn to investigating biologic markers of risk that can be tested cross-sectionally in exposed populations.

Tests of sister chromatid exchange and chromosomal aberrations have been criticized because they do not necessarily indicate increased cancer risk. However, public health decisions do not require scientific certainty—exposures linked to these effects should be reduced. A particularly attractive feature of this approach is that markers of risk should decrease after reduced exposure, thereby confirming that intervention has been appropriate. Early studies of pesticide applicators through use of sister chromatid exchange techniques have produced valuable results (33, 96, 176), and better tests will become available, such as quantification of DNA adduct levels (169). Along this same line of inquiry is the detection of genetic susceptibility to chemical exposure in developing cancer (88). The strongest potential for such testing may lie in the development of linkage analysis techniques to map "susceptibility" genes. However, it will be many years before such techniques are practicable.

Reproductive Hazards

Many studies in the past were ecological, and concentrated on general population exposure. Such studies will continue to give controversial results due to the multiple comparisons involved and the unknown exposures. That the effects of low exposures in the general population cannot be detected by epidemiologic methods must be confronted. Emphasis should be placed on high exposure groups.

Surveillance of potentially high risk groups such as manufacturers and applicators is needed, and is easy to implement for congenital defects and for birth rates (58, 95, 152, 153, 175). More sensitive indices, such as early spontaneous abortion and semen analyses, may be necessary in specific circumstances, but the cost and personal resistance in participating render use of such techniques on a large scale unpractical (175).

DBCP is the only pesticide discovered so far to have a clear reproductive effect in humans. This may be simply because occupational studies have concentrated on males. Greater participation of women in the work force should result in more epidemiologic studies of women exposed to pesticides. Future epidemiologic studies of reproductive hazards due to pesticides should concentrate on identifying exposed women, particularly in agricultural work.

Neurotoxic Hazards

Johnson & Anger (83) have emphasized the need for pragmatic standards-based research to clarify the relationship of work place chemicals to neurobehavioral deficits, particularly at levels below which routine neurologic testing or biologic monitoring may detect abnormalities. For organophosphate field exposure in particular, demonstration of neurobehavioral abnormalities during chronic low level exposure sufficient to cause mild decreases in acetylcholinesterase, but insufficient to cause symptoms, would have important implications for medical surveillance and worker protection.

Additional neurophysiologic measures, such as the EMG and sensory-evoked potential, are tools to explore the possible physiologic correlates of decrements in behavioral performance. These tools may help to disentangle the secondary psychologic effects following exposure from the organic effects. Computer-generated neurobehavioral batteries may provide cheaper and more easily administered research tools allowing for screening of larger populations.

The greatest issue surrounding the field of long-term neurobehavioral effects of chemical exposures is simply whether the problems are real, and if so how extensive they are. The former can only be assessed by careful studies including pre-exposure assessment, since it is not clear whether the behavioral measures are measures of outcome, or measures of pre-existing psychologic characteristics whereby people choose certain jobs and adopt work practices that lead them to become heavily exposed.

CONCLUSIONS

With few exceptions, the delayed effects of pesticides on human health have been difficult to detect. Perhaps the health risks are sufficiently small that they are below the power of epidemiologic studies to detect. Yet, it is possible that there are very few effects at all. Concerns may have arisen from the inevitable false positive associations of studies testing a large number of exposures and outcomes. Undoubtedly, however, the need continues for surveillance and assessment of delayed human health effects from pesticide exposure, albeit with some changes in emphasis and methods.

Literature Cited

1. Abbott, D. C., Goulding, R., Tatton, J. 1968. Organochlorine pesticide residues in human fat in Great Britain. *Br. Med. J.* 3:146–49
2. Agent Orange Program. 1985. *Mortality among Vietnam veterans in Massachusetts, 1972–1983*. Boston: Commonwealth of Massachusetts, Off. of Commissioner of Veterans' Serv.
3. Agu, V. U., Christensen, B. L., Buffler, P. A. 1980. Geographic patterns of multiple myeloma: Racial and industrial correlates, state of Texas, 1969–71. *J. Natl. Cancer Inst.* 65:735–38
4. Axelson, O., Dahlgren, E., Jansson, C. D., Rehnlund, S. O. 1978. Arsenic exposure and mortality: A case-referent study from a Swedish copper smelter. *Br. J. Indust. Med.* 35:8–15
5. Axelson, O., Sundell, L. 1974. Herbicide exposure, mortality and tumor incidence. An epidemiological investiga-

tion on Swedish railroad workers. *Work Environ. Health* 11:21–28
6. Axelson, O., Sundell, L., Andersson, K., Edling, C., Hogstedt, C., Kling, H. 1980. Herbicide exposure and tumor mortality an updated epidemiologic investigation on Swedish railroad workers. *Scand. J. Work Environ. Health* 6:73–79
7. Balarajan, R., Acheson, E. D. 1984. Soft tissue sarcomas in agriculture and forestry workers. *J. Epidemiol. Community Health* 38:113–16
8. Balarajan, R., McDowall, M. 1983. Congenital malformations and agricultural workers. *Lancet* 1:1112–13
9. Bank, W. J., Pleasure, D. E., Suzuki, K., Nigro, M., Katz, R. 1972. Thallium poisoning. *Arch. Neurol.* 26:456–64
10. Barthel, E. 1976. High incidence of lung cancer in persons with chronic pro-

fessional exposure to pesticides in agriculture. *Z. Erk. Atmungsorgane* 146: 266–74

11. Barthel, E. 1981. Increased risk of lung cancer in pesticide-exposed male agricultural workers. *J. Toxicol. Environ. Health* 8:1027–40

12. Bishop, C. M., Jones, A. H. 1981. Non-Hodgkin's lymphoma of the scalp in workers exposed to dioxins. *Lancet.* 2:369

13. Blair, A., Grauman, D. J., Lubin, J. H., Fraumeni, J. F. 1983. Lung cancer and other causes of death among licensed pesticide applicators. *J. Natl. Cancer Inst.* 71:31–37

14. Blair, A., Thomas, T. L. 1979. Leukemia among Nebraska farmers: A death certificate study. *Am. J. Epidemiol.* 110: 264–73

15. Bleeker, M. L. 1984. Clinical neurotoxicology: Detection of neurobehavioral and neurological impairments occurring in the workplace and the environment. *Arch. Environ. Health* 39:213–17

16. Bond, G. G., Ott, M. G., Brenner, F. E., Cook, R. R. 1983. Medical and morbidity surveillance findings among employees potentially exposed to TCDD. *Brit. J. Indust. Med.* 40:318–24

17. Bowers, M. B., Goodman, E., Sim, V. M. 1964. Some behavioral changes in man following anticholinesterase administration. *J. Nerv. Ment. Dis.* 138: 383–89

18. Brogan, W. F., Brogan, C. E., Dadd, J. T. 1980. Herbicides and cleft lip and palate. *Lancet* 2:597–98

19. Brown, C. C., Chu, K. C. 1983. Implications of the multistage theory of carcinogenesis applied to occupational arsenic exposure. *J. Natl. Cancer Inst.* 70:455–63

20. Bruzzi, P. 1983. Health impact of the accidental release of TCDD at Seveso. In *Accidental Exposure to Dioxins: Human Health Aspects,* ed. F. Coulston, F. Pocchiari, pp. 215–28. New York: Academic

21. Buchel, K. H. 1984. Political, economic, and philosophical aspects of pesticide use for human welfare. *Regul. Toxicol. Pharmacol.* 4:174–91

22. Buesching, D. P., Wollstadt, L. 1984. Cancer mortality among farmers. *J. Natl. Cancer Inst.* 72:503

23. Burchfiel, J. L., Duffy, F. H., Sim, V. M. 1976. Persistent effects of sarin and dieldrin upon the primate electroencephalogram. *Toxicol. Appl. Pharmacol.* 35:365–79

24. Burmeister, L. F. 1981. Cancer mortality in Iowa farmers, 1971–78. *J. Natl. Cancer Inst.* 66:461–64

25. Burmeister, L. F., Everett, G. D., van Lier, S. F., Isacson, P. 1983. Selected cancer mortality and farm practices in Iowa. *Am. J. Epidemiol.* 118:72–77

26. Burmeister, L. F., van Lier, S. F., Isacson, P. 1982. Leukemia and farm practices in Iowa. *Am. J. Epidemiol.* 115: 720–28

27. Cantor, K. P. 1982. Farming and mortality from non-Hodgkin's lymphoma: A case-control study. *Int. J. Cancer* 29: 239–47

28. Cantor, K. P., Blair, A. 1984. Farming and mortality from multiple myeloma: A case-control study with the use of death certificates. *J. Natl. Cancer Inst.* 72: 251–55

29. Coggon, D., Acheson, E. D. 1982. Do phenoxy herbicides cause cancer in man? *Lancet* 1:1057–59

30. Constable, J. D., Hatch, M. C. 1984. Agent orange and birth defects. *N. Engl. J. Med.* 310:653–54

31. Cook, R. R. 1981. Dioxin, chloracne, and soft tissue sarcoma. *Lancet* 1:618–19

32. Cook, R. R., Townsend, J. C., Ott, M. G., Silverstein, L. G. 1980. Mortality experience of employees exposed to 2,3,7,8-tetrachlorodibenzo-*p*-dioxin (TCDD). *J. Occup. Med.* 22:530–32

33. Crossen, P. E., Morgan, W. F., Horan, J. J., Stewart, J. 1978. Cytogenetic studies of pesticide and herbicide sprayers. *NZ Med. J.* 88:192–95

34. Crow, K. D. 1981. Soft tissue sarcomas and chlorinated phenols. *Lancet* 2:369

35. Cutting, R. T., Phuoc, T. H., Ballo, J. M., Benenson, M. W., Evans, C. H. 1970. In *Congenital Malformations, Hydatidiform Moles and Stillbirths in the Republic of Vietnam. 1960–1969.* Washington DC:US GPO

36. D'Ercole, A. J., Arthur, R. D., Cain, J. D., Barrentine, B. F. 1976. Insecticide exposure of mothers and newborns in a rural agriculture area. *Pediatrics* 57:869–74

37. Delzell, E., Grufferman, S. 1985. Mortality among white and nonwhite farmers in North Carolina, 1976–1978. *Am. J. Epidemiol.* 121:391–402

38. Ditraglia, D., Brown, D. P., Namekata, T., Iverson, N. 1981. Mortality study of workers employed at organochlorine pesticide manufacturing plants. *Scand. J. Work Environ. Health* 7 (Suppl. 4):140–46

39. Donna, A., Betta, P. G., Robutti, F., Crosignani, P., Berrino, F., Bellingeri, D. 1984. Ovarian mesothelial tumors and

herbicides: A case-control study. *Carcinogenesis* 5:941–42

40. Duffy, F. H., Burchfiel, J. L., Bartels, P. H., Gaon, M., Sim, V. M. 1979. Long-term effects of an organophosphate upon the human electroencephalogram. *Toxicol. Appl. Pharmacol.* 47:161–76

41. Editorial. 1982. Phenoxy herbicides, trichlorophenols, and soft-tissue sarcomas. *Lancet* 1:1051–52

42. Egnatz, D. G., Oh, M. G., Townsend, J. C., Olson, R. D., Johns, D. B. 1980. DBCP and testicular effects in chemical workers: An epidemiological survey of Midland, Michigan. *J. Occup. Med.* 22:727–32

43. Enterline, P. E., March, G. M. 1982. Cancer among workers exposed to arsenic and other substances in a copper smelter. *Am. J. Epidemiol.* 116:895–911

44. Erickson, J. D., Mulinare, J., McClain, P. W., Fitch, T. G., James, L. M., McClearn, A. B., Adams, M. J. 1984. Vietnam veterans' risk for fathering babies with birth defects. *J. Am. Med. Assoc.* 252:903–12

45. Eriksson, M., Hardell, L., Berg, N. O., Moller, T., Axelson, O. 1981. Soft-tissue sarcomas and exposure to chemical substances: A case-referent study. *Br. J. Indust. Med.* 38:27–33

46. Fasal, E., Jackson, E. W., Klauber, M. R. 1968. Leukemia and lymphoma mortality and farm residence. *Am. J. Epidemiol.* 87:267–74

47. Feldman, R. G., Ricks, N. L., Baker, E. L. 1980. Neuropsychological effects of industrial toxins: A review. *Am. J. Indust. Med.* 1:211–27

48. Field, B., Kerr, C. 1979. Herbicide use and incidence of neural-tube defects. *Lancet* 1:1341–42

49. Fingerhut, M. A., Halperin, W. E., Honchar, P. A., Smith, A. B., Groth, D. H., Russell, W. O. 1984. An evaluation of reports of dioxin exposure and soft tissue sarcoma pathology among chemical workers in the United States. *Scand. J. Work Environ. Health* 10:299–303

50. Friedlander, B. R., Hearne, F. T. 1980. Epidemilogic considerations in studying neurotoxic disorders. In *Experimental and Clinical Neurotoxicology,* ed. P. S. Spencer, H. H. Schaumberg. Baltimore: Williams & Wilkins

51. Furst, A., Radding, S. B. 1984. New developments in the study of metal carcinogenesis. *J. Environ. Sci. Health* C2:103–33

52. Gallagher, R. P., Threlfall, W. J. 1984. Cancer and occupational exposure to chlorophenols. *Lancet* 2:48

53. Gershon, S., Shaw, F. H. 1961. Psychiatric sequelae of chronic exposure to organophosphate insecticides. *Lancet* 1:1371–74

54. Glass, R. I., Lyness, R. N., Mengle, D. C., Powell, K. E., Kahn, E. 1979. Sperm count depression in pesticide applicators exposed to dibromochloropropane. *Am. J. Epidemiol.* 109:346–51

55. Golding, J., Sladden, T. 1983. Congenital malformations and agricultural workers. *Lancet* 1:1393

56. Goldsmith, J. R., Potashnik, G., Israeli, R. 1984. Reproductive outcomes in families of DBCP exposed men. *Arch. Environ. Health* 39:85–89

57. Greene, M. H., Brinton, L. A., Fraumeni, J. F., D'Amico, R. 1978. Familial and sporadic Hodgkin's disease associated with occupational wood exposure. *Lancet* 2:626–27

58. Halperin, W. E., Frazier, T. M. 1985. Surveillance for the effects of workplace exposure. *Ann. Rev. Public Health* 6:419–32

59. Hanify, J. A., Metcalf, P., Nebbs, C. L., Worsley, K. J. 1981. Aerial spraying of 2,4,5-T and human birth malformations: An epidemiological investigation. *Science* 212:349–51

60. Hanninen, H. 1985. Twenty-five years of behavioral toxicology within occupational medicine: A personal account. *Am. J. Indust. Med.* 7:19–30

61. Hardell, L. 1977. Malignant mesenchymal tumours and exposure to phenoxy acids—a clinical observation. *Lakartidningen* 74:2753–54

62. Hardell, L. 1979. Malignant lymphoma of histiocytic type and exposure to phenoxyacetic acids or chlorophenols. *Lancet* 1:55–56

63. Hardell, L. 1981. Relation of soft-tissue sarcoma, malignant lymphoma and colon cancer to phenoxy acids, chlorophenols and other agents. *Scand. J. Work Environ. Health* 7:119–30

64. Hardell, L., Axelson, O. 1982. Soft-tissue sarcoma, malignant lymphoma, and exposure to phenoxyacids or chlorophenols. *Lancet* 2:1408–9

65. Hardell, L., Bengtsson, N. O. 1983. Epidemiological study of socioeconomic factors and clinical findings in Hodgkin's disease, and reanalysis of previous data regarding chemical exposure. *Br. J. Cancer* 48:217–25

66. Hardell, L., Eriksson, M. 1981. Soft-tissue sarcomas, phenoxy herbicides, and chlorinated phenols. *Lancet* 2:250

67. Hardell, L., Eriksson, M., Lenner, P., Lundgren, E. 1981. Malignant lympho-

ma and exposure to chemicals, especially organic solvents, chlorophenols and phenoxy acids: a case-control study. *Br. J. Cancer* 43:169–76

68. Hardell, L., Johansson, B., Axelson, O. 1982. Epidemiological study of nasal and nasopharyngeal cancer and their relation to phenoxy acid or chlorophenol exposure. *Br. J. Indust. Med.* 3:247–57

69. Hardell, L., Sandstrom, A. 1979. Case-control study: Soft-tissue sarcomas and exposure to phenoxyacetic acids or chlorophenols. *Br. J. Cancer* 39:711–17

70. Harmon, G. E., Reigart, J. R., Sandifer, S. H. 1975. Long-term followup of survivors of acute pesticide poisoning. *J. SC Med. Assoc.* 26:253–57

71. Hatch, M. C. 1984. Reproductive effects of the dioxins. In *Public Health Risks of the Dioxins*, ed. W. W. Lowrance, pp. 255–74. Los Altos, Calif.: Kaufmann

72. Hay, A. 1982. Phenoxy herbicides, trichlorophenols, and soft-tissue sarcomas. *Lancet* 1:1240

73. Hayes, W. J. 1982. *Pesticides Studied in Man.* Baltimore: Williams & Wilkins

74. Hessel, S. M., Berman, E. 1982. Severe peripheral neuropathy after exposure to monosodium methyl arsenate. *J. Toxicol. Clin. Toxicol.* 19:281–87

75. Hine, C. H. 1969. Methyl bromide poisoning: A review of ten cases. *J. Occup. Med.* 11:1–10

76. Hoar, S. K., Blair, A., Holmes, F. F., Boysen, C., Robel, R. J. 1985. Herbicides and colon cancer. *Lancet* 1:1277–78

77. Honchar, P. A., Halperin, W. E. 1981. 2,4,5-T, trichlorophenol, and soft-tissue sarcoma. *Lancet* 1:268–69

78. Infante, P. F., Epstein, S. S., Newton, W. A. 1978. Blood dyscrasias and childhood tumors and exposure to chlordane and heptachlor. *Scand. J. Work Environ. Health* 4:137–50

79. International Agency for Research on Cancer. 1973. Some organochlorine pesticides. *IARC Monogr. Eval. Carcinog. Risk Chem. Hum.* 5:83–124

80. International Agency for Research on Cancer. 1980. Some metals and metallic compounds. *IARC Monogr. Eval. Carcinog. Risk Chem. Hum.* 23:39–141

81. International Agency for Research on Cancer. 1982. Chemicals, industrial processes and industries associated with cancer in humans, IARC Monographs, Volumes 1 to 29. *IARC Monogr. Eval. Carcinog. Risk Chem. Hum. Suppl.* 4:1–292

82. International Agency for Research on Cancer. 1983. Cancer epidemiology of pesticide manufacturers, formulators and users. *IARC Monogr. Eval. Carcinog. Risk Chem. Hum.* 30:37–56

83. Johnson, B., Anger, W. K. 1983. Behavioral toxicology. In *Environmental and Occupational Medicine,* ed. W. N. Rom. Boston: Little, Brown

84. Johnson, F. E., Kugler, M. A., Brown, S. M. 1981. Soft tissue sarcomas and chlorinated phenols. *Lancet* 2:40

85. Johnson, M. K. 1982. The target of initiation of delayed neurotoxicity by organophosphate esters: Biochemical studies and toxicological applications. *Rev. Biochem. Toxicol.* 4:141–212

86. Kahn, E., Whorton, D. 1980. Letters to the editor re: "Sperm count depression in pesticide applicators exposed to dibromochloropropane." *Am. J. Epidemiol.* 112:161–64

87. Kharrazi, M., Potashnik, G., Goldsmith, J. R. 1980. Reproductive effects of dibromochloropropane. *Isr. J. Med. Sci.* 16:403–6

88. King, M. C. 1984. Genetic and epidemiologic approaches to detecting genetic susceptibility to chemical exposures. In *Banbury Report 16: Genetic Variability in Responses to Chemical Exposure,* ed. G. S. Omenn, H. V. Gelboin, pp. 377–92. Cold Spring Harbor, NY: Cold Spring Harbor Lab.

89. Kunstadter, P. 1982. In *A Study of Herbicides and Birth Defects in the Republic of Vietnam: An Analysis of Hosptial Records.* Washington DC: Natl. Acad. Sci., Natl. Acad. Press

90. Lantz, G. D., Cunningham, G. R., Huckins, C., Lipshultz, L. I. 1981. Recovery from severe oligospermia after exposure to dibromochloropropane. *Fertil. Steril.* 35:46–53

91. Lathrop, G. D., Wolfe, W. H., Albanese, R. A., Moynahan, P. M. 1984. *An epidemiologic investigation of health effects in Air Force personnel following exposure to herbicides: Baseline morbidity study results.* Washington DC: Surgeon General, US Air Force

92. Lawrence, C. E., Reilly, A. A., Quickenton, P., Greenwald, P., Page, W. F., Kuntz, A. J. 1985. Mortality patterns of New York State Vietnam veterans. *Am. J. Public Health* 75:277–79

93. LeQuesne, P. M., McLeod, J. G. 1977. Peripheral neuropathy following a single exposure to arsenic. *J. Neurol. Sci.* 32:437–51

94. Levin, J. S., Rodnitzky, R. L., Mick, D. L. 1976. Anxiety associated with exposure to organophosphate compounds. *Arch. Gen. Psychiatry* 33:225–28

95. Levine, R. J., Blunden, P. B., DalCorso, R. D., Starr, T. B., Ross, C. E. 1983. Superiority of reproductive histories to sperm counts in detecting infertility at a dibromochloropropane manufacturing plant. *J. Occup. Med.* 25:591–97

96. Linnainmaa, K. 1983. Sister chromatid exchanges among workers occupationally exposed to phenoxy acid herbicides 2,4-D and MCPA. *Teratogen. Carcinog. Mutagen.* 3:269–79

97. Lipshultz, L. I., Ross, C. E., Whorton, D., Milby, T., Smith, R., Joyner, R. E. 1980. Dibromochloropropane and its effect on testicular function in man. *J. Virol.* 124:464–68

98. Lynge, E. 1985. A follow-up study of cancer incidence among workers in manufacture of phenoxy herbicides in Denmark. *Br. J. Cancer* 52:259–70

99. Mabuchi, K., Lilienfeld, A. M., Snell, L. M. 1980. Cancer and occupational exposure to arsenic: A study of pesticide workers. *Prev. Med.* 9:51–77

100. May, G. 1982. Tetrachlorodibenzodioxin: A survey of subjects ten years after exposure. *Br. J. Indust. Med.* 39:128–35

101. Melius, J. M., Schulte, P. A. 1981. Epidemiologic design for field studies: Occupational neurotoxicity. *Scand. J. Work Environ. Health* 7(Suppl 4):34–39

102. Merrill, D. G., Mihm, F. G. 1982. Prolonged toxicity of organophosphate poisoning. *Crit. Care Med.* 10:550–51

103. Meselson, M. S., Westing, A. H., Constable, J. D., Cook, R. E. 1972. Background material relevant to presentation at the 1970 AAAS Herbicide Assessment Commission. *US Congress. Rec. 92nd Congr. 2nd Session* 118:S3227–23

104. Metcalf, D. R., Holmes, J. H. 1969. EEG, psychological and neurological alterations in humans with organophosphate exposure. *Ann. NY Acad. Sci.* 160:357–65

105. Midtling, J. E., Barnett, P., Coye, M. J., Velasco, A. R., Romero, P., et al. 1985. Clinical management of field worker organophosphate poisoning. *West. J. Med.* 142:514–18

106. Milby, T. H., Whorton, D. 1980. Epidemiological assessment of occupationally related, chemically induced sperm count suppression. *J. Occup. Med.* 22:77–82

107. Milham, S. 1971. Leukemia and multiple myeloma in farmers. *Am. J. Epidemiol.* 94:307–10

108. Milham, S. 1982. Herbicides, occupation, and cancer. *Lancet* 1:1464–65

109. Morgan, D. P., Lin, L. I., Saikaly, H. H. 1980. Morbidity and mortality in workers occupationally exposed to pesticides. *Arch. Environ. Contam. Toxicol.* 9:349–82

110. Morgan, J. P. 1982. The Jamaica ginger paralysis. *J. Am. Med. Assoc.* 248:1864–67

111. Moses, M., Lilis, R., Crow, K. D., Thornton, J., Fischbein, A., Anderson, H. A., Selikoff, I. J. 1984. Health status of workers with past exposure to 2,3,7,8-tetrachlorodibenzo-p-dioxin in the manufacture of 2,4,5-trichlorophenoxyacetic acid: Comparison of findings with and without chloracne. *Am. J. Indust. Med.* 5:161–82

112. Moses, M., Selikoff, I. J. 1981. Soft tissue sarcomas, phenoxy herbicides, and chlorinated phenols. *Lancet* 1:1370

113. Mrak, E. M. 1984. Pesticides: The good and the bad. *Regul. Toxicol. Pharmacol.* 4:28–36

114. Namba, T., Nolte, C. T., Jackrel, J., Grob, D. 1971. Poisoning due to organophosphate insecticides: Acute and chronic manifestations. *Am. J. Med.* 50:475–92

115. Nelson, C. J., Holson, J. F., Green, H. G., Gaylor, D. W. 1979. Retrospective study of the relationship between agricultural use of 2,4,5-T and cleft palate occurrence in Arkansas. *Teratology* 19:377–83

116. Newell, K. W., Ross, A. D., Renner, R. M. 1984. Phenoxy and picolinic acid herbicides and small-intestinal adenocarcinoma in sheep. *Lancet* 2:1301–5

117. Nordberg, G. F., Andersen, O. 1981. Metal interactions in carcinogenesis: Enhancement, inhibition. *Environ. Health Perspect.* 40:65–81

118. O'Leary, J. A., Davies, J. E., Feldman, M. 1970. Spontaneous abortion and human pesticide residues in DDT and DDE. *Am. J. Obstet. Gynecol.* 108:1291–92

119. Olsson, H., Brandt, L. 1981. Non-Hodgkin's lymphoma of the skin and occupational exposure to herbicides. *Lancet* 2:579

120. Orris, P. 1981. Letter to the editor: Unjustified conclusion? *J. Occup. Med.* 23:7–8

121. Ott, M. G., Holder, B. B., Gordon, H. L. 1974. Respiratory cancer and occupational exposure to arsenicals. *Arch. Environ. Health* 29:250–55

122. Ott, M. G., Holder, B. B., Olson, R. D. 1980. A mortality analysis of employees engaged in the manufacture of 2,4,5-trichlorophenoxyacetic acid. *J. Occup. Med.* 22:47–50

123. Pazderova-Vejlupkova, J., Nemcova, M., Pickova, J., Jirasek, L. 1981. The

development and prognosis of chronic intoxication by tetrachlordibenzo-*p*-dioxin in men. *Arch. Environ. Health* 36:5–11
124. Pearce, N. E., Smith, A. H., Fisher, D. O. 1985. Malignant lymphoma and multiple myeloma linked with agricultural occupations in a New Zealand cancer registry-based study. *Am. J. Epidemiol.* 121:225–37
125. Pearce, N. E., Smith, A. H., Howard, J. K., Sheppard, R. A., Giles, H. J., Teague, C. A. 1986. Non-Hodgkin's lymphoma and exposure to phenoxy herbicides, chlorophenols, fencing work and meat works employment: A case-control study. *Br. J. Indust. Med.* In press
126. Perold, J. G., Bezuidenhout, D. J. J. 1980. Chronic organophosphate poisoning. *S. Afr. Med. J.* 57:7–9
127. Pershagen, G. 1981. The carcinogenicity of arsenic. *Environ. Health Perspect.* 40:93–100
128. Pershagen, G. 1983. The epidemiology of human arsenic exposure. In *Biological and Environmental Effects of Arsenic*, ed. B. A. Fowler. Amsterdam:Elsevier
129. Pershagen, G., Wall, S., Taube, A., Linnman, L. 1981. On the interaction between occupational arsenic exposure and smoking and its relationship to lung cancer. *Scand. J. Work Environ. Health* 7:302–9
130. Potashnik, G. 1983. A four year reassessment of workers with dibromochloropropane-induced testicular dysfunction. *Andrologia* 15:164–70
131. Potashnik, G., Ben-Aderet, N., Israeli, R., Yani-Inbar, I., Sober, I. 1978. Suppressive effect of 1,2-dibromo-3-chloropropane on human spermatogenesis. *Fertil. Steril.* 30:444–47
132. Potashnik, G., Yanai-Luba, I., Sarks, M. I., Israeli, R. 1979. Effect of dibromochloropropane in human testicular function. *Isr. J. Med. Sci.* 15:438–42
133. Priester, W. A., Mason, T. J. 1974. Human cancer mortality in relation to poultry population, by county, in 10 southeastern states. *J. Natl. Cancer Inst.* 53:45–49
134. Procianoy, R. S., Schvartsman, S. 1981. Blood pesticide concentrations in mothers and their newborn infants. *Acta Paediatr. Scand.* 70:925–28
135. Radomski, J. L., Astolfi, E., Deichmann, W. B., Rey, A. A. 1971. Blood levels of organochlorine pesticides in Argentine occupationally and nonoccupationally exposed adults, children and newborn infants. *Toxicol. Appl. Pharmacol.* 20:186–93
136. Reggiani, G. 1983. Anatomy of a TCDD

spill: The Seveso accident. *Hazard Assess. Chem. Curr. Dev.* 2:269–342
137. Riihimaki, V., Asp, S., Hernberg, S. 1982. Mortality of 2,4-dichlorophenoxyacetic acid and 2,4,5-trichlorophenoxyacetic acid herbicide applicators in Finland. *Scand. J. Environ. Health* 8:37–42
138. Riihimaki, V., Asp, S., Pukkala, E., Hernberg, S. 1983. Mortality and cancer morbidity among chlorinated phenoxyacid applicators in Finland. *Chemosphere* 12:779–84
139. Rodnitzky, R. L., Levin, H. S., Mick, D. L. 1975. Occupational exposure to organophosphate pesticides. *Arch. Environ. Health* 30:98–103
140. Sandifer, S. H., Wilkins, R. T., Loadholt, C. B., Lane, L. G., Eldridge, J. C. 1979. Spermatogenesis in agricultural workers exposed to dibromochloropropane (DBCP). *Bull. Environ. Contam. Toxicol.* 23:703–10
141. Sarma, P. R., Jacobs, J. 1982. Thoracic soft-tissue sarcoma in Vietnam veterans exposed to agent orange. *N. Engl. J. Med.* 306:1109
142. Saxena, M. C., Siddiqui, M. K., Seth, T. D., Krishna-Murti, C. R., Bhargava, A. K., Kutty, D. 1981. Organochlorine pesticides in specimens from women undergoing spontaneous abortion, premature or full-term delivery. *J. Anal. Toxicol.* 5:6–9
143. Saxena, M. C., Siddiqui, M. K. J., Bhargava, A. K., Seth, T. D., Krishnamurti, C. R., Kutty, D. 1980. Role of chlorinated hydrocarbon pesticides in abortions and premature labour. *Toxicology* 17:323–31
143a. Seifert, J., Casida, J. E. 1982. Possible role of microtubules and associated proteases in organophosphorus ester-induced delayed neurotoxicity. *Biochem. Pharmacol.* 31:2065–70
143b. Seifert, J., Casida, J. E. 1984. Neural microtubular and lysosomal phenyl valerate esterases and proteases in relation to organophosphate-induced delayed neurotoxicity. *Comp. Biochem. Physiol.* 78C:271–76
144. Siddiqui, M. K. J., Sanea, M. C., Bhargava, A. K., Seth, T. D., Murti, C. R. Krishna, Kutty, D. 1981. Agrochemicals in the maternal blood, milk, and cord blood: A source of toxicants for prenates and neonates. *Environ. Res.* 24:24–32
145. Singer, R., Moses, M., Valciukas, J., Lilis, R., Selikoff, I. J. 1982. Nerve conduction velocity studies of workers employed in the manufacture of phenoxy herbicides. *Environ. Res.* 29:297–311

146. Smith, A. H., Fisher, D. O., Giles, H. J., Pearce, N. E. 1983. The New Zealand soft tissue sarcoma case-control study: Interview findings concerning phenoxyacetic acid exposure. *Chemosphere* 12:565–71

147. Smith, A. H., Fisher, D. O., Pearce, N. E., Chapman, C. J. 1982. Congenital defects and miscarriages among New Zealand 2,4,5-T sprayers. *Arch. Environ. Health* 37:197–200

148. Smith, A. H., Fisher, D. O., Pearce, N. E., Teague, C. A. 1982. Do agricultural chemicals cause soft tissue sarcoma? Initial findings of a case-control study in New Zealand. *Community Health Studies* 6:114–19

149. Smith, A. H., Matheson, D. P., Fisher, D. O., Chapman, C. J. 1981. Preliminary report of reproductive outcomes among pesticide applicators using 2,4,5-T. *NZ Med. J.* 93:177–79

150. Smith, A. H., Pearce, N. E., Fisher, D. O., Giles, H. J., Teague, C. A., Howard, J. K. 1984. Soft tissue sarcoma and exposure to phenoxyherbicides and chlorophenols in New Zealand. *J. Natl. Cancer Inst.* 73:1111–17

151. Smith, P. W., Stavinoha, W. S., Ryan, L. C. 1968. Cholinesterase inhibition in relation to fitness to fly. *Aerospace Med.* 139:754–58

152. Starr, T. B., Levine, R. J. 1983. Assessing effects of occupational exposure on fertility with indirect standardization. *Am. J. Epidemiol.* 118:897–904

153. Stein, Z. A. 1984. Surveillance: Symptoms, exposure, and trust. *Prog. Clin. Biol. Res.* 160:131–38

154. Suskind, R. R., Hertzberg, V. S. 1984. Human health effects of 2,4,5-T and its toxic contaminants. *J. Am. Med. Assoc.* 251:2372–80

155. Tabershaw, I. R., Cooper, W. C. 1966. Sequelae of acute organophosphate poisoning. *J. Occup. Med.* 8:5–20

156. Taylor, J. R., Selhorst, J. B., Calabrese, V. P. 1980. Clordecone. In *Experimental and Clinical Neurotoxicology*, ed. P. S. Spencer, H. H. Schaumberg, pp. 407–21. Baltimore: Williams & Wilkins

157. Thiess, A. M., Frentzel-Beyme, R., Link, R. 1982. Mortality study of persons exposed to dioxin in a trichlorophenol-process accident that occurred in the BASF AG on November 17, 1953. *Am. J. Indust. Med.* 3:179–89

158. Thomas, H. F. 1980. 2,4,5-T use and congenital malformation rates in Hungary. *Lancet* 2:214–15

159. Tilson, H. A., Mitchell, C. L. 1984. Neurobehavioral techniques to assess the effects of chemicals on the nervous system. *Ann. Rev. Pharmacol. Toxicol.* 24:425–50

160. Tognoni, G., Bonaccorsi, A. 1982. Epidemiological problems with TCDD (a critical review). *Drug Metab. Rev.* 13:447–69

161. Townsend, J. C., Bodner, K. M., Van-Peenen, P. F. D., Olsen, R. D., Cook, R. R. 1982. Survey of reproductive events of wives of employees exposed to chlorinated dioxins. *Am. J. Epidemiol.* 115:695–713

162. US Environmental Protection Agency. 1979. *Report of assessment of a field investigation of six-year spontaneous abortion rates in three Oregon areas in relation to forest 2,4,5-T spray practices (Alsea II Report)*, Washington DC:US EPA

163. Valciukas, J. A. 1984. A decade of behavioral toxicology: Impressions of a NIOSH/WHO workshop in Cincinnati, May 1983. *Am. J. Indust. Med.* 5:405–6

164. Valciukas, J. A., Lilis, R. 1980. Psychometric techniques in environmental research. *Environ. Res.* 21:275–97

165. Walsh, R. J., Donovan, J. W., Adena, M. A., Rose, G., Battistutta, D. 1983. In *Case-control Study of Congenital Anomalies and Vietnam Service (Birth Defects Study)* Canberra: Australian Govern. Publ. Serv.

166. Wang, H. H., Grufferman, S. 1981. Aplastic anemia and occupational pesticide exposure: A case-control study. *J. Occup. Med.* 23:364–66

167. Wang, H. H., MacMahon, B. 1979. Mortality of pesticide applicators. *J. Occup. Med.* 21:741–44

168. Wang, H. H., MacMahon, B. 1979. Mortality of workers employed in the manufacture of chlordane and heptachlor. *J. Occup. Med.* 21:745–48

169. Weinstein, I. B. 1983. The monitoring of DNA adducts as an approach to carcinogen detection. *Ann. Rev. Public Health* 4:409–13

170. Whorton, D., Krauss, R. M., Marshall, S. 1977. Infertility in male pesticide workers. *Lancet* 2:1259–61

171. Whorton, D., Milby, T. H., Krauss, R. M., Stubbs, H. A. 1979. Testicular function in DBCP exposed pesticide workers. *J. Occup. Med.* 21:161–66

172. Whorton, M. D., Obrinsky, D. L. 1983. Persistence of symptoms after mild to moderate acute organophosphate poisoning among 19 farm field workers. *J. Toxicol. Environ. Health* 11:347–54

173. Wolff, M. S. 1983. Occupationally de-

rived chemicals in breast milk. *Am. J. Indust. Med.* 4:259–81

174. Wong, O., Brocker, W., Davis, H. V., Nagle, G. S. 1984. Mortality of workers potentially exposed to organic and inorganic brominated chemicals, DBCP, TRIS, PBB, and DDT. *Br. J. Indust. Med.* 41:15–24

175. Wong, O., Morgan, R. W., Whorton, M. D. 1985. An epidemiologic surveillance program for evaluating occupational reproductive hazards. *Am. J. Indust. Med.* 7:295–306

176. Yoder, J., Watson, M., Benson, W. W. 1973. Lymphocyte chromosome analysis of agricultural workers during extensive occupational exposure to pesticides. *Mutat. Res.* 21:335–40

177. Zack, J. A., Gaffey, W. R. 1983. A mortality study of workers employed at the Monsanto Company plant in Nitro, West Virginia. *Environ. Sci. Res.* 26:575–91

178. Zack, J. A., Suskind, R. R. 1980. The mortality experience of workers exposed to tetrachlorodibenzodioxin in a trichlorophenol process accident. *J. Occup. Med.* 22:11–14

Symposium on Nutrition

Ann. Rev. Public Health. 1986. 7:475–79

SYMPOSIUM ON NUTRITION:
Introduction*

Artemis P. Simopoulos

Nutrition Coordinating Committee, National Institutes of Health, Bethesda, Maryland 20892

The health of the individual and the population in general is determined by a variety of biologic (genetic), behavioral, sociocultural, and environmental factors. Nutrition is one environmental factor of great importance in determining an individual's level of health and well-being. A person's requirements for nutrients are influenced by genetics, lifestyle, the nature of diet, and the homeostatic demands under changing physiological conditions expressed as growth, reproduction, and response to stress, injury, or disease.

Information on the nutritional status of the American population is obtained through a number of surveys and complemented with information derived from epidemiologic studies and clinical trials.

The National Center for Health Statistics (NCHS) has carried out three major national surveys that have included measurements of weight and height. The National Health and Examination Survey (NHES) was carried out in 1960 to 1962; the first National Health and Nutrition Examination Survey (NHANES I) in 1971 to 1974; and NHANES II in 1976 to 1980. Both NHANES I and II collected data from a national probability sample representative of the US civilian, noninstitutionalized population, 6 months to 74 years of age.

The NCHS surveys show that:

1. Americans as a group have become heavier over the past 20 years.
2. Obesity is more prevalent in blacks than whites.
3. Black women are heavier than white women.
4. Obesity is more prevalent in lower socioeconomic groups, particularly among females.
5. Rural populations tend to be more overweight than urban populations.

The most common nutritional disorder in the United States is obesity. Obesity is an independent risk factor for cardiovascular disease (2), and death from cardiovascular disease is the most common cause of death in adults in the United States, accounting for 48% of all deaths. Both excess weight and hypertension may contribute independently to increased risk of cardiovascular disease.

In the past decade, there has been a proliferation of articles in both the scientific literature and in the lay press (newspapers and magazines), as well as coverage on talk shows, about eating disorders, particularly anorexia and bulimia. Symptoms of bulimia occur along with a continuum of weight disorders, including anorexia nervosa and obesity. All three conditions occur much more frequently in women than men, with bulimia and anorexia occurring especially among young women of college age.

Thus, in a Symposium on Nutrition for the *Annual Review of Public Health,* the following five topics are included specifically because of their public health importance to morbidity and mortality:

1. Obesity and Body Weight Standards;
2. The Importance of Obesity in the Development of Coronary Risk Factors and Disease—The Epidemiologic Evidence;
3. Dietary Aspects of the Treatment of Hypertension;
4. Public Health Approaches to Obesity and Its Management;
5. Anorexia Nervosa and Bulimia.

The first paper, "Obesity and Body Weight Standards," describes the findings of the Workshop on Body Weight, Health, and Longevity, held at the National Institutes of Health. A summary of the workshop was published in 1984 (3). The paper includes a list of definitions of various body weight standards and refers to the findings of the Framingham Heart Study population over a 26-year follow-up (1), which indicate that weights above the ranges recommended by the 1959 Metropolitan Life Insurance Table are associated with increased morbidity and mortality. Furthermore, the Framingham Heart Study data

1. validated the concept of desirable body weight as defined by the 1959 Metropolitan Life Insurance Company Table;
2. suggested that elevated mortality in low-weight American men results from the mortality risks associated with cigarette smoking;
3. showed that cigarette smoking is a potential confounder of the relationship between relative weight and long-term mortality, and statistical control for this factor requires careful consideration;
4. suggested that obesity is an independent risk factor for cardiovascular disease;
5. indicated that weight gain after the young adult years conveyed an increased risk of cardiovascular disease in both sexes.

In addition, the paper reviews the most recent findings from the NHES Cycles II and III and NHANES I and II in children, adolescents, and adults. The prevalence of obesity is increasing in all age groups. The author points out that the estimates of the prevalence of obesity from the normative data obtained from these surveys are a statistical estimate and not one based on morbidity and mortality as are the data from longitudinal studies, such as the data from the Framingham Heart Study population.

Normative data that use as a reference standard the average body weight at ages 20–29 underestimate the prevalence of obesity in the population. The use of the 1959 Metropolitan Life Insurance Company table of desirable weights is recommended for use in adults. A series of three tables based on this table are included for adult men and women, along with the calculations for the Metropolitan Relative Weight (MRW) at 100, 110, and 120.

Dr. Helen Hubert in her review on "The Importance of Obesity in the Development of Coronary Risk Factors and Disease—The Epidemiologic Evidence," points out that population-based studies indirectly suggest that increased body weight for height is independently associated with increased low density lipoprotein cholesterol and decreased high density lipoprotein cholesterol, an adverse lipoprotein pattern.

Dr. Hubert refers to her work, which has been presented but not yet published, and states that more direct evidence is found from the longitudinal Framingham Heart Study indicating that the initial degree of obesity or weight change is significantly and independently related to change in total and lipoprotein cholesterol over time. Dr. Hubert emphasizes that weight change has been found to be the strongest and most consistent lifestyle correlate of lipoprotein cholesterol change, particularly in healthy, young adult populations. Furthermore, these data suggest that obesity and weight gain, which are quite common in young adulthood, elevate coronary heart disease risk. Much may be gained from education and intervention during these years.

Similarly, a strong positive relationship of weight or obesity to systolic and diastolic blood pressure change and to the development of hypertension over time has been well documented in prospective epidemiologic studies in males and females of all ages. A review of the experimental literature further substantiates that weight loss in borderline and definite hypertensives can be an effective treatment modality and that weight reduction in controlled hypertensives may significantly improve the success of withdrawal of drug therapy.

This point is clearly made by Dr. Norman Kaplan in his review on "Dietary Aspects of the Treatment of Hypertension." Dr. Kaplan reviews extensively the role of obesity and its effects on blood pressure control. Furthermore, he reviews the role of sodium, potassium, calcium, magnesium, fat and polyunsaturated fatty acids, alcohol, and other dietary factors such as protein, garlic, and caffeine on the treatment of blood pressure and concludes: Based upon currently available evidence, a practical dietary prescription should be:

1. For the overweight, weight reduction should be the primary goal.
2. For all hypertensives, dietary sodium should be restricted to a 2 g (88 mmol/dl) level.
3. Potassium intake need not be specifically increased since it will rise with a lowered sodium intake. Those who are hypokalemic may benefit from potassium supplementation.
4. Supplemental magnesium and calcium should only be given to those who are deficient, until additional evidence of their efficacy is available. Caution is advised in not reducing the dietary sources of calcium when dietary sodium is reduced.
5. More fiber and less saturated fat are beneficial for other reasons and may also help lower blood pressure.
6. Alcohol should be limited to two ounces a day.

"The Public Health Approaches to Obesity and Its Management" are reviewed by Dr. Kelly D. Brownell. Dr. Brownell reviews the theoretical and physiologic aspects of the etiology of obesity, such as "The Set Point Theory," fat cell number and size, and fat distribution and risk and states that these ideas are relatively new and must be studied in more detail. They may be important links in explaining why obesity develops, why some individuals are at greater risk as a result of their obesity, and why some dieters struggle for a lifetime without losing much weight while others lose weight with ease.

Many investigators have developed schemes for the classification of obesity. Dr. Brownell favors the one proposed by Dr. Stunkard, who proposed three categories of overweight: Mild (0–30% overweight); Moderate (30–100% overweight); and Severe (greater than 100%). This classification scheme suggests different treatments for persons in the three categories.

Dr. Brownell reviews the clinical treatments for obesity and, under the section "Public Health Approaches," discusses an array of potential approaches, such as distribution of booklets and pamphlets on nutrition, exercise, and weight loss by government agencies, private groups, insurance companies, and television and radio stations. Self-help groups and commercial groups and their popularity are also reviewed, as are community programs and work site programs. Dr. Brownell is enthusiastic about weight loss competitions at the work site and states:

> More controlled studies are needed in this promising area. The focus of the competition on *motivation* rather than *education* may lead to new and more effective approaches to weight control. The work site may be a fruitful channel for the delivery of such programs.

Finally, Dr. Brownell proposes "A Stepped-Care Model for Obesity," which is modeled after the current approach to the management of hypertension. The stepped-care approach proposed may eventually have the greatest public health impact on obesity.

Obesity, anorexia, and bulimia are considered eating disorders. Drs. Joseph

H. Autry, Ellen S. Stover, and Natalie Reatig state: "Anorexia nervosa is increasing in public health importance and has been linked to other disorders such as depression and cardiac problems." A patient with anorexia nervosa loses body weight in excess of 25% of previous body weight. Although the disorder is seen mostly in adolescent females, it is not limited to females. The majority of the studies have assessed prevalence in college student populations. There is evidence that the disorder is less prevalent in older age groups and in males. The prevalence in the general population has been estimated to be between 1.0 and 4.2%, and the mortality rate is approximately 10%.

Autry, Stover, and Reatig reviewed the criteria for definition and state:

> It is important to differentiate anorexia nervosa as a symptom and anorexia as a syndrome with other symptoms, such as depression and sleep disturbance. A large percentage of the women who suffer from anorexia nervosa are also bulimic. Bulimia is defined as the rapid consumption of large amounts of food in a short period of time, frequently followed by self-induced vomiting or the use of cathartics or diuretics.

The authors review the current knowledge of anorexia and bulimia, the psychiatric, physiologic, metabolic, and endocrine aspects, and carry out an extensive review of studies in the treatment of this disorder. They conclude their paper with a section on "Future Research Needs," both in terms of pathogenesis and treatment.

Research on body weight, health, and longevity is an important aspect of the programs of the National Institutes of Health and the Alcohol, Drug Abuse, and Mental Health Administration. Eventually body weight standards will have to be based on specific information from data on body composition. It is hoped that we will be able to identify those at risk for developing obesity and define more precisely the range of overweight and obesity associated with increased morbidity and mortality. Furthermore, within the obese population, those susceptible to hypertension, diabetes, coronary artery disease, and some forms of cancer (e.g. cancer of the breast, endometrium, and prostate) will have to be identified and differentiated from those who are not. Eating disorders and concepts of body image will similarly be better understood and treated.

Until more information becomes available, the effort to stay within the range of the 1959 Metropolitan Life Insurance Company desirable weight table is highly recommended. Obesity and its sequelae are difficult to treat. Prevention of obesity needs to be continuously emphasized.

Literature Cited

1. Garrison, R. J., Feinleib, M., Castelli, W. P. McNamara P. M. 1983. Cigarette smoking as a confounder of the relationship between relative weight and long-term mortality. *J. Am. Med. Assoc.* 249:2199–2203
2. Hubert, H. B., Feinleib, M., McNamara P. M., Castelli, W. P. 1983. Obesity as an independent risk factor for cardiovascular disease: A 26 year follow-up of participants in the Framingham Heart Study. *Circulation.* 67:968–77
3. Simopoulos, A. P., Van Itallie, T. B. 1984. Body weight, health and longevity. *Annals of Internal Medicine.* 100: 285–95

Ann. Rev. Public Health. 1986. 7:481–92

OBESITY AND BODY WEIGHT STANDARDS*

Artemis P. Simopoulos

Nutrition Coordinating Committee, National Institutes of Health, Bethesda, Maryland 20892

INTRODUCTION

The prevalence of overweight and obesity in a population depends on the particular reference or standard of desirable weight selected for use. The standards traditionally used are the weight-for-height tables for men and women developed by the Metropolitan Life Insurance Company (12) based on the 1959 Build and Blood Pressure Study (2). Thus, the definition of overweight and obesity in adults is based on actuarial analyses that indicate the weight range for each height category that is associated with the lowest mortality rate in an insured population.

Body weight, by itself, is not a measure of obesity. Therefore, when it is used to "define" obesity, it must be related to more appropriate measures of body fat. To this end, a number of indices of body weight have been developed on the basis of varying relationships with total body fat. These indices have utilized, for the most part, body weight in some combination with height. In children, this has most commonly been the use of weight-for-height distributions (percentiles), while in adults the common index has been based on the quotient, W/H^n. Although a number of different values of n have been suggested for use in different population groups, the most commonly used power function has been 2, as in $W(kg)/H(m)^2$.

Other approaches have defined some measure of weight at a given age (such as median or mean) as the "standard" and related all other weights to this arbitrarily defined "standard." Still others have defined the "standard" within

---

the population being studied and related other weights to that value, e.g. Metropolitan Relative Weight (MRW) (see below).

DEFINITIONS

Metropolitan Relative Weight (MRW), an index used in the Framingham Heart Study, is based on the midpoint of the desirable weight range for medium frame (as given in the 1959 Metropolitan Life Table) chosen as the reference weight for a given height (Table 1). MRW is computed for each subject by forming the ratio of his body weight to the reference weight for his height. This ratio is expressed as a whole number in percent. The average Framingham man has a MRW of 115 to 121% depending on the specific height group, while the majority of adult American men are in MRW groups above 120%.

Desirable Body Weight refers to the weight associated with the lowest mortality as used by the Metropolitan Life Insurance Company in 1959. This table presented a range in weight for a given height based on small, medium, and large frame size (12).

Table 1 Desirable weight ranges—ages 25 and over[a]

Height (ft in)	Men weight range	Women[b] weight range
4 9		90–118
4 10		92–121
4 11		95–124
5 0		98–127
5 1	105–134	101–130
5 2	108–137	104–134
5 3	111–141	107–138
5 4	114–145	110–142
5 5	117–149	114–146
5 6	121–154	118–150
5 7	125–159	122–154
5 8	129–163	126–159
5 9	133–167	130–164
5 10	137–172	134–169
5 11	141–177	
6 0	145–182	
6 1	149–187	
6 2	153–192	
6 3	157–197	

[a]Adapted from the 1959 Metropolitan Desirable Weight Table. (Weight, in pounds, without clothing; height without shoes.)

[b]For women between the ages of 18–25 years, subtract one pound for each year under 25.

Body Mass Index is another approach to the estimation of the prevalence of overweight. This weight-height index is obtained by dividing weight (W) in kilograms by height (H) in meters squared $[W(Kg)/H(m)^2]$ (Quetelet's Index). The most common method has been to use a power function of 2 for both men and women. Recently, however, it has been suggested that a power function of 1.5 may be more appropriate for women; this question requires further investigation. The Body Mass Index has a relatively high correlation with body fat (as estimated from body density), particularly when age is taken into consideration (14), and a relatively low correlation with height. In the absence of skinfold measurements, it is the most satisfactory index of obesity based on weight and height that is available (10).

Skinfold Thickness is a more direct index of body fat. Hubert et al (9) have reported that in Framingham men, subscapular skinfold measurements were significantly and independently associated with increased risk of myocardial infarction, whereas MRW was not. It is quite possible that MRW may represent a somewhat different measure of body mass in each sex, since excess weight results from muscularity more often in males than in females.

Frame Size is a consideration in the Metropolitan Life 1959 Desirable Weight Table that makes a distinction between persons of small, medium, and large frame. The division of frame size in the Metropolitan Life Table was not based on any anthropometric measurement of the subjects but, rather, represents an arbitrary division of the population into the lowest quartile (small frame), the middle two quartiles (medium frame), and the highest quartile (large frame).

In theory, frame size reflects differences among individuals of the same gender and height in regard to such factors as chest breadth, hip width, bone thickness, and length of trunk relative to total height. "Frame" is a skeletal concept. The main determinants of body frame are genetics, nutrition, and level of physical activity. Few systematic studies have been made to assess frame size as a factor affecting body weight, independently of height and body fat content. Moreover, many indices of body frame size are too complex and cumbersome to use in routine examinations. For this reason, the use of frame size has been deleted from Tables 1, 3, and 4.

PREVALENCE AND HEALTH IMPLICATIONS OF OBESITY

The National Center for Health Statistics has carried out three major surveys that provide normative data on a national probability sample of the US population: the National Health Examination Survey (NHES), 1960–1962; the National Health and Nutrition Examination Survey (NHANES I), 1971–1974; and NHANES II, 1976–1980. The data have made it possible to examine the prevalence of obesity at the time of the surveys and to permit assessment of body weight trends during the three time periods. The three surveys have defined "overweight" as being a body mass index (BMI) at or higher than that which obtains at the eighty-fifth percentile for men (BMI 28 kg/m^2) and women (BMI 34 kg/m$^{1.5}$) aged 20 to 29 years studied between 1976 and 1980 (23). "Severe overweight" is defined as a BMI (32 kg/m^2 for men and 42 kg/m$^{1.5}$ for women) at or higher than the ninety-fifth percentile of the same 20- to 29-year-old reference group.

The rationale underlying use of the 20- to 29-year-old reference population is that young adults are relatively lean and the increase in body weight that usually occurs as men and women age is due almost entirely to fat accumulation. It is, of course, well known that the US population at ages 20–29, although young, is not necessarily lean; therefore, any calculation based on this "rationale" underestimates the prevalence of obesity. Furthermore, the criteria (eighty-fifth or ninety-fifth percentile) are defined statistically; they are not derived from morbidity or mortality experience of the survey population. Thus, by the NHANES BMI criteria, 32.6 million adult Americans are overweight, while 11.5 million are severely overweight.

If we calculate the prevalence of obesity on the basis of the work of Garrison (6) and Hubert (9), using criteria related to morbidity and mortality from cardiovascular disease, 80% of men and 70% of women over 40 years of age in the Framingham Heart Study are above the desirable weight range (MRW > 110%; 24.4 kg/m^2) and are at increased risk for cardiovascular disease. Studies have shown that the weights of the Framingham Heart Study cohort are similar to those in the general population of the US.

Obesity is a major health problem in the US. Data from NHES and NHANES I and II also permit assessment of body weight trends among Americans from 1960 to 1962, 1971 to 1974, and 1976 to 1980. A comparison of mean heights and weights of adults aged 18 to 74 years in the three surveys (Table 2) shows that both men and women were taller and heavier in 1971 to 1974 and 1976 to 1980 than they were in 1960 to 1962. As noted above, the survey data are based on a national probability sample and are normative.

Data from the NHANES I survey show that overweight affects a significant proportion of our population: 14% of the men and 24% of the women between ages of 20 to 74 years were found to be 20% or more above their desirable weight. (By the NHANES terminology, "desirable" weight is defined as the average weight at 20–29 years of age.) One of every three women past the age of 55 is overweight. As can be seen in Figure 1, men were most likely to be overweight during their forties, whereas overweight in women increased with age, peaking in the late fifties and sixties. Similarly, data from the second NHANES (1976 to 1980) indicate that the prevalence of obesity persists and that those in the ninetieth percentile are even heavier than in previous surveys.

Dietz et al (5) carried out an analysis of trends in the prevalence of childhood

Table 2   Mean weights and heights by age and sex in three populations[a]

Age group	Men			Women		
	HES	NHANES I	NHANES II	HES	NHANES I	NHANES II
Weight (kg)						
18–24 yr	71.7	74.8	73.9	57.6	59.9	60.8
25–34 yr	76.7	79.8	78.5	60.8	63.5	64.4
35–44 yr	77.1	80.7	80.7	64.4	67.1	67.1
45–54 yr	77.1	79.4	80.7	65.8	67.6	68.0
55–64 yr	74.4	77.6	78.9	68.0	67.6	68.0
65–74 yr	71.7	74.4	74.8	65.3	66.2	66.7
18–74 yr	75.3	78.0	78.0	63.5	64.9	65.3
Height (m)						
18–24 yr	1.74	1.77	1.77	1.62	1.63	1.63
25–34 yr	1.76	1.77	1.77	1.62	1.63	1.63
35–44 yr	1.74	1.76	1.76	1.61	1.63	1.63
45–54 yr	1.73	1.75	1.75	1.60	1.62	1.61
55–64 yr	1.71	1.73	1.74	1.58	1.60	1.60
65–74 yr	1.70	1.71	1.71	1.56	1.58	1.58
18–74 yr	1.73	1.75	1.76	1.60	1.62	1.62

[a]The three populations are from the National Health and Examination Survey, 1960 to 1962, and the National Health and Nutrition Examination Surveys I, 1971 to 1974, and II, 1976 to 1980. Two pounds were deducted from HES data to allow for weight of clothing; total weight of all clothing for NHANES I and II ranged from 0.1 to 0.3 kg and was not deducted from weights in table. Height was measured without shoes. Data are preliminary. Age-adjusted mean values and estimates of variations (standard error) are not currently available.

and adolescent obesity in the United States using data collected from the NHES Cycles II and III and NHANES I and II in 6–11-year-old children and 12–17-year-old adolescents. Dietz et al state:

> Obesity was defined as a triceps skinfold ≥ 85th percentile of 6–11 year old children studied in NHES Cycle II or 12–17 year old adolescents studied in NHES Cycle III. Superobesity was defined as a triceps skinfold ≥ 95th percentile. Over the 10–15 year period encompassed by these surveys, obesity and superobesity increased by 54% ($p < .0001$) and 98% ($p < .0001$) respectively in 6–11-year olds and by 39% ($p < .0001$) and 64% ($p < .0001$) respectively in 12–17 year olds. In both groups, the increases in prevalence were greater in blacks than whites. In 6–11 year olds, greater increases occurred in males, whereas in 12–17 year olds, greater increases occurred in females. Previously documented differentials in the prevalence of obesity by season and region of the country persisted independent of the changes in prevalence. These data indicate that obesity is epidemic in the pediatric population, and emphasize the need for more effective therapy and prevention.

The findings of Dietz et al that the prevalence of obesity and superobesity is on the increase in both children and adolescents raises great concern for the future of young adults in our population.

Obesity in the adult may be preceded by obesity during childhood, but few studies (1, 4, 13) on this association have been reported because reliable data

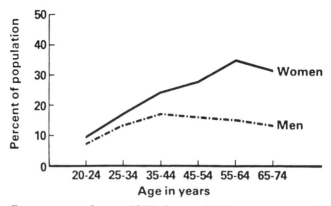

Figure 1   Fourteen percent of men and 24% of women 20–74 years of age were 20% or more above desirable weight. Men were most likely to be overweight during their forties. Overweight in women increased with age, peaking in the late fifties and early sixties.

are difficult to obtain on a longitudinal basis from childhood to adulthood. Stark et al (20) carried out an analysis of the data from the longitudinal study of obesity in the National Survey of Health and Development in England and found a positive correlation between relative weight at any two ages covered by the study; this means that the risk of being overweight as an adult is greater for overweight children and adolescents than for those of average or below average weight. The clinical impression that most severely overweight children (relative weight > 140%) are still overweight in adolescence was confirmed, but the study showed that not all overweight children and adolescents grew into overweight adults. The survey procedure did not allow assessment of the extent to which treatment of severe overweight might have influenced the natural history.

In the US, Abraham & Nordsieck (1) found that 74% and 72% of 11–13-year-old overweight boys and girls, respectively, were still overweight as adults, whereas in Stark's study 40% of the overweight 11-year-old and 50% of the 14-year-old children were still overweight at 26 years. Because of the differences used in sampling and in the methods used in assessing overweight, it is difficult to compare the results of these two studies. Stark et al concluded (20):

> The risk of being overweight in adulthood was related to the degree of overweight in childhood and was about four in ten for overweight 7-year-olds. Analysis of the data in the reverse direction showed that 7 percent and 13 percent respectively of the 25-year-old overweight men and women had been overweight at the age of 7. These results suggest that there is no optimal age during childhood for the prediction of overweight in adult life and that excessive weight gain may begin at any time. Overweight children are more likely to remain overweight than their contemporaries of normal weight are to become overweight.

Childhood obesity presents a serious health problem in the US and most other developed countries. Because treatment is difficult and long-term results often disappointing, more attention is being given to prevention.

Obesity is associated with cardiovascular disease (9), hypertension (7, 16), diabetes, and some forms of cancer (17). Elsewhere in this volume, Hubert discusses obesity as an independent risk factor for cardiovascular disease and its association with hypertension, and Kaplan further discusses the association of obesity and hypertension.

Dr. Van Itallie (22) reviewed the association between obesity and diabetes mellitus and stated:

> Epidemiological studies have disclosed a striking relationship between the average fatness among populations of certain countries and prevalence of diabetes. Prospective studies of the relationship between obesity and diabetes may reveal even more fully the strength of the association than do the more typical cross-sectional surveys relating diabetes prevalence to degree of fatness. The lesser degree of association in many cross-sectional studies is probably mainly attributable to the loss of weight that can occur with diabetes.

Furthermore, Westlund & Nicholaysen (24), in a prospective study, showed that in moderate obesity, risk of diabetes was increased about ten-fold. In those whose weights exceeded the standard by 45% or more, risk was increased about 30-fold.

The association of overweight/obesity with cancer was noted by Hoffman in 1937 in his book, *Cancer and Diet* (8), in which he concluded, "Overnutrition is common in the case of cancer patients to a remarkable and exceptional degree, and that overabundant food consumption unquestionably is the underlying cause of the root condition of cancer in modern life." It was further discussed by Tannenbaum (21) in 1940, when he reviewed the data from the Medico-Actuarial-Mortality Investigation, the Medical Impairment Study, the Metropolitan Life Insurance Company Records (1938–1939), and the New York Life Insurance Company Records:

> Although the results of experimental work with animals and the analyses of insurance statistics strongly suggest that body weight is a factor affecting cancer incidence, there are many considerations that must be critically studied and evaluated before the fundamental nature of the relationship is fully understood. The weight of an animal or a human being is the result of many complex, often interrelated factors, such as the racial and hereditary characteristics, the qualitative and quantitative composition of the diet, the hormonal balance, the basal metabolic rate, exercise, previous health, and many others. One cannot be certain that the relationship between cancer and weight as discussed in this paper is necessarily a direct, primary one. It may be, and in uncompleted experimental work there is evidence for it, that some of the factors controlling weight are of more direct significance than weight, with the latter being merely a resultant of these forces.

What is the practical significance of this apparent relationship of weight to cancer inception and incidence? If further critical, comprehensive studies should confirm the results reported here, it would appear that an important prophylactic measure has been brought to the attention of the medical profession. By establishing and maintaining weight levels at a minimum compatible with general good health [possibly 10 to 20 pounds (4.5 to 9 Kg) below present "normal" levels], cancer may be prevented in a considerable number of persons in whom it would otherwise develop; at least, the cancer process might be delayed in time of appearance. Such a regimen is already known to affect beneficially other pathologic conditions, such as diabetes, heart disease, cerebral hemorrhage and other degenerative diseases.

Thus, increases in all-cause mortality with increases in weight were recognized by the insurance companies at the beginning of this century.

Most recently, the analyses of data of the long-term prospective study conducted by the American Cancer Society over the period 1959–1972 confirmed the finding that the lowest mortality was found among those close to average weight and those 10–20% below average weight (11). It should be pointed out that the study describes the mortality according to variations in weight among 750,000 men and women drawn from the general population. Cancer mortality was elevated among those 40% or more overweight (defined in this study as 40% above average weight). Cancer of the colon and rectum was the principal site of excess cancer mortality among men, while cancer of the gall bladder and biliary passages, breast, cervix, endometrium, uterus, and ovary were the major sites of excess mortality among women.

The report on obesity from the Royal College of Physicians (15) and the recent analyses of the 26-year follow-up of the Framingham Heart Study (6) indicate that mild degrees of overweight are, on a public health basis, important. Risks associated with excess weight are not, as previously thought, only confined to those who are substantially obese, because a progressive increase in morbidity and mortality is apparent with even a small increase in weights above the upper limits of the range of the 1959 Metropolitan Life Insurance Company table (6). See Tables 3 and 4.

BODY WEIGHT, HEALTH, AND LONGEVITY

In order to define precisely the health implications of obesity and thus begin to formulate the concepts of the relationship between body weight, health, and longevity and to clarify the terminology used *(ideal, desirable, acceptable, MRW),* a workshop was held in 1982, sponsored by the National Institutes of Health Nutrition Coordinating Committee and the Centers for Disease Control. The workshop reviewed data developed by the life insurance industry, recent

Table 3 Desirable weight ranges for men—ages 25 and over[a]

Height (ft in)	Weight range	Weight[b] MRW=100	Weight[c] MRW=110	Weight MRW=120
5 1	105–134	117	129	140
5 2	108–137	120	132	144
5 3	111–141	123	135	148
5 4	114–145	126	139	151
5 5	117–149	129	142	155
5 6	121–154	133	146	160
5 7	125–159	138	152	166
5 8	129–163	142	156	170
5 9	133–167	146	161	175
5 10	137–172	150	165	180
5 11	141–177	155	170	186
6 0	145–182	159	175	191
6 1	149–187	164	180	197
6 2	153–192	169	186	203
6 3	157–197	174	191	209
BMI (all heights)		21.66	23.83	26.00

[a]Adapted from the 1959 Metropolitan Desirable Weight Table. (Weight, in pounds, without clothing; height without shoes.)
[b]Midpoint of medium frame range—used to compute MRW: MRW = [(Actual weight)/(Midpoint of medium frame range)] × 100
[c]In the US adult population over 40 years of age, 80% of men and 70% of women have weights that exceed MRW = 110, and, consequently, are at increased risk for cardiovascular disease. The average weight of the adult US population is above MRW = 120; and individual with a weight over MRW = 120 is "obese."

analyses of data from the Framingham Study (5209 subjects) (6, 9), and other studies of a variety of populations that examined the relationship of body weight to morbidity and mortality, such as the Build Study 1979 (3) and the new data from the 1959–1972 American Cancer Society Study (755, 502 subjects) (11). A summary of the workshop's proceedings, including descriptions and critiques of the studies has been published (18, 19).

The participants of the workshop concluded:

In this United States, studies based on life insurance data (for example, the Build and Blood Pressure Study, 1959; Build Study 1979; Provident Mutual Life Study), the American Cancer Society Study, and other long-term studies, such as the Framingham Heart Study and Manitoba Study, indicate that below-average weights tend to be associated with the greatest longevity, if such weights are not associated with concurrent illness or a history of significant medical impairment. Overweight persons tend to die sooner than average-weight persons, particularly those who are overweight at younger ages. The effect of obesity on mortality is delayed, so that it is not seen in short-term studies; the extensive data from the Build Study

Table 4   Desirable weight ranges for women—ages 25 and over[a]

Height (ft in)	Weight range	Weight[b] MRW=100	Weight[c] MRW=110	Weight MRW=120
4 9	90–118	100	110	120
4 10	92–121	103	113	124
4 11	95–124	106	117	127
5 0	98–127	109	120	131
5 1	101–130	112	124	134
5 2	104–134	116	128	139
5 3	107–138	120	132	144
5 4	110–142	124	136	149
5 5	114–146	128	141	154
5 6	118–150	132	145	158
5 7	122–154	136	150	163
5 8	126–159	140	154	168
5 9	130–164	144	158	173
5 10	134–169	148	163	177
BMI (all heights)		21.32	23.47	25.58

[a]Adapted from the 1959 Metropolitan Desirable Weight Table. (Weight, in pounds, without clothing; height without shoes.)

[b]Midpoint of medium frame range—used to compute MRW: MRW = [(Actual weight)/ (Midpoint of medium frame range)] × 100

[c]In the US adult population over 40 years of age, 80% of men and 70% of women have weights that exceed MRW = 110, and, consequently, are at increased risk for cardiovascular disease. The average weight of the adult US population is above MRW = 120; and individual with a weight over MRW = 120 is "obese."

Note: For women between the ages of 18–25 years, subtract one pound for each year under 25.

1979 show this delayed effect particularly well. The recent analyses of the Framingham Heart Study data emphasize that obesity is a significant independent predictor of cardiovascular disease, with smoking having a separate effect. Furthermore, the concept of "desirable weight" developed by the Metropolitan Life Insurance Company in 1959 has been validated by a recent long-term study. In addition to the age range of the population studied, the interpretation of studies on body weight, morbidity, and mortality must also carefully consider the definition of obesity used, preexisting illnesses in persons, the length of follow-up, and any confounding risk factors.

In order to develop body weight standards that reflect morbidity and mortality, the participants of the workshop recommended:

An appropriate database that relates body weight by age, sex, and possibly frame size to morbidity and mortality should be developed to permit the preparation of reference tables for defining the range of desirable body weight from morbidity and mortality statistics. Ideally, reference data should consider appropriate attributes (such as physical activity level and nature of diet) as well as possible changes in the attributes. These changes will require new observational studies to measure, in study populations, the relation of such factors to morbidity and mortality. Therefore, it is recommended that, at a minimum, the following are needed to develop a reference data table that relates body weight to health and longevity:

•The population studied should be representative of the healthy population to which the reference data will be applied.

•Data on weight and height should be analyzed and presented separately by sex, age, and duration of follow-up, with age divided by decades. This procedure takes into account age-related changes in weight and permits establishment of age-related desirable weight goals.

•Data on weight and height should also be expressed as the body mass index with a median, range, and standard deviation presented for each age and sex group. Data so presented can be converted into tables relating weight and height, although questions remain regarding the validity of the body mass index for estimating body fat in persons outside the groups for which the index was originally derived. Consequently, caution must be used in comparing the body mass index between groups with standards not validated on the groups under consideration.

• Efforts should be made to develop uncomplicated indices that correlate with the body fat content better than body mass index does.

•All statements regarding the ranges in which the morbidity and mortality rates are lowest should be based on statistically significant differences in mortality rates between the nadir of the curve and the proposed limits of the range.

• The range should be broad enough to encompass subgroups whose life expectancy is known to differ because of certain life styles, such as smoking, or whose socioeconomic status or other demographic characteristics contribute to differences in life expectancy. The expected differences contributed by such characteristics should be explicitly noted.

•The value of indices of frame size should be assessed.

Because the latest Framingham data show that obesity is a significant independent predictor for cardiovascular disease, there is a need to investigate the ways in which obesity becomes, or acts as, a "marker" for premature demise; identify the various types of obesity associated with specific diseases at different stages of the life cycle (for example, upper trunk obesity with diabetes, fat cell number and hypertension in early adulthood, and fat cell size and hypertension in middle age); and define the effect of duration of being overweight on health to ascertain the specific age (how early in life) at which obesity becomes a marker for both morbidity and mortality.

On the basis of the information at hand and until further research defines the range of body weight for least morbidity and longest survival, the recommended range of weights should conform to Table 1 based on the 1959 Metropolitian Life Insurance

Metropolitan relative weight appears to be an appropriate reference standard. Its use by epidemiologists and clinical investigators should help in comparing and interpreting various studies. Table 1 represents desirable body weight ranges for men and women over 25 years of age, weighed without clothing and shoes, for general use by the public and health professionals. For research purposes, it also includes Metropolitan Relative Weight for both men and women.

Literature Cited

1. Abraham, S., Nordsieck, M. 1960. Relationship of excess weight in children and adults. *Public Health Rep.* 75:263–73
2. *Build and Blood Pressure Study,* Vol. 1. 1959. Chicago: Soc. Actuaries
3. *Build Study 1979.* 1979. Chicago: Soc. Actuaries and Assoc. Life Insurance Med. Directors
4. Charney, E., Goodman, H. C., McBride, M. 1976. Childhood antecedents of adult obesity. Do chubby infants become obese adults? *N. Engl. J Med.* 295:6–9
5. Dietz, W. H., Gortmaker, S. L., Sobol, A. M., Wehler, C. A. 1985. Trends in the prevalence of childhood and adolescent obesity in the United States. *Pediatr. Res.* 19(4):527 (Abstr.)
6. Garrison, R. J., Feinleib, M., Castelli, W. P., McNamara, P. M. 1983. Cigarette smoking as a confounder of the relationship between relative weight and long-term mortality: The Framingham Heart Study. *J. Am. Med. Assoc.* 249:2199–2203
7. Havlik, R. J., Hubert, H. B., Fabsitz, R. R., Feinleib, M. 1983. Weight and hypertension. *Ann. Internal Med.* 98(5):855–59
8. Hoffman, F. L. 1937. *Cancer and Diet.* Baltimore: Williams & Wilkins
9. Hubert, H. B., Feinleib, M., McNamara, P. M., Castelli, W. P. 1983. Obesity as an independent risk factor for cardiovascular disease: A 26-year followup of participants in the Framingham Heart Study. *Circulation* 67:968–77
10. Keys, A., Fidanza, F., Karvonen, M. J., Kimura, N., Taylor, H. L. 1972. Indices of relative weight and obesity. *J. Chron. Dis.* 25:329–43
11. Lew, E. A., Garfinkel, L. 1979. Variations in mortality by weight among 750,000 men and women. *J. Chron. Dis.* 32:563–76
12. Metropolitan Life Insurance Company. 1959. *Stat. Bull.* 40:1–4
13. Mullins, A. G. 1958. The prognosis in juvenile obesity. *Arch. Dis. Child.* 33:307–14
14. Norgan, N. G., Ferro-Luzzi, A. 1982. Weight-height indices as estimators of fatness in men. *Human Nutr. Clin. Nutr.* 36:363–72
15. Royal College of Physicians of London. 1983. Obesity: A report of the Royal College of Physicians. *J. R. Coll. Phys.* 17:5–65
16. Simopoulos, A. P. 1985. Dietary control of hypertension and obesity and body weight standards. *J. Am. Dietetic Assoc.* 85:419–22
17. Simopoulos, A. P. 1985. The health implications of overweight and obesity. *Nutrition Rev.* 43(2):33–40
18. Simopoulos, A. P., Van Itallie, T. B. 1984. Body weight, health, and longevity. *Ann. Internal Med.* 100:285–95
19. Special Report: Body Weight, Health, and Longevity: Conclusions and Recommendations of the Workshop. 1985. *Nutrition Rev.* 43(2):61–63
20. Stark, O., Atkins, E., Wolff, O. H., Douglas, J. W. 1981. Longitudinal study of obesity in the National Survey of Health and Development. *Br. Med. J.* 283:13–17
21. Tannenbaum, A. 1940. Relationship of body weight to cancer incidence. *Arch. Pathol.* 30:509–17
22. Van Itallie, T. B. 1979. Obesity: Adverse effects on health and longevity. *Am. J. Clin. Nutrition* 32:2723–33
23. Van Itallie, T. B., Abraham, S. 1985. Some hazards of obesity and its treatment. In *Recent Advances of Obesity Research. IV. Proc. 4th Int. Congr. on Obesity,* ed. J. Hirsch, T. B. Van Itallie. London: Libby
24. Westlund, K., Nicholaysen, R. 1972. Ten-year mortality and morbidity related to serum cholesterol: A follow-up of 3,751 men aged 40–49. *Scand. J. Clin. Lab. Invest.* 30(Suppl. 127):1–24

Ann. Rev. Public Health. 1986. 7:493–502

THE IMPORTANCE OF OBESITY IN THE DEVELOPMENT OF CORONARY RISK FACTORS AND DISEASE: The Epidemiologic Evidence

Helen B. Hubert

General Health, Incorporated, 3299 K Street, NW, Washington DC 20007

INTRODUCTION

Coronary heart disease (CHD) is caused by a complex interaction of genetic and life-style factors that begin to exert their effects many years prior to diagnosis of the disease. Numerous epidemiologic studies in middle-aged populations have shown the importance of attributes such as elevated blood pressure and blood lipids in the etiology of CHD; as a result, intervention in high-risk individuals has been focused on reduction of risk factors with pharmacologic treatment and a modified-fat diet. While such approaches to risk reduction are important and can decrease mortality, it is also clear that optimal preventive strategies will require modification of early markers for the development of CHD, hypertension, and hyperlipidemia. The accumulated evidence strongly suggests that overweight or obesity is such a precursor to disease development and that prevention of CHD can be greatly promoted by the control of this attribute in overfed and sedentary populations such as those in North America.

THE MAJOR CORONARY RISK FACTORS

While it is difficult to prove causality in population-based research, there is little doubt that obesity and increased body weight for height are directly related to the development of a disadvantageous coronary risk profile. The criteria for causality, including temporal sequence of cause and effect, strength of association, dose-response, consistency of findings among studies, and biologic

493

0163-7525/86/0510-0493$02.00

plausibility, are well-satisfied. The fact that the pathogenetic mechanisms through which obesity operates are hypothesized but have not been definitively proven, should not be a barrier to acceptance of its obvious impact.

Total and Lipoprotein Cholesterol

Levels of total serum or plasma cholesterol marked by elevation in low-density lipoprotein cholesterol (LDL-C) and/or reduction in high-density lipoprotein cholesterol (HDL-C) are believed to be important predictors of future coronary events within population groups. Results of the Lipid Research Clinics Prevalence Study in ten North American populations have shown that measures of obesity (e.g. weight/height^2) are strongly and consistently associated with levels of HDL-C and LDL-C in children and adults of both sexes, even after adjustment for other factors known to influence lipoprotein cholesterols (15, 18, 33, 47). These and other population-based studies (7, 12, 49) indirectly suggest that increased body weight for height is independently associated with increased LDL-C and decreased HDL-C, i.e. an adverse lipoprotein pattern.

More direct evidence is found in longitudinal studies of men and women that have shown that initial degree of obesity or weight change is significantly related to change in total and lipoprotein cholesterols over time (1, 6, 22a). For example, in the Framingham Heart Study cohort, a 10% increase in relative weight, defined as an individual's weight compared to the median for his sex-height group, was associated with increases in total cholesterol of 11.3 mg/dl in men and 6.3 mg/dl in women. It is also important to note that weight change has been found to be one of the strongest and most consistent, independent life-style correlates of lipoprotein cholesterol change, particularly in healthy, young adult populations (22a). Among 20–29-year-old men in the Framingham Offspring Study (22a), the average change in LDL-C over eight years was 19.3 mg/dl greater in the highest compared to the lowest quintile of change in body mass index (kg/m^2). Among young women in this cohort the difference between quintiles was 8.8 mg/dl. These data suggest that obesity and weight gain, which are quite common in young adulthood, elevate CHD risk and that much may be gained from education and intervention during these years.

The impact of weight reduction on total and lipoprotein cholesterol change in men has been demonstrated in the Multiple Risk Factor Intervention Trial and the Coronary Primary Prevention Trial (2, 17, 31, 35). Although neither intervention study explicitly included weight reduction as a treatment modality, both trials showed that weight loss significantly and independently improved lipoprotein profiles in men at high risk for CHD, irrespective of the effects of lipid-lowering drugs or a modified-fat diet. Analyses done by Kuller et al (31) indicated that a one unit decrease in body mass index (kg/m^2), approximately 3 kg, was associated with a 1.2–1.3 mg/dl increase in HDL-C after adjustment for other correlates of HDL-C change. In the Coronary Primary Prevention Trial, decreases in LDL-C, influenced by weight reduction, were associated with reduced CHD incidence in both treatment and nontreatment groups (35, 36), suggesting that weight loss may be an effective intervention strategy with or without drug therapy. The favorable long-term effects of weight reduction on lipoproteins in women also have been demonstrated in recent clinical studies (3, 10).

Blood Pressure

The strong positive relationships of excess weight or weight change to systolic and diastolic blood pressure change and the development of hypertension over time have been well-documented in prospective epidemiologic studies of males and females of all ages (1, 9, 14, 19, 21, 25, 26, 29, 30, 39, 40). These data are collectively impressive and indicate that early prevention of weight gain may be an important key to the reduction of hypertension and its sequelae in the general population. Additional support for this point of view comes from recent findings of the Framingham Offspring Study, which indicated that subscapular skinfold measurements were significant independent predictors of hypertension in young adult men and women and that change in body mass index was the strongest modifiable life-style correlate of blood pressure change over eight years in the cohort initially 20–29 years of age (11, 22a). In this young, healthy group each unit change in body mass index (kg/m^2) was associated with approximately a 1 mm Hg change in systolic blood pressure in both men and women over time.

A review of the experimental literature further substantiates that weight loss in borderline and definite hypertensives can be an effective treatment modality (13, 20, 45) and that weight reduction in controlled hypertensives may significantly improve the success of withdrawal of drug therapy (32). In a summary of the results of controlled studies, Hovell (20) has shown that a decrease in weight of 3 kg, for example, may be associated with a 5–7 mm Hg decrease in systolic and a 3–4 mm Hg decrease in diastolic blood pressure. It is important to recognize that due to the large proportion of obese, hypertensive subjects in the experimental trials, the magnitude of the effects of weight loss is greater than would be inferred from observational studies of more hetergeneous populations. These findings are yet more impressive when viewed in conjunction with reports from studies such as the Hypertension Detection and Follow-up Program, which indicate that treatment of hypertension does result in significant reduction in coronary and total mortality over time (24).

CORONARY DISEASE INCIDENCE

Despite the compelling evidence that increased body weight for height or obesity is directly associated with the development of an adverse coronary profile and despite further data suggesting its independent influence on other cardiovascular processes (37, 38), considerable debate continues over the relative importance of obesity in the prevention of CHD. Controversy has been stimulated by epidemiologic studies that have found no "independent" influence of obesity on CHD risk and conclusions stating that excess weight is benign if it is unaccompanied by other risk factors for disease such as hypertension or hypercholesterolemia (27, 28). Attempts to compare the results from numerous studies, sometimes conducted in very dissimilar populations and with very different methodologies, have made consensus more difficult to achieve. Differences in length of follow-up, definition and distribution of obesity in populations, cohort ages, criteria for disease, and concommitant life style, cultural, and genetic influences have complicated comparative analysis.

In light of such difficulties, this review focuses on results from prospective studies in North American populations in which longitudinal observation was continued for a minimum of four to five years (Table 1). Published reports of these studies, conducted primarily in men, present data that consistently show a graded, linear relationship between some obesity measure and CHD morbidity or mortality or show associations that are significant ($p \leq 0.05$) or marginally significant ($p \leq 0.10$) on univariate or age-adjusted analysis (4, 5, 16, 22, 23, 27, 28, 34, 41–44, 46, 48). In the Manitoba Study (44), for example, men whose body mass index (kg/m^2) was 22.6–25.0 experienced almost twice the risk of CHD over 26 years compared to those whose body mass index was less than 22.6. Risk at indices of 25.1–27.5 and 27.5 or more was 2.4 and 2.8 times that of leaner men. The only notable exception is found in a study of the Chicago Peoples Gas Company (8), in which investigators reported a significant quadratic relationship between body mass index and CHD mortality in men.

Results of multivariate analyses that are adjusted for the influence of other CHD risk factors reveal significant independent relationships between obesity and outcomes primarily in the younger cohorts studied (Table 1; 4, 16, 22, 23, 43, 44). The Pooling Project data suggest that in 40–49-year-old men a 10% increase in Metropolitan relative weight, an individual's actual compared to his "desirable" weight defined by the 1959 Metropolitan Life Insurance Company tables, would be associated with a 13–19% increase in disease incidence (43). Analyses of Framingham and Manitoba data specifically indicate that the impact of being overweight was most evident in those who were studied prior to middle age and were followed for an extended period of time (22, 44). In Framingham, a 10% increase in Metropolitan relative weight was independently associated with a 13% increase in CHD among males and an 8% increase among females. It is particularly noteworthy that obesity in younger Framingham Study participants (i.e. those under 50 years of age) still conveyed an increased risk of CHD even when unaccompanied by borderline or definite hypertension, hypercholesterolemia, cigarette smoking, glucose intolerance.

Table 1 Obesity or overweight and CHD incidence: Results of prospective epidemiological studies in North American populations studied more than four years

Study	Population size	Age at baseline (yrs)	Weight measure	Follow-up duration (yrs)	Number of events	Linear dose-response evident	Univariate or age-adjusted analysis				Variables included	Multivariate analysis			
							Total CHD	MI	AP	CHD Dth		Total CHD	MI	AP	CHD Dth
Framingham Study (22, 23)	2252 (M)	28–62	% of 1959 MLI	26	653 CHD	yes	*	*	*	*	Age, systolic bp, cholesterol, ECG-LVH, smoking, glucose intol.	*	–	*	*
	2818 (F)		desirable W		452		*	*	*	*		*	*	*	*
	1502 (M)	34–68	subscapular skinfolds	20	375		*	*	*	*		*	*	*	*
Manitoba Study (44)	3983 (M)	15–64 (mean=31)	W/H^2	26	390 CHD	yes	*	*	–[a]	*[b]	Age, systolic bp, diastolic bp	*	*		*[b]
Minneapolis Businessmen (28)	279 (M)	47–57	sum of skinfolds	20	60 CHD 42 MI	yes	+	+[c]			Systolic bp, cholesterol, smoking, cold pressor	–	–[c]		
San Francisco Longshore-men (41)	3263 (M)	35–64	above/below mean W for H	16	291 CHD dth	no data				*					

Table 1 (continued)

Study	Population size	Age at baseline (yrs)	Weight measure	Follow-up duration (yrs)	Number of events	Linear dose-response evident	Univariate or age-adjusted analysis				Multivariate analysis				
							Total CHD	MI	AP	CHD Dth	Variables included	Total CHD	MI	AP	CHD Dth
Los Angeles Civil Servants (4)	354 (M)	30–39	H / 3√W̄	15	16 MI	yes (all ages combined)	no tests				Age, systolic bp, diastolic bp, cholesterol		*d	−a	
	382 (M)	40–49			13 AP								−d	*a	
	389 (M)	50–59			54 MI								−d	−a	
	160 (M)	60–70			32 MI								−d	−a	
Chicago Peoples Gas (8)	1233 (M)	40–59	W / H²	14	88 CHD dth	quadratic									
American Cancer Society (34)	336,442 (M)	30–89	% of average W	12–13	? CHD dth	yes	no tests								
	419,060 (F)														
Pooling Project (43)	2170 (M)	40–44	% of 1959 MLI desirable W	8.6 (average)	114 MI	yes (all ages combined)		*d			Diastolic bp, cholesterol, smoking		*d		
	2121 (M)	45–49			200			*d					*d		
	1938 (M)	50–54			225			−d							
	826 (M)	55–59			104			−d							
Western Collaborative (46)	2249 (M)	39–49	W / H²	8.5	145 CHD	no data	−				Age, systolic bp, cholesterol, smoking, exercise, Type A, education	+			
	905 (M)	50–59			112		*								

Study	N	Age	Measure of obesity		CHD outcome	Data on CHD			Variables adjusted for	
Build Study 1979 (49)	3,500,000 (M) 500,000 (F)	15–69	% of average W	6.6 (average)	25,853 CHD dth 1.338	yes		no tests		
Tecumseh (5)	3643 (M & F)	≥ 30	ratio actual to predicted W	6	45 sudden CHD dth	no data				*[b]
US Railroad (27)	2442 (M)	40–59	sum of skinfolds	5	212 CHD 79 MI	yes	*	−[c]	Age, systolic bp, cholesterol, smoking, exercise	−
Normative Aging Study (16)	1021 (M)	28–52	W/H^2	5	25 CHD	yes	*		$\triangle$ cholesterol, $\triangle$ systolic bp, cholesterol, systolic bp, smoking	*
Western Electric (42)	1989 (M)	40–55	subscapular skinfolds	4.5	88 CHD	no data	*			

Abbreviations used: *p ≤ 0.05; +p ≤ 0.10; − not statistically significant; CHD = Coronary heart disease; MI = Myocardial infarction; AP = Angina pectoris; Dth = Death; W = Weight; H = Height; M = Male; F = Female, MLI = Metropolitan Life Insurance Co.
[a]Without other CHD.
[b]Sudden CHD death only.
[c]Includes CHD death.
[d]Includes sudden CHD death.

or left ventricular hypertrophy. Further analyses indicated that weight gain between age 25 and into middle and older ages in Framingham was associated with a significantly increased risk of disease, particularly among men, which could not be attributed to either the initial weight or the levels of the risk factors that may have resulted from weight change. Increases in Metropolitan relative weight of 10 and 20% resulted in 17 and 37% increases in CHD among Framingham males. Although few other longitudinal, population-based studies are available for comparison, the accumulated evidence strongly suggests that obesity is an important risk factor for premature CHD in the general population.

DISEASE PREVENTION

Although the process that leads to the development of symptomatic CHD remains uncertain, it appears that obesity or increased body weight for height plays a major fundamental role. The available evidence concerning the pronounced effects of obesity on the major CHD risk factors; its reported independent influence on such processes as cardiovascular hemodynamics, intravascular volume, fibrinolytic activity, and plasma fibrinogen concentrations; and its contribution to premature CHD incidence cannot be overlooked. It is clear that preventive strategies that include successful weight control need to be developed and supported.

Literature Cited

1. Ashley, F. W., Kannel, W. B. 1974. Relation of weight change to changes in atherogenic traits: The Framingham Study. *J. Chron. Dis.* 27:103–14
2. Caggiula, A. W., Christakis, G., Farrand, M., Hulley, S. B., Johnson, R., et al. 1981. The Multiple Risk Factor Intervention Trial (MRFIT). IV. Intervention on blood lipids. *Prev. Med.* 10:443–75
3. Carmena, R., Ascaso, J. F., Tebar, J., Soriano, J. 1984. Changes in plasma high-density lipoproteins after body weight reduction in obese women. *Int. J. Obesity* 8:135–40
4. Chapman, J. M., Coulson, A. H., Clark, V. A., Borun, E. R. 1971. The differential effect of serum cholesterol, blood pressure and weight on the incidence of myocardial infarction and angina pectoris. *J. Chron. Dis.* 23:631–45
5. Chiang, B. N., Perlman, L. V., Fulton, M., Ostrander, L. D., Epstein, F. H. 1970. Predisposing factors in sudden cardiac death in Tecumseh, Michigan: A prospective study. *Circulation* 41:31–37
6. Criqui, M. H., Frankville, D. D., Barrett-Conner, E., Klauber, M. R., Holdbrook, M. J., et al. 1983. Change and correlates of change in high and low density lipoprotein cholesterol after six years: A prospective study. *Am. J. Epidemiol.* 118:52–59
7. Donahue, R. P., Orchard, T. J., Kuller, L. H., Drash, A. L. 1985. Lipids and lipoproteins in a young adult population: The Beaver County Lipid Study. *Am. J. Epidemiol.* 122:458–67
8. Dyer, A. R., Stamler, J., Berkson, D. M., Lindberg, H. A. 1975. Relationship of relative weight and body mass index to 14-year mortality in the Chicago Peoples Gas Company Study. *J. Chron. Dis.* 28:109–23
9. Dyer, A. R., Stamler, J., Shekelle, R. B., Schoenberger, J. A., Stamler, R., et al. 1982. Relative weight and blood pressure in four Chicago epidemiologic studies. *J. Chron. Dis.* 35:897–908
10. Follick, M. J., Abrams, D. B., Smith, T. W., Henderson, L. O., Herbert, P. N. 1984. Contrasting short- and long-term effects of weight loss on lipoprotein levels. *Arch. Intern. Med.* 144:1571–74

11. Garrison, R. J., Kannel, W. B., Stokes, J., Castelli, W. P. 1985. Incidence and precursors of hypertension in young adults: The Framingham Offspring Study. *CVD Epidemiol. Newslett.* 37:41 (Abstr.)

12. Garrison, R. J., Wilson, P. W., Castelli, W. P., Feinleib, M., Kannel, W. B., et al. 1980. Obesity and lipoprotein cholesterol in the Framingham Offspring Study. *Metabolism* 29:1053–60

13. Gillum, R. F., Prineas, R. J., Jeffery, R. W., Jacobs, D. R., Elmer, P. J., et al. 1983. Nonpharmacologic therapy of hypertension: The independent effects of weight reduction and sodium restriction in overweight borderline hypertensive patients. *Am. Heart J.* 105:128–33

14. Gillum, R. F., Taylor, H. L., Brozek, J., Polansky, P., Blackburn, H. 1982. Indices of obesity and blood pressure in young men followed 32 years. *J. Chron. Dis.* 35:211–19

15. Glueck, C. J., Taylor, H. L., Jacobs, D., Morrison, J. A., Beaglehole, R., et al. 1980. Plasma high-density lipoprotein cholesterol: Association with measurements of body mass. The Lipid Research Clinics Program Prevalence Study. *Circulation* 62 (Suppl. IV): IV-62–IV-69

16. Glynn, R. J., Rosner, B., Silbert, J. E. 1982. Changes in cholesterol and triglyceride as predictors of ischemic heart disease in men. *Circulation* 66:724–31

17. Gordon, D. J., Salz, K. M., Roggenkamp, K. J., Franklin, F. A. 1982. Dietary determinants of plasma cholesterol change in the recruitment phase of the Lipid Research Clinics Coronary Primary Prevention Trial. *Arteriosclerosis* 2:537–48

18. Heiss, G., Johnson, N. J., Reiland, S., Davis, C. E., Tyroler, H. A. 1980. The epidemiology of plasma high-density lipoprotein cholesterol levels. The Lipid Research Clinics Program Prevalence Study. Summary. *Circulation* 62 (Suppl. IV): IV-116–IV-136

19. Higgins, M. W., Keller, J. B., Metzner, H. L., Moore, F. E., Ostrander, L. D. 1980. Studies of blood pressure in Tecumseh, Michigan. II. Antecedents in childhood of high blood pressure in young adults. *Hypertension* 2 (Suppl. I): I-117–I-123

20. Hovell, M. F. 1982. The experimental evidence for weight-loss treatment of essential hypertension: A critical review. *Am. J. Public Health* 72:359–68

21. Hsu, P. H., Mathewson, F. A. L., Rabkin, S. W. 1977. Blood pressure and body mass index patterns—a longitudinal study. *J. Chron. Dis.* 30:93–113

22. Hubert, H. B., Castelli, W. P. 1985. Obesity as a predictor of coronary heart disease. In *Dietary Treatment and Prevention of Obesity,* ed. R. T. Frankle, J. Dwyer, L. Moragne, A. Owen, pp. 125–35. London: Libbey

22a. Hubert, H. B., Eaker, E. D., Garrison, R. J., Castelli, W. P. 1986. Life-style correlates of risk factor change in young adults: An eight year study of coronary heart disease risk factors in the Framingham offspring. Submitted for publication

23. Hubert, H. B., Feinleib, M., McNamara, P. M., Castelli, W. P. 1983. Obesity as an independent risk factor for cardiovascular disease: A 26-year follow-up of participants in the Framingham Heart Study. *Circulation* 67:968–77

24. Hypertension Detection and Follow-up Program Cooperative Group. 1979. Five-year findings of the Hypertension Detection and Follow-up Program. I. Reduction in mortality of persons with high blood pressure, including mild hypertension. *J. Am. Med. Assoc.* 242:2562–71

25. Johnson, B. C., Karunas, T. M., Epstein, F. H. 1973. Longitudinal change in blood pressure in individuals, families and social groups. *Clin. Sci. Mol. Med.* 45:35s–45s

26. Kannel, W. B., Brand, N., Skinner, J. J., Dawber, T. R., McNamara, P. M. 1967. The relation of adiposity to blood pressure and development of hypertension: The Framingham Study. *Ann. Intern. Med.* 67:48–59

27. Keys, A., Aravanis, C., Blackburn, H., Van Buchem, F. S. P., Buzina, R., et al. 1972. Coronary heart disease: Overweight and obesity as risk factors. *Ann. Intern. Med.* 77:15–27

28. Keys, A., Taylor, H. L., Blackburn, H., Brozek, J., Anderson, J. T., et al. 1971. Mortality and coronary heart disease among men studied for 23 years. *Arch. Intern. Med.* 128:201–14

29. Kotchen, J. M., Kotchen, T. A., Guthrie, G. P., Cottrill, C. M., McKean, H. E. 1980. Correlates of adolescent blood pressure at five-year follow-up. *Hypertension* 2 (Suppl. I):I-124–I-129

30. Kuller, L. H., Crook, M., Almes, M. J., Detre, K., Reese, G., et al. 1980. Dormont High School (Pittsburgh, Pennsylvania) Blood Pressure Study. *Hypertension* 2 (Suppl. I):I-109–I-116

31. Kuller, L. H., Hulley, S. B., LaPorte, R. E., Neaton, J., Dai, W. S. 1983. Environmental determinants, liver function, and high density lipoprotein cholesterol levels. *Am. J. Epidemiol.* 117:406–18

32. Langford, H. G., Blaufox, M. D., Ober-

man, A., Hawkins, C. M., Curb, J. D., et al. 1985. Dietary therapy slows the return of hypertension after stopping prolonged medication. *J. Am. Med. Assoc.* 253:657–64

33. Laskarzewski, P., Morrison, J. A., Mellies, M. J., Kelly, K., Gartside, P. S., et al. 1980. Relationships of measurements of body mass to plasma lipoproteins in schoolchildren and adults. *Am. J. Epidemiol.* 111:395–406

34. Lew, E. A., Garfinkel, L. 1979. Variations in mortality by weight among 750,000 men and women. *J. Chron. Dis.* 32:563–76

35. Lipid Research Clinics Program. 1985. Relationships between changes in diet and changes in total and low density lipoprotein cholesterol in hypercholesterolemic men: The diet plus placebo group of the Lipid Research Clinics Coronary Primary Prevention Trial. *CVD Epidemiol. Newslett.* 37:29 (Abstr.)

36. Lipid Research Clinics Program. 1985. Relationships between reductions in coronary heart disease and in low density lipoprotein cholesterol in hypercholesterolemic men: The diet plus placebo group of the Lipid Research Clinics Coronary Primary Prevention Trial. *CVD Epidemiol. Newslett.* 37:28 (Abstr.)

37. Meade, T. W., Chakrabarti, R., Haines, A. P., North, W. R. S., Stirling, Y. 1979. Characteristics affecting fibrinolytic activity and plasma fibrinogen concentrations. *Br. Med. J.* 1:153–56

38. Messerli, F. H., Sundgaard-Riise, K., Reisin, E., Dreslinski, G., Dunn, F. G., et al. 1983. Disparate cardiovascular effects of obesity and arterial hypertension. *Am. J. Med.* 74:808–12

39. Noppa, H. 1980. Body weight change in relation to incidence of ischemic heart disease and change in risk factors for ischemic heart disease. *Am. J. Epidemiol.* 111:693–704

40. Oberman, A., Lane, N. E., Harlan, W. R., Graybiel, A., Mitchell, R. E. 1967. Trends in systolic blood pressure in the Thousand Aviator cohort over a twenty-four-year period. *Circulation* 36:812–22

41. Paffenbarger, R. S., Laughlin, M. E., Gima, A. S., Black, R. A. 1970. Work activity of longshoremen as related to death from coronary heart disease and stroke. *N. Engl. J. Med.* 282:1109–14

42. Paul, O., Lepper, M. H., Phelan, W. H., Dupertuis, G. W., MacMillan, A., et al. 1963. A longitudinal study of coronary heart disease. *Circulation* 28:20–31

43. Pooling Project Research Group. 1978. Relationship of blood pressure, serum cholesterol, smoking habit, relative weight and ECG abnormalities to incidence of major coronary events: Final report of the Pooling Project. *J. Chron. Dis.* 31:201–306

44. Rabkin, S. W., Mathewson, F. A. L., Hsu, P. H. 1977. Relation of body weight to development of ischemic heart disease in a cohort of young North American men after a 26 year observation period: The Manitoba Study. *Am. J. Cardiol.* 39: 452–58

45. Reisin, E., Frohlich, E. D. 1982. Effects of weight reduction on arterial pressure. *J. Chron. Dis.* 35:887–91

46. Rosenman, R. H., Brand, R. J., Sholtz, R. I., Friedman, M. 1976. Multivariate prediction of coronary heart disease during 8.5 year follow-up in the Western Collaborative Group Study. *Am. J. Cardiol.* 37:903–10

47. Schwarz, W., Trost, D. C., Reiland, S. L., Rifkind, B. M., Heiss, G. 1982. Correlates of low density lipoprotein cholesterol: Associations with physical, chemical, dietary, and behavioral characteristics. The Lipid Research Clinics Prevalence Study. *Arteriosclerosis* 2: 513–22

48. Society of Actuaries and Association of Life Insurance Medical Directors of America. 1980. *Build Study 1979.* Chicago: Soc. Actuaries

49. Wilson, P. W. F., Garrison, R. J., Abbott, R. D., Castelli, W. P. 1983. Factors associated with lipoprotein cholesterol levels: The Framingham Study. *Arteriosclerosis* 3:273–81

Ann. Rev. Public Health. 1986. 7:503–19

DIETARY ASPECTS OF THE TREATMENT OF HYPERTENSION

Norman M. Kaplan

Department of Internal Medicine, University of Texas Southwestern Medical School, Dallas, Texas 75235

Hypertension may or may not be more common today than in the past, distant or recent. Regardless, it is the most prevalent risk factor for premature cardiovascular disease, and, since cardiovascular diseases are the leading cause of death in the United States and all industrialized countries, hypertension can correctly be called our major public health problem (24).

As seen in Figure 1, the total estimated hypertensive population in the United States now numbers some 30 million people. Though some would add another 20 or more million to this number by including all with diastolic levels between 90 and 95 mm Hg, as well as those between 85 and 90, I believe the criteria used in the NHANES study—systolic above 160 and/or diastolic above 95 mm Hg—are more appropriate, since as many as one third of those with diastolic readings above 95 mm Hg are below 90 mm Hg on repeated readings (25). I do not address further the issue about variability of the blood pressure. I raise the issue simply to remind all interested in Public Health that there is no benefit and a great deal of potential harm in the use of such loose criteria as to label and treat many who are not and never will be hypertensive.

Beyond the number of hypertensives, the percentages given in Figure 1 on the number of hypertensives on therapy and under adequate control must disturb all who have been lulled into assuming that the war on hypertension has been won because of the marked fall in death rates for both heart attack and stroke that have occurred since 1968. Despite all of the efforts expended against it over the past 25 years, hypertension remains frequently untreated and infrequently well controlled.

503

0163-7525/86/0510-0503$02.00

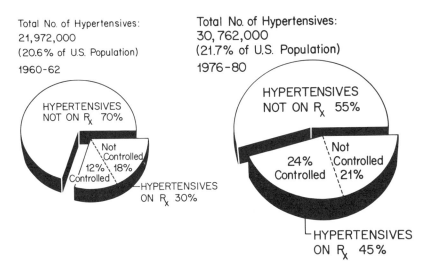

Total No. of Hypertensives:
21,972,000
(20.6% of U.S. Population)
1960-62

HYPERTENSIVES
NOT ON R$_X$ 70%

Not
Controlled
12% 18%
Controlled

HYPERTENSIVES
ON R$_X$ 30%

Total No. of Hypertensives:
30,762,000
(21.7% of U.S. Population)
1976-80

HYPERTENSIVES
NOT ON R$_X$ 55%

Not
24% Controlled
Controlled 21%

HYPERTENSIVES
ON R$_X$ 45%

Figure 1   The estimated total number of hypertensive people aged 18 to 74 in the United States in 1960–1962 (based on the National Health Examination Survey I) and in 1976–1980 (based on the National Health and Nutrition Examination Survey II). Hypertension was defined as systolic blood pressure equal to or greater than 160 mm Hg, and/or diastolic blood pressure equal to or greater than 95 mm Hg, and/or taking antihypertensive medication. Hypertension was defined as "controlled" if systolic blood pressure was below 160 mm Hg and diastolic below 95. These readings were the first one taken in each survey.

THE SEARCH FOR A CAUSE

Much of this effort has been directed toward the search for a cause for what is called *essential, primary,* or *idiopathic hypertension,* the diagnosis in over 95% of those found to have a persistently elevated blood pressure. Though a great deal has been learned about the pathophysiology of primary hypertension and plausible sets of hypotheses have been put forward to explain its pathogenesis, we are still unable to remove the adjective "idiopathic" from its description. Nonetheless, evidence continues to accrue that points toward dietary factors, both in pathogenesis and in therapy. The evidence concerning pathogenesis is still not strong enough to mandate dietary changes in the population at large, since we still lack a method to identify the 20% who are destined to become hypertensive.

Changes in diet are increasingly advocated for those who are hypertensive, however, not only because of the evidence that certain changes lower the blood pressure but also because of concern about the ever increasing use of preventative medications that present additional risks while reducing the risk from elevated blood pressure.

THE USE OF DIETARY CHANGE FOR THERAPY

In this paper I review the current status of dietary factors in the treatment of hypertension, leaving discussion of the role of diet in pathogenesis for the future, when it is hoped that knowledge will be sufficient to mandate preventative changes in diet. In the meantime, those who advocate dietary change both for therapy and for prevention need not apologize for their advocacy in the absence of such certainty. What is being advocated is simply a return toward what our ancestors consumed, which the human physiology has likely evolved over millenia to handle (11) (Table 1). From Table 1, notice how much modern man has altered his protein, fat, sodium, potassium, and calcium intake. Most of this change has probably occurred over the last few hundred years since less natural and more processed foods have been in our diets. These alterations have played a significant role in the rather recent epidemic of coronary disease. A return to a more natural diet can only be of benefit (61).

As I have observed elsewhere (26), the advocacy of these dietary changes can be defended against the claim, valid though it may be, that there is little proof that they will maintain a lower blood pressure and no proof that they will protect against premature cardiovascular disease. Such changes should do no harm to those who do not need them and they may provide a great deal of benefit to those who do.

Before examining the specific recommended dietary changes, two more general aspects about their use should be noted. One is the rather common feeling among practitioners that they are both ineffectual and difficult to implement. As I noted (26),

The lack of confidence in the effectiveness of non-drug therapies also represents a reaction by physicians against the overly-enthusiastic advocacy of these maneuvers by 'true believers,' quacks, and health gurus who promise major benefits, with no supporting evidence. Most

Table 1 Comparison of the late Paleolithic diet and the current American diet[a]

	Late Paleolithic diet (assuming 35% meat)	Current American diet
Total dietary energy (%)		
Protein	34	12
Carbohydrate	45	46
Fat	21	42
P : S ratio	1.41	0.44
Sodium (mg)	690	3500
Potassium (mg)	11000	2400
K/Na ratio	16:1	0.7:1
Calcium	1580	740

[a] (Data from Ref. 11).

physicians are suspicious of the claims of long-term benefits from non-drug therapies and are unwilling to spend the time and effort needed to implement non-drug therapies in the absence of proof of their efficacy.

The second point relates to the first: Most of the evidence about the anti-hypertensive efficacy of dietary changes is methodologically weak, with relatively small numbers of patients studied for short periods under uncontrolled circumstances. Even when comparisons are made between a dietary change and the current diet, few studies have used random assignment of patients carefully screened over a six-week or longer run-in period and some type of blinding of both subjects and investigators.

Here again, I "will not address further the more philosophical issues about the intrinsic value of self-help and the need for a re-structured physician-patient relationship which are involved in the use of non-drug therapies. These arguments are strong justifications for their use but they remain purely theoretical in the absence of evidence that these therapies work in the real world" (26).

CALORIC RESTRICTION

Blood pressure usually increases with a gain in weight. People with a body weight 20% or more above ideal have a frequency of hypertension about two times higher than do the nonobese (17). The manner by which weight gain induces hypertension is unknown, though cardiac output tends to be elevated more than peripheral resistance. Blood pressure usually falls with a loss in weight.

Though the evidence concerning the effect of weight loss on hypertension is generally considered to be very strong (49), few controlled studies have documented the effects (26). Of ten studies reported since 1954, eight were parallel in design but only one (49) involved a group randomly assigned to a diet and managed similarly to another group not given a diet.

In only four of the studies was weight loss clearly dissociated from dietary sodium restriction (50, 9. 13. 36). In two studies, significant weight loss without sodium restriction was accompanied by either no fall in blood pressure (9) or less of a fall (13) than when sodium was restricted. The study that most clearly demonstrated the effectiveness of weight loss without sodium restriction (49) unfortunately did not monitor the sodium intake closely and used a low calorie diet that was not designed to maintain a fixed level of sodium intake. Two more recent studies, however, showed that weight loss is antihypertensive in the absence of dietary sodium restriction (50, 36).

Weight loss, then, likely exerts an independent antihypertensive effect. Unfortunately, the achievement and maintenance of significant weight loss is rare (63). In all studies published from 1966 to 1977, the average weight loss was 5.4 kg and only about 20% lost more than 9 kg. Though perhaps more people have successfully lost weight than those involved in special weight-loss programs, the overall long-term success rate is probably no better than 20% even with multidisciplinary programs (45). The problem may relate to diminished energy requirements in obese patients after they have lost weight.

In summary, weight loss, though fairly easy to achieve, seldom lasts; however, even small amounts of weight loss will often lower the blood pressure. It seems logical to use the likelihood of a fall in blood pressure to further motivate obese hypertensives to reduce their calorie intake. The observation of a falling blood pressure along with the falling weight should help keep them on a diet (26).

SODIUM RESTRICTION

The epidemiological and experimental evidence relating a high sodium intake to the development of hypertension is strong; a marked reduction of sodium intake has long been known to decrease blood pressure significantly (7). In the 1970s, more modest sodium restriction was shown to reduce the blood pressure, but the studies were, in general, poorly controlled, neither randomized nor blinded, and often admixed with diuretic therapy (26).

More carefully controlled trials have been published recently (14, 37, 51, 10, 1) (Table 2). Two (34, 62) were similar in design, with small groups of patients initially placed on a diet containing 60 to 100 mmol per day of sodium and then randomly assigned in a double-blind, cross-over design to take either sodium chloride capsules to return sodium intake back to the pre-study level or identical-appearing placebo capsules.

In both studies, the average blood pressure fell significantly during the lower sodium periods, 12/6 mm Hg in MacGregor et al's (34), 10/5 in Watt et al's study (62). The pressures returned almost to the pre-study level when sodium chloride was added in MacGregor et al's study, whereas the pressures were the same during both the lower and higher sodium periods in the study by Watt et al. The different results could reflect different patients and protocols. Overall, MacGregor et al's study was methodologically stronger. In a similar manner, the overall failure to observe an antihypertensive effect of moderate sodium restriction reported in the study by Richards et al (52) may also reflect weaknesses in the experimental design, including the small number of subjects (26).

On the other hand, the other two studies shown in Table 2 involved a parallel design, with patients randomly placed into a lower-sodium or a control group. In the study by Silman et al (57), significant falls in blood pressure were noted over the 52 weeks, but the differences between the two groups were not statistically different. Once again, methodological problems may have been responsible, including the marked variability in the infrequently measured blood pressures, since the difference of 9/7 mm Hg in this study was statistically

Table 2 Studies of moderate sodium restriction in mild hypertension

Ref.	No. patients	Pre-therapy BP monitoring	Design	Urinary sodium Low sodium	Urinary sodium High sodium	Blood pressure (mm Hg) Initial	Change Low sodium	Change High sodium
(34)	19	2 mo.	random, crossover, blind (4-wk periods)	86	162	156/98	−12/6	−2/1
(62)	13	2 wk	random, crossover, blind (4-wk periods)	59	139	150/91	−10/5	−10/5
(52)	12	> 10 d	random, crossover (4–6-wk periods)	80	180	150/92	−5/2	
(57)								
Diet	12	1 mo.	parallel (52 wk)	117		165/98	−29/18	
Control	16				159	160/98		−20/11
(3)								
Diet + R_x	45	none	parallel (12 wk)	37		142/88	−11/6[a]	
Diet + R_x	45				161	139/86		−6/3[a]

[a] The diet group were able to reduce their daily total number tablets of antihypertensive drugs from 163 to 75, whereas the control group reduced theirs only from 146 to 140.

insignificant but a difference of 10/5 mm Hg in MacGregor's shorter and more frequently monitored study was significant at the $p < 0.01$ level (34).

The study by Beard et al (3) involved 90 hypertensives who remained on various antihypertensive drugs for 12 weeks, during which time half sharply reduced their dietary sodium intake to an average of only 37 mmol per day. This group had a greater fall in blood pressure despite the purposeful discontinuation of more than half of their daily total number of antihypertensive tablets, whereas the control group had to remain on almost the full amount of medication to achieve a lesser fall in blood pressure.

Not all hypertensives have a fall in blood pressure on a reduced sodium intake diet. Though there may be two populations, one sodium sensitive, the other sodium resistant (29), there is more likely a continuum of responsiveness, with a greater response usually observed in older people, in those with higher levels of blood pressure, and in those who have a lesser rise in renin-aldosterone levels (31).

Even if blood pressure does not fall, there is no apparent potential for harm from moderate sodium restriction to a level of 75 to 100 mmol per day, which should be easily achieved by deleting most high sodium foods from the diet and adding no extra sodium at the table or in the cooking. More rigid sodium restriction, to a level below 50 mmol per day, may be impractical for patients to achieve; it may also stimulate the renin-angiotensin and sympathetic nervous systems and therefore limit both the antihypertensive and potassium-sparing effects of more moderate sodium restriction (48).

Adherence to a diet moderately restricted in sodium should be helped by convenient monitoring of urinary sodium chloride levels (28) and the increasing availability of processed foods that either are low in sodium or list sodium content on their labels. Of particular interest is the finding that the taste preference for sodium decreases after three months of such a moderately reduced (77 mmol per day) intake (4), so such a diet should be more acceptable with time.

Potential for Prevention

In addition to the likelihood that moderate sodium restriction will lower the blood pressure of those with hypertension, there is hope that it might prevent the development of the disease if started early enough. In a study of almost 500 infants in Belgium, the half given one half as much sodium as usual for the first six months of life had a significantly lower blood pressure at the end of the six months than did those given the usual amount (20). Moreover, a group of young, borderline hypertensives given a diet with 50 to 85 mmol of sodium per day for six weeks had a decrease in two features that may be involved in the pathogenesis of the disease: the intracellular concentration of sodium and the pressor responsiveness to stress (2).

In summary, then, moderate restriction of sodium intake may prevent or delay the development of hypertension; however, even if that turns out not to be true, there seems good reason to encourage all hypertensives to reduce the unnaturally high levels of sodium intake that we have only recently begun to consume. Since the taste preference we acquire for sodium has been shown to diminish after a few months of dietary restriction, there should be no permanent discomfort and, potentially, considerable benefit from moderate sodium reduction (26).

POTASSIUM SUPPLEMENTATION

Many of the reported benefits of a reduced sodium intake may reflect an increased potassium intake, since whenever sodium is deleted from the diet by the substitution of natural foods for processed products, potassium intake will increase. Some have long held that the high ratio of sodium to potassium in the diet is the important factor in the development of hypertension, and that the reversal of this ratio back to that consumed by more primitive man would both prevent and relieve hypertension (39). Some evidence supports this view: blood pressure was inversely correlated with dietary intake and urinary excretion of potassium in blacks (but not whites) living in Evans County, Georgia (16). Among 91 hypertensive patients, an inverse correlation was noted among plasma, exchangeable and total body potassium, and the blood pressure (33). The lower blood pressure of vegetarians has been ascribed to their large intake of potassium (42).

Controlled Trials

The intake of additional potassium has been shown to lower the blood pressure—some time ago in rather poorly controlled trials, more recently in somewhat better controlled ones (52, 41, 21, 35, 59, 43) (Table 3). MacGregor et al used a long run-in period and a random, cross-over, double-blind design, but most of these studies were of short duration and open design. They show a uniform, albeit limited, fall in blood pressure by the addition of from 64 to 175 mmol of extra potassium a day. However, half of the 12 patients studied by Richards et al had some rise in their intra-arterial diastolic blood pressures after potassium supplementation. More recently, the addition of 64 mmol per day of potassium was found to have no additive antihypertensive effect beyond that observed when the patients were given a diet moderately restricted in sodium (58).

Even more recently, we have found that the correction of diuretic-induced hypokalemia by the intake of 60 mmol of KCl per day for six weeks did have a significant antihypertensive effect in 9 of 16 hypokalemic hypertensives (27). Regardless of the results of this carefully controlled trial and the other data shown in Table 3, "the potential hazards and considerable cost of large amounts of potassium supplements make this practice unacceptable. A more sensible

Table 3 Studies of potassium supplementation in mild hypertension

Ref.	No. patients	Pre-therapy BP monitoring	Design	Urinary excretion of potassium		Blood pressure (mm Hg)	
				Control	Added KCL	Initial	Change
(21)	20	2 wk	open; 10 d of diet with 25 or 175 mmol KCL	41	123	114 (MAP)	−11 (MAP)
(41)	8	4 wk	open; 2 wk of 70 mmol KCl	46	113	158/101	−10/8
(35)	23	2 mo	random, crossover, double-blind; 4 wk each of placebo or 64 mmol KCl	68	118	154/99	−6/4 vs +1/0 placebo
(59)	10	1 wk	open; 12 d of 96 mmol KCl	65	128	156/93	−8/2
(43)	16	4 wk	open, 8 wk of 100 mmol KCl	66	153	152/98	−17/10
(52)	12	> 10 d	random, crossover; 4–6 wk each of control, low sodium or extra potassium	@60	@200	150/92	−2/1

approach is to reduce the intake of high sodium–low potassium processed foods and increase the intake of low sodium–high potassium natural foods. In addition, KCl should be partially substituted for NaCl in cooking and at the table" (26).

CALCIUM SUPPLEMENTATION

Too much calcium in the blood or vascular tissue may be involved in the pathogenesis of hypertension. The increased peripheral vascular tone of essential hypertension may be the consequence of increased intracellular calcium. The free calcium level within blood platelets of patients with essential hypertension, elevated in close correlation to the level of the blood pressure, fell after successful lowering of the blood pressure by various antihypertensive agents (12).

Nonetheless, the intake of too little, not too much, calcium may be associated with hypertension, and oral calcium supplements may lower, not raise, the blood pressure (37). The blood pressure fell after supplementation of the diet with 1 g per day of elemental calcium, both in normal pregnant women (6) and in normal young adults (5). When data obtained from a one-day diet recall performed in the National Health and Nutrition Examination Survey were analyzed, the hypertensives were found to have a 19.6% lower estimated calcium intake (38). However, the validity of these data, despite their large number, has been questioned (14), particularly in view of some other inexplicable findings, including a progressively lower caloric intake among those with increasingly greater obesity, and an average reported sodium intake about one half of that found by more accurate 24 hour urine measurements.

Preliminary data suggest an antihypertensive effect of supplemental calcium in patients with essential hypertension (37, 51). In Resnick et al's study, 15 subjects were given 2 g per day of calcium carbonate for five months. In McCarron & Morris' study, 32 hypertensives took either 1 g per day of elemental oral calcium or placebo for eight weeks each in a randomized, double-blind, cross-over trial. In both studies, about half of the patients given calcium had a significant fall in blood pressure.

The evidence remains incomplete. A number of possible abnormalities in calcium homeostasis may be at work in essential hypertension, and much more evidence is needed. "For now, the wisest course may be to ensure that, in the attempt to reduce dietary sodium and cholesterol, the dietary sources of calcium, mainly milk and cheese, not be reduced but the lower-fat and lower-sodium forms of these should be used. Since many people are likely not ingesting an adequate amount of calcium, some increase in calcium intake should be helpful in reducing osteoporosis if not hypertension" (26).

MAGNESIUM SUPPLEMENTATION

The administration of magnesium may also lower the blood pressure (45). In one study, 39 hypertensive patients were randomly assigned to receive 15 mmol per day of magnesium as aspartate hydrochloride for six months, or to serve as controls. Nineteen of the 20 given magnesium had a fall in supine blood pressure, averaging 12/8 mm Hg, whereas the average fell 0/4 mm Hg in the controls.

Magnesium plays a major role in the control of vascular tone. When extracellular magnesium is lowered, the influx of calcium into cells is enhanced, causing contraction (1), and when magnesium is infused into human subjects, vasodilation is induced that is comparable to that seen with calcium entry blockade (22).

Based upon the experimental evidence, there is obviously a need for more clinical data. In the meantime, hypomagnesemia, which is frequently induced by diuretic therapy, should be avoided and corrected. Whether the chronic administration of extra magnesium to people with presumably normal magnesium levels will lower the blood pressure remains to be seen (26).

OTHER DIETARY CHANGES

There is no convincing evidence for a role of trace elements in the pathogenesis or treatment of hypertension (55) beyond rare instances of the induction of hypertension by exposure to toxic heavy metals.

Fat and Fatty Acids

A few controlled studies have shown that the blood pressure may fall in response to a decrease in total fat along with an increase in polyunsaturated fat. In North Karelia, Finland, 57 couples were randomly allocated to three different diets for six-week intervals: one group continued their usual diet, the second reduced their daily sodium intake from 192 mmol to 77 mmol, the third reduced daily total fat intake from 108 g to 52 g and increased the polyunsaturated-to-saturated-fat ratio from 0.27 to 0.98 (47). In each group, about half of the subjects were hypertensive. There was little change in body weight or potassium excretion. The systolic and diastolic pressures fell significantly in both normotensive and hypertensive subjects on the low saturated fat diet, whereas only the diastolic pressures fell in the other two hypertensive groups on the control and low sodium diets.

A few other studies in man and a number of studies in hypertensive animals have shown an antihypertensive effect of increased intake of polyunsaturated fatty acids such as linoleic acid (60). The effect has been assumed to be mediated by way of an increased synthesis of vasodilatory prostaglandins.

Vegetarian Diets

A vegetarian diet may lower the blood pressure. A group of 59 healthy omnivorous subjects were randomly assigned to a control group whose diet was unchanged or to either a vegetarian or an omnivorous diet for six weeks and then crossed-over to the other diet for another six weeks. With the vegetarian diet, the blood pressures fell an average of 5 to 6 mm Hg systolic and 2 to 3 mm Hg diastolic (54). The ingredients of a vegetarian diet that may lower the blood pressure are unknown. Possibilities include its increased content of polyunsaturated fat, fiber, vegetable protein, potassium, and magnesium.

Others

Neither variations in dietary protein intake (40) nor in dietary carbohydrate intake (19) seem to have a persistent effect on the blood pressure.

Garlic extract has a potent though transient antihypertensive effect in animals (15). Despite its wide use as a folk remedy, no controlled trials of its use in man have been reported.

Caffeine raises the blood pressure acutely but its intake has not been clearly associated with induction of permanent hypertension, likely because of the development of tolerance to its hemodynamic effects (53). Patients should be advised to avoid caffeine for an hour before blood pressure measurements are taken, but it seems unlikely that more sustained avoidance will have much of an antihypertensive effect.

The long-term value of these diverse dietary changes in the practical management of hypertension remains largely unknown but multiple changes in diet may make a major difference, as shown in the study by Pacy et al (44) upon 50 hypertensive diabetics randomly assigned to either a daily dose of a diuretic or a low sodium, low fat, high fiber diet (Table 4).

Table 4 Changes after three months of therapy with diuretic or diet[a]

	Weight kg	Blood pressure mm Hg[b]	Total cholesterol mg/dl	HDL$_2$ cholesterol mg/dl	Glycosylated hemoglobin %
Diuretic[c]					
Bendrofluazide 10 mg	−1.6	−20.9/−6.4	+8	+4	+0.9
Diet[c]					
High fiber (30–45 g)					
Low fat (15%),	−2.9	−15.5/−8.6	−4	+8	−1.6
Low sodium (40-50 mmol)					

[a]From Ref. (44).
[b]Systolic/diastolic.
[c]Twenty-five diabetic hypertensives in each group.

Not only did the diet lower the mean blood pressure equally as well as did the diuretic, but it also favorably changed the blood lipids and diabetic control which were adversely affected by the diuretic. Thus, for many hypertensive patients, a major overhaul of the diet may be an effective and safe way to lower the blood pressure (26).

ALCOHOL

The last of the dietary factors to be considered may be, in practice, the most important: in moderate amounts, alcohol appears to protect against coronary heart disease; but, even in moderate amounts, alcohol may elevate the blood pressure. The epidemiological evidence for a cardioprotective effect of moderate alcohol intake against CHD is quite strong and consistent (18), despite the deleterious effects of larger amounts of alcohol on myocardial cells.

On the other hand, the evidence that even a little alcohol will raise the blood pressure has become equally convincing (30, 8, 46), as seen in the report on 20,920 persons not receiving antihypertensive therapy screened at the Sydney, Australia Hospital (8). Blood pressures were progressively higher with increasing alcohol consumption, and the relationship was even closer after statistical correction for age, obesity, and smoking.

Beyond such epidemiological evidence, the administration of alcohol, under controlled conditions has been shown to raise the blood pressure of hypertensive men (32). Chronic alcohol intake may exert chronic pressor actions, which cannot be tightly connected to known pressor mechanisms (46). Among patients admitted to a hospital who drank three or more ounces of ethanol per day, 52% were hypertensive but only 9% remained hypertensive when they quit drinking while hospitalized (56) (Figure 2). Almost all who remained abstinent for the next six months remained normotensive, whereas many of those who went back to drinking alcohol became hypertensive again. All things considered, alcohol in more than moderate amounts, i.e. more than two ounces per day, may raise the blood pressure enough to make it the most prevalent cause of reversible hypertension.

Those who drink more should be firmly counseled to cut back, both for their blood pressure and for multiple other reasons.

SUMMARY

Based upon currently available evidence, a practical dietary prescription should be:

1. For the overweight, weight reduction should be the primary goal.
2. For all hypertensives, dietary sodium should be restricted to a 2 g (88 mmol/d) level.
3. Potassium intake need not be specifically increased since it will rise with a lowered sodium intake. Those who are hypokalemic may benefit from potassium supplementation.

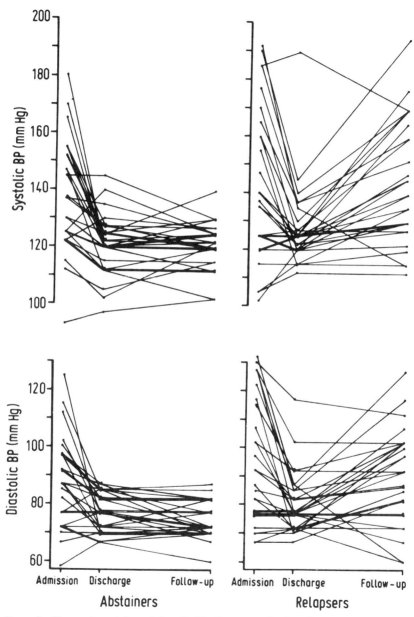

Figure 2 Changes in systolic and diastolic blood pressure after detoxification and following continued abstention (*n*=28) or relapse (*n*=28) among patients who drank three or more ounces of ethanol daily prior to admission. (From Ref. 56.)

4. Supplemental magnesium and calcium should only be given to those who are deficient, until additional evidence of their efficacy is available. Caution is advised in not reducing the dietary sources of calcium when dietary sodium is reduced.

5. More fiber and less saturated fat are beneficial for other reasons and may also help to lower the blood pressure.

6. Alcohol should be limited to two ounces per day.

The 1984 report of the Joint National Committee (23) recommends that "nonpharmacologic approaches [be] used both as definitive intervention and as an adjunct to drug therapy." In addressing the 40% of all hypertensives who are in the 90 to 94 mmHg range, the report states, "Nonpharmacologic therapy should be pursued aggressively while blood pressures are carefully monitored."

Dietary changes are the major components of nondrug therapy. They should be enthusiastically offered to all hypertensives, while providing the various motivational tools and follow-up procedures that are readily available to maximize their acceptance and effectiveness.

Literature Cited

1. Altura, B. M., Altura, B. T. 1981. Role of magnesium ions in contractility of blood vessels and skeletal muscles. *Magnesium Bull.* 1a:102–14

2. Ambrosioni, E., Costa, E. V., Borghi, C., Montebugnoli, L., Giordani, M. R., et al. 1982. Effects of moderate salt restriction on intralymphocytic sodium and pressor response to stress in borderline hypertension. *Hypertension* 4:789–94

3. Beard, T. C., Cooke, H. M., Gray, W. R., Barge, R. 1982. Randomised controlled trial of a no-added-sodium diet for mild hypertension. *Lancet* 2:455–58

4. Beauchamp, G. K., Bertino, M., Engelman, K. 1983. Modification of salt taste. *Ann. Intern. Med.* 98(Part 2):763–69

5. Belizan, J. M., Villar, J., Pineda, O., et al. 1983. Reduction of blood pressure with calcium supplementation in young adults. *J. Am. Med. Assoc.* 249:1161–65

6. Belizan, J. M., Villar, J., Zalazar, A., Rojas, L., Chan, D., et al. 1983. Preliminary evidence of the effect of calcium supplementation on blood pressure in normal pregnant women. *Am. J. Obstet. Gynecol.* 146:175–80

7. Chapman, C. B., Gibbons, T. B. 1949. The diet and hypertension: A review. *Medicine* 29:29–69

8. Cooke, K. M., Frost, G. W., Stokes, G. S. 1983. Blood pressure and its relationship to low levels of alcohol consumption. *Clin. Exp. Pharmacol. Physiol.* 10:229–33

9. Dahl, L. K., Silver, L., Christie, R. W. 1958. The role of salt in the fall of blood pressure accompanying reduction in obesity. *N. Engl. J. Med.* 258:1186–92

10. Dyckner, T., Wester, P. O. 1983. Effect of magnesium on blood pressure. *Br. Med. J.* 286:1847–49

11. Eaton, S. B., Konner, M. 1985. Paleolithic nutrition: A consideration of its nature and current implications. *N. Engl. J. Med.* 312:283–89

12. Erne, P., Bolli, P., Burgisser, E., Buhler, F. R. 1984. Correlation of platelet calcium with blood pressure: Effect of antihypertensive therapy. *N. Engl. J. Med.* 310:1084–88

13. Fagerberg, B., Andersson, O. K., Isaksson, B., Bjorntorp, P. 1984. Blood pressure control during weight reduction in obese hypertensive men: Separate effects of sodium and energy restriction. *Br. Med. J.* 288:11–14

14. Feinleib, M., Lenfant, C., Miller, S. A. 1984. Hypertension and calcium. *Science* 226:384–89

15. Foushee, D. B., Ruffin, J., Banerjee, U. 1982. Garlic as a natural agent for the treatment of hypertension: A preliminary report. *Cytobios* 34:145–52

16. Grim, C. E., Luft, F. C., Miller, J. Z., et al. 1980. Racial differences in blood pressure in Evans County, Georgia: Re-

lationship to sodium and potassium intake and plasma renin activity. *J. Chron. Dis.* 33:87–94

17. Havlik, R. J., Hubert, H. B., Fabsitz, R. R., Feinleib, M. 1983. Weight and hypertension. *Ann. Intern. Med.* 98(Pt. 2):855–59

18. Hennekens, C. H. 1983. Alcohol. In *Prevention of Coronary Heart Disease,* ed. N. M. Kaplan, J. Stamler, pp. 130–38. Philadelphia: Saunders

19. Hodges, R. E., Rebello, T. 1983. Carbohydrates and blood pressure. *Ann. Intern. Med.* 98(Pt. 2):838–41

20. Hofman, A., Hazebroek, A., Valkenburg, H. A. 1983. A randomized trial of sodium intake and blood pressure in newborn infants. *J. Am. Med. Assoc.* 250:370–73

21. Iimura, O., Kijima, T., Kikuchi, K., et al. 1981. Studies on the hypotensive effect of high potassium intake in patients with essential hypertension. *Clin. Sci.* 61:77s–80s

22. Ji, B. H., Erne, P., Kiowski, W., Buhler, F. R., Bolli, P. 1983. Magnesium-induced vasodilation is comparable to that induced by calcium entry blockade. *J. Hypertension* 1(Suppl. 2):368–71

23. Joint National Committee on Detection, Evaluation, and Treatment of High Blood Pressure, 1984. The 1984 report of the Joint National Committee on Detection, Evaluation, and Treatment of High Blood Pressure. *Arch. Intern. Med.* 144:1045–57

24. Kaplan, N. M. 1983. An overview of hypertension: The individual and the public challenge. In *Clinical Hypertension,* ed. N. M. Kaplan, pp. 1–41. Baltimore: Williams & Wilkins. 454 pp.

25. Kaplan, N. M. 1983. Hypertension: Prevalence, risks, and effect of therapy. *Ann. Intern. Med.* 98(Pt. 2):705–9

26. Kaplan, N. M. 1985. Non-drug treatment of hypertension. *Ann. Intern. Med.* 102:359–73

27. Kaplan, N. M., Carnegie, A., Raskin, P., Heller, J. A., Simmons, M. 1985. Potassium supplementation in hypertensive patients with diuretic-induced hypokalemia. *N. Engl. J. Med.* 312:746–49

28. Kaplan, N. M., Simmons, M., McPhee, C., Carnegie, A., Stefanu, C., et al. 1982. Two techniques to improve adherence to dietary sodium restriction in the treatment of hypertension. *Arch. Intern. Med.* 142:1638–41

29. Kawasaki, T., Delea, C. S., Bartter, F. C., Smith, H. 1978. The effect of high-sodium and low-sodium intakes on blood pressure and other related variables in human subjects with idiopathic hypertension. *Am. J. Med.* 64:193–98

30. Klatsky, A. L., Friedman, G. D., Siegelaub, A. B., Gerard, M. J. 1977. Alcohol consumption and blood pressure: Kaiser-Permanente multiphasic health examination data. *N. Engl. J. Med.* 296:1194–1200

31. Koolen, M. I., van Brummelen, P. 1984. Sodium sensitivity in essential hypertension: Role of the renin-angiotension-aldosterone system and predictive value of an intravenous frusemide test. *J. Hypertension* 2:55–59

32. Kupari, M. 1983. Acute cardiovascular effects of ethanol: A controlled noninvasive study. *Br. Heart J.* 49:174–82

33. Lever, A. F., Beretta-Piccoli, C., Brown, J. J., Davies, D. L., Fraser, R., Robertson, J. I. S. 1981. Sodium and potassium in essential hypertension. *Br. Med. J.* 283:463–68

34. MacGregor, G. A., Markandu, N., Best, F., et al. 1982. Double-blind randomised crossover trial of moderate sodium restriction in essential hypertension. *Lancet* 2:351–55

35. MacGregor, G. A., Smith, S. J., Markandu N. D., Banks, R. A., Sagnella, G. A. 1982. Moderate potassium supplementation in essential hypertension. *Lancet* 2:567–70

36. Maxwell, M. H., Kushiro, T., Dornfeld, L. P., Tuck, M. L., Waks, A. U. 1984. Blood pressure changes in obese hypertensive subjects during rapid weight loss: Comparison of restricted versus unchanged salt intake. *Arch. Int. Med.* 144:1581–84

37. McCarron, D. A., Morris, C. 1984. Oral Ca^{2+} in mild to moderate hypertension: A randomized, placebo-controlled trial. *Clin. Res.* 32:335A (Abstr.)

38. McCarron, D. A., Morris, C. D., Henry, H. J., Stanton, J. L. 1984. Blood pressure and nutrient intake in the United States. *Science* 224:1392–98

39. Meneely, G. R., Battarbee, H. D. 1976. High sodium-low potassium environment and hypertension. *Am. J. Cardiol.* 38:768–85

40. Meyer, T. W., Anderson, S., Brenner, B. M. 1983. Dietary protein intake and progressive glomerular sclerosis: The role of capillary hypertension and hyperperfusion in the progression of renal disease. *Ann. Intern. Med.* 98(Pt. 2):832–38

41. Morgan, T. O. 1982. The effect of potassium and bicarbonate ions on the rise in blood pressure caused by sodium chloride. *Clin. Sci.* 63:407s–9s

42. Ophir, O., Peer, G., Gilad, J., Blum, M., Aviram, A. 1983. Low blood pressure in vegetarians: The possible role of potassium. *Am. J. Clin. Nutr.* 37:755–62

43. Overlack, A., Muller, H. M., Kolloch, R., et al. 1983. Long-term antihypertensive effect of oral potassium in essential hypertension. *J. Hypertension* 1(Suppl. 2):165–67

44. Pacy, P. J., Dodson, P. M., Kubicki, A. J., Fletcher, R. F., Taylor, K. G. 1984. Comparison of the hypotensive and metabolic effects of bendrofluazide therapy and a high fibre, low fat, low sodium diet in diabetic subjects with mild hypertension. *J. Hypertension* 2:215–20

45. Palgi, A., Bistrian, B. R., Blackburn, G. L. 1984. Two to seven year maintenance of weight loss. *Clin. Res.* 32:632A (Abstr.)

46. Potter, J. F., Beevers, D. G. 1984. Pressor effect of alcohol in hypertension. *Lancet* 1:119–22

47. Puska, P., Iacono, J. M., Nissinen, A., et al. 1983. Controlled, randomised trial of the effect of dietary fat on blood pressure. *Lancet* 1:1–5

48. Ram, C. V. S., Garrett, B. N., Kaplan, N. M. 1981. Moderate sodium restriction and various diuretics in the treatment of hypertension: Effects of potassium wastage and blood pressure control. *Arch. Intern. Med.* 141:1015–19

49. Reisin, E., Abel, R., Modan, M., Silverberg, D. S., Eliahou, H. E., et al. 1978. Effect of weight loss without salt restriction on the reduction of blood pressure in overweight hypertensive patients. *N. Engl. J. Med.* 298:1–5

50. Reisin, E., Frohlich, E. D., Messerli, F. H., et al. 1983. Cardiovascular changes after weight reduction in obesity hypertension. *Ann. Intern. Med.* 98:315–19

51. Resnick, L., Nicholson, J. P., Laragh, J. H. 1984. Outpatient therapy of essential hypertension with dietary calcium supplementation. *J. Am. Coll. Cardiol.* 3:616 (Abstr.)

52. Richards, A. M., Nicholls, M. G., Espiner, E. A., et al. 1984. Blood-pressure response to moderate sodium restriction and to potassium supplementation in mild essential hypertension. *Lancet* 1:757–61

53. Robertson, D., Wade, D., Workman, R., Woosley, R. L., Oates, J. A. 1981. Tolerance to the humoral and hemodynamic effects of caffeine in man. *J. Clin. Invest.* 67:1111–17

54. Rouse, I. L., Beilen, L. J., Armstrong, B. K., Vandongen, R. 1983. Blood-pressure-lowering effect of a vegetarian diet: Controlled trial in normotensive subjects. *Lancet* 1:5–9

55. Saltman, P. 1983. Trace elements and blood pressure. *Ann. Int. Med.* 98(Pt. 2):823–27

56. Saunders, J. B., Beevers, D. G., Paton, A. 1981. Alcohol-induced hypertension, *Lancet* 2:653–56

57. Silman, A. J., Locke, C., Mitchell, P., Humpherson, P. 1983. Evaluation of the effectiveness of a low sodium diet in the treatment of mild to moderate hypertension. *Lancet* 1:1179–82

58. Smith, S. J., Markandu, N. D., Sagnella, G. A., McGregor, G. A. 1985. Moderate potassium chloride supplementation in essential hypertension: Is it additive to moderate sodium restriction? *Br. Med. J.* 290:110–13

59. Smith, S. J., Markandu, N. D., Sagnella, G. A., Poston, L., Hilton, P. J. et al. 1983. Does potassium lower blood pressure by increasing sodium excretion? A metabolic study in patients with mild to moderate essential hypertension. *J. Hypertension* 1(Suppl. 2):27–30

60. Smith-Barbaro, P. A., Pucak, G. J. 1983. Dietary fat and blood pressure. *Ann. Intern. Med.* 98(Pt. 2):828–31

61. Stamler, J., Liu, K. 1983. The benefits of prevention. In *Prevention of Coronary Heart Disease,* ed. N. M. Kaplan, J. Stamler, pp. 188–207. Philadelphia: Saunders. 219 pp.

62. Watt, G. C. M., Edwards, C., Hart, J. T., Hart, M., Walton, P., Foy, C. J. W. 1983. Dietary sodium restriction for mild hypertension in general practice. *Br. Med. J.* 286:432–36

63. Wing, R. R., Jeffery, R. W. 1979. Outpatient treatments of obesity: A comparison of methodology and clinical results. *Int. J. Obesity* 3:261–79

Ann. Rev. Public Health. 1986. 7:521–33

PUBLIC HEALTH APPROACHES TO OBESITY AND ITS MANAGEMENT

Kelly D. Brownell

Department of Psychology, University of Pennsylvania School of Medicine, Philadelphia, Pennsylvania 19104

Three aspects of obesity combine to make it a compelling public health problem: its seriousness, prevalence, and resistance to change (1–5). The medical risks are substantial. These have been reviewed elsewhere (1–3, 6). Often ignored in this concept of "risk" are the social and psychological hazards of obesity. These can be serious, permanent, and sometimes disabling (5, 7), and are more prominent in the eyes of obese persons than are physical complications.

The prevalence of obesity depends on the criteria used to define the condition, but no less than 15% of adult Americans are obese, with estimates ranging as high as 50% (1, 2). It is not a disorder that yields easily to treatment. The most intensive and costly programs delivered in clinical settings produce significant weight losses in less than half the patients (5, 8). Large-scale public health approaches reach more people, but the impact on individuals is weaker.

This gloomy picture has prevailed for years, but the mood is changing. Exciting developments are taking place in conceptual approaches to obesity, in studies of hunger, satiety, and body weight regulation, and in methods for weight reduction, both in the clinic and the community.

THEORY AND PHYSIOLOGY

The Set Point Theory

The most popular, and perhaps most thoroughly studied theory of obesity rests on the concept of a body weight set point (9, 10). This concept proposes an ideal biological weight which the organism is "set" to defend against weight loss or

0163-7525/86/0510-0521$02.00

gain. Some internal, physiological mechanism regulates weight much the way a thermostat regulates temperature in the home.

If the set point exists, the ideal biological weight in some humans may be considerably above (or below) the cultural ideal. To attain society's thin standard, such persons may fight a physiology that defends a higher weight by exerting pressure to gain. Bennett & Gurin (10) feel the challenge between a dieter and the set point is not a fair fight: "The set point is a tireless opponent. The dieter's only allies are willpower and whatever incentives there are that make chronic physical discomfort worthwhile" (p. 7).

Does the set point exist? I believe so. Does it have practical implications? Not yet. Some compelling arguments refute the set point concept (11), but many arguments support it. Keesey (9) reviewed the literature, including studies by his group, and showed precise defense of body weight in many species in response to several challenges.

As work on physiology continues, it may be possible to determine whether a set point exists. We may learn methods for its specification, biological and psychological mediators and consequences, and, ultimately, methods for its alteration.

There has been much speculation on ways to change the set point. Among the suggested methods for resetting the set point are lesions in the hypothalamus and other areas of the brain (9), exercise (10), diet (9), certain drugs (12), and surgery (13). These are likely possibilities, but none has been proven definitively.

Fat Cells

Obesity can occur from increased size or number of fat cells. Hirsch & Knittle (14) first proposed that increased fat cell number (hyperplastic obesity) occurred in childhood-onset obese persons, because cell proliferation could not occur after adolescence. A corollary of the fat cell theory was that attaining ideal weight would be difficult for such persons because cell size can decrease but not cell number. Even when cells reached normal size, a person might still be obese if cell number were increased. Further weight loss could occur from lean tissue or by further depleting fat cells of their normal amount of lipid, thus creating a state of semi-starvation.

It is now clear that adults *can* add fat cells, but only when a significant degree of obesity is reached. It appears that cells have a maximum size, and that an energy surplus at this point stimulates recruitment of "pre-adipocytes" into true fat cells (15, 16). Even so, fat cell size and number may be one factor that determines the limits of weight loss.

Bjorntorp and colleagues (17) reported fascinating results in a study of fat cell changes in obese women losing weight. At the point weight loss ceased, fat cells had reached normal size, even though some women were still obese by virtue of increased cell number. It was as though a biological factor (perhaps a set point), dictated by cell size, presented a barrier to weight loss.

This study by Bjorntorp et al (17) was the first of its kind; two other studies (18, 19) have shown less convincing findings. It is not clear, therefore, whether fat cell size plays the central role in limiting weight loss as the initial study suggested. If the finding is replicated, it may be possible someday to do fat cell measurements before weight loss to determine the weight at which an individual will encounter this hypothesized barrier. Fat cell size may set the limit on weight loss and cell number may determine the weight at which the limit occurs.

FAT DISTRIBUTION AND RISK   An important new development is the discovery that the size of fat cells and the distribution of body fat determine at least part of the risk of obesity. Bjorntorp & Sjostrom (20) found that increased cell size is associated with greater metabolic complications than a similar degree of obesity resulting from increased cell number. This stimulated work on distribution of fat in various parts of the body.

Men and women differ in the complications from their obesity and in their fat distribution (15). Obese men tend to store their fat in the abdominal region (upper body obesity), whereas women distribute fat on the thighs, hips, and buttocks (lower body obesity). Bjorntorp has noted (15):

> Obese men have more pronounced hyperinsulinemia, decreased glucose tolerance, overt diabetes mellitus, hypertriglyceridemia, and hypertension than obese women at comparable degrees of moderate obesity. Women have to be much more severely obese to reach the degree of complicating disorders that the obese men suffer at a moderate increase of total body fat. These sex differences are at least partly associated with the distribution of body fat, because obese women with male type of adipose tissue distribution (much abdominal fat) are more prone to complications that obese women with female type of adipose distribution.

The relationship of upper body obesity to risk has been confirmed in prospective epidemiology trials. Such a study of men in Goteborg, Sweden found no relationship between risk for ischemic heart disease and body weight per se, the body mass index (weight/height^2), or other indices of obesity (21). However, fat distribution, measured by waist-to-hip circumference, had a strong association with the complications of obesity, including several coronary risk factors. Similar results have been reported in the Paris Prospective Study (22). This may occur because the abdominal fat depot is lipolytically sensitive, making the fat easy to mobilize. This may influence insulin sensitivity and glucose transport, and may increase the likelihood of hypertriglyceridemia (15).

Like the set point theory, these ideas about fat cells are relatively new and must be studied in more detail. They may be important links in explaining why obesity develops, why some individuals are at greater risk as a result of their obesity, and why some dieters struggle for a lifetime without losing much weight while others lose with ease.

A CLASSIFICATION SCHEME FOR OBESITY

Garrow (23, 24) was among the first to classify obesity. He proposed four types of obesity, defined by degree of overweight. This and other classification schemes were debated at a National Institute of Health conference on the topic, the results of which were reported in the *International Journal of Obesity* (1984, Vol. 8, No. 5). No one scheme has been accepted, but one suggested by Stunkard (13) is appealing because of its logic and implications for treatment.

Stunkard (13) proposed three categories of obesity. The categories vary by percentage overweight: Mild (0–30% overweight); Moderate (30–100%); and Severe (greater than 100%). Most overweight persons fall into the first two categories. Until obesity reaches at least the Moderate level, it is created by increased fat cell size. At the upper range of the Moderate category and in the full range of the Severe category, individuals have increased cell size and number. As mentioned above, the risk of obesity depends more on cell size and fat distribution than on weight per se (15), but for the purposes of the classification scheme, the increase in risk begins somewhere in the Moderate category and becomes worse as weight increases.

The classification scheme suggests different treatments for persons in the three categories. Large-scale public health programs, which include a great many approaches (see below), are most effective for mildly overweight persons, and are sometimes effective in the Moderate category (25). More intensive clinical, dietary, commercial, and self-help approaches are indicated for the Moderate category, and surgery may be the treatment of choice for severely overweight persons who have failed at more conventional programs. The stepped-care approach proposed later in this chapter will show how these approaches to weight reduction can be used from a public health perspective.

This classification scheme will certainly undergo further refinement. For example, the Moderate category is very broad and includes persons with varying degrees of pathology, risk, and response to treatment, so further division of this category may be helpful. For now, the three-part scheme is helpful because it suggests different approaches for each category.

CLINICAL TREATMENTS FOR OBESITY

Following the classification scheme presented above, intensive clinical programs would be the focus of a discussion of the Moderate category, and would also apply to some persons in the Mild and Severe categories. The focus of this chapter, however, is on public health approaches, so I refer readers to other reviews on clinical programs (4, 5, 8, 13, 24, 26).

PUBLIC HEALTH APPROACHES

Many diet programs, clinics, and approaches have been used on a large scale. Only three such approaches have been evaluated at all: self-help and commercial groups; community interventions; and work site programs. These are discussed below. The remaining approaches have potential, but little is known about their effectiveness.

The Array of Potential Approaches

The number of available treatments for obesity is enormous. There would be many options if one considered only the diet guides available in book stores. One common approach is the distribution of booklets and pamphlets on nutrition, exercise, and weight loss by government agencies, private groups like the American Heart Association, insurance companies, and even food companies. No systematic evaluation has been done on the impact of this distribution of information.

Television and radio stations have aired diet specials in which a commentator guides viewers through a weight loss program, but, again, no evaluations are available. Perhaps the most widespread approach is advice from diet books, magazines, and newspapers. The quality of advice varies from scientifically validated to dangerous. The public health impact of these approaches is unknown.

These areas are ripe for research by program evaluators. Television stations, newspapers, diet books, and well-meaning agencies have the potential for large impact. More needs to be known about the groups these programs reach, whether the impact is significant and enduring, and whether these approaches can be improved.

Self-Help and Commercial Groups

The best known commercial group for weight reduction is Weight Watchers, and the most popular self-help groups are Overeaters Anonymous and TOPS (Take Off Pounds Sensibly). There are dozens of other programs. More than 500,000 people each week attend Weight Watchers alone (25). Such programs are important because they are self-supporting, widely available, and highly attractive to dieters.

Considering the potential and popularity of self-help and commercial groups, it is discouraging that so little evaluation has been done. Some groups, like Overeaters Anonymous, are difficult to evaluate because the anonymity guaranteed participants prevents long-term tracking. The commercial programs are notoriously unwilling to permit external evaluation. Even where some evaluation is done, as Levitz & Stunkard (27) did with TOPS, the information may not be used in planning programs.

What information exists suggests modest weight losses from these programs

(25, 27–29), but grouping the programs does a disservice to some and flatters others. Ashwell (28) evaluated several slimming groups in the United Kingdom and Australia, including the Australian Weight Watchers. The weight losses varied, but the most striking finding was the high attrition. Over half the participants dropped out within the first six weeks. Volkmar et al (29) reported similar results from an American group; attrition reached 80% within 24 weeks.

The most promising report of a self-help group is from Norway, where one program has enrolled 80,000 persons of a population of 4 million (30). Attrition was less than 10% and the average weight loss was 14 pounds. This suggests that great improvement may still be made in self-help approaches (25).

The precise role that commercial and self-help groups can play in a public health approach to obesity remains to be defined. Attrition complicates interpretation of the weight losses reported by most groups, because reports are based only on the "survivors" who remain in a program. Undoubtedly certain programs will succeed with certain types of people better than others. It is important to determine the types of dieters who will respond to a given program, to convey this information to individuals, and to develop a system for matching individuals to programs.

Community Programs

Several large-scale community programs have been launched to reduce morbidity and mortality from coronary disease. The hope is that the social environment of an entire community can be changed to alter health practices and lifestyle patterns. This approach offers great hope for large-scale changes. The two earliest programs, and thus the programs with the greatest time for evaluation, are the Stanford Three Community Study in California (31) and the North Karelia Study in Finland (32).

The Stanford study was an attempt to reduce risk in two small towns with an intensive educational program delivered primarily through the media. One of these towns also received an intensive, face-to-face counseling program aimed at high-risk individuals. These two towns were compared with a control community that received no program. There were changes in the intervention towns in the major coronary risk factors of smoking, cholesterol, and blood pressure.

Obesity was not a major target of the Stanford study but some evidence is available on weight changes (31). Mean weights did not change in the intervention communities during the two-year program or at a one-year follow-up. The control community, however, showed a gain of one pound, a statistically significant increase. Thus, the program had only a marginal effect on weight (25).

The North Karelia project evaluated an educational campaign in a large community of 180,000 persons. Risk factors were reduced, as was morbidity and mortality from coronary disease. However, obesity occurred with low prevalence and was not a target for the program. No data on weight were reported.

If there is potential for community programs to affect weight status, it has not been realized. One reason is that weight has not been targeted. Other risk factors have changed, so weight might follow the same course. This notion is open for testing.

Work-Site Programs

The work site offers many unique opportunities for public health approaches to weight reduction (25, 33–36). Many people can be screened, treated, and evaluated over months and even years. Some or all of the cost may be born by employers, and work-related factors such as morale, productivity, and absenteeism are possible to measure.

Perhaps the greatest potential of work site programs lies in the social bonds that can exist among co-workers. Social support plays an important role in susceptibility to and recovery from disease (37, 38), and appears to be influential in weight control (5, 39, 40). It is, for example, one of the few correlates of long-term success in diet programs (40). The frequent and sometimes influential social contacts at the work site might be exploited to encourage people to join and complete weight loss programs.

Many companies have attempted weight loss and nutrition programs (33, 36, 41), but little is known about their effects because program implementation has taken precedence over evaluation. The first controlled study was reported by Stunkard & Brownell (42) and involved a behavioral program conducted through the United Storeworkers Union in New York City for the employees of the main Gimbels Department Store. The same behavioral program that produced reliable effects in the clinic (5) had disappointing effects in the work site. Attrition was 50% compared to 15% in the clinic and weight losses were half the expected level.

Several subsequent studies produced remarkably similar results. Another report on programs with the storeworkers, this time including employees of the main Bloomingdales store, still found high attrition and small weight losses (43). Two studies by Abrams, Follick, and colleagues (44, 45) found the same 50% attrition with hospital workers in Rhode Island. These authors did, however, report promising long-term results using a program designed specifically to prevent relapse. Another study with employees of an electronics manufacturing firm again found high attrition (46). These controlled studies are joined by several descriptive reports of the weight-loss efforts of hospital workers (47) and bank employees (48).

What is consistent across these programs, using different approaches with different populations, is the 50% attrition and the small weight losses. The high attrition may result from programs that are convenient and are offered at low cost; neither factor screens out people who are not highly motivated. People who are not highly motivated are likely to drop out and to do poorly. It appears that programs developed in the clinic do not work as well in the work site. This argues for a new approach.

WEIGHT LOSS COMPETITIONS AT THE WORK SITE   Brownell et al (49) reported the results of weight loss competitions held in three types of business and industry. The first was between three banks with approximately 200 employees each. The presidents of the banks challenged the other banks to a weight loss contest. Employees who joined were weighed and given weight loss goals, calculated as their ideal weight subtracted from actual weight, to a maximum of 20 pounds (to discourage crash dieting). Each person paid $5, which formed the prize for the winning team. The only "program" consisted of weekly installments of a weight control manual (50) and a weekly weigh-in. Unlike the previous programs based on clinical models, there were no professionally conducted group meetings.

The results from the competition were much better than for previous programs. Attrition was less than 5% and the weight losses averaged 5 kg for women and 8.5 kg for men. Two replications of this program were conducted and were reported in the same paper (49). One was a competition between persons assigned randomly to teams in a small manufacturing plant, and the other was between divisions of a large manufacturing company with 1200 employees. The results were also positive. A six-month follow-up was conducted in the bank competition, and the average participant had maintained 80% of the weight lost during the program.

The results of these competitions were also striking when considering the cost-effectiveness and response of both employees and management. Figure 1 shows the cost per pound lost for the competition, other work site programs, and a university clinic. The cost-effectiveness favors the competition. Our costs have been reduced further and are now half that shown in Figure 1 (49).

Questionnaires were given to employees and managers (presidents, vice presidents, and personnel managers) before and after the program to evaluate reactions to the competitions. In the first 200 questionnaires, only one person reported a negative reaction. The others were either neutral or positive, with the vast majority endorsing the program. These businesses have since initiated new competitions, and 25 or more businesses and industries in the community have undertaken programs.

I have had contact with a number of other businesses across the country who have now used the competition approach. The reports have been positive, but are not published. Supporting data for the concept have emerged from a study by Jeffery et al (51) using payroll deductions as incentive to lose weight.

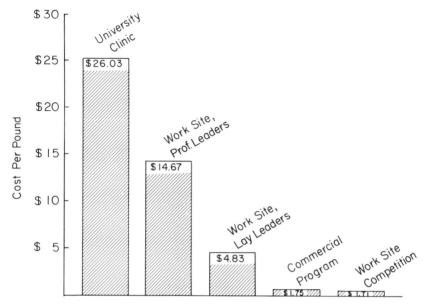

Figure 1   The cost per pound lost for different weight loss programs. Estimates were obtained for a university clinic, for a popular self-help program, and for several work-site programs. Reprinted from Brownell et al (49).

Several smoking cessation competitions have been reported, each with encouraging results. Pechacek and colleagues (52, 53) used community-based competitions in which people who stopped smoking could qualify for prizes such as merchandise and vacation trips. In four competitions held in two cities, involving more than 2000 participants, the average estimated cessation rate at a three-month follow-up was approximately 35%. This is a striking result, particularly considering the low cost.

A study by Klesges, Vasey & Glasgow (54) tested a smoking competition among five banks, modeled after the weight loss competitions described above (49). Four banks were involved in the competition, and the fifth received a clinical program delivered by professionals. Both the competition banks and the control bank had equivalent cessation rates, but there were large differences in recruitment rates when the program began. In the control bank, 53% of the smoking employees joined the program, compared to 88% in the competition banks. With equivalent cessation rates, the higher recruitment produced by the competition yielded a far greater public health impact.

More controlled studies are needed in this promising area. The focus of the competition on *motivation* rather than *education* may lead to new and more effective approaches to weight control. The work site may be a fruitful channel for the delivery of such programs.

A STEPPED-CARE MODEL FOR OBESITY

The challenge in the weight reduction area is not to determine which treatment is best—all approaches work for at least a small percentage of dieters. The challenge is to specify approaches to individuals and to reserve the most costly programs for those who do not respond to previous programs.

I propose a stepped-care approach to weight reduction (Figure 2). This is modeled after the current approach to the management of hypertension. The first step is an inexpensive motivational and educational approach, like a weight loss competition, media programs, popular books, widely distributed educational materials, and interventions in the schools. None of these possibilities has been studied enough to warrant widespread use, but preliminary results in several areas are promising.

The second level would comprise commercial and self-help groups. These bring greater cost, but the structure and social support can be helpful for some persons. There are, however, wide differences in the nature, cost, and effectiveness of such programs. This is another area where more research is needed, to identify individuals who will succeed at various programs.

The third level is an intensive clinical program delivered by professionals. This usually takes the form of weekly meetings conducted in groups for two to six months, followed by regular "booster" sessions scheduled over one year or more. Depending on a person's degree of obesity, an aggressive diet such as a very-low-calorie diet (5, 8) could be combined with the behavioral program. The group behavioral program is the most thoroughly tested approach to dieting (5, 13). However, the cost is high and clinics are not available in some areas. This option is best reserved for individuals who have not succeeded in through the earlier steps.

One option at the fourth and final level is individual counseling by a highly trained professional, be it psychologist, nutritionist, dietitian, or exercise

STEPPED-CARE MODEL FOR OBESITY

Step I	Step 2	Step 3	Step 4
Media Programs	Commercial Programs	Clinical Groups	Individual Programs
Competitions	Self-Help Groups	Aggressive Diets	Residential Programs
Popular Books			Surgery
Brochures			
Self-Diet			

Figure 2   A stepped-care model for the management of obesity. As the steps progress, cost and intensity increase.

specialist. Such a program might involve inpatient treatment if necessary or a residential program where people would be removed from their typical environment. The cost of any such approach is high, and the effectiveness has not been demonstrated. The final step may be surgery, but this should be reserved for massively obese persons who have not responded to other approaches.

This stepped care model is presented as a foundation upon which further refinement is needed. Other low-cost motivational approaches than the competition must be developed. More needs to be known about matching an individual to a self-help or commercial program. Clinical programs must be improved. Professional counseling along with inpatient and residential programs have not been studied systematically. These provide pressing questions for further research.

Literature Cited

1. Bray, G. A. 1976. *The Obese Patient.* Philadelphia: Saunders
2. Van Itallie, T. B. 1979. Obesity: Adverse effects on health and longevity. *Am. J. Clin. Nutr.* 32:2723–33
3. Simopoulos, A. P., Van Itallie, T. B. 1983. Body weight, health, and longevity. *Ann. Int. Med.* 100:285–95
4. Stunkard, A. J., ed. 1980. *Obesity.* Philadelphia: Saunders
5. Brownell, K. D. 1982. Obesity: Understanding and treating a serious prevalent, and refractory disorder. *J. Consult. Clin. Psychol.* 50:820–40
6. Hubert, H. B., Feinleib, M., McNamara, P. M., Castelli, W. P. 1983. Obesity as an independent risk factor for cardiovascular disease: A 26-year follow-up of participants of the Framingham Heart Study. *Circulation* 67:968–77
7. Wadden, T. A., Stunkard, A. J. 1985. Adverse social and psychological consequences of obesity. *Ann. Int. Med.* 103:1062–67
8. Wadden, T. A., Stunkard, A. J., Brownell, K. D. 1983. Very-low-calorie diets: Their efficacy, safety, and future. *Ann. Int. Med.* 99:675–84
9. Keesey, R. E. 1986. A set point theory of obesity. In *The Physiology, Psychology, and Treatment of the Eating Disorders,* ed. K. D. Brownell, J. P. Foreyt. New York: Basic
10. Bennett, W., Gurin, J. 1982. *The Dieter's Dilemma: Eating Less and Weighing More.* New York: Basic
11. Wirtshafter, D., Davis, J. D. 1977. Set points, settling points, and the control of body weight. *Physiol. Behav.* 19:75–78
12. Stunkard, A. J. 1982. Anorectic agents lower a body weight set point. *Life Sci.* 30:2043–55
13. Stunkard, A. J. 1984. The current status of treatment of obesity in adults. *Eating and Its Disorders,* ed. In A. J. Stunkard, E. Stellar. New York: Raven
14. Hirsch, J., Knittle, J. L. 1979. Cellularity of obese and nonobese human adipose tissue. *Fed. Proc.* 29:1516–21
15. Bjorntorp, P. 1985. Fat cells and obesity. See Ref. 9
16. Sjostrom, L. 1980. Fat cells and body weight. See Ref. 4
17. Bjorntorp, P., Carlgren, G., Isaksson, B., Krotkiewski, M., Larsson, M., Sjostrom, L. 1975. Effect of an energy-reduced dietary regimen in relation to adipose tissue cellularity in obese women. *Am. J. Clin. Nutr.* 28:445–52
18. Bosello, O., Ostuzzi, R., Rossi, F. A., Armelli, F., Cigolini, M., Micciolo, R., Scuro, L. A. 1980. Adipose tissue cellularity and weight reduction forecasing. *Am. J. Clin. Nutr.* 33:776–82
19. Strain, G. W., Strain, J. J., Zumoff, B., Knittle, J. 1984. Do fat cell morphometrics predict weight loss maintenance? *Int. J. Obesity* 8:53–59
20. Bjorntorp, P., Sjostrom, L. 1971. Number and size of adipose tissue fat cells in relation to prognosis for weight reduction. *Metabolism* 20:703–13
21. Krotkiewski, M., Bjorntorp, P., Sjostrom, L., Smith, U. 1983. Impact of obesity on metabolism in men and women—importance of regional adipose tissue distribution. *J. Clin. Invest.* 72:1150–62
22. Ducimetiere, P., Avons, P., Cambien,

F., Richard, J. L. 1983. Corpulence history and fat distribution in CHD etiology—The Paris Prospective Study. *Europ. Heart. J.* 4(Suppl.):8

23. Garrow, J. S. 1978. *Energy Balance and Obesity in Man.* Amsterdam: Elsevier. 2nd ed.

24. Garrow, J. S. 1981. *Treat obesity seriously: A clinical manual.* London: Churchill Livingstone

25. Stunkard, A. J. 1986. The control of obesity: Social and community perspectives. See Ref. 9

26. Brownell, K. D., Foreyt, J. P., Eds. 1986. *The Physiology, Psychology, and Treatment of the Eating Disorders.* New York: Basic

27. Levitz, L. S., Stunkard, A. J. 1974. A therapeutic coalition for obesity: Behavior modification and patient self-help. *Am. J. Psychiatr.* 131:423–27

28. Ashwell, M. 1978. Commercial weight loss groups. In *Recent Advances in Obesity Research: II*, ed. G. A. Bray. London: Newman

29. Volkmar, F. R., Stunkard, A. J., Woolston, J., Bailey, B. A. 1981. High attrition rates in commercial weight reduction programs. *Arch. Int. Med.* 141:426–28

30. Grimsmo, A., Helgesen, G., Borchgrevink, C. F. 1981. Short-term and long-term effects of lay groups on weight reduction. *Br. Med. J.* 283:1093–95

31. Farquhar, J. W., Maccoby, N., Wood, P. D., et al. 1977. Community education for cardiovascular disease. *Lancet* 1: 1192–95

32. Puska, P., Nissinen, A., Salonen, J. T. 1983. Ten years of the North Karelia Project: Results with community based prevention of coronary heart disease. *Scand. J. Soc. Med.* 11:65–68

33. Fielding, J. E. 1984. *Corporate Health Management.* Reading, Mass.: Addison-Wesley

34. Fielding, J. E. 1982. Effectiveness of employee health improvement programs. *J. Occup. Med.* 24:907–16

35. Brownell, K. D. 1985. Weight control at the worksite: The power of social and behavioral factors. In *Behavioral Medicine in Industry,* ed. M. F. Cataldo, T. J. Coates. New York: Wiley

36. Foreyt, J. P., Scott, L. W., Gotto, A. M. 1980. Weight control and nutrition education in occupational settings. *Public Health Rep.* 95:127–36

37. Cobb, S. 1976. Social support as a moderator of life stress. *Psychosom. Med.* 38:300–14

38. Berkman, L. F., Syme, S. L. 1979. Social networks, host resistance resistance, and mortality: A nine-year follow-up of Alameda County residents. *Am. J. Epidemiol.* 109:186–204

39. Colletti, G., Brownell, K. D. 1982. The physical and emotional benefits of social support: Applications to obesity, smoking, and alcoholism. *Progr. Behav. Modificat.* 13:110–79

40. Brownell, K. D. 1985. Behavioral, psychological, and environmental predictors of success at weight reduction. *Int. J. Obesity* 8:543–51

41. Fielding, J. E., Breslow, L. 1983. Health promotion programs sponsored by California employers. *Am. J. Public Health* 73:538–42

42. Stunkard, A. J., Brownell, K. D. 1980. Work site treatment for obesity. *Am. J. Psychiatr.* 137:252–53

43. Brownell, K. D., Stunkard, A. J., McKeon, P. E. 1984. Weight reduction at the work site: A promise partially fulfilled. *Am. J. Psychiatr.* 142:47–52

44. Abrams, D. B., Follick, M. J. 1983. Behavioral weight loss intervention at the worksite: Feasibility and maintenance. *J. Consult. Clin. Psychol.* 51:226–33

45. Follick, M. J., Fowler, J. L., Brown, R. 1986. Attrition in work site interventions. *J. Consult. Clin. Psychol.* In press

46. Peterson, G., Abrams, D. B., Elder, J. P., Beaudin, P. A. 1985. Weight loss at the worksite: The challenge of making a public health impact. *Behav. Therapy* 16:213–22

47. Sangor, M. R., Bichanich, P. 1977. Weight reducing program for hospital employees. *J. Am. Dietetic Assoc.* 71: 535–36

48. Fisher, E. B. Jr., Lowe, M. R., Levenkron, J. C., Newman, A. 1982. Reinforcement and structural support of maintained risk reduction. In *Adherence, Compliance and Generalization in Behavioral Medicine,* ed. R. B. Stuart. New York: Brunner/Mazel

49. Brownell, K. D., Cohen, R. Y., Stunkard, A. J., Felix, M. J., Cooley, N. B. 1984. Weight loss competitions at the work site: Impact on weight, morale, and cost-effectiveness. *Am. J. Public Health* 74:1283–85

50. Brownell, K. D. 1979. *Behavior therapy for obesity: A treatment manual.* Unpublished manuscript, Univ. of Penn., Philadelphia

51. Jeffery, R. W., Forster, J. L., Snell, M. K. 1986. Promoting weight control at the worksite: A program based on self-mo-

tivation using payroll based incentives. *Prev. Med.* In press

52. Pechacek, T. P., Mittelmark, M., Jeffery, R. W., Loken, B., Luepker, R. 1985. Quit and win: Direct incentives for smoking cessation. Submitted for publication

53. Pechacek, T. P., Siller, C., Glasgow, R., Mittelmark, M., Jeffery. R. W., Loken, B., Luepker, R. 1985. Quit and win: A replication. Submitted for publication

54. Klesges, R. C., Vasey, M. W., Glasgow, R. E. 1986. A worksite smoking modification competition: Potential for public health impact. *Am. J. Public Health* 76:198–200

Ann. Rev. Public Health. 1986. 7:535–43

ANOREXIA NERVOSA AND BULIMIA*

Joseph H. Autry

Office of Policy Analysis and Coordination, National Institute of Mental Health, Rockville, Maryland 20857

Ellen S. Stover

Division of Basic Sciences, National Institute of Mental Health, Rockville, Maryland 20857

Natalie Reatig

Division of Education and Service Systems Liaison, National Institute of Mental Health, Rockville, Maryland 20857

Regina Casper

Department of Psychiatry, Pritzker School of Medicine, University of Chicago, Chicago, Illinois 60637

INTRODUCTION

Anorexia nervosa is a heterogeneous disorder of self-starvation primarily found in adolescent females. It is characterized by profound weight loss; denial of illness; an overriding and irrational fear of becoming overweight; distorted body image; increased physical activity; and metabolic changes and disturbances in endocrine function, reflected in prolonged amenorrhea (7). Studies have indicated that the incidence of anorexia nervosa has doubled over the past two decades. In a retrospective study in Monroe County, New York, it was found that the incidence increased from a rate of 0.35 per 100,000 population in

---

1960–1969 to 0.64 per 100,000 from 1970–1976. A study in Switzerland found that from the 1950s to the 1970s, the incidence of treated cases increased from 0.38 to 1.12 per 100,000. It remains uncertain whether these figures represent a true increase in incidence or an increase in awareness. More recent studies estimate the prevalence in the general population to be between 1.0 and 4.2% (15). The majority of the studies have assessed prevalence in college student populations; there is evidence that the disorder is less prevalent in older age groups and in males (21).

We review ongoing research to understand and define the syndrome as well as current therapeutic approaches. Anorexia nervosa is increasing in public health importance and has been associated with both mental and physical disorders such as depression and cardiac problems.

REVIEW OF CURRENT KNOWLEDGE

Anorexia nervosa, a disorder involving severe weight loss in excess of 25% of previous body weight, is primarily seen in adolescent females. Many patients indicate psychological, interpersonal, and family difficulties, as well as related physiological problems (9). The current *Diagnostic and Statistical Manual of Mental Disorders* (DSM-III)[1] (6) lists these criteria: "an intense fear of becoming obese, disturbance of body image, significant weight loss, refusal to maintain a minimal normal body weight . . . no known physical illness that would account for the weight loss." Recent studies suggest that some of the DSM III criteria require revision (11). Halmi notes that there is little consensus among researchers on several exclusion criteria, such as age, degree of weight loss, the relationship to major affective disorders, and inclusion of amenorrhea, lanugo, bradycardia, and bulimia, or self-induced vomiting.

It is likely that there may be associated disorders, and researchers now refer to subgroups within the disorder. It is important to differentiate anorexia nervosa as a syndrome and anorexia as a symptom with other symptoms, such as depression and sleep disturbance. A large percentage of the women who suffer from anorexia nervosa are also bulimic. Bulimia is defined as the rapid consumption of large amounts of food in a short period of time, frequently followed by self-induced vomiting or the use of cathartics or diuretics. Although there has been substantial speculation that bulimia is a highly prevalent disorder, very few studies have attempted to document the incidence. Studies conducted among college and high school students indicate that between 5.9 and 13% meet the essential DSM III criteria for a probable diagnosis of bulimia; the variance in percentages is related to differences in criteria used relative to the frequency of self-induced vomiting and/or purging. Those

---

[1]A classification system for psychiatric disorders.

studies with most rigorous sampling criteria support that the incidence is approximately 5% among high school and college female students and 1.5% among male students. Further prevalence studies are needed to overcome the limitations of self-reported data, sampling biases, and clinically significant episodes. Depressive symptoms have been reported in the emaciated state, and tend to decrease with weight gain. How anorexia nervosa and affective disorder differ requires further investigation.

There is agreement that in addition to the severe weight loss, psychological difficulties emerge as part of this syndrome. A possible role of genetic factors is suggested by some researchers, who report an increased incidence of affective disorders in relatives of anorexics and bulimics. Evidence also exists that patients with anorexia nervosa (primarily those with bulimia) and patients with affective disorder share common features. Katz describes a subgroup of patients who show sleep abnormalities, which may be indicative of current affective disorder (15).

The more psychoanalytic viewpoint sees the difficulties as arising out of conflict with the mother. It has been hypothesized that the pressures resulting from a changing environment have created difficulties for some young women and have affected their ability to cope. Others suggest that changing norms have required young women to deal with conflicting role expectations.

Anorexia nervosa patients often come from upper middle-class families with high achievement orientation. One of the parents, usually the mother, tends to be dominant and over-protective, while the other parent is weak, submissive, and often absent from the home for long periods of time. Prior to the illness, these adolescents have been described as academically successful, well-liked, athletic, achievement oriented, and dependent (9).

Various personality disorder diagnoses such as schizoid, borderline, histrionic, and antisocial personality have been made in this patient population. In addition to psychological, social, and family difficulties, anorexia nervosa is accompanied by physiological changes. These include irregular cardiac rhythms, abnormalities in temperature regulation, thyroid function, and the secretion of gonadotropin, cortisol, growth hormone, and vasopressin (9, 20). A diagnosis of anorexia nervosa is suggested when a thin young woman has leukopenia, a relative lymphocytosis, a low fasting serum glucose level, and an elevated serum cholesterol. A return to physiological normal range occurs with weight gain. A low serum potassium level and a low serum chloride level could indicate that the patient is engaging in self-induced vomiting or laxative or diuretic abuse. Some investigators also believe that there may be a hypothalamic disorder (3). Investigators have shown that pituitary function is normal in anorexia nervosa (3).

It is currently assumed that endocrine changes are not primary in anorexia nervosa but occur during the course of the illness. According to Casper, several factors seem to contribute to endocrine dysfunction in anorexia nervosa: (*a*) reduced caloric intake; (*b*) a selective food intake, leading to different types of malnutrition (for example, trace metal deficiencies)(3a) leading to metabolic changes, depending upon individual preferences; (*c*) weight loss; and (*d*) unknown factors, some of which may be specific to anorexia nervosa.

Casper notes that the first three factors exert the strongest influence and that nearly every endocrine system undergoes some changes in anorexia nervosa. Endocrine dysfunction seems to occur in sequential order, for example, species survival is affected first: The hypothalamic-pituitary-gonadal axis undergoes a gradual regression from a mature adult Luteinizing Hormone (LH) and Follicle Stimulating Hormone (FSH) secretion pattern to a midpubertal and ultimately to a prepubertal secretion pattern, when LH and FSH levels are no longer sufficient to stimulate ovarian or testicular function. Consequently, levels of estrogen (female) and testosterone (male) are low and progesterone levels are virtually absent in acute anorexia nervosa. The clinical manifestation of this system's dysfunction is amenorrhea (either primary or secondary) in females and impotence in males. If patients with anorexia nervosa who had secondary amenorrhea recover, they will undergo puberty a second time (R. Casper, unpublished paper, 1985).

Changes in the hypothalamic-pituitary-adrenal axis (HYPAC) occur later in the course of the disorder than gonadal axis changes and involve increased 24-hour mean plasma cortisol concentrations, not suppressed by dexamethasone. Current knowledge suggests that the reasons for these changes are two-fold: (*a*) the half-life of cortisol in plasma is increased and its metabolic clearance is delayed; and (*b*) activation of the HYPAC axis occurs in anorexia nervosa. Whether and to what extent, however, the findings are simply a reflection of the above-mentioned factors or whether they represent a constellation unique to anorexia nervosa is difficult to determine, since control groups, subject to the same caloric restrictions and degree of weight loss, are difficult to obtain.[2]

A consensus has not been reached regarding the inclusion of amenorrhea as a necessary criterion for the diagnosis of anorexia nervosa. Amenorrhea occurs in 1/5 to 1/3 of anorexia patients before a substantial weight loss occurs, and therefore the amehorrea cannot be attributed solely to the patient's emaciation. Also, after nutritional rehabilitation, the return of normal menstrual cycles lags behind the return to a normal body weight. Several studies have shown that the

---

[2]An example of a system that seems unperturbed in anorexia nervosa is the prolactin system; prolactin levels remain generally within the normal range during anorexia nervosa.

Casper notes that all endocrine abnormalities are reversible when weight is restored to a normal age-and-sex appropriate weight and that this coincides generally with recovery from anorexia nervosa.

return of menses in anorexia nervosa is associated with marked psychological improvement. In a follow-up study, Halmi demonstrated that one year after treatment, the amenorrheic normal-weight patients had similar psychological difficulties to the underweight patients. Halmi concludes that sufficient evidence exists to include amenorrhea as a criterion for anorexia nervosa (11).

TREATMENT STUDIES

Research studies have attempted to assess the relative efficacy of both behavioral or psychosocial and pharmacologic approaches. Generally a treatment approach attempts to restore normal nutrition and body weight, as well as to address psychiatric abnormalities and maintain body weight over a long-term period. In a recent review of therapies, Halmi notes that "a variety of methods of shaping . . . behavior have appeared" (11). Operant conditioning approaches utilize social reinforcements that are contingent on weight gain. Several studies suggest that if reinforcements are tied to the eating behavior, it is possible to stop weight loss and decrease vomiting. Agras found that providing regular feedback regarding weight as well as positive reinforcements had a strong effect in increasing weight gain (1).

Halmi states that only two randomly assigned controlled treatment studies have evaluated behavior therapy (11). One showed that patients receiving an operant conditioning program gained weight three times as fast as those who received a program of strict isolation, appetite-stimulating drugs, and psychotherapy (25).

The second study, supported by The National Institute of Mental Health (NIMH) over a ten-year period, compared behavior therapy with drug therapy (12). Patients were randomly assigned to: (*a*) behavior modification and placebo; (*b*) behavior modification and the drug, cyproheptadine; (*c*) ward milieu and placebo; or (*d*) ward milieu and cyproheptadine. The findings indicated no significant difference in weight gain in the groups, in that all groups gained weight. A shortcoming in this study was the large number of variables affecting outcome. The following predictors were not controlled: age, onset of illness, presence of vomiting, number of previous hospitalizations, and previous treatment failures. These variables need to be controlled in any future treatment assessment studies (12).

Psychodynamic as well as behavior therapy has also been utilized as an adjunct to the medical management of these patients. Some therapists stress the denial of the condition and believe that awareness is necessary in the therapeutic process to reduce the anorexic symptoms. Minuchin et al stress the importance of the dysfunctional family unit and the necessity of addressing this in treatment (17).

The majority of treatment studies have involved the use of pharmacologic agents in small samples. Neuroleptic drugs were initially tried with a view toward their antipsychotic effects targeting the anorectic delusional body image distortion and obsessive-compulsive symptomatology. Observed similarities between eating disorders and depression on measures of symptomatology, family histories of affective disorders, and responses to the Dexamethasone Suppression Test (DST) and Thyroid Releasing Hormone (TRH) probes have led clinicians to attempt treatment with antidepressant drugs. Also, psychopharmacologic agents have been utilized because their pharmacologic properties frequently enhance food intake. Patients might also benefit from the "side effect" of inducing weight gain.

Treatment results as measured by the two major outcome criteria, weight gain and changes in anorectic perceptions and behaviors, have been equivocal. Chlorpromazine was reported to facilitate some short-term weight gain but only about half of those who improved sustained the recovery at follow-up (4, 5). Pimozide succeeded in improving weight gain for an older, more severely ill subgroup, but a later study with sulpiride failed to demonstrate significant superiority for the drug against placebo on these outcome measures (22, 23).

Treatment response to tricyclic antidepressants in achieving weight gain has been reported primarily from uncontrolled trials. The drugs were reported successful in elevating the mood of patients with depressive symptomatology. Evidence from a controlled trial of clomipramine, showing improvement on weight maintenance (though not weight gain), has not been followed up, and recent controlled studies of amitriptyline found no significant differences favoring the drug (2, 12, 16). These investigators reported poor tolerance of tricyclics by anorectic patients, in that response was slower and they suffered from anticholinergic side effects. This finding was confirmed further by Hudson and colleagues (13).

Case reports of weight gain from using lithium therapy were not borne out by a placebo-controlled study. Gross et al note that the drug "may augment weight gain in patients also treated with behavior modification" (10). Lithium treatment did produce attitude changes and decreases in denial, somatization, depression, and obsessive-compulsive behaviors. The use of lithium is somewhat problematic due to its potential toxicity, and constant monitoring for electrolyte imbalance is necessary in this patient population.

Cyproheptadine, a serotonin and histamine antagonist, has been the most rigorously studied drug treatment. A three-hospital NIMH collaborative investigation compared the drug against placebo and a behavioral therapy. Analysis of the 105 patients completing the study failed to show any main effects of cyproheptadine on weight gain but did find significant improvement for a subgroup characterized as having a history of complications while delivering children, a 41 to 52% weight loss from normal, and a history of prior outpatient treatment failures. Cyproheptadine improved anorectic attitudes and reduced preoccupation with thinness, as well as increased general sociability. All patients became less depressed; weight gain was correlated with a decrease in depression; and in comparison to pretreatment attitudinal variables, patients showed less fear of becoming fat, less denial of illness, and a less pejorative attitude about food. Items predictive of poor short-term outcome were: early age of onset of illness, a greater number of hospitalizations, self-induced vomiting, greater body distortion, and greater denial of illness. The drug seems to be well tolerated, with only minimal and reversible side-effects reported.

Most investigators believe that admission to a hospital is necessary for initial weight gain. This serves to remove the patient from the home environment, provides nursing care, and allows the initiation of psychotherapy. Starvation causes psychological disorganization, and in the malnourished state, it is difficult to accomplish effective psychotherapy. Halmi (11) has suggested that initial outpatient therapy may be successful for patients who have had anorexia nervosa for less than four months, are not binging or vomiting, and have parents who are cooperative in family therapy.

There appears to be agreement among investigators that most patients gain weight on admission to the hospital irrespective of the treatment modality utilized. However, patients' initial response to in-hospital treatment does not predict the ultimate outcome. Garner & Garfinkel (8) developed a self-report Eating Attitudes Test (EAT), which appears to be a reliable objective measure of the symptomatology of anorexia nervosa. They suggest that both the initial EAT score and the score after treatment can be used as a prognostic index. The EAT may be a useful instrument in evaluating outcome after discharge from the hospital.

Anorexia nervosa tends to be a chronic condition, and long-term psychotherapy and follow-up are required even after apparent improvement.

FUTURE RESEARCH NEEDS

Research studies are needed to address the following:

1. Psychological factors that influence the development and maintenance of anorexia nervosa and bulimia;
2. Cognitive and psychological dysfunction that may be the result of prolonged starvation;
3. The relationship between psychiatric illnesses (e.g. depression) and eating disorders (e.g. anorexia and bulimia);
4. Genetic, endocrine, and psychosocial studies that might elucidate why the phenomena are more prevalent in females;
5. The influence of cultural factors and the family on an individual's eating habits and food beliefs.

Treatment studies are needed to explore:

1. The evaluation of differential outcome from earlier-treatment interventions;
2. The long-term management of patients with these disorders;
3. The efficacy of different psychotherapeutic applications (cognitive, interpersonal, group, and family) in the treatment of anorexia and bulimia;
4. Further exploration of different pharmacological approaches used in the treatment of anorexia nervosa and bulimia;
5. Systematic studies of combined pharmacologic and behavioral interventions or comparisons between the two;
6. Studies of the influence on course, outcome, and treatment response of various psychiatric disturbances associated with anorexia and bulimia.

Anorexia nervosa and bulimia are becoming more prevalant and are of increasing significance as an issue of public health importance. Although research in these areas has been increasing, and there are numerous valuable reports in the scientific literature, significant gaps in knowledge remain. Much of the research has been conducted on small samples, primarily adolescent and college-age females, and has been concerned with specific treatment modalities that have been evaluated in terms of short-term effects. Research has been hampered by a lack of standardized instruments to assess initial behavior and follow-up assessment, and few studies have involved comprehensive outcome measures related to a wide range of variables. Further research is needed not only to elucidate diagnostic criteria; the validity of subgroups within the anorexia population; the efficacy of various treatment modalities, singly and in combination; and the assessment of outcome over extended periods of time; but also to integrate and assess psychological, behavioral, and physiological relationships as interrelated aspects of the syndrome. Such research is difficult and complex and can be carried out successfully only through intensive long-range interdisciplinary research.

ACKNOWLEDGMENTS

We would like to thank Mr. Edward Flynn for his assistance in preparing this report.

Literature Cited

1. Agras, S. W., Kraemer, H. C. 1984. The treatment of anorexia nervosa: Do different treatments bare different outcomes. In *Eating and Its Disorders*, ed. A. J. Stunkard, E. Stellar. New York: Raven
2. Biederman, J., Herzog, D. V., Rivinus, T. M., Harper, G. P., et al. 1985. Amitriptyline in the treatment of anorexia nervosa: A double-blind, placebo-controlled study. *J. Clin. Psychopharmacol.* 5(1): 10–16
3. Casper, R. H. 1984. Hypothalmic dysfunction and symptoms of anorexia nervosa. *Psychiatr. Clinics North Am.* 7(2)
3a. Casper, R. C., Kirschner, B., Sandstead, H. H., Jacob, R. A., Davis, J. M. 1980. An evaluation of trace metals, vita-

mins, and taste function in anorexia nervosa. *Am. J. Clin. Nutr.* 33:1801–8
4. Crisp, A. H. 1965. Some aspects of the evolution, presentation and follow-up of anorexia nervosa. *Proc. R. Soc. Med.* 58:814–20
5. Dally, P. J., Sargant, W. A. 1960. A new treatment for anorexia nervosa. (chlorpromazine). *Br. Med. J.* 1:1770–73
6. *Diagnostic and Statistical Manual of Mental Disorders.* 1980. Am. Psychiatric Assoc. 3rd ed.
7. Falk, J. R., Halmi, K. A., Eckert, E., Casper, R. 1985. *Proc. Soc. Menstrual Cycle Res.: Menarche, an Interdisciplinary Review,* ed. Golub. New York: Springer. In press
8. Garner, D., Garfinkel, P. 1979. The Eating Attitudes Test: An index of the symptoms of anorexia nervosa. *Psychol. Med.* 9:273–79
9. Golden, N., Sacker, I. 1984. An overview of the etiology, diagnosis, and mistreatment of anorexia nervosa. *Clin. Pediatr.* April, pp. 209–14
10. Gross, H. A., Ebert, M. H., Faden, V. B., et al. 1981. A double-blind controlled trial of lithium carbonate in primary anorexia nervosa. *J. Clin. Psychopharmacol.* 1:376–81
11. Halmi, K. A. 1983. The state of research in anorexia nervosa and bulimia. *Psychiatr. Dev.* 3:247–62
12. Halmi, K. A., Eckert, E., Falk, J. R. 1982. Cyproheptadine, an antidepressant and weight-inducing drug for anorexia nervosa. *Lancet* 1:1357–58
13. Hudson, J. I., Pope, H. G., Jonas, J. M., Yurgelun-Todd, D. 1985. Treatment of anorexia nervosa with antidepressants. *J. Clin. Psychopharmacol.* 5(1):17–23
14. Hudson, J. I., Pope, H. G. Jr., Jonas, J. M. 1984. Treatment of bulimia with antidepressants: Theoretical considerations and clinical findings. See Ref. 1, pp. 259–73
15. Katz, J. L., Kuperberg, A., Pollack, C.

P., Walsh, T. B., et al. 1984. *Am. J. Psychiatry* 141:6
16. Lacey, J. H., Crisp, A. H. 1980. Hunger, food intake and weight: The impact of clomipramine on a refeeding anorexia nervosa population. *Post-grad. Med. J.* 56:79–85
17. Minuchin, S., Rosman, B. L., Baker, L. 1979. *Psychosomatic Families: Anorexia Nervosa in Context.* Cambridge, Mass.: Harvard Univ. Press
18. Mitchell, J. E., Groat, R. 1984. A placebo-controlled, bouble-blind trial of amitriptyline in bulimia. *J. Clin. Psychopharmacol.* 4(4):186–93
19. Pope, H. G. Jr., Hudson, J. I., Jonas, J. M., Yurgulen-Todd, D. 1983. Bulimia treated with imipramine: A placebo-controlled double-blind study. *Am. J. Psychiatry* 140:554–58
20. Powers, P. 1982. Heart failure during treatment of anorexia nervosa. *Am. J. Psychiatry* 139:9
21. Vandereycken, W., Van den Brouke, S. 1984. Anorexia nervosa in males. *Acta Psychiatr. Scand.* Nov., pp. 447–54
22. Vandereycken, W. 1984. Neuroleptics in the short-term treatment of anorexia nervosa: A double-blind placebo-controlled study with sulpiride. *Br. J. Psychiatry* 144:288–92
23. Vandereycken, W., Pierloot, R. 1982. Pimozide combined with behavior therapy in the short term treatment of anorexia nervosa: A double-blind placebo-controlled cross-over study. *Acta Psychiatric Scand.* 60:446–51
24. Walsh, B. T., Stewart, J. W., Roose, S. P., Gladis, M., Glassman, A. H. 1984. Treatment of bulimia with phenelzine: A double-blind, placebo-controlled study. *Arch. Gen. Psychiatry* 41:1105–9
25. Wulliemer, F., Rossel, F., Sinclair, K. 1975. La Therapy Comportementale de l'anorexia nervouse *J. Psychosom. Res.* 19:267–72

SUBJECT INDEX

Women
  life expectancy of, 61
Workers' compensation
  asbestos exposure and, 185-88
  occupational health and, 338-
    40
Work-Factor, 82
Working Group on Risks and
  High Blood Pressure, 208
Work measurement
  ergonomics and, 81-83
  traditional
    limitations of, 83
Workmen's Compensation Act
  (1897), 185

Workplace
  asbestos and, 180-88
  smoking restrictions and, 133-
    34
  weight reduction and, 527-29
World Health Assembly, 10,
  224
World Health Organization, 3,
  115, 128, 130, 199, 331,
  362, 375-76, 431
  drug regulation and, 224, 227,
    230-32
World Health Organization/
  International Society of
  Hypertension Review, 198

X

Xeroderma pigmentosum
  cancer and, 164

Y

Yellow fever
  nuclear war and, 429
  relocation diffusion and, 324

Z

Zomax
  withdrawal from market, 225

CUMULATIVE INDEXES

CONTRIBUTING AUTHORS VOLUMES 1–7

Lave, J. R., 5:193–213
Lebowitz, M. D., 4:203–21
Leaf, A., 7:411–40
Leaning, J., 7:411–40
Lee, G. M., 5:1–52
Lee, P. R., 7:217–35
Leonard, C. O., 2:219–51
Levin, L. S., 4:181–201
Levy, R. I., 2:49–70
Lewis, C. E., 4:259–83
Lewis, M. A., 4:259–83
Lindheim, R., 2:1-39; 4:335–59
Louis, T. A., 4:25–46; 6:1–20
Lynch, B. S., 7:267–91

M

Maccoby, N., 6:147–93
Makuc, D., 2:159–82
Mandula, B., 6:195–221
Marmot, M., 2:253–76
Marsland, D., 7:357–89
Mayo, F., 7:357–89
McAlister, A., 6:147–93
McIntyre, K. M., 3:101–28
McNeil, B. J., 5:135–61
Meade, M. S., 7:313–35
Meilahn, E., 3:153–78
Moolgavkar, S. H., 7:151–69
Morrison, P. R., 6:325–32
Moses, L. E., 5:267–92
Mosteller, F., 6:1–20
Murnaghan, J. H., 2:299–361
Murt, H. A., 5:107–33

N

Needleman, H. L., 2:277–98
Nelson, N., 4:363–65
Nissinen, A., 6:147–93
Norman, M., 4:131–54

O

Ockene, J. K., 3:101–28
Okun, D. A., 4:47–67
Omenn, G. S., 6:107–30
Ongerth, H. J., 3:419–44
Ongerth, J. E., 3:419–44

Osterman-Golkar, S., 4:397–402
Ouslander, J. G., 3:50–83

P

Pagano, M., 6:325–32
Pauker, S. G., 5:135–61
Pearlman, L. A., 3:225–48
Perine, P. L., 6:85–106
Porter, I. H., 3:277–319
Prentice, R. L., 7:35–58
Puska, P., 6:147–93

R

Rao, K. S., 3:1–27
Reatig, N., 7:535–43
Richardson, W. C., 1:95–119
Robbins, F. C., 7:105–25
Robbins, J. B., 7:105–25
Robertson, L. S., 7:13–34
Rogan, W. J., 4:381–84
Room, R., 5:293–317
Rosenfield, P. L., 4:311–34
Rosenstock, L., 7:337–56

S

Sacco, C., 6:131–46
Salonen, J. T., 6:147–93
Sanazaro, P. J., 1:37–68
Schaffarzick, R. W., 7:391–409
Schoen, M. H., 2:71–92
Schwetz, B. A., 3:1–27
Scitovsky, A. A., 7:59–75
Shapiro, A. P., 4:285–310
Shapiro, S. H., 4:25–46
Sharp, D. S., 7:411–71
Shonick, W., 5:53–81
Siegel, J. M., 5:343–67
Simopoulos, A. P., 7:475–79; 7:481–92
Smith, A. H., 7:411–71
Socholitzky, E., 2:117–43
Sondik, E., 7:267–91
Sorsa, M., 4:403–7
Spinner, N. B., 5:1–52
Stallones, R. A., 1:69–82

Starfield, B., 6:21–40
Stason, W. B., 6:41–63
Stokes, M. E., 1:163–225
Stoll, J. G., 2:431–71
Stover, E. S., 7:535–43
Sullivan, J., 3:249–76
Syme, S. L., 3:179–99; 4:335–59

T

Terris, M., 1:323–44
Thomson, G., 5:1–52
Torrens, P. R., 6:65–83
Townsend, M., 3:153–78
Tuomilehto, J., 6:147–93
Tyler, C. W. Jr., 4:223–58

V

Vainio, H., 4:403–7
Vogt, T. M., 2:31–47

W

Walsh, D. C., 7:127–49
Ware, J. H., 4:1–23
Warner, K. E., 5:107–33
Warren, K. S., 2:101–15
Watts, C. A., 1:95–119
Wegman, D. H., 6:363–65
Wehrle, P. F., 2:363–95
Weill, H., 7:171–92
Weinberg, G., 3:153–78
Weinstein, I. B., 4:409–13
Weinstein, M. C., 6:41–63
Wennberg, J. E., 1:277–95
Whittemore, A. S., 2:397–429
Wilkins, J., 2:363–95
Wilson, R. W., 1:1–36; 5:83–106
Wingard, D. L., 5:433–58
Winkelstein, W. Jr.,2:253–76
Wolman, A., 7:1–12
Wood, M., 7:357–89
Wrensch, M. R., 5:1–52

Y

Yankauer, A., 3:249–76

CHAPTER TITLES, VOLUMES 1–7

AGE AND DISEASE SPECIFIC

Long-Term Care: Can Our Society Meet the Needs of its Elderly? R. L. Kane, R. A. Kane 1:227–53

The Decline in Cardiovascular Disease Mortality R. I. Levy 2:49–70

Prevention of Dental Disease: Caries and Periodontal Disease M. H. Schoen, J. R. Freed 2:71–92

The Control of Helminths: Nonreplicating Infectious Agents of Man K. S. Warren 2:101–15

Recent Trends in Infant Feeding D. B. Jelliffe, E. F. P. Jelliffe 2:145–58

Maternal Behavior and Perinatal Risks: Alcohol, Smoking, and Drugs I. M. Cushner 2:201–18

Issues in Antenatal and Neonatal Screening and Surveillance for Hereditary and Congenital Disorders N. A. Holtzman, C. O. Leonard, M. R. Farfel 2:219–51

Primary Prevention of Ischemic Heart Disease: Evaluation of Community Interventions W. Winkelstein, Jr., M. Marmot 2:253–76

Immunizing Agents: Potential for Controlling or Eradicating Infectious Disease P. F. Wehrle, J. Wilkins 2:363–95

Defining the Health Problems of the Elderly J. G. Ouslander, J. C. Beck 3:50–83

Control of Hereditary Disorders I. H. Porter 3:277–319

The Chronically Medically Disabled and "Deinstitutionalization" J. Archer, E. M. Gruenberg 3:445–68

Health Consequences of the Experience of Migration S. V. Kasl, L. Berkman 4:69–90

Deinstitutionalization: Health Consequences for the Mentally Ill M. Greenblatt, M. Norman 4:131–54

Schistosomiasis Control: Past, Present, and Future P. Jordan, P. L. Rosenfield 4:311–34

Mortality and Morbidity from Injuries in Sports and Recreation J. F. Kraus, C. Conroy 5:163–92

Alcohol Control and Public Health R. Room 5:293–317

Vision Disorders in Public Health R. N. Kleinstein 5:369–84

Postneonatal Mortality B. Starfield 6:21–40

Epidemiology of the Sexually Transmitted Diseases P. L. Perine, H. H. Handsfield, K. K. Holmes, J. H. Blount 6:85–106

Legal Aspects of Human Genetics R. B. Dworkin, G. S. Omenn 6:107–30

Behavioral and Environmental Interventions for Reducing Motor Vehicle Trauma L. S. Robertson 7:13–34

Medical Care at the End of Life: The Interaction of Economics and Ethics A. A. Scitovsky, A. M. Capron 7:59–75

International Drug Regulation P. R. Lee, J. Herzstein 7:217–35

Monitoring for Congenital Malformations N. A. Holtzman, M. J. Khoury 7:237–66

Diet and Chemoprevention in NCI's Research Strategy to Achieve National Cancer Control Objectives P. Greenwald, E. Sondik, B. S. Lynch 7:267–91

Public Health Aspects of Nuclear War J. Leaning, A. Leaf 7:411–40

BEHAVIORAL ASPECTS OF HEALTH

Public Health and Individual Liberty D. E. Beauchamp 1:121–36

Behavioral Interventions and Compliance to Treatment Regimes R. C. Benfari, E. Eaker, J. G. Stoll 2:431–71

562

Annual Reviews Inc.

A NONPROFIT SCIENTIFIC PUBLISHER

ORDER FORM

4139 El Camino Way, Palo Alto, CA 94306-9981, USA • (415) 493-4400

Annual Reviews Inc. publications are available directly from our office by mail or telephone (paid by credit card or purchase order), through booksellers and subscription agents, worldwide, and through participating professional societies. Prices subject to change without notice.

- **Individuals:** Prepayment required on new accounts by check or money order (in U.S. dollars, check drawn on U.S. bank) or charge to credit card — American Express, VISA, MasterCard.
- **Institutional buyers:** Please include purchase order number.
- **Students:** $10.00 discount from retail price, per volume. Prepayment required. Proof of student status must be provided (photocopy of student I.D. or signature of department secretary is acceptable). Students must send orders direct to Annual Reviews. Orders received through bookstores and institutions requesting student rates will be returned.
- **Professional Society Members:** Members of professional societies that have a contractual arrangement with Annual Reviews may order books through their society at a reduced rate. Check with your society for information.

Regular orders: Please list the volumes you wish to order by volume number.
Standing orders: New volume in the series will be sent to you automatically each year upon publication. Cancellation may be made at any time. Please indicate volume number to begin standing order.
Prepublication orders: Volumes not yet published will be shipped in month and year indicated.
California orders: Add applicable sales tax.
Postage paid (4th class bookrate/surface mail) **by Annual Reviews Inc.** Airmail postage extra.

ANNUAL REVIEWS SERIES		Prices Postpaid per volume USA/elsewhere	Regular Order Please send:	Standing Order Begin with:
			Vol. number	Vol. number
Annual Review of **ANTHROPOLOGY** (Prices of Volumes in brackets effective until 12/31/85)				
[Vols. 1-10	(1972-1981)	$20.00/$21.00]		
[Vol. 11	(1982)	$22.00/$25.00]		
[Vols. 12-14	(1983-1985)	$27.00/$30.00]		
Vols. 1-14	(1972-1985)	$27.00/$30.00		
Vol. 15	(avail. Oct. 1986)	$31.00/$34.00	Vol(s). _____	Vol. _____
Annual Review of **ASTRONOMY AND ASTROPHYSICS** (Prices of Volumes in brackets effective until 12/31/85)				
[Vols. 1-2, 4-19	(1963-1964; 1966-1981)	$20.00/$21.00]		
[Vol. 20	(1982)	$22.00/$25.00]		
[Vols. 21-23	(1983-1985)	$44.00/$47.00]		
Vols. 1-2, 4-20	(1963-1964; 1966-1982)	$27.00/$30.00		
Vols. 21-23	(1983-1985)	$44.00/$47.00		
Vol. 24	(avail. Sept. 1986)	$44.00/$47.00	Vol(s). _____	Vol. _____
Annual Review of **BIOCHEMISTRY** (Prices of Volumes in brackets effective until 12/31/85)				
[Vols. 30-34, 36-50	(1961-1965; 1967-1981)	$21.00/$22.00]		
[Vol. 51	(1982)	$23.00/$26.00]		
[Vols. 52-54	(1983-1985)	$29.00/$32.00]		
Vols. 30-34, 36-54	(1961-1965; 1967-1985)	$29.00/$32.00		
Vol. 55	(avail. July 1986)	$33.00/$36.00	Vol(s). _____	Vol. _____
Annual Review of **BIOPHYSICS AND BIOPHYSICAL CHEMISTRY** (Prices of Vols. in brackets effective until 12/31/85)				
(*Formerly* Annual Review of Biophysics and Bioengineering)				
[Vols. 1-10	(1972-1981)	$20.00/$21.00]		
[Vol. 11	(1982)	$22.00/$25.00]		
[Vols. 12-14	(1983-1985)	$47.00/$50.00]		
Vols. 1-11	(1972-1982)	$27.00/$30.00		
Vols. 12-14	(1983-1985)	$47.00/$50.00		
Vol. 15	(avail. June 1986)	$47.00/$50.00	Vol(s). _____	Vol. _____
Annual Review of **CELL BIOLOGY**				
Vol. 1	(1985)	$27.00/$30.00		
Vol. 2	(avail. Nov. 1986)	$31.00/$34.00	Vol(s). _____	Vol. _____
Annual Review of **COMPUTER SCIENCE**				
Vol. 1	(avail. late 1986)	**Price not yet established**	Vol. _____	Vol. _____
Annual Review of **EARTH AND PLANETARY SCIENCES** (Prices of Volumes in brackets effective until 12/31/85)				
[Vols. 1-9	(1973-1981)	$20.00/$21.00]		
[Vol. 10	(1982)	$22.00/$25.00]		
[Vols. 11-13	(1983-1985)	$44.00/$47.00]		
Vols. 1-10	(1973-1982)	$27.00/$30.00		
Vols. 11-13	(1983-1985)	$44.00/$47.00		
Vol. 14	(avail. May 1986)	$44.00/$47.00	Vol(s). _____	Vol. _____

ANNUAL REVIEWS SERIES		Prices Postpaid per volume USA/elsewhere	Regular Order Please send:	Standing Order Begin with:
Annual Review of ECOLOGY AND SYSTEMATICS (Prices of Volumes in brackets effective until 12/31/85)				
[Vols. 1-12	(1970-1981)	$20.00/$21.00]		
[Vol. 13	(1982)	$22.00/$25.00]		
[Vols. 14-16	(1983-1985)	$27.00/$30.00]		
Vols. 1-16	(1970-1985)	$27.00/$30.00		
Vol. 17	(avail. Nov. 1986)	$31.00/$34.00	Vol(s). _____	Vol. _____
Annual Review of ENERGY (Prices of Volumes in brackets effective until 12/31/85)				
[Vols. 1-6	(1976-1981)	$20.00/$21.00]		
[Vol. 7	(1982)	$22.00/$25.00]		
[Vols. 8-10	(1983-1985)	$56.00/$59.00]		
Vols. 1-7	(1976-1982)	$27.00/$30.00		
Vols. 8-10	(1983-1985)	$56.00/$59.00		
Vol. 11	(avail. Oct. 1986)	$56.00/$59.00	Vol(s). _____	Vol. _____
Annual Review of ENTOMOLOGY (Prices of Volumes in brackets effective until 12/31/85)				
[Vols. 9-16, 18-26	(1964-1971; 1973-1981)	$20.00/$21.00]		
[Vol. 27	(1982)	$22.00/$25.00]		
[Vols. 28-30	(1983-1985)	$27.00/$30.00]		
Vols. 9-16, 18-30	(1964-1971; 1973-1985)	$27.00/$30.00		
Vol. 31	(avail. Jan. 1986)	$31.00/$34.00	Vol(s). _____	Vol. _____
Annual Review of FLUID MECHANICS (Prices of Volumes in brackets effective until 12/31/85)				
[Vols. 1-5, 7-13	(1969-1973; 1975-1981)	$20.00/$21.00]		
[Vol. 14	(1982)	$22.00/$25.00]		
[Vols. 15-17	(1983-1985)	$28.00/$31.00]		
Vols. 1-5, 7-17	(1969-1973; 1975-1985)	$28.00/$31.00		
Vol. 18	(avail. Jan. 1986)	$32.00/$35.00	Vol(s). _____	Vol. _____
Annual Review of GENETICS (Prices of Volumes in brackets effective until 12/31/85)				
[Vols. 1-15	(1967-1981)	$20.00/$21.00]		
[Vol. 16	(1982)	$22.00/$25.00]		
[Vols. 17-19	(1983-1985)	$27.00/$30.00]		
Vols. 1-19	(1967-1985)	$27.00/$30.00		
Vol. 20	(avail. Dec. 1986)	$31.00/$34.00	Vol(s). _____	Vol. _____
Annual Review of IMMUNOLOGY				
Vols. 1-3	(1983-1985)	$27.00/$30.00		
Vol. 4	(avail. April 1986)	$31.00/$34.00	Vol(s). _____	Vol. _____
Annual Review of MATERIALS SCIENCE (Prices of Volumes in brackets effective until 12/31/85)				
[Vols. 1-11	(1971-1981)	$20.00/$21.00]		
[Vol. 12	(1982)	$22.00/$25.00]		
[Vols. 13-15	(1983-1985)	$64.00/$67.00]		
Vols. 1-12	(1971-1982)	$27.00/$30.00		
Vols. 13-15	(1983-1985)	$64.00/$67.00		
Vol. 16	(avail. August 1986)	$64.00/$67.00	Vol(s). _____	Vol. _____
Annual Review of MEDICINE (Prices of Volumes in brackets effective until 12/31/85)				
[Vols. 1-3, 5-15, 17-32	(1950-52; 1954-64; 1966-81)	$20.00/$21.00]		
[Vol. 33	(1982)	$22.00/$25.00]		
[Vols. 34-36	(1983-1985)	$27.00/$30.00]		
Vols. 1-3, 5-15, 17-36	(1950-52; 1954-64; 1966-85)	$27.00/$30.00		
Vol. 37	(avail. April 1986)	$31.00/$34.00	Vol(s). _____	Vol. _____
Annual Review of MICROBIOLOGY (Prices of Volumes in brackets effective until 12/31/85)				
[Vols. 18-35	(1964-1981)	$20.00/$21.00]		
[Vol. 36	(1982)	$22.00/$25.00]		
[Vols. 37-39	(1983-1985)	$27.00/$30.00]		
Vols. 18-39	(1964-1985)	$27.00/$30.00		
Vol. 40	(avail. Oct. 1986)	$31.00/$34.00	Vol(s). _____	Vol. _____
Annual Review of NEUROSCIENCE (Prices of Volumes in brackets effective until 12/31/85)				
[Vols. 1-4	(1978-1981)	$20.00/$21.00]		
[Vol. 5	(1982)	$22.00/$25.00]		
[Vols. 6-8	(1983-1985)	$27.00/$30.00]		
Vols. 1-8	(1978-1985)	$27.00/$30.00		
Vol. 9	(avail. March 1986)	$31.00/$34.00	Vol(s). _____	Vol. _____